Clinical Neuroscience

Clinical Neuroscience

Edited by **Robin Deaver**

hayle
medical

New York

Published by Hayle Medical,
30 West, 37th Street, Suite 612,
New York, NY 10018, USA
www.haylemedical.com

Clinical Neuroscience
Edited by Robin Deaver

International Standard Book Number:978-1-63241-407-6 (Hardback)

The publisher's policy is to use permanent paper from mills that operate a sustainable forestry policy. Furthermore, the publisher ensures that the text paper and cover boards used have met acceptable environmental accreditation standards.

Trademark Notice: Registered trademark of products or corporate names are used only for explanation and identification without intent to infringe.

Printed in the United States of America.

Contents

Preface

The world is advancing at a fast pace like never before. Therefore, the need is to keep up with the latest developments. This book was an idea that came to fruition when the specialists in the area realized the need to coordinate together and document essential themes in the subject. That's when I was requested to be the editor. Editing this book has been an honour as it brings together diverse authors researching on different streams of the field. The book collates essential materials contributed by veterans in the area which can be utilized by students and researchers alike.

Neuroscience is the branch of science that deals with the detailed study of the central nervous system. It is an interdisciplinary field that encompasses cognitive science, computer science, mathematics, medicine, genetics, and also combines disciplines such as psychology, philosophy and physics. The composite structure of the brain is more complex than any other part of the body. This discipline tries to study the structure, working, changes and malfunctions of brain. This text sheds light on the unexplored concepts and applications of neuroscience. It presents researches performed by experts across the globe which cover significant aspects related to all branches of this field. This book contains some path-breaking studies in the field of clinical neuroscience. It aims to serve as a resource guide for students and experts alike and contribute to the growth of the discipline.

Each chapter is a sole-standing publication that reflects each author's interpretation. Thus, the book displays a multi-facetted picture of our current understanding of applications and diverse aspects of the field. I would like to thank the contributors of this book and my family for their endless support.

Editor

Neurocognitive Basis of Schizophrenia: Information Processing Abnormalities and Clues for Treatment

André Aleman[1,2]

[1] Department of Neuroscience, University Medical Center Groningen, University of Groningen, 9700 RB Groningen, The Netherlands
[2] Department of Psychology, University of Groningen, 9712 CP Groningen, The Netherlands

Correspondence should be addressed to André Aleman; a.aleman@med.umcg.nl

Academic Editor: Daniela Schulz

Schizophrenia is a chronic and severe psychiatric disorder that affects all aspects of patients' lives. Over the past decades, research applying methods from psychology and neuroscience has increasingly been zooming in on specific information processing abnormalities in schizophrenia. Impaired activation of and connectivity between frontotemporal, frontoparietal, and frontostriatal brain networks subserving cognitive functioning and integration of cognition and emotion has been consistently reported. Major issues in schizophrenia research concern the cognitive and neural basis of hallucinations, abnormalities in cognitive-emotional processing, social cognition (including theory of mind), poor awareness of illness, and apathy. Recent findings from cognitive neuroscience studies in these areas are discussed. The findings may have implications for treatment, for example, noninvasive neurostimulation of specific brain areas. Ultimately, a better understanding of the cognitive neuroscience of schizophrenia will pave the way for the development of effective treatment strategies.

1. Introduction: Schizophrenia

Schizophrenia belongs to the most severe psychiatric disorders. It is characterized by hallucinations, delusions, cognitive impairment, and social withdrawal [1]. In most cases, people with this diagnosis might have difficulty to think clearly, to distinguish reality from fantasy, to react in an emotionally appropriate way, and to interact with others. One of the most tragic features of the disorder is the early appearance of the symptoms, usually between ages 20 and 35, with devastating effects on social relationships, education, and starting a professional career, thereby ruining all promises of early adulthood. Approximately 15% of patients with schizophrenia commit suicide. The general population lifetime prevalence of schizophrenia is approximately 1.0%, and the annual incidence rate is between 0.16 and 0.42/1000 persons at risk [2]. Although textbooks used to state that schizophrenia affects men and women equally (e.g., Kaplan et al. [3]), evidence is accumulating that men are at higher risk for schizophrenia [4], especially during adolescence and young adulthood and especially for schizophrenia with negative symptoms.

Symptoms of schizophrenia include delusions, hallucinations, disorganized speech, grossly disorganized or catatonic behavior, affective flattening, alogia, and avolition [5]. None of these symptoms is pathognomonic for schizophrenia [6]. Symptoms of schizophrenia have been characterized to be "waxing and waning", referring to the acute and chronic phases in which symptoms can be present. Acute symptoms are usually so-called "positive" symptoms (which are present in schizophrenia but not in healthy individuals), such as delusions and hallucinations. On the other hand, negative symptoms (the absence of functions that are present in healthy individuals), such as affective flattening and avolition, are more persistent and have stronger prognostic importance [7, 8].

2. Cognitive Dysfunction

It is surprising that cognitive dysfunction, although it is widely recognized to be a hallmark of schizophrenia, is not listed among the symptoms of schizophrenia in the American Psychiatric Association's Diagnostic and Statistical Manual, be it version DSM-IV or the new DSM 5. Indeed, numerous neuropsychological investigations have established that patients with schizophrenia suffer from significant deficits in attention, memory, executive functioning, and general intellectual abilities [9, 10]. Large and stable effect sizes have been reported for memory impairment [11]. In a recent meta-analysis, Reichenberg and Harvey [10] presented a quantitative integration of the published literature showing that the most severe impairments are apparent in episodic memory and executive control processes (with effect sizes around 1 SD in magnitude), evident against a background of a generalized cognitive deficit. This was recently confirmed in yet another meta-analysis that concluded that there is a large and stable, general cognitive deficit that is similar across the world and has not changed over the past decades, despite some changes in diagnostic criteria [12]. The neuropsychological impairments potentially represent genetic liability to the disorder: similar, yet milder, impairments are evident in schizophrenia patients even before the onset of psychotic symptoms, as well as in the nonpsychotic relatives of schizophrenia patients. In relatives, meta-analyses have established effect sizes of medium magnitude (around 0.5 SD), with strongest impairment in executive functioning and memory [13, 14]. However, this effect size also implies that a considerable proportion of relatives have no neuropsychological impairment.

Another meta-analysis of studies conducted with patients identified processing speed inefficiency as the largest single cognitive impairment in schizophrenia [15]. However, in a meta-analysis of moderator variables affecting processing speed in patients with schizophrenia, Knowles et al. [16] showed that the processing speed impairment is substantially affected by several moderating factors, in particular antipsychotic medication dosage.

It should be noted that studies of cognitive impairment in schizophrenia have used a large number of different neuropsychological tests. Such heterogeneity of measurement poses problems for interpretation as comparison between different studies is difficult when the measures have different characteristics (e.g., slight differences in cognitive processes that are targeted, but also differences in duration of the test, reliability, validity, etc.). Therefore, the consensus battery MATRICS [17] that was proposed by a team of investigators coordinated by the National Institutes of Mental Health (NIMH) is a laudable development that can improve comparability which is especially needed for treatment studies in which the effect of an intervention (be it pharmacotherapy or psychotherapy) is assessed on cognitive functioning. MATRICS is an abbreviation of "Measurement and Treatment Research to Improve Cognition in Schizophrenia." The consensus cognitive battery includes tests with adequate reliability and validity in the following domains: speed of processing, attention/vigilance, working memory, verbal learning and memory, visual learning and memory, reasoning and problem solving, and social cognition (see http://www.matricsinc.org/MCCB.htm).

Another important point to be aware of concerns the heterogeneity of the cognitive impairment itself among patients. That is, although on a group level patients consistently perform worse than healthy control subjects, this is not necessarily the case at an individual level. Thus, a small subgroup of patients is neuropsychologically normal; that is, their performance on neuropsychological tests of attention, memory

and executive functioning is in the normal range of age- and education-matched samples [18]. However, a study by Wilk et al. [19] revealed that, even after matching schizophrenia patients to control subjects on IQ, patients still exhibited performance deficits in memory and speed visual processing.

With regard to brain regions underlying these deficits in cognitive functioning, it is now clear that frontal and temporal cortices are strongly involved. For example, the classic finding by Weinberger et al. [20] of reduced DLPFC activation has been widely replicated [21]. On the other hand several studies have reported increased prefrontal activation during working memory tasks [22, 23]. However, this may be observed primarily in tasks that are difficult for patients, but which they are still able to perform. When the task becomes too difficult and their performance is worse than that of comparison subjects, patients will typically show less activation. With regard to the temporal cortex, its involvement in functional scans during episodic memory has also consistently been reported with compromised activation in schizophrenia [24].

Even though the importance of the frontal and temporal cortex is well recognized, compromised frontostriatal and frontoparietal function is also well established in schizophrenia [25]. To summarize, cognitive dysfunction is a hallmark of schizophrenia that is increasingly being recognized [26] and should be taken into account when considering issues of etiology, course of illness, and treatment. Indeed, it has been argued that neuroimaging of cognitive dysfunction in schizophrenia will prove to be useful in characterizing the genetic and environmental risk factors that are likely to be causally related to the disorder [27].

In the treatment of cognitive dysfunction in schizophrenia, an important question is whether cognitive training can remediate impairments. Antipsychotic medication is not very successful in improving cognitive function, but neither does it deteriorate cognition, when adequately dosed [28–30]. Medication with weak dopamine antagonists could be associated with increased activation of frontal areas in schizophrenia patients [31]. Over the past years, several meta-analyses have shown that cognitive training can improve cognitive functioning in patients, above and beyond improvement on a specific cognitive task that was trained [32, 33]. Cognitive training may consequently also improve brain function as measured with neuroimaging methods [34]. A typical cognitive training program consists of several weeks of training with several sessions a week in which the patient receives instruction to improve strategy and extensively practices computer-based cognitive tasks.

3. Cognitive and Neural Basis of Hallucinations

Hallucinations are a frequent symptom of psychosis and may occur (lifetime) in 60–70% of patients with schizophrenia [35]. Although hallucinations can occur in any sensory modality (visual, auditory, somatosensory, olfactory, gustatory), auditory hallucinations are most common in schizophrenia. Specifically, most patients are bothered by auditory-verbal hallucinations (AVH), or "hearing voices."

Typically, they hear disturbing comments on their behavior, or abusive language. Most hallucinations have a negative content and distract patients from their daily tasks. The frequency can differ widely, with some patients only hearing brief comments a few times a week to others with continuous hallucinations. Approximately half of the patients experience the voices as coming from outside the head, the other half experiences them as coming from inside the head—but not being their own voice [36]. Antipsychotics are generally effective in reducing hallucinations but fail to reduce the symptom in up to 30% of patients. In order to measure brain activity that directly correlates with the ongoing experience of hallucinations, investigators using functional MRI have asked patients to indicate with the aid of button-presses the occurrence of hallucinations in the scanner. For this, patients are needed who experience intermittent hallucinatory episodes. This allows the investigator to contrast scans made during the hallucinatory episodes with those made in the absence of hallucinations. A drawback of this method is that only small groups can generally be included in such studies, as this method requires that patients experience several discrete periods of hallucinations during their stay in the scanner (typically an hour). Thus, the power of such studies tends to be limited, and their results should be interpreted with some caution. These studies typically involve the superior temporal gyrus in the left, but occasionally also right, hemisphere [37–40]. Other cortical areas that have been shown to activate during hallucinations include the anterior cingulate cortex and the inferior frontal gyrus (e.g., Broca's area and its homologue in the right hemisphere). Activation of subcortical areas such as thalamus and basal ganglia has also been reported regularly. Two meta-analyses have summarized the brain activation studies on hallucination-related activation during scanning [41, 42]. The meta-analysis reported by Jardri et al. integrated findings from 10 studies, including a total of 68 patients diagnosed with a disorder in the schizophrenia spectrum. Analyses involved the stereotactic coordinates of 129 significant foci. AVH were associated with increased activation likelihoods in a bilateral neural network that included Broca's area, the anterior insula, the precentral gyrus, the frontal operculum, the middle and superior temporal gyri, the inferior parietal lobule, and the hippocampal/parahippocampal region. Six out of eight activation clusters were found in the left hemisphere. The authors concluded that not only frontotemporal speech areas are involved in the mediation of AVH, but also medial temporal areas associated with verbal memory. The other meta-analysis, by Kühn and Gallinat [42], distinguished between "state" versus "trait" aspects of AVH. "State" refers to the hallucinatory state, that is, the activation of brain regions during the experience of hallucinations (e.g., with the button-press method). "Trait," in contrast, refers to the comparison of brain activity between patients with and without hallucinations in the preceding week or month, and thus concerns the tendency to hallucinate or liability for hallucinations. Kühn and Gallinat [42] found that the state of experiencing AVH is primarily related to speech production regions such as Broca's area, whereas the trait that may render an individual prone to hallucinations is related to brain regions involved in auditory processing

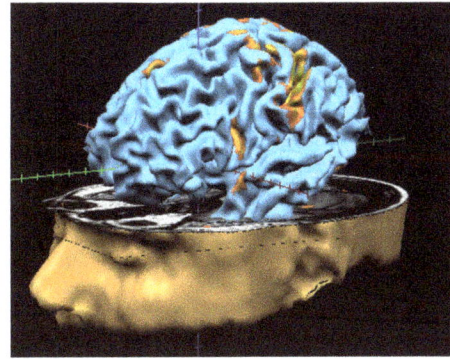

FIGURE 1: Activation of brain areas during language processing as measured with an fMRI scan (Philips 3T, Neuroimaging Center Groningen). Such language-related regions in the inferior frontal gyrus (Broca's area), temporoparietal cortex (Wernicke's area), and anterior cingulate are also seen to be active during auditory-verbal hallucinations.

and speech perception. Thus, aberrant activation of speech processing circuitry is essential to AVH (see Figure 1).

Treatment of hallucinations in schizophrenia consists mainly of prescription of antipsychotics. However, for the patients in which medication does not ameliorate hallucinations sufficiently (about 30% of patients with hallucinations), cognitive therapy can be useful. In addition, noninvasive neurostimulation by means of repetitive transcranial magnetic stimulation (rTMS) has been used to reduce hallucinations [43–45]. Most studies apply daily 1 Hz stimulation over the left temporoparietal junction for 15–30 min. during 1–3 weeks. Bilateral stimulation of the temporoparietal region has also been tried, but did not yield better effects [46]. A recent meta-analysis revealed a moderate effect size (in the order of $d = 0.40$) for rTMS as compared to sham in improving auditory-verbal hallucinations in schizophrenia [47].

Research into the cognitive basis of hallucinations has revealed three factors to be of importance (for a recent overview of relevant cognitive processes, see [48]). One refers to the role of intrusions and the lack of cognitive inhibition. More specifically, studies that have used tasks demanding the volitional suppression of memory events and irrelevant memories have shown that AVH in schizophrenia are associated with a deficit in intentional cognitive inhibition [49–51]. A second factor concerns top-down influences on perception. Besides "bottom-up" influences (data coming in from the senses), perception is also guided by internally generated elements. These are referred to as "top-down factors." In bottom-up processes, the focus is on physical characteristics of a stimulus that drive perception. Top-down factors, in contrast, include prior knowledge, perceptual expectations, and mental imagery. The role of memory and thought in shaping perception is acknowledged. Put another way, this refers to processes that contribute to perception but do not originate directly from the external world but from the mind/brain of the perceiver. Several theoretical suggestions have been made implying an overreliance on top-down factors at the cost of bottom-up factors in driving hallucinatory perception (cf. [52]). For example, Grossberg [53] suggested that strong top-down excitation can create conscious experiences in the absence of bottom-up information. In this way, conscious mental imagery can arise. Grossberg then proposes a mechanism by which this top-down excitation becomes chronically hyperactive, through which sensory expectations can generate conscious experiences (through the activation of mental images) that are not under volitional control of the subject—in other words, hallucinations. The hypothesis that people with hallucinatory propensity may be characterized by strong top-down expectations has been put to the test empirically. Vercammen and Aleman [54] investigated the role of semantic expectations on perception in nonclinical individuals (i.e., without a psychiatric disorder or psychiatric symptoms that need treatment) with a disposition towards hallucination (as established with the revised Launay-Slade Hallucination Scale, LSHS). Studying people without a psychiatric disorder, but with a predisposition for hallucinations has several advantages. Specifically, the data are not contaminated by the possible effects of medication, hospitalization, or severity of psychopathology. The study involved 40 subjects selected from 350 undergraduates with the help of the LSHS to ensure sufficient variation regarding the experience of hallucination-like events (i.e., people with high scores and low scores were selected along with people with intermediate scores). Semantic expectation was manipulated by presenting sentences and leaving out the last word. That is, the last word was not clearly audible as it was embedded in white noise. Stimuli consisted of short sentences of 5–7 words, such as "The unfortunate carpenter hit his . . . ." A predictable word would then be "thumb," but the actually presented word was "toe." Another example: "The thief reported to the . . . .," where the word "owner" was presented instead of the more expected "police." The distinction between expected and unexpected words was validated in a separate pilot study. Subjects were asked to press the appropriate response button to indicate whether or not they heard a word and subsequently to identify this word out loud. Subjects were encouraged to identify the word only if they were positively convinced, and otherwise to state that they were uncertain of its identity. Results revealed that LSHS scores were correlated with the number of semantically primed errors. More specifically, subjects with higher levels of hallucination proneness were more likely to report hearing a word that fits the sentence context, when it was not actually presented. This effect remained significant after controlling of general performance on the task. Thus, these results support the conclusion that aberrant top-down processing, particularly in the form of strong semantic expectations, may contribute to the experience of auditory-verbal hallucinations.

In a follow-up study, Daalman et al. [55] investigated the same task for semantically primed top-down errors in patients with schizophrenia, people from the general population reporting auditory-verbal hallucinations, and healthy control subjects. They replicated the finding by Vercammen and Aleman [54] for the nonpsychotic individuals with AVH: they made significantly more top-down errors compared to healthy controls, while overall accuracy was similar. Notably, the severity of hallucination proneness correlated with the number of top-down errors. Thus, the results confirmed

that nonpsychotic individuals with AVH are influenced more strongly by top-down processing (i.e., perceptual expectations) than healthy controls. In the patient group, however, the number of top-down errors, corrected for overall accuracy was in between those of the other two groups and did not differ significantly from either the nonpsychotic individuals with AVH or the healthy controls. The seemingly lack of a role for semantic expectations in the patient group suggests different cognitive mechanisms for pathological and nonpathological hallucinations, which not only calls for further comparison of cognitive mechanisms underlying different forms of hallucination, but also challenges the notion of a continuity between psychotic-like experiences in people without a psychiatric diagnosis and psychotic phenomena in patients [56].

With regard to the neural basis of top-down processing, secondary perceptual areas are of importance. A study of verbal speech imagery [57] revealed activation of speech perception cortex (Wernicke's area). Activation in such areas has also been shown to be strong during hallucinations (as reviewed above). Interestingly, the temporoparietal region in the left hemisphere (converging with Wernicke's area) has been shown to have reduced connectivity in the resting states to the cingulate cortex and the bilateral amygdala [58]. The cingulate has been shown to play a key role in self-referent processing and attentional control (monitoring), whereas the temporoparietal cortex has been implied in sense of agency and the amygdalae in emotional salience. Finally, a study using functional magnetic resonance imaging with dynamic causal modeling for the analysis of directionality in activated networks revealed reduced connectivity from Wernicke's to Broca's area in patients with auditory-verbal hallucinations [59]. This may suggest that activity in Broca's area may be less constrained by perceptual information received from the temporal cortex and Broca may subsequently actively generate spurious activity in a search for meaningful linguistic percepts.

The third, and most researched, cognitive factor involved in hallucinations concerns source-monitoring. This refers to the ability to discriminate between imagined and perceived information, that is, between internal and external sources driving the perceptual experience [60]. More specifically, it has been suggested that a difficulty to differentiate between information that has been perceived from the outside world and information that has been imagined may explain the genesis of hallucinations [61]. These symptoms suggest that the patient has difficulty in maintaining the distinction between internally- and externally-generated events, which have been referred to as manifestations of *autonoetic agnosia*, meaning literally "the inability to identify self-generated mental events" [62]. Therefore, these symptoms could be caused by a deficit in monitoring the self-generation of thoughts [63] or a bias towards misattributing internal thoughts to external sources [64].

Autonoetic agnosia has been measured with various cognitive tests, including the assessment of source monitoring [65]. A meta-analysis of studies investigating accuracy of self-attribution in schizophrenia revealed a significant impairment in patients as compared to age and education matched control subjects [66]. There was also a relationship with hallucinations: patients with hallucinations made more errors than patients without hallucinations. The systematic review included 23 published studies that contrasted the performance of schizophrenia patients with healthy controls (with a total of 1370 participants) and 9 studies that directly compared patients with and without auditory hallucinations (315 participants). The authors noted that the homogeneity in results across studies was remarkable. That is, the self-recognition difficulties were found regardless of the action modality, timing delay, and design used to measure self-recognition. Some tasks involved voice recognition, others source memory for words or pictures.

The neural basis of source monitoring has also been studied. For example, Simons et al. [67] used fMRI to investigate the brain areas associated with this ability in healthy subjects, who were to remember whether information had previously been perceived or imagined, or whether information had been presented on the left or right of a monitor screen (control condition). Their results indicated a role of the medial anterior prefrontal cortex, thalamus, and cerebellum in reality monitoring. These regions have also been implicated in schizophrenia. Morever, reduced prefrontal activation was associated with the same misattribution error that has been observed in schizophrenia. Allen et al. [68] investigated neural activation differences between patients with and without hallucinations during a verbal self-monitoring task. They hypothesized that patients with a history of auditory verbal hallucinations would misattribute their own speech as external and show differential activation in brain areas implicated in hallucinations. Subjects listened to prerecorded words while being scanned with fMRI. The source (self/nonself) and acoustic quality (undistorted/distorted) of the presented words were varied across trials. The hallucinator group made more external misattributions (indicating that their own, slightly distorted speech was that of another person) and showed altered activation in the superior temporal gyrus and anterior cingulate compared with both other groups. The authors interpreted the reduced activation of the anterior cingulate as evidence it impaired self-monitoring.

4. Emotional Processing Abnormalities: Perception and Regulation

Although several authors have maintained that schizophrenia is primarily a cognitive disorder [26, 69, 70], research in recent decades has been accumulating to certainly also support the view of schizophrenia as an *emotional* disorder [71, 72]. Indeed, this may seem surprising as schizophrenia has always been considered to be a "nonaffective" psychosis in psychiatry. However, the term "nonaffective" was primarily used to indicate that mood disturbance is not a key feature of schizophrenia, in contrast to bipolar disorder or psychotic depression. The evidence for emotional abnormalities in schizophrenia comes from studies investigating emotional perception, emotional experience, and emotion regulation. A large and robust deficit in emotion perception was quantified for patients with schizophrenia, irrespective of task type, in a meta-analysis of facial emotion perception studies [73]. Not only emotion perception from facial expressions is impaired,

recognition of emotional prosody (from tone of voice) is equally impaired [74]. A meta-analysis of studies investigating deficits in emotion perception and their relationship to outcome measures documented a significant association between poor emotion perception and worse outcome in schizophrenia [75]. The authors included 25 studies and reported medium to large range positive correlations between emotion identification and functional outcome domains involving social problem solving, social skills, and community functioning. Li et al. [76] reported a meta-analysis of 15 activation studies during facial emotion processing in schizophrenia and found reduced activation in bilateral amygdala, parahippocampal gyrus, and fusiform gyrus, right superior frontal gyrus and lentiform nucleus of patients as compared to healthy controls. In contrast, Anticevic et al. [77] reported a meta-analysis of neuroimaging studies that investigated amygdala recruitment in response to aversive emotional stimuli in schizophrenia and reported that patients activate the amygdala similarly to healthy controls. This could suggest that the emotion perception deficit may be more related to early processing deficits in perceptual regions or late processing deficits in association with cortex or frontal regions (involved in categorization) than to diminished responsivity of emotional circuitry, though this remains a question for further research. Notably, in a study of social perception, in which subjects rated the trustworthiness of faces during fMRI, we observed reduced amygdala activation to untrusworthy faces in patients with schizophrenia as compared to age- and education-matched healthy control subjects [78]. Thus, in certain circumstances the amygdala response might be compromised in schizophrenia, maybe especially when subtle social cues are involved. The studies using aversive emotional stimulation generally used very explicit and strong negative stimuli.

Recent emerging work with functional imaging is providing key insights in the neural correlates of cognitive influences on the emotion control. Ochsner et al. [79] examined the ability to cognitively transform the emotional experience of a negative affect, which has been termed "reappraisal." Generating a more positive interpretation (or less negative interpretation) for an image showing people in pain, which initially triggers negative affect, is an instance of reappraisal. Strategies people can use to reappraise involve telling themselves that people in the photo are not really in that much trouble, that things will not turn out all that badly, or that things are not quite as bad as they seem [80]. In case human injury is portrayed one could imagine that it is a scene from a movie and no real injury was involved, and so forth. Numerous psychological studies have shown this to be an effective way of reducing emotion-induced distress [81]. Ochsner et al. [79] proposed that reappraisal would be mediated by interactions between cognitive control and emotion-processing systems. Concerning cognitive-processing systems, they proposed the involvement of three major areas: (1) the LPFC, implicated in generating a strategy for cognitively reframing an emotional event in unemotional terms and keeping that in mind by working memory processes; (2) the dorsal anterior cingulate cortex, regarding the interference between top-down reappraisals that neutralize affect and bottom-up evaluations that continue to generate an affective response and consequently signaling the need for reappraisal to continue; and (3) the dorsal regions of the MPFC, involved in reevaluating the relationship between internal states and external stimuli used to monitor changes in one's emotional state during reappraisal. With respect to emotion-processing systems, the amygdala and medial orbital frontal cortex (MOFC) are associated with differentially encoding and representing the affective properties of stimuli [82].

Participants in Ochsner et al.'s [79] study were shown aversive and neutral photos in order to compare reappraisal to another condition that could draw on processes invoked by reappraisal but which would not be related to regulation of affect per se. For that purpose, they employed two conditions: (1) "attend", where participants were asked to let themselves respond emotionally to each photo by being aware of their feelings without trying to alter them and (2) "reappraise", where subjects had to interpret photos in such a way that they felt less negative in response to them. As both conditions involved attention to emotion, regions with greater activation when reappraising than attending were thought to reflect processes used to exert cognitive control. In contrast, regions more active for attend than reappraise trials were hypothesized to be important for emotion processing that would be deactivated by reappraisal. According to their findings, reappraisal of negative photos successfully diminished negative affect, and the neural correlates were (1) activation in the regions of the LPFC and MPFC essential for working memory, cognitive control, and self-monitoring and (2) decreased activation in the MOFC and the amygdala, which are involved in emotion processing [79]. This has subsequently been confirmed in other studies, although the decrease in amygdala activation was only reported in half of the studies. Nevertheless, a recent meta-analysis of 48 neuroimaging studies reported that reappraisal consistently activated cognitive control regions in frontal cortex and lateral temporal cortex and modulated the bilateral amygdala [83].

We investigated the neural correlates of reappraisal in people with a predisposition towards psychosis. To this end, 600 undergraduate students completed the Community Assessment of Psychic Experiences Questionnaire (CAPE), positive symptom subscale. We subsequently selected two groups, one from each extreme end of the distribution (total $N = 34$). We expected less effective emotion regulation strategies in the high psychosis proneness group, but observed equal performance, that is, both groups reported successful diminishment of experienced negative emotion. However, high psychosis-prone subjects showed stronger activation than low subjects in a number of prefrontal regions (anterior cingulate, left dorsomedial PFC, and right ventrolateral PFC) during reappraisal, relative to only attending to negative pictures. The amygdala response to negative stimuli was decreased through reappraisal only in the low group. Functional connectivity analysis revealed less prefrontal-amygdala coupling in high psychosis-prone subjects. Thus, the evidence from neural activation patterns points towards less efficient interaction between regions involved in cognitive control and emotion processing. In patients with schizophrenia, reduced levels of reappraisal have been reported [84, 85],

suggesting dysfunction in regions subserving cognitive control of emotion. However, only one study has been reported as yet using the above mentioned neuroimaging task in patients [86]. Schizophrenia patients showed that prefrontal hypoactivation of the right VLPFC occurred during downregulation, compared to control subjects, and showed no coupling between prefrontal cortex and amygdala, in contrast to control subjects.

5. Social Cognition, Theory of Mind, and Empathy

Social cognition concerns the cognitive functions underlying social perception and interaction. Besides emotion recognition, understanding other people is crucial for this. Theory of mind (ToM) can be defined as the ability to correctly attribute feelings, knowledge, intentions, and goals to other people and is of crucial importance for proper social interaction [87]. It has been suggested to be involved in positive symptoms of schizophrenia, for example, paranoid delusions [88, 89]. A deficit in overruling the automatic response and hence wrongfully maintaining a positive self-image may result in an impaired ToM, leading to an inappropriate attribution of threatening thoughts, intentions, or behaviors to others. Two main brain regions are found to play a crucial part in ToM, the temporoparietal junction and the prefrontal cortex. The temporoparietal junction is thought to be recruited selectively for the attribution of mental states to others [90, 91]. Furthermore, several neuroimaging studies have shown frontal lobe activation in healthy subjects while reasoning about other people's mental states (e.g., [92]) as well as an impaired theory of mind in people with frontal lobe lesions (e.g., [93]). At least three possible contributions of the frontal lobe to the ability to have a theory of mind have been formulated. First, the frontal lobe is thought to contribute to the theory of mind concerning the control processes supporting complex reasoning [94]. Second, the frontal lobes may be involved in holding two separate perspectives simultaneously [95]. A third possible contribution of the frontal lobes to theory of mind was put forward by Ruby and Decety [92]. They suggest that the frontal lobes are of crucial importance in inhibiting one's own perspective of the world while inferring someone else's perspective.

In an experiment by Vogeley and colleagues [96], short stories were administered in which subjects themselves were featured (high self-perspective), compared with stories in which the subject did not play any part (low self-perspective). In both types of stories, the subject had to infer the perspective of another person. However, only in the high self-perspective condition, the subject had to take his/her own perspective into account. This enabled the isolation of inhibition of one's own perspective and showed right inferior frontal gyrus activation. Consistent with these findings, Samson et al. [91, 94] developed an elegant paradigm which enables the direct comparison of a low inhibition self-perspective condition with a high inhibition self-perspective condition. This task is particularly interesting since it allows for the selective measurement of the inhibition of self-perspective in a nonemotional setting. The task was administered to a patient who suffered from a right hemisphere stroke, resulting in a lesion in the right inferior and middle frontal gyrus extending to the right superior temporal gyrus and showed a specific deficit in the high inhibition self-perspective task as compared to the low-inhibition self-perspective task. Following these results, Samson et al. [94] suggest that theory of mind consists of two components, which are confounded in classic theory of mind tasks. They propose that taking someone else's perspective may be a serial process in which the inhibition of self-perspective is a first and necessary step before someone else's perspective can be inferred. The brain region that is thought to be of critical importance for this process is the right inferior prefrontal cortex. This inference is confirmed by the findings that the right inferior prefrontal cortex is necessary for the inhibition of responses in nonsocial tasks [97].

With regard to insight, it could be hypothesized that due to a lack of inhibitory control rational, explicit self-processing cannot proceed and will therefore not be able to overrule the automatic response preserving the positive self-image. Psychotic patients who lack insight may show an impaired self-inhibition as compared to psychotic patients who do have insight into their condition, leading to the inability to use the feedback provided by the environment to adapt their wrongfully preserved self-image.

Theory of mind may further be decomposed into different mechanisms for the *cognitive* and the *affective* aspects of mentalizing, which may be differentially impaired in schizophrenia patients [98]. In order to study the role of PFC cortices for these different ToM aspects, Shamay-Tsoory and Aharon-Peretz [99] designed an interesting task that allowed evaluation of affective and cognitive mentalizing abilities based on verbal and nonverbal information. The task involves the ability to judge mental states based on verbal and eye gaze cues, with stimuli divided into three main conditions: affective, cognitive, and physical. Additionally, different aspects of ToM can be assessed: (1) first order ToM, requiring the attribution of a mental state (cognitive) or an emotion (affective) to a character and (2) second order ToM, based on understanding beliefs about others' beliefs and desires (cognitive) or understanding emotions about others' emotions (affective). Results showed that patients with schizophrenia (especially those with negative symptoms) and patients with ventromedial (VM) prefrontal damage were significantly less accurate in their response to affective 2nd order ToM conditions compared to controls. We investigated differences in prefrontal cortex activation between subjects with high versus low psychosis proneness scores during mentalizing to further delineate the role of PFC regions in vulnerability towards psychosis. Using the same task as Shamay-Tsoory and Aharon-Peretz [99], we observed stronger prefrontal activation in psychosis-prone subjects than in subjects without this proneness during first and second order mentalizing [100]. For first order mentalizing, this excessive recruitment of PFC was localized in the anterior prefrontal cortex (BA 10), whereas for second order mentalizing lateral prefrontal regions were hyperactivated (BA 46/49). A limitation of the task may be that the stimuli are rather artificial, schematic drawings, which may compromise ecological validity.

Other ToM paradigms allow for measurement of inhibition of self-perspective, a key component of ToM, and belief reasoning being another important component. Samson et al. [94] showed that inhibition of self-perspective can be selectively impaired in patients with frontal brain damage. Using neuroimaging in healthy volunteers, with the same theory of mind task as Samson et al. [94], we found activation of bilateral inferior frontal gyrus for inhibition of self-perspective, while belief reasoning was mediated by the left superior and middle temporal gyri [101]. We also investigated brain activation during this task in participants with psychosis-proneness as established by high scores on the CAPE psychosis subscale [102]. A stop-signal task was included additionally, to measure simple response inhibition. Thus, we could test the hypothesis that the reduced inhibition of self-perspective is not due to a general reduction in the inhibitory function of the frontal cortex. A stronger activation of the left inferior frontal gyrus was found for psychosis-prone subjects, when compared to subjects without psychosis-proneness. Such a difference was not observed on the simple response inhibition task, however. Therefore, the results indicate that, at a neural level, psychosis-prone subjects need a stronger recruitment of neural resources in order to inhibit self-perspective. Indeed, the distinction between self-inhibition and belief reasoning needs further investigation in patient populations.

Research has also been directed at a concept that is related to ToM: empathy. Rather than concerning the ability to understand what others think, empathy refers to the ability to feel what others *feel*. Several studies have reported reduced levels of empathy in patients with schizophrenia [103]. Social cognition also encompasses other processes than the higher-order cognitive processes involved in theory of mind. More specifically, the investigation of perception and interpretation of social cues deserves more attention. For example, patients with schizophrenia may be impaired in detecting facial cues associated with trustworthiness [78, 104]. Other aspects of social cues involve signals of approach and avoidance. In schizophrenia, perception of such cues has been tested using a visual distance illusion in which two cartoon figures that are running and looking towards each other look more close to each other than two figures running and looking away from each other, even when the actual physical distance is the same [105, 106]. Patients with schizophrenia are less sensitive to this illusion [106], as are patients with autism [105] and Klinefelter syndrome [106], who also have social-emotional deficits.

6. Reduced Insight/Awareness of Illness

Lack of insight (unawareness of illness) is a common and clinically relevant feature of psychosis [107]. It can be subdivided into three components: (1) awareness of having an illness, (2) recognizing psychotic symptoms as abnormal, and (3) acceptance of prescribed treatment [108]. Lack of insight has been associated with poor treatment compliance and medical adherence, poorer global functioning, severity of psychopathology, recurrence, and poorer outcome [109]. This is not only inconvenient for the patient, it can also lead to considerable distress in family members, friends and treating clinicians since it hampers their attempt to help and impedes with solutions to the problems engendered by the symptoms of the patient (e.g., believes he is being poisoned and refuses to eat). The cognitive and neural bases of insight in psychosis remain unclear, however, rendering it a scientific mystery. Although associations have been established between poor insight in psychosis and reduced cognitive functioning, especially with regard to cognitive set-shifting thought to be mediated by the frontal cortex, the modest magnitude of the association suggests that cognitive factors can not sufficiently explain impaired insight (see meta-analysis by Aleman et al., [110]). Indeed, in a replication and extension of this meta-analysis (based on data from 72 studies and a total population of 5429 patients), Nair et al. [111] reported that there is a small but significant relationship between clinical insight, some aspects of cognitive insight, and neurocognition. This underlines the complexity of the insight construct and may imply that while the neurocognitive model is important, cognitive impairment is likely to be the only one of several contributing factors. A study by Quee et al. [112] in 270 patients with nonaffective psychosis points to one of these factors: phase of illness. Neurocognitive impairment was associated with reduced insight, but only in patients with multiple episode or chronic psychosis. Social cognition, that is, recognition of emotional expressions and mentalizing, was also related to insight. No relationship between cognitive impairment and reduced insight was found in patients with recent-onset psychosis.

A framework is needed that can account for the above mentioned observations, that is, the role of impaired cognitive flexibility and other cognitive impairments, but that at the same time moves beyond these factors, as they can only provide partial explanations at best. Insight in psychosis could be hypothesized to depend on self-evaluation, where self-evaluation is conceptualized along the lines of Epstein's [113] cognitive-experiential self theory (CEST). According to CEST, people respond to the world on two levels, rational and experiential. These ways of responding are conceived of as two distinct mental systems for adapting to the demands of our environment. The rational system is thought to operate primarily on a conscious level, involving working memory and language (though the latter not by definition). In contrast, the experiential self has a stronger emotional input. It is thought to operate largely at an unconscious level and processes information fast and holistically. The rational system will be slower than the experiential system and will require more effort. It is important to note that, although the two systems are thought of as independent, they are assumed to interact with each other and will both influence behavior. This account can be complemented by the model of dual attitudes, proposed by Wilson et al. [114]. This model highlights the complex interplay between implicit and explicit evaluations and posits that people may simultaneously possess different evaluations towards the same attitude object. Such dual attitudes will then become represented at an explicit level, where they are readily accessible to self-reporting. However, the activation of these newly formed attitudes has not yet become automatic and, hence, requires a fair amount of cognitive capacity and motivation. At the same time, people's original attitudes are assumed to continue to exist in

memory, albeit at an implicit level. When there is sufficient capacity and motivation, people will effortfully retrieve their newly formed, explicit attitudes from memory. By contrast, when capacity and motivation are lacking, people's original, implicit attitudes may reemerge. It is important to note that several quantitative measures have been developed to target aspects of implicit and explicit self-processing (e.g., [114, 115]).

In short, consistent with CEST, one can presume that implicit, experiential self-processing is biased towards maintaining a positive self-image (which excludes severe mental illness). To obtain insight in psychosis, rational, explicit self-processing must overrule this automatic response. This will only occur in the face of sufficient cognitive capacity and motivation. However, a large number of psychotic patients lack both, which hampers the development of insight.

A number of studies have focused on the hypothesis that reduced insight may arise from abnormalities in brain circuits subserving self-evaluation. Self-evaluation involves the ability to think about and make judgments regarding one's own cognitive, personality, physical, and emotional characteristics. Thus, patients with reduced insight are hypothesized to have difficulties in evaluating their own behavior and mental processes in relationship to their environment, and to implicit and explicit sociocultural rules and expectations. An important component of self-awareness is the ability to reflect on your personal abilities, characteristics, and personal situation. The underlying neurocognitive processes for such self-evaluation are still unclear but potentially relevant for understanding insight in psychosis. Johnson et al. [116] studied brain activation during self-evaluation in healthy subjects, who were asked to respond to a variety of statements requiring knowledge of and reflection on their own abilities, traits, and attitudes (e.g., "I forget important things", "I am a good friend"). Reponses were compared to those of statements requiring a basic level of semantic knowledge (e.g., "ten seconds is more than a minute", "you need water to live"), used as a control condition for auditory comprehension, attentional demands, decision-making, the motoric response, and any common retrieval processes. The results showed involvement of the medial prefrontal cortex and posterior cingulate during self-evaluation. This is consistent with lesion locations in patients with impaired self-awareness, as well as with other functional imaging studies involving mentalizing about the self or others [117]. Thus, one could hypothesize reduced activation of self-related regions in patients with poor insight as compared to patients with intact insight.

Van der Meer et al. [118] provided a quantitative integration of the neuroimaging evidence regarding self-evaluation, which yielded two areas within the medial prefrontal cortex (MPFC), namely the ventral and dorsal MPFC. In a study that contrasted schizophrenia patients with good versus poor insight on a task of self-evaluation and other evaluations, better insight (as measured with the Schedule of Assessment of Insight Expanded [119]) was associated with greater response in the inferior frontal gyrus, anterior insula, and inferior parietal lobule during self-reflection [120]. In addition, better cognitive insight (as measured with the Beck Cognitive Insight Scale [121]) was associated with higher activation in the ventromedial prefrontal cortex during self-reflection.

The cognitive regulation of emotion may also be regarded to be of relevance for insight. Patients with reduced insight seem to have more difficulties in accepting the emotional consequences of a threatening experience to the self, as is becoming aware of having a mental illness. Several studies have found that many forms of psychopathology revolve around failures to adaptively regulate emotional responses, with consequences ranging from personal distress to socially maladaptive and self-destructive behaviors [122]. Empathy may also be of relevance. We hypothesized a relationship between reduced levels of empathy and less insight in psychosis, based on the rationale that being touched by the emotional state of others will facilitate the accommodation of their perspective and will therefore make a contribution to insight over and above emotion perception and perspective taking. Consistent with this prediction, a regression analysis involving several cognitive and affective measures showed the strongest unique contribution to be from empathy [123]. For this study, forty-six patients with a diagnosis of schizophrenia and fifty-three healthy controls were assessed with a test battery consisting of tests of social cognition (a self-rating scale for affective empathy, a ToM task assessing both cognitive and affective ToM, and two tests of emotion perception), verbal memory, executive functioning, psychomotor speed, and intelligence. Being able to empathize with others at both the affective and cognitive level may enhance insight in schizophrenia. Brain research could focus on regions known to be involved in empathy, for example, anterior insula, cingulate cortex, and regions subserving action simulation and mentalizing [124].

7. Apathy

Besides psychotic symptoms such as hallucinations on the one hand and cognitive impairment on the other, lack of initiative and social withdrawal are key symptoms of schizophrenia. Apathy or lack of will (also termed avolition or abulia) refers to markedly reduced levels of interest in daily activities and a lack of initiative. It may present as indifference. Profound levels of apathy are common in schizophrenia patients, and have been suggested to be the most central feature of negative symptoms, representing the critical component, particularly with regard to functional outcome [125]. Understanding apathy has important implications, as apathy is the strongest predictor of poor functioning, unemployment, severity of illness, and worse outcome in routine clinical practice [126, 127]. Indeed, apathy is arguably one of the most important clinical and scientific problem for schizophrenia researchers to tackle. Surprisingly, though, studies into the cognitive and neural substrate of apathy are scarce, even though a number of studies have addressed the brain basis of negative symptoms of schizophrenia, that largely reflect apathy (e.g., affective flattening, diminished levels of interest, social withdrawal, and lack of energy). However, there is also a paucity of research into the cognitive and neural basis of negative symptoms in general. Positive symptoms, such as delusions and hallucinations, may dominate in acute phases of the illness and draw more attention due to their bizarre nature. In addition, there has been a lack of theorizing with regard to negative symptoms

such as apathy. Apathy should be studied in its own right. Indeed, accumulating evidence supports apathy as a distinct syndrome with an identifiable neurobiology [128].

Different forms of apathy have been distinguished on clinical grounds. For example, Stuss et al. [129] proposed multiple subtypes, depending on which neural circuit is affected. Involvement of the oculomotor circuit would yield a different form of apathy (e.g., based on neglect) than the involvement of the supplementary motor circuit (reduced motor output). They also distinguished between apathy as a consequence of orbitofrontal impairment, which would be associated with a reduction in motivational response due to lack of limbic-affective input and "social apathy," which would result from disturbance in sense of self and social awareness due to anterior frontal lesions. Levy and Dubois [130] distinguished between three subtypes: "emotional-affective," "cognitive," and "auto-activation." The first would be characterized by deficient linkage of emotional-affective signals and ongoing behavior, the second by difficulties in elaborating action plans necessary for goal-directed behavior, and the third by the inability to self-activate thoughts and actions. The different forms of apathy are not primarily due to depression, but like depression, involve a reduction in behavioral activation.

The conceptualisation of different types of apathy has not been taken to schizophrenia as yet, but research is ongoing at the University Medical Center Groningen to investigate this in detail. Initial evidence for apathy subtypes in schizophrenia receives support from factor analyses on the structure of negative symptoms. Negative symptoms of schizophrenia are normally grouped into a single category. We recently carried out two factor analyses on large independent data sets that confirmed the distinction between two factors [131]. First, an exploratory factor analysis was carried out based on interviews with the Positive and Negative Syndrome Scale (PANSS) in a sample of 664 schizophrenia patients from the north of the Netherlands (provinces Groningen, Friesland, and Drenthe). Only items related to negative symptoms in earlier studies were included and categorized into one or more negative symptom dimensions. In a second step, the acquired symptom structure was subsequently tested for stability by confirmatory factor analysis of PANSS interviews in a large separate cohort of 2172 schizophrenia patients, from the GROUP study, that involves 13 research centers from all regions in the Netherlands. Item selection and exploratory factor analysis resulted in a two-factor structure of negative symptoms. The first factor consisted of PANSS items N1 flat affect (lack of expressivity), N3 poor rapport, N6 lack of spontaneity, G5 mannerisms and posturing, G7 motor retardation and G13 avolition. The second factor consisted of items N2 emotional withdrawal, N4 passive/apathetic social withdrawal, and G16 active social avoidance.

We interpreted the first factor as being related to core negative symptoms of schizophrenia, reflecting loss of initiation of action. It could be described as a "loss of initiative" factor. The second factor could be described as a social-emotional withdrawal factor, in particular "loss of interest" in these areas. Apathy is central to most of these items (e.g., avolition or passive/apathetic social withdrawal), which supports extrapolation to apathy proper.

Depression can pose a source of clinical and conceptual confusion, as it may be difficult to differentiate it from apathy. However, although apathy can be an expression of depression, it is independent from the symptoms associated with depression [130]. For example, key symptoms of depression as defined by the World Health Organization's international classification of diseases (ICD) include loss of confidence, excessive guilt, recurrent thoughts of death, poor concentration, sleep disturbance, and change in appetite or weight. These symptoms are not part of the concept of apathy, although some of them may be correlated, such as poor concentration. Indeed, the apathy evaluation scale [131] has been shown to correlate only weakly with depression. To avoid confusion through possible overlap with clinical depression, it is advisable to exclude a diagnosis of depression (defined as DSM-IV major depressive disorder, dysthymic disorder, depressive disorder not otherwise specified or bipolar disorder) in patients that are included in studies of apathy in schizophrenia, Parkinson's Disease or Alzheimer's Disease.

One could hypothesize different neural circuits to underlie different forms of apathy. For example, a lack of initiative could be linked to a deficient frontoparietal action network, whereas a lack of interest could be linked to a deficient ventral striatal—orbital-medial frontal saliency network. Few studies have as yet investigated the neural basis of apathy in schizophrenia, however. One study reported reduced frontal lobe volumes and more pronounced cognitive deficits in schizophrenia patients with high levels of apathy compared to schizophrenia patients with low levels of apathy [132]. Callicott et al. [133] reported an association between negative symptoms and reduced levels of N-acetyl-aspartate in DLPFC, using magnetic resonance spectroscopy, suggesting reduced neuronal integrity in that area. With regard to motivational processing, a recent fMRI study [134] showed that higher anhedonia was associated with reduced activation to positive versus negative stimuli in bilateral amygdala and right ventral striatum in patients with schizophrenia. In a similar vein, Simon et al. [135] recently reported a negative correlation between apathy levels and ventral-striatal activation during reward *anticipation* in schizophrenia patients, while activation during *receipt* of reward was negatively correlated with severity of depressive symptoms. These studies did not distinguish between subtypes of apathy, however, which are in need of further investigation.

In terms of treatment, apathy is notoriously difficult to improve. Novel pharmacotherapeutical approaches are being tested, such as sarcosine, a compound that targets glutamatergic transmission in the frontal cortex. Sarcosine is a selective inhibitor of the glycine transporter 1 [GlyT1] that has shown promise in improving negative symptoms of schizophrenia [136]. Other compounds that modulate glutamatergic signalling are being investigated [137]. Noninvasive neurostimulation with rTMS may also be a promising treatment option. Most studies apply daily 10 Hz stimulation over the left dorsolateral prefrontal cortex. A meta-analysis of nine trials published by 2008 yielded a significant effect (with moderate effect size) of rTMS as compared to sham TMS in improving negative symptoms [138]. Studies with daily stimulation for three weeks or more showed a larger effect size than trials of shorter duration. This was confirmed recently in a meta-analysis that included 12 studies, published up to 2011 [139]. It would be of interest to use fMRI before and after rTMS trials for improving apathy to evaluate whether increased activation of the dorsolateral prefrontal cortex can account for clinical improvement. Future research will also benefit from the development of brief, reliable, and valid standardized measures of negative symptoms (especially apathy/avolition) which will aid its assessment in multicenter trials [140].

8. Concluding Remarks

Although etiology and treatment of schizophrenia remain poorly understood, recent decades have shown progress in delineating cognitive and emotional processing abnormalities and elucidating their neural basis. Impaired activation of and connectivity between frontotemporal, frontoparietal, and frontostriatal brain networks subserving cognitive functioning and integration of cognition and emotion has been consistently reported. A distributed network of cortical and subcortical regions is activated during hallucinations [141]. Language circuitry has been shown to be involved in auditory-verbal hallucinations, and rTMS over language regions may reduce severity of hallucinations in some patients. The effects on brain activation of such treatments deserve further investigation [142]. Top-down attentional processing in perception may be dysregulated in people with a disposition towards hallucination. Perception of emotion is impaired in schizophrenia patients and emotion regulation may be compromised due to reduced cognitive control of emotion (connectivity between frontal areas and limbic areas). Social cognition and especially theory of mind processes have been the subject of intensive study. These processes are highly relevant for social functioning, an important target outcome for treatment of schizophrenia. Impaired self-evaluation, mediated by midline cortical areas (medial frontal and posterior cingulate) may contribute to poor awareness of illness, and more specifically insight into psychosis. Finally, future research should focus on pervasive negative symptoms such as apathy and underlying neural systems. This will pave the way for better treatment options and ultimately a better quality of life for people suffering from schizophrenia.

Conflict of Interests

The author declares that there is no conflict of interests regarding the publication of this paper.

Acknowledgment

The author was supported by a VICI Grant no. 016.128.606 from the Netherlands Organisation for Scientific Research (N.W.O.).

References

[1] K. T. Mueser and S. R. McGurk, "Schizophrenia," *The Lancet*, vol. 363, no. 9426, pp. 2063–2072, 2004.

[2] A. Jablensky, "Schizophrenia: the epidemiological horizon," in *Schizophrenia*, S. R. Hirsch and D. R. Weinberger, Eds., Blackwell, Oxford, UK, 1995.

[3] H. I. Kaplan, B. J. Sadock, and J. A. Grebb, *Synopsis of Psychiatry*, William and Wilkins, Baltimore, Md, USA, 1994.

[4] A. Aleman, R. S. Kahn, and J.-P. Selten, "Sex differences in the risk of schizophrenia: evidence from meta-analysis," *Archives of General Psychiatry*, vol. 60, no. 6, pp. 565–571, 2003.

[5] The American Psychiatric Association, *Diagnostic and Statistical Manual of Mental Disorders*, The American Psychiatric Association, Arlington, Va, USA, 5th edition, 2013.

[6] W. T. Carpenter Jr., J. S. Strauss, and S. Muleh, "Are there pathognomonic symptoms in schizophrenia? An empiric investigation of Schneider's first rank symptoms," *Archives of General Psychiatry*, vol. 28, no. 6, pp. 847–852, 1973.

[7] N. C. Andreasen, M. Flaum, V. W. Swayze II, G. Tyrrell, and S. Arndt, "Positive and negative symptoms in schizophrenia: a critical reappraisal," *Archives of General Psychiatry*, vol. 47, no. 7, pp. 615–621, 1990.

[8] H. Häfner and W. An der Heiden, "Course and outcome of schizophrenia," in *Schizophrenia*, S. R. Hirsch and D. R. Weinberger, Eds., Blackwell, London, UK, 2nd edition, 2003.

[9] R. W. Heinrichs and K. K. Zakzanis, "Neurocognitive deficit in schizophrenia: a quantitative review of the evidence," *Neuropsychology*, vol. 12, no. 3, pp. 426–445, 1998.

[10] A. Reichenberg and P. D. Harvey, "Neuropsychological impairments in schizophrenia: integration of performance-based and brain imaging findings," *Psychological Bulletin*, vol. 133, no. 5, pp. 833–858, 2007.

[11] A. Aleman, R. Hijman, E. H. F. De Haan, and R. S. Kahn, "Memory impairment in schizophrenia: a meta-analysis," *The American Journal of Psychiatry*, vol. 156, no. 9, pp. 1358–1366, 1999.

[12] J. Schaefer, E. Giangrande, D. R. Weinberger, and D. Dickinson, "The global cognitive impairment in schizophrenia: consistent over decades and around the world," *Schizophrenia Research*, vol. 150, no. 1, pp. 42–50, 2013.

[13] M. M. Sitskoorn, A. Aleman, S. J. H. Ebisch, M. C. M. Appels, and R. S. Kahn, "Cognitive deficits in relatives of patients with schizophrenia: a meta-analysis," *Schizophrenia Research*, vol. 71, no. 2-3, pp. 285–295, 2004.

[14] B. E. Snitz, A. W. MacDonald III, and C. S. Carter, "Cognitive deficits in unaffected first-degree relatives of schizophrenia patients: a meta-analytic review of putative endophenotypes," *Schizophrenia Bulletin*, vol. 32, no. 1, pp. 179–194, 2006.

[15] D. Dickinson, M. E. Ramsey, and J. M. Gold, "Overlooking the obvious: a meta-analytic comparison of digit symbol coding tasks and other cognitive measures in schizophrenia," *Archives of General Psychiatry*, vol. 64, no. 5, pp. 532–542, 2007.

[16] E. E. M. Knowles, A. S. David, and A. Reichenberg, "Processing speed deficits in schizophrenia: reexamining the evidence," *The American Journal of Psychiatry*, vol. 167, no. 7, pp. 828–835, 2010.

[17] S. R. Marder and W. Fenton, "Measurement and treatment research to improve cognition in schizophrenia: NIMH MATRICS initiative to support the development of agents for improving cognition in schizophrenia," *Schizophrenia Research*, vol. 72, no. 1, pp. 5–9, 2004.

[18] B. W. Palmer, R. K. Heaton, J. Kuck et al., "Is it possible to be schizophrenic yet neuropsychologically normal?" *Neuropsychology*, vol. 11, no. 3, pp. 437–446, 1997.

[19] C. M. Wilk, J. M. Gold, R. P. McMahon, K. Humber, V. N. Iannone, and R. W. Buchanan, "No, it is not possible to be schizophrenic yet neuropsychologically normal," *Neuropsychology*, vol. 19, no. 6, pp. 778–786, 2005.

[20] D. R. Weinberger, K. F. Berman, and R. F. Zec, "Physiologic dysfunction of dorsolateral prefrontal cortex in schizophrenia. I. Regional cerebral blood flow evidence," *Archives of General Psychiatry*, vol. 43, no. 2, pp. 114–124, 1986.

[21] M. J. Minzenberg, A. R. Laird, S. Thelen, C. S. Carter, and D. C. Glahn, "Meta-analysis of 41 functional neuroimaging studies of executive function in schizophrenia," *Archives of General Psychiatry*, vol. 66, no. 8, pp. 811–822, 2009.

[22] J. H. Callicott, A. Bertolino, V. S. Mattay et al., "Physiological dysfunction of the dorsolateral prefrontal cortex in schizophrenia revisited," *Cerebral Cortex*, vol. 10, no. 11, pp. 1078–1092, 2000.

[23] D. S. Manoach, D. Z. Press, V. Thangaraj et al., "Schizophrenic subjects activate dorsolateral prefrontal cortex during a working memory task, as measured by fMRI," *Biological Psychiatry*, vol. 45, no. 9, pp. 1128–1137, 1999.

[24] A. M. Achim and M. Lepage, "Episodic memory-related activation in schizophrenia: meta-analysis," *British Journal of Psychiatry*, vol. 187, pp. 500–509, 2005.

[25] D. M. Barch and A. Ceaser, "Cognition in schizophrenia: core psychological and neural mechanisms," *Trends in Cognitive Sciences*, vol. 16, no. 1, pp. 27–34, 2012.

[26] R. S. Kahn and R. S. Keefe, "Schizophrenia is a cognitive illness: time for a change in focus," *JAMA Psychiatry*, 2013.

[27] A. Meyer-Lindenberg, "From maps to mechanisms through neuroimaging of schizophrenia," *Nature*, vol. 468, no. 7321, pp. 194–202, 2010.

[28] A. Aleman, E. H. F. de Haan, S. A. Castner, G. V. Williams, and P. S. Goldman-Rakic, "Antipsychotics and working memory in Schizophrenia," *Science*, vol. 289, no. 5476, pp. 56–58, 2000.

[29] A. L. Mishara and T. E. Goldberg, "A meta-analysis and critical review of the effects of conventional neuroleptic treatment on cognition in schizophrenia: opening a closed book," *Biological Psychiatry*, vol. 55, no. 10, pp. 1013–1022, 2004.

[30] R. S. E. Keefe, J. A. Sweeney, H. Gu et al., "Effects of olanzapine, quetiapine, and risperidone on neurocognitive function in early psychosis: a randomized, double-blind 52-week comparison," *The American Journal of Psychiatry*, vol. 164, no. 7, pp. 1061–1071, 2007.

[31] E. J. Liemburg, H. Knegtering, H. C. Klein, R. Kortekaas, and A. Aleman, "Antipsychotic medication and prefrontal cortex activation: a review of neuroimaging findings," *European Neuropsychopharmacology*, vol. 22, no. 6, pp. 387–400, 2012.

[32] L. Krabbendam and A. Aleman, "Cognitive rehabilitation in schizophrenia: a quantitative analysis of controlled studies," *Psychopharmacology*, vol. 169, no. 3-4, pp. 376–382, 2003.

[33] T. Wykes, V. Huddy, C. Cellard, S. R. McGurk, and P. Czobor, "A meta-analysis of cognitive remediation for schizophrenia: methodology and effect sizes," *The American Journal of Psychiatry*, vol. 168, no. 5, pp. 472–485, 2011.

[34] S. M. Eack, G. E. Hogarty, R. Y. Cho et al., "Neuroprotective effects of cognitive enhancement therapy against gray matter loss in early schizophrenia: results from a 2-year randomized controlled trial," *Archives of General Psychiatry*, vol. 67, no. 7, pp. 674–682, 2010.

[35] A. Aleman and F. Laroi, *Hallucinations: The Science of Idiosyncratic Perception*, The American Psychological Association, Washington, DC, USA, 2008.

[36] S. McCarthy-Jones, T. Trauer, A. Mackinnon, E. Sims, N. Thomas, and D. L. Copolov, "A new phenomenological survey of auditory hallucinations: evidence for subtypes and implications for theory and practice," *Schizophrenia Bulletin*, 2013.

[37] D. A. Silbersweig, E. Stern, C. Frith et al., "A functional neuroanatomy of hallucinations in schizophrenia," *Nature*, vol. 378, no. 6553, pp. 176–179, 1995.

[38] S. S. Shergill, M. J. Brammer, S. C. R. Williams, R. M. Murray, and P. K. McGuire, "Mapping auditory hallucinations in schizophrenia using functional magnetic resonance imaging," *Archives of General Psychiatry*, vol. 57, no. 11, pp. 1033–1038, 2000.

[39] B. R. Lennox, S. B. G. Park, I. Medley, P. G. Morris, and P. B. Jones, "The functional anatomy of auditory hallucinations in schizophrenia," *Psychiatry Research*, vol. 100, no. 1, pp. 13–20, 2000.

[40] I. E. C. Sommer, K. M. J. Diederen, J.-D. Blom et al., "Auditory verbal hallucinations predominantly activate the right inferior frontal area," *Brain*, vol. 131, no. 12, pp. 3169–3177, 2008.

[41] R. Jardri, A. Pouchet, D. Pins, and P. Thomas, "Cortical activations during auditory verbal hallucinations in schizophrenia: a coordinate-based meta-analysis," *The American Journal of Psychiatry*, vol. 168, no. 1, pp. 73–81, 2011.

[42] S. Kühn and J. Gallinat, "Quantitative meta-analysis on state and trait aspects of auditory verbal hallucinations in schizophrenia," *Schizophrenia Bulletin*, vol. 38, no. 4, pp. 779–786, 2012.

[43] R. E. Hoffman, R. Gueorguieva, K. A. Hawkins et al., "Temporoparietal transcranial magnetic stimulation for auditory hallucinations: safety, efficacy and moderators in a fifty patient sample," *Biological Psychiatry*, vol. 58, no. 2, pp. 97–104, 2005.

[44] A. Aleman, I. E. Sommer, and R. S. Kahn, "Efficacy of slow repetitive transcranial magnetic stimulation in the treatment of resistant auditory hallucinations in schizophrenia: a meta-analysis," *Journal of Clinical Psychiatry*, vol. 68, no. 3, pp. 416–421, 2007.

[45] A. Aleman, "Use of repetitive transcranial magnetic stimulation for treatment in psychiatry," *Clinical Psychopharmacology and Neuroscience*, vol. 11, no. 2, pp. 53–59, 2013.

[46] A. Vercammen, H. Knegtering, R. Bruggeman et al., "Effects of bilateral repetitive transcranial magnetic stimulation on treatment resistant auditory-verbal hallucinations in schizophrenia: a randomized controlled trial," *Schizophrenia Research*, vol. 114, no. 1–3, pp. 172–179, 2009.

[47] C. W. Slotema, A. Aleman, Z. J. Daskalakis, and I. E. Sommer, "Meta-analysis of repetitive transcranial magnetic stimulation in the treatment of auditory verbal hallucinations: update and effects after one month," *Schizophrenia Research*, vol. 142, no. 1–3, pp. 40–45, 2012.

[48] F. Waters, P. Allen, A. Aleman et al., "Auditory hallucinations in schizophrenia and nonschizophrenia populations: a review and integrated model of cognitive mechanisms," *Schizophrenia Bulletin*, vol. 38, no. 4, pp. 683–693, 2012.

[49] J. C. Badcock, F. A. V. Waters, M. T. Maybery, and P. T. Michie, "Auditory hallucinations: failure to inhibit irrelevant memories," *Cognitive Neuropsychiatry*, vol. 10, no. 2, pp. 125–136, 2005.

[50] F. A. V. Waters, J. C. Badcock, P. T. Michie, and M. T. Maybery, "Auditory hallucinations in schizophrenia: intrusive thoughts and forgotten memories," *Cognitive Neuropsychiatry*, vol. 11, no. 1, pp. 65–83, 2006.

[51] M. F. Soriano, J. F. Jiménez, P. Román, and M. T. Bajo, "Intentional inhibition in memory and hallucinations: directed forgetting and updating," *Neuropsychology*, vol. 23, no. 1, pp. 61–70, 2009.

[52] R.-P. Behrendt, "Underconstrained perception: a theoretical approach to the nature and function of verbal hallucinations," *Comprehensive Psychiatry*, vol. 39, no. 4, pp. 236–248, 1998.

[53] S. Grossberg, "How hallucinations may arise from brain mechanisms of learning, attention, and volition," *Journal of the International Neuropsychological Society*, vol. 6, no. 5, pp. 583–592, 2000.

[54] A. Vercammen and A. Aleman, "Semantic expectations can induce false perceptions in hallucination-prone individuals," *Schizophrenia Bulletin*, vol. 36, no. 1, pp. 151–156, 2010.

[55] K. Daalman, S. Verkooijen, E. M. Derks, A. Aleman, and I. E. Sommer, "The influence of semantic top-down processing in auditory verbal hallucinations," *Schizophrenia Research*, vol. 139, no. 1–3, pp. 82–86, 2012.

[56] A. S. David, "Why we need more debate on whether psychotic symptoms lie on a continuum with normality," *Psychological Medicine*, vol. 40, no. 12, pp. 1935–1942, 2010.

[57] A. Aleman, E. Formisano, H. Koppenhagen, P. Hagoort, E. H. F. de Haan, and R. S. Kahn, "The functional neuroanatomy of metrical stress evaluation of perceived and imagined spoken words," *Cerebral Cortex*, vol. 15, no. 2, pp. 221–228, 2005.

[58] A. Vercammen, H. Knegtering, J. A. denBoer, E. J. Liemburg, and A. Aleman, "Auditory hallucinations in schizophrenia are associated with reduced functional connectivity of the temporo-parietal area," *Biological Psychiatry*, vol. 67, no. 10, pp. 912–918, 2010.

[59] B. Curcic-Blake, E. Liemburg, A. Vercammen et al., "When broca goes uninformed: reduced information flow to Broca's area in Schizophrenia patients with auditory hallucinations," *Schizophrenia Bulletin*, vol. 39, no. 5, pp. 1087–1095, 2013.

[60] M. K. Johnson, S. Hashtroudi, and D. Stephen Lindsay, "Source monitoring," *Psychological Bulletin*, vol. 114, no. 1, pp. 3–28, 1993.

[61] M. K. Johnson and C. L. Raye, "Reality monitoring," *Psychological Review*, vol. 88, no. 1, pp. 67–85, 1981.

[62] R. S. E. Keefe, "The neurobiology of disturbances of the self: autonoetic agnosia in schizophrenia," in *Insight and Psychosis*, X. F. Amador and A. David, Eds., Oxford University Press, New York, NY, USA, 1998.

[63] C. D. Frith and D. J. Done, "Towards a neuropsychology of schizophrenia," *British Journal of Psychiatry*, vol. 153, pp. 437–443, 1988.

[64] R. P. Bentall, G. A. Baker, and S. Havers, "Reality monitoring and psychotic hallucinations," *British Journal of Clinical Psychology*, vol. 30, no. 3, pp. 213–222, 1991.

[65] R. S. E. Keefe, M. C. Arnold, U. J. Bayen, J. P. McEvoy, and W. H. Wilson, "Source-monitoring deficits for self-generated stimuli in schizophrenia: multinomial modeling of data from three sources," *Schizophrenia Research*, vol. 57, no. 1, pp. 51–67, 2002.

[66] F. Waters, T. Woodward, P. Allen, A. Aleman, and I. Sommer, "Self-recognition deficits in schizophrenia patients with auditory hallucinations: a meta-analysis of the literature," *Schizophrenia Bulletin*, vol. 38, no. 4, pp. 741–750, 2012.

[67] J. S. Simons, S. W. Davis, S. J. Gilbert, C. D. Frith, and P. W. Burgess, "Discriminating imagined from perceived information engages brain areas implicated in schizophrenia," *NeuroImage*, vol. 32, no. 2, pp. 696–703, 2006.

[68] P. Allen, E. Amaro, C. H. Y. Fu et al., "Neural correlates of the misattribution of speech in schizophrenia," *British Journal of Psychiatry*, vol. 190, pp. 162–169, 2007.

[69] B. Elvevåg and T. E. Goldberg, "Cognitive impairment in schizophrenia is the core of the disorder," *Critical Reviews in Neurobiology*, vol. 14, no. 1, pp. 1–21, 2000.

[70] R. W. Heinrichs, "The primacy of cognition in schizophrenia," *The American Psychologist*, vol. 60, no. 3, pp. 229–242, 2005.

[71] A. Aleman and A. S. David, "How to fill a half-full glass: emotion and schizophrenia," *The American Psychologist*, vol. 61, no. 1, pp. 75–76, 2006.

[72] A. Aleman and R. S. Kahn, "Strange feelings: do amygdala abnormalities dysregulate the emotional brain in schizophrenia?" *Progress in Neurobiology*, vol. 77, no. 5, pp. 283–298, 2005.

[73] C. G. Kohler, J. B. Walker, E. A. Martin, K. M. Healey, and P. J. Moberg, "Facial emotion perception in schizophrenia: a meta-analytic review," *Schizophrenia Bulletin*, vol. 36, no. 5, pp. 1009–1019, 2010.

[74] M. Hoekert, R. S. Kahn, M. Pijnenborg, and A. Aleman, "Impaired recognition and expression of emotional prosody in schizophrenia: review and meta-analysis," *Schizophrenia Research*, vol. 96, no. 1–3, pp. 135–145, 2007.

[75] F. Irani, S. Seligman, V. Kamath, C. Kohler, and R. C. Gur, "A meta-analysis of emotion perception and functional outcomes in schizophrenia," *Schizophrenia Research*, vol. 137, no. 1–3, pp. 203–211, 2012.

[76] H. Li, R. C. K. Chan, G. M. McAlonan, and Q.-Y. Gong, "Facial emotion processing in schizophrenia: a meta-analysis of functional neuroimaging data," *Schizophrenia Bulletin*, vol. 36, no. 5, pp. 1029–1039, 2010.

[77] A. Anticevic, J. X. Van Snellenberg, R. E. Cohen, G. Repovs, E. C. Dowd, and D. M. Barch, "Amygdala recruitment in schizophrenia in response to aversive emotional material: a meta-analysis of neuroimaging studies," *Schizophrenia Bulletin*, vol. 38, no. 3, pp. 608–621, 2012.

[78] D. Baas, A. Aleman, M. Vink, N. F. Ramsey, E. H. F. de Haan, and R. S. Kahn, "Evidence of altered cortical and amygdala activation during social decision-making in schizophrenia," *NeuroImage*, vol. 40, no. 2, pp. 719–727, 2008.

[79] K. N. Ochsner, S. A. Bunge, J. J. Gross, and J. D. E. Gabrieli, "Rethinking feelings: an fMRI study of the cognitive regulation of emotion," *Journal of Cognitive Neuroscience*, vol. 14, no. 8, pp. 1215–1229, 2002.

[80] K. McRae, B. Ciesielski, and J. J. Gross, "Unpacking cognitive reappraisal: goals, tactics, and outcomes," *Emotion*, vol. 12, no. 2, pp. 250–255, 2012.

[81] J. J. Gross, "Antecedent- and response-focused emotion regulation: divergent consequences for experience, expression, and physiology," *Journal of Personality and Social Psychology*, vol. 74, no. 1, pp. 224–237, 1998.

[82] A. Bechara, H. Damasio, A. R. Damasio, and G. P. Lee, "Different contributions of the human amygdala and ventromedial prefrontal cortex to decision-making," *Journal of Neuroscience*, vol. 19, no. 13, pp. 5473–5481, 1999.

[83] J. T. Buhle, J. A. Silvers, T. D. Wager et al., "Cognitive reappraisal of emotion: a meta-analysis of human neuroimaging studies," *Cereb Cortex*, 2013.

[84] D. Kimhy, J. Vakhrusheva, L. Jobson-Ahmed, N. Tarrier, D. Malaspina, and J. J. Gross, "Emotion awareness and regulation in individuals with schizophrenia: implications for social functioning," *Psychiatry Research*, vol. 200, no. 2-3, pp. 193–201, 2012.

[85] L. van der Meer, M. V. Wout, and A. Aleman, "Emotion regulation strategies in patients with schizophrenia," *Psychiatry Research*, vol. 170, no. 2-3, pp. 108–113, 2009.

[86] R. W. Morris, A. Sparks, P. B. Mitchell, C. S. Weickert, and M. J. Green, "Lack of cortico-limbic coupling in bipolar disorder and schizophrenia during emotion regulation," *Translational Psychiatry*, vol. 2, article e90, 2012.

[87] R. M. Seyfarth and D. L. Cheney, "Affiliation, empathy, and the origins of theory of mind," *Proceedings of the National Academy of Sciences of the USA*, vol. 110, supplement 2, pp. 10349–10356, 2013.

[88] L. Harrington, R. Langdon, R. J. Siegert, and J. McClure, "Schizophrenia, theory of mind, and persecutory delusions," *Cognitive Neuropsychiatry*, vol. 10, no. 2, pp. 87–104, 2005.

[89] R. Corcoran, G. Mercer, and C. D. Frith, "Schizophrenia, symptomatology and social inference: investigating "theory of mind" in people with schizophrenia," *Schizophrenia Research*, vol. 17, no. 1, pp. 5–13, 1995.

[90] R. Saxe and N. Kanwisher, "People thinking about thinking people: the role of the temporo-parietal junction in 'theory of mind'," *NeuroImage*, vol. 19, no. 4, pp. 1835–1842, 2003.

[91] D. Samson, I. A. Apperly, C. Chiavarino, and G. W. Humphreys, "Left temporoparietal junction is necessary for representing someone else's belief," *Nature Neuroscience*, vol. 7, no. 5, pp. 499–500, 2004.

[92] P. Ruby and J. Decety, "What you believe versus what you think they believe: a neuroimaging study of conceptual perspective-taking," *European Journal of Neuroscience*, vol. 17, no. 11, pp. 2475–2480, 2003.

[93] A. D. Rowe, P. R. Bullock, C. E. Polkey, and R. G. Morris, "'Theory of mind' impairments and their relationship to executive functioning following frontal lobe excisions," *Brain*, vol. 124, pp. 600–616, 2001.

[94] D. Samson, I. A. Apperly, U. Kathirgamanathan, and G. W. Humphreys, "Seeing it my way: a case of a selective deficit in inhibiting self-perspective," *Brain*, vol. 128, no. 5, pp. 1102–1111, 2005.

[95] H. L. Gallagher and C. D. Frith, "Functional imaging of 'theory of mind'," *Trends in Cognitive Sciences*, vol. 7, no. 2, pp. 77–83, 2003.

[96] K. Vogeley, P. Bussfeld, A. Newen et al., "Mind reading: neural mechanisms of theory of mind and self-perspective," *NeuroImage*, vol. 14, no. 1, pp. 170–181, 2001.

[97] A. R. Aron, T. W. Robbins, and R. A. Poldrack, "Inhibition and the right inferior frontal cortex," *Trends in Cognitive Sciences*, vol. 8, no. 4, pp. 170–177, 2004.

[98] S. G. Shamay-Tsoory, J. Aharon-Peretz, and Y. Levkovitz, "The neuroanatomical basis of affective mentalizing in schizophrenia: comparison of patients with schizophrenia and patients with localized prefrontal lesions," *Schizophrenia Research*, vol. 90, no. 1–3, pp. 274–283, 2007.

[99] S. G. Shamay-Tsoory and J. Aharon-Peretz, "Dissociable prefrontal networks for cognitive and affective theory of mind: a lesion study," *Neuropsychologia*, vol. 45, no. 13, pp. 3054–3067, 2007.

[100] G. Modinos, R. Renken, S. G. Shamay-Tsoory, J. Ormel, and A. Aleman, "Neurobiological correlates of theory of mind in psychosis proneness," *Neuropsychologia*, vol. 48, no. 13, pp. 3715–3724, 2010.

[101] L. van der Meer, N. A. Groenewold, W. A. Nolen, M. Pijnenborg, and A. Aleman, "Inhibit yourself and understand the other: neural basis of distinct processes underlying Theory of Mind," *NeuroImage*, vol. 56, no. 4, pp. 2364–2374, 2011.

[102] L. van der Meer, N. A. Groenewold, M. Pijnenborg, and A. Aleman, "Psychosis-proneness and neural correlates of self-inhibition in theory of mind," *PLoS ONE*, vol. 8, no. 7, Article ID e67774, 2013.

[103] B. Derntl, A. Finkelmeyer, T. K. Toygar et al., "Generalized deficit in all core components of empathy in schizophrenia," *Schizophrenia Research*, vol. 108, no. 1–3, pp. 197–206, 2009.

[104] D. Baas, M. Van't Wout, A. Aleman, and R. S. Kahn, "Social judgement in clinically stable patients with schizophrenia and healthy relatives: behavioural evidence of social brain dysfunction," *Psychological Medicine*, vol. 38, no. 5, pp. 747–754, 2008.

[105] T. Jellema, J. Lorteije, S. van Rijn et al., "Involuntary interpretation of social cues is compromised in autism spectrum disorders," *Autism Research*, vol. 2, no. 4, pp. 192–204, 2009.

[106] M. van 't Wout, S. van Rijn, T. Jellema, R. S. Kahn, and A. Aleman, "Deficits in implicit attention to social signals in schizophrenia and high risk groups: behavioural evidence from a new illusion," *PLoS ONE*, vol. 4, no. 5, Article ID e5581, 2009.

[107] X. F. Amador and A. S. David, Eds., *Insight and Psychosis: awareness of Illness in Schizophrenia and Related Disorders*, Oxford University Press, Oxford, UK, 2nd edition, 2004.

[108] A. S. David, "Insight and psychosis," *British Journal of Psychiatry*, vol. 156, pp. 798–808, 1990.

[109] A. S. David, "The clinical importance of insight: an overview," in *Insight and Psychosis: Awareness of Illness in Schizophrenia and Related Disorders*, X. F. Amador and A. S. David, Eds., Oxford University Press, Oxford, UK, 2nd edition, 2004.

[110] A. Aleman, N. Agrawal, K. D. Morgan, and A. S. David, "Insight in psychosis and neuropsychological function: meta-analysis," *British Journal of Psychiatry*, vol. 189, pp. 204–212, 2006.

[111] A. Nair, E. C. Palmer, A. Aleman, and A. S. David, "Relationship between cognitive functioning and clinical and cognitive insight in psychotic disorders: a review and meta-analysis," *Schizophrenia Research*, vol. 152, no. 1, pp. 191–200, 2014.

[112] P. J. Quee, L. van der Meer, R. Bruggeman et al., "Insight in psychosis: relationship with neurocognition, social cognition and clinical symptoms depends on phase of illness," *Schizophrenia Bulletin*, vol. 37, no. 1, pp. 29–37, 2011.

[113] S. Epstein, "Integration of the cognitive and the psychodynamic unconscious," *The American Psychologist*, vol. 49, no. 8, pp. 709–724, 1994.

[114] T. D. Wilson, S. Lindsey, and T. Y. Schooler, "A model of dual attitudes," *Psychological Review*, vol. 107, no. 1, pp. 101–126, 2000.

[115] S. L. Koole, A. Dijksterhuis, and A. van Knippenberg, "What's in a name: implicit self-esteem and the automatic self," *Journal of Personality and Social Psychology*, vol. 80, no. 4, pp. 669–685, 2001.

[116] S. C. Johnson, L. C. Baxter, L. S. Wilder, J. G. Pipe, J. E. Heiserman, and G. P. Prigatano, "Neural correlates of self-reflection," *Brain*, vol. 125, no. 8, pp. 1808–1814, 2002.

[117] D. T. Stuss, G. G. Gallup Jr., and M. P. Alexander, "The frontal lobes are necessary for 'theory of mind'," *Brain*, vol. 124, no. 2, pp. 279–286, 2001.

[118] L. van der Meer, S. Costafreda, A. Aleman, and A. S. David, "Self-reflection and the brain: a theoretical review and meta-analysis of neuroimaging studies with implications for schizophrenia," *Neuroscience and Biobehavioral Reviews*, vol. 34, no. 6, pp. 935–946, 2010.

[119] R. Kemp and A. S. David, "Insight and compliance," in *Treatment Compliance and the Therapeutic Alliance*, pp. 61–84, Harwood Academic Publishers, Amsterdam, The the Netherlands, 1997.

[120] L. van der Meer, A. E. de Vos, A. P. Stiekema et al., "Insight in schizophrenia: involvement of self-reflection networks?" *Schizophrenia Bulletin2013*, vol. 39, no. 6, pp. 1288–1295.

[121] A. T. Beck, E. Baruch, J. M. Balter, R. A. Steer, and D. M. Warman, "A new instrument for measuring insight: the beck cognitive insight scale," *Schizophrenia Research*, vol. 68, no. 2-3, pp. 319–329, 2004.

[122] R. J. Davidson, "Affective style, psychopathology, and resilience: brain mechanisms and plasticity," *The American Psychologist*, vol. 55, no. 11, pp. 1196–1214, 2000.

[123] G. H. Pijnenborg, J. M. Spikman, B. F. Jeronimus, and A. Aleman, "Insight in schizophrenia: associations with empathy," *European Archives of Psychiatry and Clinical Neurosciences*, vol. 263, no. 4, pp. 299–307, 2013.

[124] H. G. Engen and T. Singer, "Empathy circuits," *Current Opinion in Neurobiology*, vol. 23, no. 2, pp. 275–282, 2013.

[125] G. Foussias and G. Remington, "Negative symptoms in schizophrenia: avolition and occam's razor," *Schizophrenia Bulletin*, vol. 36, no. 2, pp. 359–369, 2010.

[126] M. Kiang, B. K. Christensen, G. Remington, and S. Kapur, "Apathy in schizophrenia: clinical correlates and association with functional outcome," *Schizophrenia Research*, vol. 63, no. 1-2, pp. 79–88, 2003.

[127] R. Bottlender, A. Strauss, and H.-J. Möller, "Social disability in schizophrenic, schizoaffective and affective disorders 15 years after first admission," *Schizophrenia Research*, vol. 116, no. 1, pp. 9–15, 2010.

[128] R. van Reekum, D. T. Stuss, and L. Ostrander, "Apathy: why care?" *Journal of Neuropsychiatry and Clinical Neurosciences*, vol. 17, no. 1, pp. 7–19, 2005.

[129] D. T. Stuss, R. van Reekum, and K. J. Murphy, "Differentiation of states and causes of apathy," in *The Neuropsychology of Emotion*, J. Borod, Ed., Oxford University Press, New York, NY, USA, 2000.

[130] R. Levy and B. Dubois, "Apathy and the functional anatomy of the prefrontal cortex-basal ganglia circuits," *Cerebral Cortex*, vol. 16, no. 7, pp. 916–928, 2006.

[131] E. Liemburg, S. Castelein, R. Stewart et al., "Two subdomains of negative symptoms in psychotic disorders: established and confirmed in two large cohorts," *Journal of Psychiatric Research*, vol. 47, no. 6, pp. 718–725, 2013.

[132] R. M. Roth, L. A. Flashman, A. J. Saykin, T. W. McAllister, and R. Vidaver, "Apathy in schizophrenia: reduced frontal lobe volume and neuropsychological deficits," *The American Journal of Psychiatry*, vol. 161, no. 1, pp. 157–159, 2004.

[133] J. H. Callicott, A. Bertolino, M. F. Egan, V. S. Mattay, F. J. P. Langheim, and D. R. Weinberger, "Selective relationship between prefrontal N-acetylaspartate measures and negative symptoms in schizophrenia," *The American Journal of Psychiatry*, vol. 157, no. 10, pp. 1646–1651, 2000.

[134] E. C. Dowd and D. M. Barch, "Anhedonia and emotional experience in schizophrenia: neural and behavioral indicators," *Biological Psychiatry*, vol. 67, no. 10, pp. 902–911, 2010.

[135] J. J. Simon, A. Biller, S. Walther et al., "Neural correlates of reward processing in schizophrenia: relationship to apathy and depression," *Schizophrenia Research*, vol. 118, no. 1–3, pp. 154–161, 2010.

[136] G. E. Tsai and P.-Y. Lin, "Strategies to enhance N-Methyl-D-Aspartate receptor-mediated neurotransmission in schizophrenia, a critical review and meta-analysis," *Current Pharmaceutical Design*, vol. 16, no. 5, pp. 522–537, 2010.

[137] M. J. Noetzel, C. K. Jones, and P. J. Conn, "Emerging approaches for treatment of schizophrenia: modulation of glutamatergic signaling," *Discovery Medicine*, vol. 14, no. 78, pp. 335–343, 2012.

[138] J. J. Dlabač-de Lange, R. Knegtering, and A. Aleman, "Repetitive transcranial magnetic stimulation for negative symptoms of schizophrenia: review and meta-analysis," *Journal of Clinical Psychiatry*, vol. 71, no. 4, pp. 411–418, 2010.

[139] R. Prikryl and H. P. Kucerova, "Can repetitive transcranial magnetic stimulation be considered effective treatment option for negative symptoms of schizophrenia?" *The Journal of ECT*, vol. 29, no. 1, pp. 67–74, 2013.

[140] G. P. Strauss, W. R. Keller, R. W. Buchanan et al., "Next-generation negative symptom assessment for clinical trials: validation of the Brief Negative Symptom Scale," *Schizophrenia Research*, vol. 142, no. 1–3, pp. 88–92, 2012.

[141] P. Allen, F. Larøi, P. K. McGuire, and A. Aleman, "The hallucinating brain: a review of structural and functional neuroimaging studies of hallucinations," *Neuroscience and Biobehavioral Reviews*, vol. 32, no. 1, pp. 175–191, 2008.

[142] A. Vercammen, H. Knegtering, E. J. Liemburg, J. A. D. Boer, and A. Aleman, "Functional connectivity of the temporo-parietal region in schizophrenia: effects of rTMS treatment of auditory hallucinations," *Journal of Psychiatric Research*, vol. 44, no. 11, pp. 725–731, 2010.

Improving Cognitive Function from Children to Old Age: A Systematic Review of Recent Smart Ageing Intervention Studies

Rui Nouchi[1,2] and Ryuta Kawashima[2,3]

[1] Human and Social Response Research Division, International Research Institute of Disaster Science, Tohoku University, 4-1 Seiryo-cho, Aoba-ku, Sendai 980-8575, Japan

[2] Department of Advanced Brain Science, Smart Ageing International Research Center, Institute of Development, Aging and Cancer, Tohoku University, 4-1 Seiryo-cho, Aoba-ku, Sendai 980-8575, Japan

[3] Department of Functional Brain Imaging, Institute of Development, Aging and Cancer, Tohoku University, 4-1 Seiryo-cho, Aoba-ku, Sendai 980-8575, Japan

Correspondence should be addressed to Rui Nouchi; rnouchi@idac.tohoku.ac.jp

Academic Editor: Daniela Schulz

Background. Cognitive functions are important for daily life at any age. One purpose of *Smart Ageing* is to investigate how to improve cognitive functions. This systematic review evaluates beneficial effects of the intervention on cognitive functions. *Method.* We conducted a systematic review of intervention studies of improvements of cognitive functions published or in press before December 2013. Because of the heterogeneity of the intervention programs, a systematic and critical review of the interventions and outcomes was conducted instead of a meta-analysis. *Results.* We identified nine completed and published studies, which were divided into four categories: cognitive training using video game, cognitive training using PC, cognitive training using paper and pencil, and exercise training. Review results showed that various intervention programs can improve cognitive functions such as executive functions, working memory, episodic memory, processing speed, and general cognitive ability/IQ. *Conclusions.* The systematic review demonstrated that some intervention programs can be effective for improving various aspects of cognitive functioning at any age. Some limitations to this review include its small sample size and heterogeneity of programs and cognitive function measures, in addition to unresolved issues such as transfer of everyday skills and effectiveness for nonhealthy people.

1. Background

Cognitive function includes a variety of mental processes such as perception, attention, memory, decision making, and language comprehension. Cognitive function serves a critical role in everyday behavior and social behavior. For instance, when one goes shopping, it is necessary to memorize information about what to buy, how to make a proper judgment to buy, and how to have a conversation with shop assistants. Considering communication with a friend, we identify the friend by looking at faces or hearing a voice and sharing information with the friend.

Our cognitive functions change during our lifetimes [1–4]. Cognitive functions improve from childhood to young adulthood. Some cognitive functions such as executive functions and working memory reach a peak during 20s or

30s [5]. However, semantic knowledge (semantic memory) develops to the age of 60 or 70 [6]. An elderly person might experience a decline of several cognitive functions, including memory [3, 7], attention [8], executive functions [9, 10], and processing speed [11]. Previous studies have demonstrated that higher cognitive functions in children and young adults are positively correlated with higher academic achievements [12–17]. A decline in the cognitive abilities of older people has been shown to engender difficulty in performing basic activities of daily living [18–23]. Consequently, improvements of cognitive functions using intervention programs are attracting attention at all age levels.

Confirming expectations of society and scientific fields related to improvement of cognitive functions, we have undertaken Smart Ageing research (http://www2.idac.tohoku.ac.jp/dep/sairc/index.html). The Smart Ageing concept includes a positive acceptance of later stages in life and a perspective of aging as a series of "developmental stages toward intellectual maturity." Smart Ageing is a revolutionary paradigm shift away from negative concepts, such as anti-aging, which imply an unwillingness to accept or face later stages of life. One purpose of Smart Ageing research is to investigate how to develop the cognitive functions of healthy children, how to retain them in healthy adults, and how to improve them in community-dwelling seniors because cognitive functions serve a critical role in everyday life. To achieve that purpose, we have conducted widely varied intervention studies. Ours is a rare case of one laboratory that has conducted intervention studies to assess cognitive functions in subjects from children to older people.

Previous review papers demonstrated that some intervention programs can improve cognitive functions in healthy and nonhealthy children, young adults, and older adults [24–38]. Intervention programs were divided into interventions of two main types: cognitive training and exercise training. Cognitive training was defined as an intervention that provides structured practice on tasks related to aspects of cognitive functioning such as memory, attention, language, and executive function. There are many types of cognitive training such as working memory training [28, 39, 40], processing speed training [38, 41], memory strategic training [24, 42–44], and brain training game [45–47]. Some cognitive training intervention studies using randomized controlled trials (RCT) have shown improvements of cognitive functions [44, 45, 47–51]. There are two types of exercise training such as aerobic exercise training and strength exercise training [36]. Aerobic exercise training is defined as structured exercise programs involving the use of large muscle groups for extended periods of time in activities that are rhythmic in nature, including but not limited to walking, stepping, running, swimming, cycling, and rowing [32]. Strength exercise training uses resistance against the force of muscular contraction to build strength, anaerobic endurance, and skeletal muscle mass. Strength exercise training often uses gravity to oppose muscle contraction [34, 52, 53]. Earlier studies using RCT have revealed that aerobic exercise training alone and strength exercise training alone improved cognitive functions [32, 53, 54].

Given that the research area of intervention for improvements of cognitive function is growing rapidly, it is important to review evidence of recent intervention studies and to ascertain the methodological quality of intervention studies. For intervention studies, transfer effects especially are important phenomena. A transfer effect is defined as "the ability to extend what has been learned in one context to new contexts" [55]. Additionally, the transfer effect is classifiable in terms of a near transfer effect and a far transfer effect [56–59]. The near transfer effect refers to improvements in cognitive domains that are related closely to the trained cognitive processes. In contrast, the far transfer effect refers to improvements in cognitive domain that are not closely related to the trained cognitive processes. It is necessary to evaluate whether intervention programs had near or far transfer effects. Consequently, in the systematic review, we evaluate the beneficial effects of the intervention on cognitive functions and the methodological quality of recent intervention studies for Smart Ageing.

2. Methods

2.1. Search Strategy. In accordance with the preferred reporting items for systematic reviews and meta-analysis (PRISMA) statement [60], we conducted a systematic review of intervention studies of improvements of cognitive functions for Smart Ageing published or in press before December 2013. To identify relevant studies, we searched PubMed, Google Scholar, and PsycINFO using the following key words for cognitive function: "cognitive," "cognitive abilities," "cognition," "memory," and "speed of processing"; for interventions: "treatment," "training," "intervention," "randomized controlled trials," or "RCT"; for author: "kawashima" and "ryuta." We searched references of included papers and relevant systematic reviews. We also asked experts in the field if they knew of other related papers meeting inclusion criteria. Supporting PRISMA checklist is available as Supplemental Materials (see Supplementary Material available online at http://dx.doi.org/10.1155/2014/235479).

2.2. Inclusion and Exclusion Criteria. We included studies in healthy participants who had no diagnosis such as developmental disorder, depression, posttraumatic stress disorder (PTSD), dementia, mild cognitive impairment, or Alzheimer's disease. Studies must have been published in English and must have used standardized psychological tests or tools to measure cognitive functions. We excluded single case reports, dissertations, meeting abstracts, study protocols, and review papers. We also excluded studies which measured no cognitive functions.

2.3. Quality Assessment. The quality of each study was assessed using a modified Delphi list [61]. To enhance the quality of assessment, additional elements were considered, including details of random allocation methods, adequate description of the control/comparison group, between-group statistical comparison, reporting dropouts, and reporting consolidated standards of reporting trials (CONSORT) statement (http://www.consort-statement.org/). These quality assessment criteria were based on a previous systematic review paper. The total score (Max = 14) is reported in Table 1.

2.4. Statistical Analysis. Because of the heterogeneity of the intervention programs, types of participants, outcomes assessed, and measurement tools used, a systematic and critical review of the interventions and outcomes was conducted instead of a meta-analysis.

3. Results

The database search strategy initially yielded 25 journal articles (20 articles from PubMed, Google Scholar, and PsycINFO and 5 articles from an expert's suggestions). Based on the stated inclusion and exclusion criteria, 9 of the 25

TABLE 1: Scores of methodological quality.

Authors	Q1	Q2	Q3	Q4	Q5	Q6	Q7	Q8	Q9	Q10	Q11	Q12	Q13	Q14	Total score (MAX = 14)
Uchida and Kawashima [66]	Y	Y	Y	Y	Y	N	N	Y	N	Y	?	Y	Y	N	9
Nouchi et al. [45]	Y	Y	Y	Y	Y	?	N	Y	N	Y	Y	Y	Y	Y	11
Nouchi et al. [47]	Y	Y	Y	Y	Y	?	N	Y	Y	Y	Y	Y	Y	Y	12
Nouchi et al. [65]	Y	Y	Y	Y	Y	N	N	Y	Y	Y	?	Y	Y	Y	11
Tachibana et al. [79]	Y	Y	Y	Y	Y	N	N	Y	N	Y	?	Y	Y	Y	10
Takeuchi et al. [38]	Y	Y	Y	Y	Y	?	Y	Y	N	N	?	Y	Y	N	9
Takeuchi et al. [62]	Y	Y	Y	Y	Y	?	Y	Y	N	N	Y	Y	Y	N	10
Takeuchi et al. [63]	Y	Y	Y	Y	Y	?	Y	Y	N	N	?	Y	N	N	8
Takeuchi et al. [64]	Y	Y	Y	Y	Y	?	Y	Y	N	N	?	Y	Y	N	9
Total score across studies	9	9	9	9	9	0	4	9	2	5	3	9	8	4	

Q1: random allocation; Q2: treatment allocation concealed; Q3: groups/subjects similar at baseline regarding important prognostic values; Q4: eligibility criteria specified; Q5: blinded outcome assessor; Q6: care provider blinded; Q7: patient blinded; Q8: point estimates and measures of variability presented for the primary outcome measures; Q9: intention-to-treat analysis; Q10: details of random allocation methods; Q11: adequate description of the control/comparison group; Q12: between-group statistical comparison; Q13: reporting dropouts; Q14: reporting CONSORT statement.
Y: yes; the study met the criteria of the question, N: no; the study did not meet the criteria of the question, and ?: no information or the study was not the case with the question.
Takeuchi et al. [38], who used processing speed training, published their findings in Journal of Neuroscience. Takeuchi et al. [62], who used working memory training with mental calculation, published their findings in PLoS One.

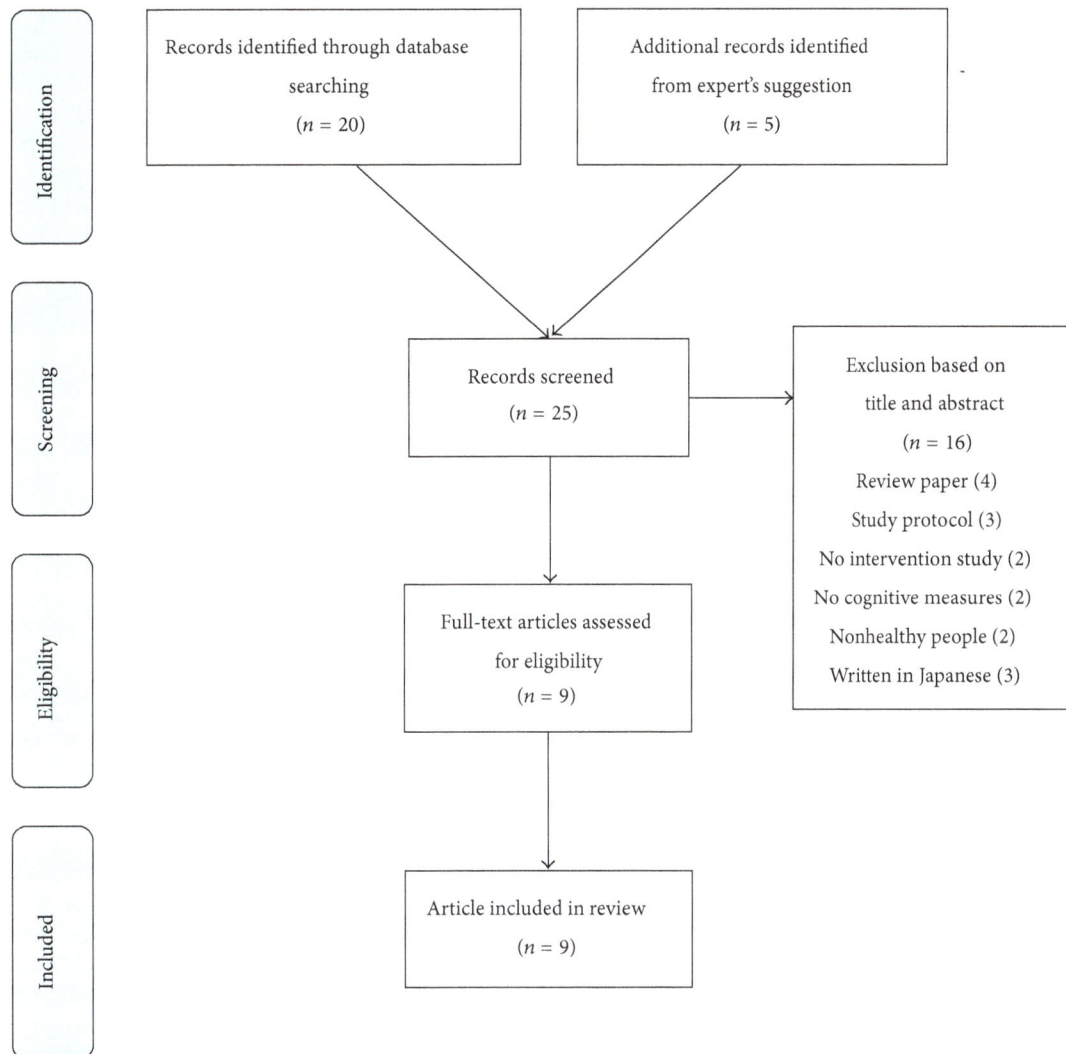

FIGURE 1: Flow diagram of search results.

publications [38, 45, 47, 62–67] were eligible for the current review (Figure 1). We present details of these interventions in short descriptions.

Of the 16 excluded articles, four articles were review articles discussing cognitive intervention [28, 68–70]. Three articles were excluded because they were protocols for intervention [71–73]. Two articles were not intervention studies [74, 75]. Two articles did not measure any cognitive functions [76, 77]. Two articles were excluded because the participants had been diagnosed as having dementia or autism spectrum disorder [78, 79]. Three articles were written in Japanese [80–82].

3.1. Quality Assessment. An assessment of the methodological quality of the included studies is presented in Table 1. The quality assessment ranged from 8 to 12, with an average of 9.89 (SD = 1.27). All included studies had sufficient good methodological quality. A study by Nouchi et al. [65] had the highest methodological quality. The score of item 6 (care-provider blinded) was low among the included studies

because no care providers were involved in six studies that used PC-based training programs or video games [38, 45, 47, 62–64]. The score of item 11 (adequate description of the control/comparison group) was also low because of the use of a passive control or a waiting list control group [38, 63–67]. Four studies [38, 62–64] investigated changes of brain structure or neural mechanisms though cognitive training. Therefore, the studies did not use an intention-to-treat (ITT) analysis. Consequently, the score of item 9 (using ITT analysis) was low. However, all studies met the methodological qualities of item of 1, 2, 3, 4, 5, 8, and 12.

3.2. Participants, Sample Size, and Duration of Intervention. Among the nine studies, one study included preschool children (4–6 years old) [67], five studies included young adults (undergraduate and graduate students) [38, 47, 62–64], and three studies included elderly people (over 60 years old) [45, 65, 66]. The numbers of participants in the nine studies were from 32 [45, 47] to 236 [67]. The durations of intervention were from 6 days [38, 62] to 23 weeks [66].

A six-day intervention was used in two studies [38, 62]. A four-week intervention was used in five studies [45, 47, 63–65]. Two studies used intervention periods of longer than 3 months [66, 67].

3.3. Methods of Intervention Programs. Table 2 presents characteristics of the intervention programs. Two studies used video games such as the popular brain training game (Brain Age) and popular puzzle games (Tetris) [45, 47]. Four studies used PC-based cognitive training such as working memory training, processing speed training, and multitask training [38, 62–64]. Two studies used paper-pencil-based intervention programs [66, 67]. One study used exercise training [65]. Four studies used an active control condition [45, 47, 62, 66], where the other five used a waiting list or no-training control group [38, 63–65, 67].

3.4. Cognitive Function Measures, Analysis Methods, and Significant Findings. To evaluate the beneficial effects of intervention on cognitive functions, a wide variety of cognitive functions measures was used. Most measures were standardized psychological measures. They showed high reliability and validity. Measures of the cognitive functions were divided into seven domains: general cognitive functions/intelligence quotient (IQ), executive functions, episodic memory, working memory/short-term memory, attention, processing speed, and others (Table 3).

To measure general cognitive functions/IQ, five studies for young people [38, 47, 63, 64] used Raven's advanced progressive matrices test. Two studies of elderly people [45, 66] used the minimental state examination as a measure of general cognitive function/IQ. To measure executive functions, the Stroop test was widely used [38, 47, 63–65]. To measure working memory/short-term memory, seven studies used digit span [38, 45, 47, 63–65]. Three studies used digit cancellation task as a measure of attention [45, 47, 65]. Five studies used symbol coding as a measure of processing speed [45, 47, 62, 65, 66].

Seven studies used analysis of covariance (ANCOVA) with a change score (posttest minus pretest scores) to detect group differences [38, 45, 47, 62–65]. Two studies used t-tests to investigate the group differences [66, 67]. Table 4 shows the significant effects after interventions. Despite the methodological heterogeneity of the interventions, eight studies found the beneficial effects of the interventions on the cognitive functions compared to control groups [38, 45, 47, 62–65, 67]. One study found no significant improvements of cognitive functions but showed significant improvement of cognitive functions in the target intervention group compared to control groups.

3.5. Short Descriptions of Eligible Articles. Next we present a short description of the intervention study. Based on the intervention programs, the included studies were divided into four categories (cognitive training using video game, cognitive training using PC programs, cognitive training using paper-pencil programs, and exercise training).

3.5.1. Cognitive Training Using Video Game Training Game. Video game training is one type of cognitive training. Two studies [45, 47] investigated the beneficial effects of brain training games on the cognitive functions. These studies used the same training periods (15 min per day, 5 days per week for 4 weeks) and the same brain training games (Brain Age) as a target intervention. Brain Age is a popular brain training game. Based on earlier neuroscience evidence, Brain Age was developed by Ryuta Kawashima. Most games in Brain Age include elements of these reading aloud and simple arithmetic calculations. For example, in the calculation 20 game, participants must answer 20 simple arithmetic calculations as quickly as possible. The questions include problems of mathematical addition, subtraction, and multiplication. In reading aloud, participants must read aloud excerpts from Japanese classical literature. In syllable count, some sentences written in a combination of kanji and kana are presented. Participants must count the kana letters after translating kanji to kana. These studies used a popular puzzle game (Tetris) as active control groups. In Tetris, players rotate and move blocks descending from the top of the screen so that these blocks form lines at the bottom of the screen. After a complete line with no gaps is formed, the line disappears and points are awarded. If no line is formed, then the blocks pile higher and higher until the block pile reaches the top of the screen, at which point the game ends and the player loses. The goal is to keep the game going as long as possible by forming complete lines with the descending blocks. As the game progresses, the descending blocks give players less time to choose where to place each block. For elderly people [45], the brain training game improved executive functions measured using the frontal assessment battery and trail making test and processing speed measured by symbol coding and symbol search measured processing speed compared to the puzzle game. For young people [47], the brain training game led to improved executive functions measured using the Wisconsin card sorting test and Stroop test, working memory measured by the operation span, letter-number sequence, and arithmetic, and processing speed measured by symbol coding and symbol search compared to the puzzle game. However, the puzzle game improved attention measured by the simple reaction task and visuospatial ability measured by mental rotation.

3.5.2. Cognitive Training Using PC Programs. There were several types of cognitive training using PC. Two studies were working memory training [62, 63]. One study was processing speed training [38]. One study was multitask training [64]. Participants of all included studies were young people. These studies also measured changes of brain structure and functions after interventions. We specifically examined the improvement of cognitive functions. Therefore, this report describes only results of cognitive functional change. Our other reviews have reported effects of cognitive intervention on neural systems [28, 69].

The processing speed training program consisted of adaptive training of processing speed tasks [77]. Training tasks involved eight tasks using computer buttons and two tasks using paper and pencil. In all, eight training tasks using

TABLE 2: Characteristics of the included intervention programs.

Study	Population	Sample size	Intervention and control groups (N)	Length of intervention	Frequency of intervention
Uchida and Kawashima [66]	Elderly people	124	(a) Reading and solving arithmetic problem (N = 64) (b) No intervention (N = 64)	23 weeks	At classroom: about 15 min once a week At home: about 15 min per day, 4–6 days per week
Nouchi et al. [45]	Elderly people	32	(a) Playing Brain Age (N = 16) (b) Playing Tetris (N = 16)	4 weeks	About 15 min per day, at least 5 days per week
Nouchi et al. [47]	Young people	32	(a) Playing Brain Age (N = 16) (b) Playing Tetris (N = 16)	4 weeks	About 15 min per day, at least 5 days per week
Nouchi et al. [65]	Elderly people	64	(a) Combination exercise training (N = 32) (b) Waiting list control group (N = 32)	4 weeks	About 30 min per day, 3 days per week
Tachibana et al. [79]	Children	238	(a) Mother-child play activity Program (N = 124) (b) Waiting list control group (N = 114)	3 months	About 10 min per a day, 5 days per week
Takeuchi et al. [38]	Young people	44	(a) Processing speed training (N = 23) (b) No intervention (N = 21)	6 days	About 4 hr per day, 5 days within a 6-day period
Takeuchi et al. [62]	Young people	55	(a) Intensive adaptive training of working memory using mental calculation (N = 18) (b) Nonadaptive training of working memory using mental calculation (placebo intervention) (N = 18) (c) No intervention (N = 19)	6 days	About 4 hours per a day, 5 days within a 6-day period
Takeuchi et al. [63]	Young people	61	(a) Working memory training (N = 41) (b) No intervention (N = 20)	4 weeks	At laboratory: about 20–60 min per day, 2 days per week At home: about 20–60 min per day, everyday
Takeuchi et al. [64]	Young people	40	(a) Multitask training (N = 41) (b) No intervention (N = 20)	4 weeks	At laboratory: about 20–60 min per day, 2 days per week At home: about 20–60 min per day, everyday

Takeuchi et al. [38], who used processing speed training, published their findings in Journal of Neuroscience. Takeuchi et al. [62], who used working memory training with mental calculation, published their findings in PLoS One.

TABLE 3: Summary of cognitive functional measures in the included studies.

General cognitive functions/IQ

Full name	Studies
Minimental state examination	Uchida and Kawashima [66]; Nouchi et al. [45]
Raven's advanced progressive matrices test	Nouchi et al. [47]; Takeuchi et al. [62]; Takeuchi et al. [63]; Takeuchi et al. [64]
Cattell culture fair test	Takeuchi et al. [38]
Tanaka B type intelligence test	Takeuchi et al. [38]; Takeuchi et al. [63]
Bochumer Matrizen test	Takeuchi et al. [63]; Takeuchi et al. [64]
Kyodai SX test	Takeuchi et al. [63]; Takeuchi et al. [64]

Executive functions

Full name	Studies
Frontal assessment battery	Uchida and Kawashima [66]; Nouchi et al. [45]
Trail making test	Nouchi et al. [45]; Takeuchi et al. [62]
Wisconsin card sorting test	Nouchi et al. [47]
Stroop test	Nouchi et al. [47]; Takeuchi et al. [38]; Takeuchi et al. [62]; Takeuchi et al. [63]
Verbal fluency task	Nouchi et al. [65]
Episodic memory	Nouchi et al. [65]; Takeuchi et al. [64]
Logical memory	Nouchi et al. [65]
First and second names	Nouchi et al. [65]

Working memory/short-term memory

Full name	Studies
Digit (letter) span	Nouchi et al. [45]; Nouchi et al. [65]; Takeuchi et al. [38]; Takeuchi et al. [62]; Takeuchi et al. [63]
Operation span	Nouchi et al. [47]
Letter-number sequence	Nouchi et al. [47]
Arithmetic	Nouchi et al. [47]; Takeuchi et al. [62]
Spatial span	Nouchi et al. [47]; Takeuchi et al. [38]; Takeuchi et al. [63]; Takeuchi et al. [64]

Attention

Full name	Studies
Digit cancellation task	Nouchi et al. [45]; Nouchi et al. [65]
Simple reaction task	Nouchi et al. [47]

Others

Full name	Studies
Processing speed	
Symbol coding	Uchida and Kawashima [66]; Nouchi et al. [45, 71, 72]; Takeuchi et al. [62]
Symbol search	Nouchi et al. [45]; Nouchi et al. [47]; Takeuchi et al. [62]
Japanese reading test	Nouchi et al. [47]; Nouchi et al. [65]
Mental rotation	Nouchi et al. [47]; Takeuchi et al. [62]
Simple arithmetic	Takeuchi et al. [38]; Takeuchi et al. [63]; Takeuchi et al. [64]
Complex arithmetic	Takeuchi et al. [38]; Takeuchi et al. [63]; Takeuchi et al. [64]
S-A creativity test	Takeuchi et al. [38]; Takeuchi et al. [63]; Takeuchi et al. [64]

Takeuchi et al. [38], who used processing speed training, published their findings in Journal of Neuroscience. Takeuchi et al. [62], who used working memory training with mental calculation, published their findings in PLoS One.

TABLE 4: Summary of improvements of cognitive function after intervention programs.

Study	Measures of cognitive functions	Significant effect of target intervention group
Uchida and Kawashima [66]	MMSE	0
	FAB	0
	Cd	0
Nouchi et al. [45]	MMSE	0
	FAB	+
	Trail making test	+
	D-CAT	0
	DS-F	0
	DS-B	0
	Cd	+
	SS	+
Nouchi et al. [47]	RAPMT	0
	WCST	+
	rST	+
	ST	+
	OpS	+
	LNS	+
	Ari	+
	DS-F	0
	DS-B	0
	SpS-F	0
	SpS-B	0
	D-CAT	0
	SRT	−
	Cd	+
	SS	+
	JART	0
	MR	−
Nouchi et al. [65]	LFT	+
	CFT	+
	rST	+
	ST	+
	LM	+
	FSN	0
	DS-F	0
	DS-B	0
	D-CAT	0
	Cd	+
	SS	+
	JART	0
Tachibana et al. [79]	DAM	+
	Understanding relationships between things	0
	Counting and comparing the numbers	0
	Calculation	0
	Completion of the pictures	0
	Working memory	+
	Processing speed	+
	Total score	0

TABLE 4: Continued.

Study	Measures of cognitive functions	Significant effect of target intervention group
Takeuchi et al. [38]	RAPM	0
	Cattell culture fair test	0
	DS	0
	SpS	0
	Tanaka B-type intelligence test	+
	ST	0
	rST	0
	Simple arithmetic	0
	Complex arithmetic	+
	S-A creativity test	0
	Word-color task	+
	Color-word task	+
Takeuchi et al. [62]	RAPM	0
	Arithmetic	0
	Cd	0
	rST	+
	ST	0
	S-A creativity test	−
	Simple arithmetic	0
	Complex arithmetic	+
	Letter mental rotation	0
	Trail making test B-A	0
	Letter span	+
Takeuchi et al. [63]	RAPM	+
	BOMAT	0
	DS	+
	SpS	+
	Tanaka B-type intelligence test	+
	Reverse Stroop interference	0
	ST interference	+
	Simple arithmetic	0
	Complex arithmetic	0
	Kyodai SX test	0
	S-A creativity test	0
Takeuchi et al. [64]	RAPM	0
	BOMAT	0
	DS	0
	SpS	0
	Tanaka B-type intelligence test	0
	Word-color Task	+
	Color-word task	0
	rST	0
	ST	+
	Simple arithmetic	0
	Complex arithmetic	0
	Kyodai SX test	0
	S-A creativity test	+

MMSE: minimental state examination; RAPMT: Raven's advanced progressive matrices test; BOMAT: Bochumer Matrizen test; DAM (Goodenough draw-a-man intelligence test); FAB: frontal assessment battery; WCST: Wisconsin card sorting test; ST: Stroop test; rST: reverse Stroop test; VFT: verbal fluency task; LM: logical memory; FSN: first and second names; DS: digit span; OpS: operation span; LNS: letter-number sequence; Ari: arithmetic; SpS: spatial span; D-CAT: digit cancellation task; SRT: simple reaction task; Cd: symbol coding; SS: symbol search; JART: Japanese reading test; MR: mental rotation.
0: no significant difference was found between the target intervention and control (intervention) groups; +: the target intervention group improved cognitive functions compared to the control (intervention) group; −: the control (intervention) group improved cognitive functions compared to the target intervention group.
Takeuchi et al. [38], who used processing speed training, published their findings in Journal of Neuroscience. Takeuchi et al. [62], who used working memory training with mental calculation, published their findings in PLoS One.

computer buttons and difficulties (stimulus presentation rates) were modulated based on the subject performance. In some training tasks using computer buttons, a certain type of stimulus was presented successively. In each trial, subjects had to push buttons that corresponded with the presented stimuli before the next trial (before the next stimuli were presented). Stimuli were presented randomly as visual numbers (one, two, three, and four), visual locations (a mark was presented in one of four corners of the interface), auditory numbers (one, two, three, and four), and auditory locations (a pure tone was presented in either the left ear or the right ear). In one paper and pencil task, rows of pairs of number strings containing three single-digit numbers (zero to nine) were printed on paper. Participants had to decide whether the strings were the same when reordered. Participants were instructed to answer as many of these questions as possible in 1 min. After a 6-day intervention period, the processing speed training group improved general cognitive ability/IQ measured by Tanaka B-types intelligence test, complex arithmetic, and processing speed measured by Word-Color and Color-Word tasks compared to the waiting list control group.

One working memory training study used mental calculations [62]. The study examined subjects in three groups: an intensive adaptive working memory training using mental calculation (adaptive working memory group), a nonadaptive working memory training using mental calculation (placebo group), and a no training group. In the adaptive working memory group, there were mental multiplication and mental addition tasks. For mental multiplication, participants were asked to solve mental multiplication problems in a normal way as participants do computations on paper in their minds and not to solve problems in any other way. Participants must continue the task until they get the correct answer. If participants answer correctly, then the problems become more difficult (the task starts from two-digit times two-digit multiplication and then becomes two-digit times three-digit multiplication and then three-digit times three-digit multiplication and then three-digit times four-digit mental multiplication). For mental addition task, ten two-digit numbers are presented one by one and the subjects are asked to add them. If they get the correct answer, the interstimulus interval (ISI) becomes shorter. In the placebo group, participants performed the similar tasks, except that the difficulty of the tasks does not change from the initial points (two-digit times two-digit multiplication in the mental multiplication task, ten-second ISI in the mental addition task). In the no training group, participants did not perform any training tasks. Results showed that the adaptive working memory training improved executive functions measured by Stroop test, working memory measured by letter span, and complex arithmetic. The adaptive working memory training decreased creativity measured by SA creativity test.

Another study used traditional working memory training tasks [63]. There were four working memory tasks: one visuospatial working memory, two types of dual working memory task, and one auditory backward operation span task. In all training tasks, the difficulties (number of items to be remembered) were modulated based on subjects'

performance. For example, in the visuospatial working memory task, circles were presented one at a time at a 1/s rate in an interface where 10 squares were distributed irregularly (circles are presented in one of these squares). After stimuli presentation, the subjects indicated the location and order of the presented stimuli by clicking on a computer screen with a mouse. After 4 weeks of working memory training, general cognitive functions/IQ was measured by Raven's advanced progressive matrices test and Tanaka B-type intelligence test, working memory was measured by digit span and spatial span, and executive functions were measured by the Stroop test.

One study used multitask training [64]. Multitasking constituted simultaneous engagement in two or more cognitive activities. Six multitask training tasks existed. In all of these tasks, a certain type of stimulus was presented successively and randomly. In each trial, the subjects had to push multiple buttons on a keyboard that corresponded to the stimuli presented before the next trial (the next stimulus) was initiated. In all six training tasks, difficulties (stimulus presentation rates) were modulated based on the subjects' performance. For example, an auditory-visual dual task in which in each trial, one auditory stimulus (1, 2, 3, or 4) is presented in English to both ears as well as one visual stimulus (a mark in one of four locations in a vertical row). The subjects must push "S" on the keyboard when they register stimulus 1, "D" for 2, "F" for 3, and "G" for 4. For the visual stimuli, the subjects must push "H" for the leftmost stimulus, "J" for the stimulus immediately after the first, and then "K" and "L" for the last two stimuli. Results showed that multiple training improved processing speed as measured by word-color task, executive functions measured by the Stroop test, and creativity measured by the S-A creativity test.

3.5.3. Exercise Training. One study examined combination exercise training for older people [65]. In the study, the combination exercise combined training of three types: aerobic, strength, and stretching. Participants performed the combination exercise training 3 days per week throughout the 4 weeks (12 workouts total). For the strength-training parts, participants were informed of the proper use of all of the equipment. They were instructed to complete as many repetitions as possible in a 30 s time period. There were twelve machines to exercise the whole body parts (chest press/seated row, squat, shoulder press/lat pull, leg extension/leg curl, abdominal crunch/back extension, lateral lift, elbow flexion/extension, horizontal leg press, pectoral deck, oblique, hip abductor/adductor, and gluteus). In a continuous interval fashion, participants performed floor-based aerobic training (e.g., running/skipping in place and arm circles) on recovery pads for a 30 s time period after each resistance exercise in an effort to maintain a consistent exercise heart rate corresponding to 60–80% of their heart maximum heart rate. Finally, participants did standardized whole-body stretching training (6 min). Whole-body stretching training consists of 12 stretching exercises (Achilles' tendon, sole of the foot, thigh, armpit, shoulder, shoulder/upper arm, chest/arm, shoulder/chest/arm, waist, back of knee, base of thigh, and back). Results of the combination exercise training for the older people demonstrated that the combination exercise training improved executive functions measured by verbal fluency task and the Stroop test, episodic memory measured by logical memory, and processing speed measured by symbol coding and symbol search compared to a waiting list control group.

3.5.4. Cognitive Training Using Paper-Pencil Programs.

There were two studies using cognitive training with paper-pencil programs. One study was a reading aloud and simple calculation intervention program for older people [66]; the other study was a play intervention program for children [67]. Intervention programs aimed to improve functions of prefrontal cortex functions and created previous neuroimaging findings. Both studies used long-term intervention periods (3 or 6 months) and a waiting list control group.

One study for elderly people used simple cognitive intervention programs (learning therapy), which involved solving arithmetic and Japanese language problems [66]. These problems were used in everyday classes of first-grade to fourth-grade elementary school students. The problems were printed on both sides of an A4-size paper (210×297 mm). As for the arithmetic problems, the lowest level of difficulty was single-digit addition, and the highest level was three-digit division. As for the Japanese language problems, the lowest level of difficulty was reading and writing simple sentences, and the highest level was reading fairy tales aloud. The participants were asked to go to classes once a week. They were then instructed to complete five sheets of each task prepared for each for that day, which were then assessed by the staff. The subjects were also asked to do their homework of two tasks for 4–6 days a week. As for their homework, the subjects were asked to complete five sheets of each task prepared for each individual. The results obtained using a paired t-test showed that learning therapy improved executive functions measured by frontal assessment battery and processing speed measured by symbol coding, but not the waiting list control group.

One study for the children used a play intervention program as cognitive training [67]. The play intervention programs consisted of a set of play activities based on standard cognitive tasks used in previous neuroimaging studies. The contents of the play activities were updated monthly (four play activities per month). The play intervention programs included the following five components. (1) For joint problem solving, the mothers and children developed mutual objectives through the play activities in our program. (2) The mothers and children were asked to alternate roles in the play activities to foster intersubjectivity. (3) To encourage warmth and responsiveness, the mothers were asked to be pleasant, warm, and responsive during the play activities. (4) To keep the children in the zone of proximal development (ZPD), which is the distance between the actual developmental level as determined by independent problem solving and the level of potential development as determined through problem solving under adult guidance or in collaboration with more capable peers, the difficulty levels of the play activities can

be adjusted according to the children's ability levels. (5) To promote self-regulation, we asked mothers to be responsive to the children's contributions and to build on them according to children's initiative in the play activities. The results showed that children in the play intervention programs improved general cognitive function/IQ measured by the Goodenough draw-a-man intelligence test, working memory measured by the new S-S intelligence test, and processing speed measured by the new S-S intelligence test compared to the waiting list control group.

4. Discussion

In this systematic review, we evaluated the effectiveness of the intervention program on cognitive functions in healthy people. The review showed that various intervention programs conducted by our laboratory can improve cognitive functions such as executive functions, working memory, episodic memory, processing speed, and general cognitive ability/IQ.

A critical comparison between different intervention studies is difficult because of the heterogeneity of the intervention programs, participants, and outcome measures. However, results of this review suggest the following important things. First, cognitive functions can be improved by some intervention programs at any age. In this review, we identified improvements of cognitive functions in children [67], young people [38, 47, 63, 64], and older people [45, 65]. Although several studies investigated younger and older people (5 studies for young people and 3 studies for older people), only one study examined children. To elucidate important issues in this field, more research is needed using children. Second, cognitive functions can be changed rapidly through interventions. Two studies for young people demonstrated improvements of cognitive functions after 6 days of intervention [38, 62]. However, it is important to note that the training time per day of these studies was quite long (4 hr) and that the total training time was 20 hr through intervention periods. No short-term intervention studies (e.g., 6 days) have been made of children and older people. Additional studies must be undertaken to elucidate the mechanisms of this issue. Third, a systematic review showed that near transfer effects can often occur but not far transfer effects (see Table 4). For instance, brain training game intervention studies [45, 47], which require participants to use executive functions and processing speed, improved executive functions and processing speed but did not improve short-term memory. However, some studies have demonstrated near and far transfer effects. Two studies for the young people [38, 63] showed improvements of general cognitive function/IQ. Two studies for young people [62, 64] showed changes of creativity after cognitive intervention. The results indicated that the far transfer effects can occur after some cognitive training intervention. It is difficult to find and conclude the common characteristics of the far transfer effects among studies because of the heterogeneity of the intervention programs. It is expected to be necessary to find a critical component of the far transfer effects after interventions.

For methodological quality, the average of the score of quality assessment was 9.89 (SD = 1.27, Max = 14). That score denotes that the methodological quality of included studies was high. However, only four studies reported the CONSORT state [45, 47, 65, 67]. The CONSORT statement is an evidence-based, minimum set of recommendations for reporting RCTs. The CONSORT statement includes a 25-item checklist, which specifically examines reporting of how the trial was designed, analyzed, and interpreted. Therefore, future studies should use and report the CONSORT statement. Use of CONSORT might improve methodological quality and facilitate a meta-analysis study.

Recent study has recommended the use of an active control group [83]. Using the active control group can control or reduce effects of social interactions and new experiences of joining the intervention programs. A recent study demonstrated that waiting list control conditions may overestimate beneficial effects of interventions [84]. Given these facts, we must use the active control group instead of a no-intervention group or a waiting-list control group. When examining the studies included studies in the review, three studies used the active control group [45, 47, 62]. These studies clearly revealed improvements of cognitive functions compared to the active control group. Based on those results, it may be concluded that intervention programs using a brain training game and working memory training can have positive effects on cognitive functions. It remains unclear how beneficial effects of interventions on cognitive functions in children compared to an active control group because of few studies have used an active control group. In the future, additional studies using an active control group for children are needed.

It is important to consider sample size in intervention programs. For the clinical trial, some phases are used to test the effectiveness and evidence of a new intervention program. Clinical trials involving new intervention programs are commonly classified into four phases (Phases 1–4) [85]. In Phase 1 trials, researchers test an intervention program in a very small group of people (20–80) to evaluate its safety, to determine an intervention a period, and to identify side effects. In Phase 2 trials, the experimental treatment is administered to a somewhat larger group of people (100–300) to elucidate whether it is effective compared with a placebo or a no-intervention control group or not and to further evaluate its safety. In Phase 3 trials, the treatment is given to large groups of people (1,000–3,000) to confirm its effectiveness, to monitor side effects, to compare it to other effective intervention programs, and to collect information that will allow it to be used safely. In Phase 4 trials, postmarketing studies delineate additional information, including the treatment's risks, benefits, and optimal use. Studies of intervention programs for improvements of cognitive functions may not fit into a single phase. For example, some may blend from Phase 1 to Phase 2 or from Phase 2 to Phase 3. When looking at the included studies in the review, the purpose of some studies met the study of Phase 2 or the blend study of Phases 2 and 3. However, several studies examined a small sample (fewer than 60). The sample sizes differed among the included studies (from 32 to 238, average = 76.67, SD = 66.66).

To generalize the effectiveness of the intervention program (Phases 3 or 4), we should conduct a large sample study.

An important limitation is the following. We did not conduct a meta-analysis of the effect size among the included studies because of the heterogeneity of intervention programs and cognitive measures. For future research, inclusion of a core set of outcome measures would be necessary to compare the effectiveness of different cognitive intervention programs. Outcome measures for basic cognitive functions such as subscales of WAIS should be part of this core set of outcome measures.

This systematic review showed that unresolved issues exist. First, the issue of whether the effects of some interventions programs generalize to improvement in everyday life activities such as driving skill is still unresolved and needs to be addressed more explicitly in future research. Second, it remains unclear whether intervention programs can improve cognitive functions in people who have any diagnosis such as developmental disorder, depression, post-traumatic stress disorder (PTSD), dementia, mild cognitive impairment, or Alzheimer's disease. Our previous studies showed that cognitive training using reading aloud improved cognitive functions in older people with dementia [78] and children with autism spectrum disorder [79]. To confirm the issue, we should conduct the intervention study with nonhealthy people as well as healthy people.

5. Conclusion

Cognitive functions are important for our daily life in any age. Consequently, we started the Smart Ageing research, which investigates how to improve cognitive functions. The conclusion of this systematic review was summarized as follows. (1) The intervention programs for Smart Ageing can be effective for improving various aspects of cognitive function (executive functions, working memory, episodic memory, processing speed, and general cognitive ability) in the healthy children, young people, and older people. (2) The cognitive functions can be changed rapidly by the short-term intervention such as 6 days. (3) The near transfer effects can often occur but not the far transfer effects. (4) The methodological quality of the included studies was high. The systematic review also indicated the following limitations and unresolved issues. (1) We did not conduct a meta-analysis for the effect size due to the heterogeneity of methods and outcome measures. (2) It is unresolved whether our intervention programs have beneficial effects on the everyday activities such as driving skill. (3) It remains unclear whether our intervention programs could improve cognitive function in the nonhealthy populations such as children with developmental disorders and older people with dementia. To overcome these problems, Smart Ageing research must be continued.

Conflict of Interests

The authors declare that there is no conflict of interests regarding the publication of this paper.

Acknowledgments

The authors thank Haruka Nouchi for searching for papers and all their other colleagues at IDAC, Tohoku University, for their support. This study was supported by JST/RISTEX and JST/CREST.

References

[1] T. Hedden and J. D. E. Gabrieli, "Insights into the ageing mind: a view from cognitive neuroscience," *Nature Reviews Neuroscience*, vol. 5, no. 2, pp. 87–96, 2004.

[2] S. Mejia, D. Pineda, L. M. Alvarez, and A. Ardila, "Individual differences in memory and executive function abilities during normal aging," *International Journal of Neuroscience*, vol. 95, no. 3-4, pp. 271–284, 1998.

[3] L. G. Nilsson, "Memory function in normal aging," *Acta Neurologica Scandinavica, Supplement*, vol. 107, supplement 179, pp. 7–13, 2003.

[4] R. C. Petersen, G. Smith, E. Kokmen, R. J. Ivnik, and E. G. Tangalos, "Memory function in normal aging," *Neurology*, vol. 42, no. 2, pp. 396–401, 1992.

[5] S. Blakemore and S. Choudhury, "Development of the adolescent brain: Implications for executive function and social cognition," *Journal of Child Psychology and Psychiatry and Allied Disciplines*, vol. 47, no. 3-4, pp. 296–312, 2006.

[6] D. C. Park, G. Lautenschlager, T. Hedden, N. S. Davidson, A. D. Smith, and P. K. Smith, "Models of visuospatial and verbal memory across the adult life span," *Psychology and Aging*, vol. 17, no. 2, pp. 299–320, 2002.

[7] T. A. Salthouse, "Memory aging from 18 to 80," *Alzheimer Disease and Associated Disorders*, vol. 17, no. 3, pp. 162–167, 2003.

[8] N. N. Yakhno, V. V. Zakharov, and A. B. Lokshina, "Impairment of memory and attention in the elderly," *Neuroscience and Behavioral Physiology*, vol. 37, no. 3, pp. 203–208, 2007.

[9] A. K. Coppin, A. Shumway-Cook, J. S. Saczynski et al., "Association of executive function and performance of dual-task physical tests among older adults: analyses from the InChianti study," *Age and Ageing*, vol. 35, no. 6, pp. 619–624, 2006.

[10] D. R. Royall, R. Palmer, L. K. Chiodo, and M. J. Polk, "Declining executive control in normal aging predicts change in functional status: the freedom house study," *Journal of the American Geriatrics Society*, vol. 52, no. 3, pp. 346–352, 2004.

[11] T. A. Salthouse, "The processing-speed theory of adult age differences in cognition," *Psychological Review*, vol. 103, no. 3, pp. 403–428, 1996.

[12] H. L. Swanson and M. Beebe-Frankenberger, "The relationship between working memory and mathematical problem solving in children at risk and not at risk for serious math difficulties," *Journal of Educational Psychology*, vol. 96, no. 3, pp. 471–491, 2004.

[13] H. L. Swanson and C. Sachse-Lee, "Mathematical problem solving and working memory in children with learning disabilities: both executive and phonological processes are important," *Journal of Experimental Child Psychology*, vol. 79, no. 3, pp. 294–321, 2001.

[14] T. E. Rohde and L. A. Thompson, "Predicting academic achievement with cognitive ability," *Intelligence*, vol. 35, no. 1, pp. 83–92, 2007.

[15] W. S. Barnett, "Long-term cognitive and academic effects of early childhood education on children in poverty," *Preventive Medicine*, vol. 27, no. 2, pp. 204–207, 1998.

[16] F. A. Campbell, E. P. Pungello, S. Miller-Johnson, M. Burchinal, and C. T. Ramey, "The development of cognitive and academic abilities: growth curves from an early childhood educational experiment," *Developmental Psychology*, vol. 37, no. 2, pp. 231–242, 2001.

[17] H. W. Stevenson, J. W. Stigler, S. Y. Lee, G. W. Lucker, S. Kitamura, and C. C. Hsu, "Cognitive performance and academic achievement of Japanese, Chinese, and American children," *Child Development*, vol. 56, no. 3, pp. 718–734, 1985.

[18] P. Barberger-Gateau and C. Fabrigoule, "Disability and cognitive impairment in the elderly," *Disability and Rehabilitation*, vol. 19, no. 5, pp. 175–193, 1997.

[19] D. A. Cahn-Weiner, P. F. Malloy, P. A. Boyle, M. Marran, and S. Salloway, "Prediction of functional status from neuropsychological tests in community-dwelling elderly individuals," *Clinical Neuropsychologist*, vol. 14, no. 2, pp. 187–195, 2000.

[20] M. C. Carlson, L. P. Fried, Q. Xue, K. Bandeen-Roche, S. L. Zeger, and J. Brandt, "Association between executive attention and physical functional performance in community-dwelling older women," *Journals of Gerontology B: Psychological Sciences and Social Sciences*, vol. 54, no. 5, pp. S262–S270, 1999.

[21] J. Grigsby, K. Kaye, J. Baxter, S. M. Shetterly, and R. F. Hamman, "Executive cognitive abilities and functional status among community-dwelling older persons in the San Luis Valley health and aging study," *Journal of the American Geriatrics Society*, vol. 46, no. 5, pp. 590–596, 1998.

[22] Y. Lee, J. H. Kim, K. J. Lee, G. Han, and J. L. Kim, "Association of cognitive status with functional limitation and disability in older adults," *Aging Clinical and Experimental Research*, vol. 17, no. 1, pp. 20–28, 2005.

[23] C. Owsley and G. McGwin Jr., "Association between visual attention and mobility in older adults," *Journal of the American Geriatrics Society*, vol. 52, no. 11, pp. 1901–1906, 2004.

[24] P. Verhaeghen, A. Marcoen, and L. Goossens, "Improving memory performance in the aged through mnemonic training: a meta-analytic study," *Psychology and Aging*, vol. 7, no. 2, pp. 242–251, 1992.

[25] S. Colcombe and A. F. Kramer, "Fitness effects on the cognitive function of older adults: a meta-analytic study," *Psychological Science*, vol. 14, no. 2, pp. 125–130, 2003.

[26] C. Lustig, P. Shah, R. Seidler, and P. A. Reuter-Lorenz, "Aging, training, and the brain: a review and future directions," *Neuropsychology Review*, vol. 19, no. 4, pp. 504–522, 2009.

[27] C. S. Green and D. Bavelier, "Exercising your brain: a review of human brain plasticity and training-induced learning," *Psychology and Aging*, vol. 23, no. 4, pp. 692–701, 2008.

[28] H. Takeuchi, Y. Taki, and R. Kawashima, "Effects of working memory training on cognitive functions and neural systems," *Reviews in the Neurosciences*, vol. 21, no. 6, pp. 427–449, 2010.

[29] M. Valenzuela and P. Sachdev, "Can cognitive exercise prevent the onset of dementia? Systematic review of randomized clinical trials with longitudinal follow-up," *The American Journal of Geriatric Psychiatry*, vol. 17, no. 3, pp. 179–187, 2009.

[30] K. V. Papp, S. J. Walsh, and P. J. Snyder, "Immediate and delayed effects of cognitive interventions in healthy elderly: a review of current literature and future directions," *Alzheimer's and Dementia*, vol. 5, no. 1, pp. 50–60, 2009.

[31] L. Jean, M. Bergeron, S. Thivierge, and M. Simard, "Cognitive intervention programs for individuals with mild cognitive impairment: systematic review of the literature," *The American Journal of Geriatric Psychiatry*, vol. 18, no. 4, pp. 281–296, 2010.

[32] P. J. Smith, J. A. Blumenthal, B. M. Hoffman et al., "Aerobic exercise and neurocognitive performance: a meta-analytic review of randomized controlled trials," *Psychosomatic Medicine*, vol. 72, no. 3, pp. 239–252, 2010.

[33] C.-N. Tseng, B.-S. Gau, and M.-F. Lou, "The effectiveness of exercise on improving cognitive function in older people: a systematic review," *Journal of Nursing Research*, vol. 19, no. 2, pp. 119–131, 2011.

[34] Y.-K. Chang, C.-Y. Pan, F.-T. Chen, C.-L. Tsai, and C.-C. Huang, "Effect of resistance-exercise training on cognitive function in healthy older adults: a review," *Journal of Aging and Physical Activity*, vol. 20, no. 4, pp. 497–517, 2012.

[35] M. N. McDonnell, A. E. Smith, and S. F. MacKintosh, "Aerobic exercise to improve cognitive function in adults with neurological disorders: a systematic review," *Archives of Physical Medicine and Rehabilitation*, vol. 92, no. 7, pp. 1044–1052, 2011.

[36] J. G. Z. van Uffelen, M. J. M. Chin A Paw, M. Hopman-Rock, and W. van Mechelen, "The effects of exercise on cognition in older adults with and without cognitive decline: a systematic review," *Clinical Journal of Sport Medicine*, vol. 18, no. 6, pp. 486–500, 2008.

[37] L. Clare and R. T. Woods, "Cognitive training and cognitive rehabilitation for people with early-stage Alzheimer's disease: a review," *Neuropsychological Rehabilitation*, vol. 14, no. 4, pp. 385–401, 2004.

[38] H. Takeuchi, Y. Taki, H. Hashizume et al., "Effects of training of processing speed on neural systems," *The Journal of Neuroscience*, vol. 31, no. 34, pp. 12139–12148, 2011.

[39] T. Klingberg, "Training and plasticity of working memory," *Trends in Cognitive Sciences*, vol. 14, no. 7, pp. 317–324, 2010.

[40] L. L. Richmond, A. B. Morrison, J. M. Chein, and I. R. Olson, "Working memory training and transfer in older adults," *Psychology and Aging*, vol. 26, no. 4, pp. 813–822, 2011.

[41] J. D. Edwards, V. G. Wadley, D. E. Vance, K. Wood, D. L. Roenker, and K. K. Ball, "The impact of speed of processing training on cognitive and everyday performance," *Aging & Mental Health*, vol. 9, no. 3, pp. 262–271, 2005.

[42] B. Carretti, E. Borella, and R. De Beni, "Does strategic memory training improve the working memory performance of younger and older adults?" *Experimental Psychology*, vol. 54, no. 4, pp. 311–320, 2007.

[43] D. F. Bjorklund, P. H. Miller, T. R. Coyle, and J. L. Slawinski, "Instructing children to use memory strategies: Evidence of utilization deficiencies in memory training studies," *Developmental Review*, vol. 17, no. 4, pp. 411–441, 1997.

[44] H. W. Mahncke, B. B. Connor, J. Appelman et al., "Memory enhancement in healthy older adults using a brain plasticity-based training program: a randomized, controlled study," *Proceedings of the National Academy of Sciences of the United States of America*, vol. 103, no. 33, pp. 12523–12528, 2006.

[45] R. Nouchi, Y. Taki, H. Takeuchi et al., "Brain training game improves executive functions and processing speed in the elderly: a randomized controlled trial," *PLoS ONE*, vol. 7, no. 1, Article ID e29676, 2012.

[46] D. J. Miller and D. P. Robertson, "Using a games console in the primary classroom: Effects of 'Brain Training' programme on computation and self-esteem," *British Journal of Educational Technology*, vol. 41, no. 2, pp. 242–255, 2010.

[47] R. Nouchi, Y. Taki, H. Takeuchi et al., "Brain training game boosts executive functions, working memory and processing speed in the young adults: a randomized controlled trial," *PLoS ONE*, vol. 8, no. 2, Article ID e55518, 2013.

[48] S. Bergman Nutley, S. Söderqvist, S. Bryde, L. B. Thorell, K. Humphreys, and T. Klingberg, "Gains in fluid intelligence after training non-verbal reasoning in 4-year-old children: a controlled, randomized study," *Developmental Science*, vol. 14, no. 3, pp. 591–601, 2011.

[49] D. J. Miller and D. P. Robertson, "Educational benefits of using game consoles in a primary classroom: a randomised controlled trial," *British Journal of Educational Technology*, vol. 42, no. 5, pp. 850–864, 2011.

[50] J. L. Mozolic, A. B. Long, A. R. Morgan, M. Rawley-Payne, and P. J. Laurienti, "A cognitive training intervention improves modality-specific attention in a randomized controlled trial of healthy older adults," *Neurobiology of Aging*, vol. 32, no. 4, pp. 655–668, 2011.

[51] K. Ball, D. B. Berch, K. F. Helmers et al., "Effects of cognitive training interventions with older adults: a randomized controlled trial," *Journal of the American Medical Association*, vol. 288, no. 18, pp. 2271–2281, 2002.

[52] R. C. Cassilhas, V. A. R. Viana, V. Grassmann et al., "The impact of resistance exercise on the cognitive function of the elderly," *Medicine & Science in Sports and Exercise*, vol. 39, no. 8, pp. 1401–1407, 2007.

[53] P. Perrig-Chiello, W. J. Perrig, R. Ehrsam, H. B. Staehelin, and F. Krings, "The effects of resistance training on well-being and memory in elderly volunteers," *Age and Ageing*, vol. 27, no. 4, pp. 469–475, 1998.

[54] C. L. Davis, P. D. Tomporowski, J. E. McDowell et al., "Exercise improves executive function and achievement and alters brain activation in overweight children: a randomized, controlled trial," *Health Psychology*, vol. 30, no. 1, pp. 91–98, 2011.

[55] J. D. Bransford, A. L. Brown, and R. R. Cocking, *How People Learn*, National Academy Press, Washington, DC, USA, 2000.

[56] S. M. Barnett and S. J. Ceci, "When and where do we apply what we learn? A taxonomy for far transfer," *Psychological Bulletin*, vol. 128, no. 4, pp. 612–637, 2002.

[57] E. M. Zelinski, "Far transfer in cognitive training of older adults," *Restorative Neurology and Neuroscience*, vol. 27, no. 5, pp. 455–471, 2009.

[58] J. D. Edwards, V. G. Wadley, R. S. Myers, D. L. Roenker, G. M. Cissell, and K. K. Ball, "Transfer of a speed of processing intervention to near and far cognitive functions," *Gerontology*, vol. 48, no. 5, pp. 329–340, 2002.

[59] J. Karbach and J. Kray, "How useful is executive control training? Age differences in near and far transfer of task-switching training," *Developmental Science*, vol. 12, no. 6, pp. 978–990, 2009.

[60] A. Liberati, D. G. Altman, J. Tetzlaff et al., "The PRISMA statement for reporting systematic reviews and meta-analyses of studies that evaluate health care interventions: explanation and elaboration," *Annals of Internal Medicine*, vol. 151, no. 4, pp. 65–94, 2009.

[61] A. P. Verhagen, H. C. W. De Vet, R. A. De Bie et al., "The Delphi list: a criteria list for quality assessment of randomized clinical trials for conducting systematic reviews developed by Delphi consensus," *Journal of Clinical Epidemiology*, vol. 51, no. 12, pp. 1235–1241, 1998.

[62] H. Takeuchi, Y. Taki, Y. Sassa et al., "Working memory training using mental calculation impacts regional gray matter of the frontal and parietal regions," *PLoS ONE*, vol. 6, no. 8, Article ID e23175, 2011.

[63] H. Takeuchi, Y. Taki, R. Nouchi et al., "Effects of working memory training on functional connectivity and cerebral blood flow during rest," *Cortex*, vol. 49, no. 8, pp. 2106–2125, 2013.

[64] H. Takeuchi, Y. Taki, R. Nouchi et al., "Anatomical correlates of quality of life: evidence from voxel-based morphometry," *Human Brain Mapping*, vol. 35, no. 5, pp. 1834–1846, 2014.

[65] R. Nouchi, Y. Taki, H. Takeuchi et al., "Four weeks of combination exercise training improved executive functions, episodic memory, and processing speed in healthy elderly people: evidence from a randomized controlled trial," *AGE*, vol. 36, no. 2, pp. 787–799, 2014.

[66] S. Uchida and R. Kawashima, "Reading and solving arithmetic problems improves cognitive functions of normal aged people: a randomized controlled study," *AGE*, vol. 30, no. 1, pp. 21–29, 2008.

[67] Y. Tachibana, A. Fukushima, H. Saito, S. Yoneyama, K. Ushida, and R. Kawashima, "A new mother-child play activity program to decrease parenting stress and improve child cognitive abilities: a cluster randomized controlled trial," *PLoS ONE*, vol. 7, no. 7, Article ID e38238, 2012.

[68] R. Kawashima, "Mental exercises for cognitive function: clinical evidence," *Journal of Preventive Medicine and Public Health*, vol. 46, supplement 1, pp. S22–S27, 2013.

[69] H. Takeuchi and R. Kawashima, "Effects of processing speed training on cognitive functions and neural systems," *Reviews in the Neurosciences*, vol. 23, no. 3, pp. 289–301, 2012.

[70] Y. Tachibana, Y. Akitsuki, and R. Kawashima, "Cognitive interventions to imporve prfrontal functions," *Brain Research Journal*, vol. 3, no. 3-4, pp. 185–205, 2011.

[71] R. Nouchi, Y. Taki, H. Takeuchi et al., "Beneficial effects of short-term combination exercise training on diverse cognitive functions in healthy older people: study protocol for a randomized controlled trial," *Trials*, vol. 13, article 200, 2012.

[72] R. Nouchi, Y. Taki, H. Takeuchi et al., "Beneficial effects of reading aloud and solving simple arithmetic calculations (learning therapy) on a wide range of cognitive functions in the healthy elderly: study protocol for a randomized controlled trial," *Trials*, vol. 13, article 32, 2012.

[73] Y. Tachibana, J. Yoshida, M. Ichinomiya et al., "A GO intervention program for enhancing elementary school children's cognitive functions and control abilities of emotion and behavior: study protocol for a randomized controlled trial," *Trials*, vol. 13, article 8, 2012.

[74] N. Maïonchi-Pino, Y. Taki, S. Yokoyama et al., "Is the phonological deficit in developmental dyslexia related to impaired phonological representations and to universal phonological grammar?" *Journal of Experimental Child Psychology*, vol. 115, no. 1, pp. 53–73, 2013.

[75] H. Takeuchi, M. Sugiura, Y. Sassa et al., "Neural correlates of the difference between working memory speed and simple sensorimotor speed: an fMRI study," *PLoS ONE*, vol. 7, no. 1, Article ID e30579, 2012.

[76] S. Kanoh, Y. M. Murayama, K. Miyamoto, T. Yoshinobu, and R. Kawashima, "A NIRS-based brain-computer interface system during motor imagery: system development and online feedback training," in *Proceedings of the Annual International Conference of the IEEE Engineering in Medicine and Biology Society*, vol. 2009, pp. 594–597, 2009.

[77] H. Takeuchi, A. Sekiguchi, Y. Taki et al., "Training of working memory impacts structural connectivity," *Journal of Neuroscience*, vol. 30, no. 9, pp. 3297–3303, 2010.

[78] R. Kawashima, K. Okita, R. Yamazaki et al., "Reading aloud and arithmetic calculation improve frontal function of people with dementia," *Journals of Gerontology A: Biological Sciences and Medical Sciences*, vol. 60, no. 3, pp. 380–384, 2005.

[79] Y. Tachibana, Y. Hwang, Y. Abe, S. Goto, K. Sugai, and R. Kawashima, "Reading aloud improves executive function of children with autism spectrum disorder: a pilot randomized controlled trial," *International Journal on Disability and Human Development*, vol. 12, no. 1, pp. 91–101, 2013.

[80] R. Kawashima, "A new intervention program for improvement of cognitive functions of senile dementia patients," *Seishin Shinkeigaku Zasshi*, vol. 107, no. 12, pp. 1305–1309, 2005.

[81] R. Kawashima, "Cognitive rehabilitation for Alzheimer disease—the learning therapy," *Rinsho Shinkeigaku*, vol. 45, no. 11, pp. 864–866, 2005.

[82] A. Sekiguchi and R. Kawashima, "Cognitive rehabilitation—the learning therapy for the senile dementia," *Brain and Nerve*, vol. 59, no. 4, pp. 357–365, 2007.

[83] Z. Shipstead, T. S. Redick, and R. W. Engle, "Is working memory training effective?" *Psychological Bulletin*, vol. 138, no. 4, pp. 628–654, 2012.

[84] J. A. Cunningham, K. Kypri, and J. McCambridge, "Exploratory randomized controlled trial evaluating the impact of a waiting list control design," *BMC Medical Research Methodology*, vol. 13, no. 1, article 150, 2013.

[85] L. M. Friedman, C. Furberg, and D. L. DeMets, *Fundamentals of Clinical Trials*, Springer, New York, NY, USA, 1998.

3

Rett Syndrome: Coming to Terms with Treatment

Alan Percy

Civitan International Research Center, University of Alabama at Birmingham, 1720 2nd Avenue South, CIRC 320E, Birmingham, AL 35294-0021, USA

Correspondence should be addressed to Alan Percy; apercy@uab.edu

Academic Editor: Ronald L. Klein

Rett syndrome (RTT) has experienced remarkable progress over the past three decades since emerging as a disorder of worldwide proportions, particularly with discovery of the linkage of RTT to *MECP2* mutations. The advances in clinical research and the increasing pace of basic science investigations have accelerated the pattern of discovery and understanding. Clinical trials are ongoing and others are planned. A review of these events and the prospects for continued success are highlighted below. The girls and women encountered today with RTT are, overall, in better general, neurologic, and behavioral health than those encountered earlier. This represents important progress worldwide from the concerted efforts of a broadly based and diverse clinical and basic research consortium as well as the efforts of parents, family, and friends.

1. Introduction: Early History of Rett Syndrome

Rett syndrome (RTT; Online Mendelian Inheritance in Man #312750; http://www.ncbi.nlm.nih.gov/omim/) was first recognized by Andreas Rett, a neurodevelopmental pediatrician in Vienna, more than fifty years ago when he observed two girls in his clinic simultaneously engaged in hand stereotypies [1, 2]. His attempts to raise awareness of this observation among physicians in Europe met with little success in creating interest in expanding understanding of this unique neurodevelopmental disorder. As it happened, most of his written efforts were in German and were not widely circulated beyond Austria. Bengt Hagberg, a Swedish child neurologist, had also identified young girls with virtually identical features, but unlike Rett, he did not report these observations or extend his information beyond Sweden. Rett's single major English publication appeared in the *Handbook of Clinical Neurology* in 1977 [3]. However, a series of extensive metabolic tests on blood and urine in his participants with this disorder had identified hyperammonemia, the subject of this *Handbook* volume. Fortunately, this finding turned

out to be spurious. At a gathering of child neurologists in Europe near the end of the 1970s, Hagberg became aware of this change in the association of these clinical features and hyperammonemia, realized that they were observing the same disorder, and planned together with Jean Aicardi, Karin Dias, and Ovidio Ramos to publish their own combined experiences. Shortly thereafter in 1981, Hagberg had a chance meeting with Rett in Toronto and following this discussion elected to name the disorder Rett syndrome. At the time, RTT was scarcely known outside of Europe, but with the 1983 publication in the *Annals of Neurology* this disorder gained immediate prominence as the leading cause of significant cognitive disability among females [4]. Rett led a series of international meetings in Vienna with representatives from throughout the world and energized this group to develop appropriate diagnostic criteria and to identify a causal relationship [5]. Vanja Holm, Hugo Moser, and Alan Percy [6] attended the 1984 meeting which saw the first effort in development of consensus criteria for diagnosis and created the first broad scale efforts worldwide in clinical and research activity [7].

2. Initial Studies

Following this initial clinical exposure to RTT, investigations began to intensify, spurred by efforts of Hugo Moser to convene an international meeting at Johns Hopkins Medical School in 1985 and the subsequent creation of the International Rett Syndrome Association (IRSA) through the leadership of three parents, Kathy Hunter, Gail Smith, and Jane Brubaker. This energized clinical studies at the Baylor College of Medicine led by Alan Percy, Daniel Glaze, and Huda Zoghbi, and Johns Hopkins led by Hugo Moser and Sakkubai Naidu. Important results emerged almost immediately with the identification of reductions in spinal fluid metabolites of the biogenic amines [8, 9], studies on prevalence from a survey of Texas residents [10], and the initiation of broad scale growth assessments by the Baylor group and the corresponding development of PET scanning analyses at Johns Hopkins [11]. This culminated among others in the first large scale growth measurement study from Baylor assessing height, weight, and head circumference [12] and, subsequently, hands and feet [13]. These results clearly demonstrated the profound failure of growth and initiated a long-term effort at defining areas of responsibility including nutrition and gastrointestinal function. In the years leading up to identification of the causal gene, considerable effort was expended in developing a clear understanding of the potential mechanisms. Similarly, significant attention was given to identifying the electrophysiological underpinnings of the common notations of epilepsy [14–18] and periodic breathing [19–21]. These early studies in the US were supported by the efforts of IRSA and the subsequent lobbying of Congress to promote funding streams through the National Institutes of Health. Program projects emerged both at Johns Hopkins and at the Baylor College of Medicine and continuing training grants from IRSA spurred these clinical advances as well as to the successful gene identification. At the same time, prevalence studies emerged ranging from 1 : 10,000 to 1 : 22,000 [10]. More recently, a population-based study from Australia indicated an incidence of about 1 : 10,000 female births [22]. As international interest grew, it became quite evident that RTT occurs worldwide, affecting all racial and ethnic groups with similar frequency.

At the same time, clinical studies identified the existence of atypical forms of RTT including the delayed onset and preserved speech variants among those with better overall function and the early onset seizure and congenital variants among those with poorer overall function [23–27].

Throughout the next decade considerable attention concentrated on identifying a causal mechanism. Among the possibilities, the speculation regarding environmental or medical causes failed to match with the striking occurrence of RTT virtually exclusively in females. This alone suggested a genetic etiology based on an X-linked dominant mechanism. Thus, a series of studies gradually focused attention to Xq28, a very gene-rich region associated with several important human disorders [28–35], culminating in the identification of mutations in the *MECP2* (*methyl-CpG-binding protein 2*) gene [36]. This discovery then led to vigorous and productive basic science investigations.

3. Mutation Analyses

Due to restriction of the initial features of RTT to young girls, the presumption had been made that the molecular abnormality represented an X-linked dominant disorder. Although not uniformly accepted [37], extensive efforts were directed at the X chromosome among girls and their families. The area of interest was narrowed to Xq28 based on DNA samples obtained through the efforts of Dan Glaze, Huda Zoghbi, and Alan Percy at Baylor [34] and Carolyn Schanen [30] at Stanford and from a large family in Argentina who were studied at Johns Hopkins [38]. This region is one very rich in genes associated with human conditions including the genes for adrenoleukodystrophy, X-linked muscular dystrophy, and color blindness. While *MECP2*, which is located at Xq28, was well known having been described previously in the cancer literature as an epigenetic modulator [39], it was not initially regarded as the primary candidate. Nevertheless, as the result of intense efforts by Ruthie Amir in the laboratory of Huda Zoghbi at the Baylor College of Medicine, the association between mutations in *MECP2* and RTT was firmly established [36]. At present, more than 250 different mutations associated with RTT have been identified in this gene [40]. However, as will be described below, these mutations not only have provided the molecular basis for almost all girls with RTT, but also have uncovered a rich and complex array of previously unanticipated disorders [41–43].

4. Clinical Diagnosis

RTT, characterized by partial or complete loss of fine motor and communication skills, remarkable stereotypic movements, principally of the hands, significant cognitive impairment, and pervasive growth failure, has its onset during the first 6–30 months of life following a period of what is considered to be normal development. Intense efforts to establish a biologic marker were uniformly unsuccessful. Although hy- perammonemia was initially described by Andy Rett and colleagues, these findings were not confirmed on subsequent testing. Indeed, it was this early metabolic finding that seemed to differentiate the separate observations of Rett and Hagberg.

With the establishment of obligate requirements for diagnosis in 1984 [7], the diagnosis of RTT was based on meeting specific clinical criteria. A series of revisions in the diagnostic criteria have emerged subsequently, as understanding of RTT has advanced, most notably through the identification of *MECP2* mutations [44–47]. An important reason for these continued revisions is the need to provide precise definitions and avoid any misunderstandings related to nuances of different languages so that application is practiced similarly throughout the world. As such, the most recent revision [46] based on an international consensus panel occurred in 2010 (Table 1). The early periods of pre- and perinatal history are typically normal. Initial development is regarded by families as normal for the first several months of life, but it is clear that the acquisition of early development milestones is often delayed beyond the period accepted as the upper limit of normal. After age of six months, continued developmental

TABLE 1: Rett Syndrome (consensus criteria—2010) (typical or classic).

Regression followed by recovery or stabilization
Must fulfill all main criteria and all exclusion criteria
Supportive criteria while present not required
Main Criteria
Partial or complete loss of purposeful hand skills
Partial or complete loss of spoken language
Gait abnormalities: dyspraxic or absent
Stereotypic hand movements
Exclusion Criteria
Traumatic brain injury
Neurometabolic disease
Severe infection
Very abnormal development in first 6 months of life

TABLE 2: Rett syndrome timing of regression period.

| Age at regression | Classic RTT | Variant RTT | |
		Higher functioning	Lower functioning
<6 months	13 (1.7%)	3 (4.4%)	27 (38%)
6–<12 months	54 (7.0%)	2 (2.9%)	9 (12%)
12–<18 months	281 (36%)	2 (2.9%)	15 (21%)
18–30 months	351 (46%)	26 (38%)	10 (14%)
>30 months	74 (9.6%)	35 (52%)	11 (15%)
Total	773	68	72

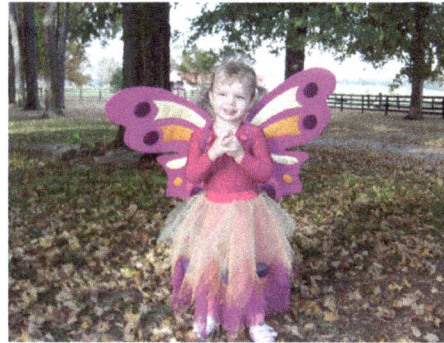

FIGURE 1: A 3-year-old girl with Rett syndrome demonstrating midline hand stereotypy and preserved ambulatory skills.

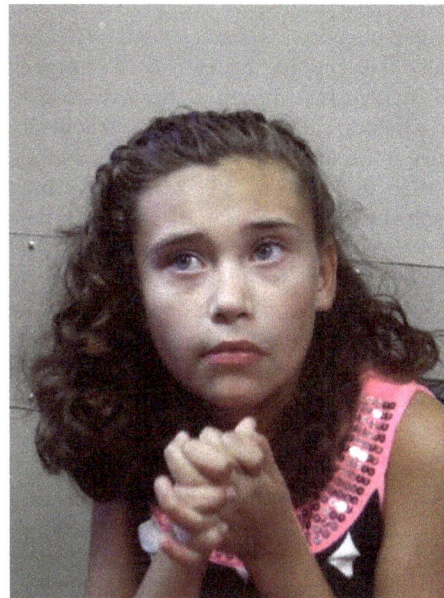

FIGURE 2: A 13-year-old ambulatory girl with Rett syndrome showing intense eye gaze and prominent midline hand stereotypy.

progress stagnates and thereafter a frank regression occurs. During this regression period, the partial or complete loss of fine motor skills and the virtually simultaneous occurrence of stereotypic movements are noted along with delays in cognitive development and abnormalities in communication including eye contact and responsiveness to attempts at socialization. The girls ignore spoken language or even loud noises, and profound irritability including inconsolable crying for prolonged periods without apparent explanation is common. It is during this phase that some are regarded as autistic. The typical period of regression is between 12 and 30 months but may be seen as early as age of 6 months age or beyond 30 months (Table 2).

Deceleration in the rate of head growth is often the first clinical sign of RTT. This was noted by Rett and described further in the context of microcephaly [1, 48]. While it is now clear that deceleration in the rate of head growth may be profound and microcephaly is evident in 70% or more, not all have head circumference deceleration to that level and not all girls actually have a remarkable change in rate of head growth such that this deceleration has been removed as an obligate criterion. Based on data from the US Natural History study, abnormal deceleration may be noted as early as one to two months of age [49]. However, the later and nearly simultaneous occurrence of reduction

or loss of fine motor hand function and the appearance of stereotypic movements is often the pivotal point of diagnostic significance. The stereotypies are typically first noted between ages of 1 and 3 years and predominantly involve the hands but may also be seen in the orofacial region and the feet, particularly if the hand movements are suppressed. Hand movements consist principally of hand-washing, hand-wringing, or hand-clapping/hand-patting and may dominate hand function to the exclusion of any effective motor skills (Figures 1–3). In some, prominent hand mouthing or picking at the hair or clothes is the predominant stereotypic movement. These stereotypies typically are noted in the midline but may be asymmetric with one hand in the mouth and the other patting, finger rubbing, or hair twirling. In rare instances, the hand-wringing may occur behind the back. Ambulation is acquired by most (~80%) girls (Figure 1). However, between age of 1 and 4 years the gait is punctuated by significant truncal ataxia and apraxia demonstrating a broad-based,

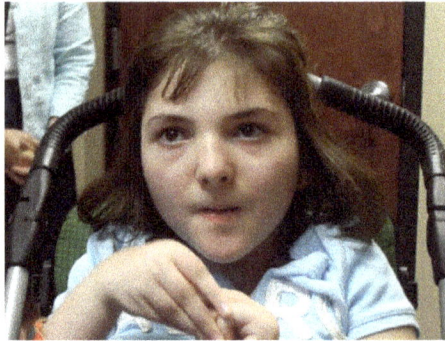

FIGURE 3: A 12-year-old girl with Rett syndrome who is nonambulatory but has excellent eye contact and a prominent midline hand stereotypy.

wandering, and purposeless character and is often initiated by retropulsion (first stepping backwards). Prominent to-and-fro truncal rocking is common, either side-to-side or back and forth, whether sitting or standing. About 30–40% of those acquiring the ability to walk will lose this independent capability, such that, overall, about 50% have independent gait. The majority of those no longer walking independently are able to walk with assistance. In some this requires only minimal guidance whereas others may require substantial support. Ambulation, whether independent or supported, should be encouraged indefinitely. Anxiety regarding fear of falling, changes in floor pattern or surface, or changes in terrain is evident and simply providing a steadying hand may be sufficient.

The clinical evaluation for RTT rests on a thorough history and current assessment including a neurological evaluation. In particular, careful attention must be accorded to the course of developmental progress from birth and a comprehensive evaluation of growth parameters (height, weight, and head circumference). Particular importance should be given to the temporal sequence of the child's developmental history noting delay in achieving specific developmental milestones, loss of motor or communicative skills, and appearance of hand stereotypies. Comprehensive laboratory tests should assess the complete chemistry profile including triglyceride and cholesterol measures and vitamin D levels. An EEG is recommended both to assess the background activity and to evaluate the presence of epileptiform features. Typically, the EEG may remain normal for the first two years of life but thereafter is marked by profound slowing of background activity and the presence of epileptiform characteristics. Frequently, the EEG may be particularly epileptiform in character during periods of sleep, but definitive seizures may not occur. Behavioral events, occurring daily or several times per week, may resemble clinical seizures. It is essential to corroborate these events by video-EEG assessment as in many cases they are not based on epileptiform activity. Careful attention to this evaluation is essential. Routine neuroimaging (cranial CT or MRI) has not been informative in general in RTT.

Confirmation of the clinical diagnosis of RTT should be based on determination of *MECP2* mutations [50–61].

Initial emphasis should be placed on sequencing the four exons of *MECP2*. In approximately 10% of individuals with the clinical diagnosis of RTT, sequence analysis is normal. Secondary analysis utilizing techniques such as multiplex ligation-dependent probe amplification (MLPA) is required to reveal large deletions involving one or more of the exons. Standard sequence determination will miss these mutations. MLPA testing will also be informative for duplications of *MECP2*, as will be discussed below. In 4-5% of individuals meeting clinical criteria for RTT, no *MECP2* mutation may be found. These individuals may represent phenocopies of RTT or may be the result of currently undefined abnormalities in the *MECP2* gene.

5. Variant Phenotypic Expression

More than twenty years ago, Hagberg recognized the occurrence of variant phenotypic expressions of RTT [23, 24]. Since then, a number of reported variances have been noted. In these, the girls meet some but not all criteria for RTT and are considered to have *atypical* RTT with definite and discernible patterns of involvement. Others have *MECP2* mutations but lack the clinical features of RTT. In these instances, both females and males may be involved. Individuals who function at level higher than that seen in typical RTT may have preservation of some speech and are most commonly associated with a specific *MECP2* mutation, namely, R133C [25]. Others may not have identifiable features consistent with RTT until age of 8–10 years and are termed delayed onset variant or *formes fruste* [23]. Quite distinct from both this group with better function and those with typical RTT, individuals may function at a lower level and generally fall into two groups, a congenital form demonstrating little or no developmental progress and an early onset seizure form featuring a relatively severe epileptic encephalopathy that produces markedly abnormal early development. Criteria [46] for these variant RTT phenotypes are based on fulfilling at least 2 of 4 main criteria and at least 5 of 11 associated features for RTT (Table 3). Hagberg noted that 107/130 (82%) girls with RTT in Sweden fulfilled the classic criteria, 16/130 (12%) displayed formes fruste, and the remaining 7 were either preserved speech or congenital forms [24]. In the RTT Natural History study funded by the National Institutes of Health, of more than 1000 participants meeting criteria for RTT, 85% were classic or typical RTT and 15% were atypical. Of those with atypical RTT, the higher and lower functioning variants were virtually equivalent in number.

Other females with *MECP2* mutations do not meet any criteria for RTT. Some of these have significant cognitive and behavioral problems with autistic features [62, 63]. These individuals generally have mutations in the 3′-region of *MECP2* and may have favorable skewing of X chromosome inactivation (XCI). Others are quite normal or have mild cognitive impairment or learning difficulties and include families in which a mother expressing the abnormal *MECP2* has skewed XCI. Her offspring may include females with classic RTT and males with variable phenotypes as described

TABLE 3: Rett syndrome (consensus criteria—2010) (atypical or variant).

Regression followed by recovery or stabilization
Meet at least 3 of 6 main criteria
Meet at least 5 of 11 supportive criteria
Main criteria
Partial or complete loss of purposeful hand skills
Partial or complete loss of spoken language
Gait abnormalities: dyspraxic or absent
Stereotypic hand movements

Supportive criteria	
Awake breathing problems	Growth retardation
Bruxism	Small hands and feet
Impaired sleep	Scoliosis and/or kyphosis
Abnormal muscle tone	Increased pain tolerance
Peripheral vasomotor abnormalities	Intense eye contact
Inappropriate laughter or screaming	

below, namely, a rapidly progressive encephalopathy or simply cognitive impairment with or without motor difficulties [64].

6. RTT in Males

Few males have been reported meeting obligate criteria for RTT. These have occurred under two distinctly different scenarios and appear not to exceed 10 males. Males with Klinefelter syndrome (47, XXY) [65–67] and *MECP2* mutations and males with somatic mosaicism [68], that is, two cell populations, and *MECP2* mutations in one cell population may have clinical features typical for RTT. Among males with mutations in *MECP2* who do not meet obligate criteria for RTT, a somewhat larger number has been identified [69]. One group numbering, less than twenty, displays a rapidly progressive encephalopathy and significant apneic episodes leading to markedly shortened (1-2 years) survival [70]. A quite separate group of similar size involves individuals presenting with mutations in the $3'$-region of *MECP2*. These males demonstrate a developmental disorder that may include only cognitive delays and inappropriate behaviors or may display developmental delay and a quite significant and steadily progressive dystonia leading to remarkable limitation of motor function [42, 64, 71]. Most of these males failing to meet RTT criteria have only been identified due to the presence of RTT in female siblings. Otherwise, they would have escaped detection in all likelihood because they display a set of developmental abnormalities distinct from RTT.

Although not demonstrating a sequence abnormality in *MECP2*, a separate group of males totaling more than 150 have a completely different defect [41, 72–74]. This group has duplication of the *MECP2* gene, not a mutation. Each duplication is rather unique in terms of its size and the number of other genes involved. Prior animal studies had demonstrated that *MECP2* is tightly regulated with either a loss or gain resulting in unique neurodevelopmental consequences so that the identification of these individuals is not surprising. Males with a *MECP2* duplication demonstrate cognitive impairment, absence of spoken language, epilepsy, and an abnormal shuffling gait and rarely display the growth retardation or hand stereotypies typical for RTT [75–77]. Frequent upper respiratory infections or chronic sinusitis events in some males are felt to relate to a separate gene among those duplicated. Many mothers of these males have the same *MECP2* duplication but appear remarkably normal due to XCI. More detailed analysis reveals that some of these mothers acknowledge depression or obsessive-compulsive behaviors [76].

7. Clinical Profile

Already in 1986, Hagberg had developed a staging system to characterize the clinical progression of RTT [78]. This staging system however was created at a time when current practices regarding nutrition, physical and occupational therapies, and surgical management of orthopedic issues were not broadly emphasized. As greater experience has been gained, it is now recognized that clinical progression requires a different view [79]. It is recognized that motor development and function evolve steadily from initial hypotonia progressing to normal tone and then to an increasing pattern of hypertonia and rigidity reminiscent of parkinsonian features. On the other hand, interpersonal interaction and communication perspectives seem to remain quite stable over time. Therefore, a developmental pattern emerges that fits a clear temporal profile: (1) a period of apparently normal early development, (2) then an arrest of developmental progress typically between age of 6 and 18 months, (3) followed by a period of regression involving a partial or complete loss of social contact and fine motor skills generally between age of 12 and 30 months, and (4) finally a prolonged period of stabilization with markedly improved social interaction, eye contact, and socialization (Figures 2 and 3) contrasting with the gradual evolution of motor function marked by increasing muscle tone, rigidity, and significant dystonic posturing, particularly of the feet, hands, and occasionally the trunk. With the recognition of *MECP2* mutations, a basis was provided for understanding the broad range of clinical involvements associated with the specific *MECP2* mutations and with other genetic factors. Further, the application of broadly based treatment programs for physical and occupational therapy, for dystonic positioning, and for orthopedic concerns has altered the long-term outlook sufficiently that utilization of the original staging system has been clouded and its implementation as structured is not currently recommended. Certainly, the clinical staging format offered a means of assessing clinical progress, but subsequent advances have rendered it less useful.

8. Clinical Issues

Specific systemic problems may alter the landscape of RTT considerably (Table 4). In order to maintain the optimal functional level, proper attention to these is essential recognizing that each individual may be quite variable with respect to the

TABLE 4: Rett syndrome (clinical issues).

Cognitive impairment	
Epilepsy	
Breathing Irregularities	
Hyperventilation, breathholding, or both	
Gastrointestinal dysfunction	
Poor chewing and swallowing	Gastroesophageal reflux
Delayed gastric emptying	Constipation
Gallbladder dysfunction	
Growth	
Sleep	
Ambulation	
Self-abuse	
Quality of Life	
Longevity	
Other associated features	
Hypertonia	Progressive dystonia
Prolonged QTc interval	Bruxism
Vasomotor disturbances	

specific medical issue. Therefore, the following guidelines are recommended for consideration and include cognitive impairment, epilepsy, breathing irregularities, gastrointestinal function, growth failure, scoliosis, sleep difficulties, ambulation, self-abuse, quality of life, and life expectancy.

Growth failure is pervasive having been recognized early on as a fundamental concern. We now understand that survival may be quite prolonged albeit less than normal. Nevertheless, this raises fundamental issues. Efforts to identify a consistent metabolic abnormality have been fruitless in spite of concerted efforts regarding standard blood chemistries, the amino and organic acids, mitochondrial function, and urea cycle metabolism. In addressing each of the potential clinical concerns, it is important to be cognizant of maintaining an open dialogue with the parents or principal caregivers. For additional information, the International Rett Syndrome Foundation (IRSF), successor to IRSA, is an excellent resource for individuals and families. IRSF provides effective guidance to interested individuals and supports both basic and clinical research investigations (http://www.rettsyndrome.org/). In recent years, patient advocacy groups have developed worldwide offering similar levels of support. These organizations are critical to maintaining a platform for exchanging relevant clinical information and providing updates on scientific advances in support of more effective treatment.

8.1. Cognitive Impairment.

Cognitive function in RTT cannot be assessed effectively due to the inability of these girls to demonstrate purposeful hand skills and effective communication. Despite these limitations, available measures provided estimates of mental developmental age at the 8–10-month level and gross motor function ranging from 12 to 18 months.

Application of modalities based on visual response has not proved more effective. More recently, advances in computer-based technology utilizing eye gaze tracking have provided a means of communication that suggests a level of interaction and comprehension not previously recognized [80–82]. It is possible that such methodology will provide an effective, reliable assessment of cognitive function in RTT. An important aspect of such modalities is appropriate consideration of the slow response time. More than a few seconds and often as long as half a minute are required to elicit a response to specific requests. Failure to allocate proper response time is likely to doom attempts at determining comprehension. Assessing cognitive function in girls with RTT remains extremely problematic and will require objective assessment of these techniques.

The acquisition of feeding, dressing, and toileting skills is poor at best, requiring assistance from others throughout their lives. Nevertheless, occupational, cognitive, and speech therapies form necessary elements of effective therapeutic management. Utilization of the advanced computer technologies noted above is an essential component of this plan where feasible. The objective assessment of this methodology will be required to substantiate its efficacy.

8.2. Epilepsy.

Seizure frequency in RTT has been reported across a broad range from 30 to 80% [83–85]. The electroencephalogram (EEG) is invariably abnormal after age of 2 years marked by slowing of background activity with a reduction or loss of posterior dominant rhythm and recurrent spike and slow spike and wave activity. Particularly during sleep in the young child, the epileptiform pattern may be nearly continuous suggesting hypsarrhythmia or nearly continuous slow spike and wave abnormalities. However, despite these findings, clinical seizure activity may be minimal or absent in the majority of girls. This represents a major challenge particularly when the child demonstrates unusual behaviors resembling clinical epilepsy. The challenge is to differentiate these behavioral patterns or possibly brainstem events from clinical seizures. This requires video-EEG monitoring to provide a satisfactory resolution and is best accomplished when these events occur relatively frequently. In the US Natural History study, 85% of girls were noted to have clinical epilepsy by age of 16, but only 30–35% required medication for their management at any given time. In addition, it was noted that new-onset epilepsy is rarely noted after age of 20 and in many instances the epileptiform EEG pattern is no longer present.

Control of clinical epilepsy in individuals with RTT is usually attained rather easily with single agents such as carbamazepine, oxcarbazepine, sodium valproate, or lamotrigine. While levetiracetam, topiramate, and clobazam have been used with increasing frequency, no evidence of superior control has been noted whereas undesirable side-effects of decreased appetite, irritability, and dull affect have been. When control of epilepsy becomes more challenging, the use of multiple medications together or the addition of alternative strategies such as the vagal nerve stimulator and the ketogenic diet has been employed with efficacy in many instances.

8.3. Breathing Irregularities. Rett noted early on the occurrence of irregular breathing during wakefulness consisting of hyperventilation or breathholding or both as a common feature. In general, this periodic breathing has its onset in early childhood (3–5 years) but is most problematic between age of 5 and 15 years and is commonly worsened by activities that increase anxiety or agitation. Periods of breathholding may be prolonged exceeding one minute and may be accompanied by air swallowing (aerophagia) leading to significant abdominal distension or bloating. The distension tends to subside, particularly during sleep. The periodic breathing may dominate periods of wakefulness and create problems with feeding and other activities. In some girls, the periodic breathing may be very subtle and actually unrecognized by parents and other caregivers. One sign can be the oral expulsion of air or saliva as in a sigh or harsh expiration. After the mid-teenage years, the breathing irregularities may tend to diminish in frequency and intensity. Efforts to arrest or modify the periodic breathing have met with limited success [86]. Buspirone, magnesium citrate, and the opiate antagonist, naltrexone, have been of limited efficacy and nothing has been uniformly beneficial [87, 88]. The selective serotonin reuptake antagonist antianxiety medications, particularly escitalopram, have been effective although not in all girls.

When patterns of irregular breathing or snoring occur during sleep, a sleep study to assess the presence of obstructive apnea or other sleep-related abnormalities is warranted as these are not features typically noted by parents [89].

8.4. Gastrointestinal Function. As stated above, growth is a major issue in RTT. Nutrition is often a specific contributor to this problem. Therefore, we recommend utilization of a nutritionist to assist with this process. Previous studies have suggested that girls with RTT have increased calorie and protein requirements, but beyond that specific issues with chewing and swallowing, recurrent aspiration, prominent gastroesophageal reflux, abnormally slow gastric emptying, and constipation require additional strategies including high calorie liquid supplements and occasionally alternative feeding via gastrostomy tubes (G-tubes) [90–94]. That is, G-tubes may be required to provide sufficient daily caloric intake, to supplement appropriate amounts of fluids, or in the case of recurrent aspiration, to by-pass oral feedings altogether to protect the health of the child. Periodic breathing and aerophagia may also be so prominent as to affect the maintenance of adequate oral intake adversely. In the US Natural History study, about 30% of girls with RTT have required gastrostomy tube placement for preservation of nutrition, adequate fluid intake, or protection of the airway [94].

Gastroesophageal reflux (GERD) is extremely common in RTT. In some instances this may lead to esophagitis, but more commonly, recurrent GERD is so significant to produce unexplained irritability or apparent distress. In these instances, it is essential to refer to a gastroenterologist for evaluation and treatment as indicated. Proton-pump inhibitors have been the most effective medication for GERD, although H2-blockers may provide temporary benefit. One

should also be alert to the possibility of *H. pylori* infection. Delayed gastric emptying has also been noted in which case bethanechol or erythromycin has proven efficacious. Marked caution should be observed with implementation of metoclopramide as the occurrence of profound movement disorders represents a potentially serious adverse consequence.

Constipation occurs virtually uniformly in RTT [93]. This relates to the general issue of poor GI function in this disorder and may also result from the tendency for these girls to have poor fluid intake. While multiple strategies including the use of high-fibre foods, enemas, mineral oil, and milk of magnesia have been employed, success has been quite variable. In addition, these strategies may be associated with adverse consequences such as the reliance on enemas leading to dependency on this treatment plan or the interference of mineral oil with proper absorption of the fat-soluble vitamins. In addition, many girls resist even flavored milk of magnesia. Miralax (polyethylene glycol) can be quite effective provided that it is given with adequate fluid volumes as it is tasteless and odorless and may be dissolved in juice. The presence of a G-tube will greatly facilitate its use as well as that of milk of magnesia.

Gallbladder dysfunction has been recognized relatively recently, although the frequency of ~3% is relatively low. It may cause marked agitation and discomfort and has been identified as early as age of 2 years. Assessment by abdominal ultrasound may reveal gallstones, but more commonly the HIDA scan is required to substantiate significant dysfunction with an ejection fraction less than 35–40%. At this point, cholecystectomy should be considered.

8.5. Growth. Growth failure in RTT is pervasive, first noted as early as 1-2 months of age with progressive, abnormal deceleration in the rate of head growth, the median head circumference approaching the second percentile for the normal population by age of 1.5 to 2 years [49]. This is followed by a decline in weight near the end of the first year of life, the median value falling below the 2nd percentile for the normal population between age of 12 and 13 years. Decline in height or length is then noted around 15 months of age, the median values declining to the 2nd percentile for the normal population around age of 12 years. Already in early childhood and continuing into adolescence, acquisition of weight gain is problematic for girls with RTT. Following menstruation weight tends to increase abnormally representing a major shift in concern for mobility and ease of transfer. Therefore, attention is required to maintain acceptable weight gain throughout childhood, during adolescence, and beyond. Similar declines in hand and foot growth are also evident, with the feet ultimately more affected than the hands. The reduction in rate of foot growth appears to parallel that of height. Growth of the hands tends to be more preserved.

8.6. Scoliosis. Scoliosis in RTT demonstrates a profound increase with age [95–101]. It is typically evident by age of 4 when it is noted in ~8% of preschoolers. By age of 16, more than 80% of girls will have some degree of scoliosis. Onset may occur as late as age of 8. Progression of the scoliosis thereafter may be of sufficient clinical significance to warrant medical or surgical attention. Progression is generally evident through the primary school years and is much more likely to be noted in girls who are nonambulatory and spend most of the day in a seating device. It is essential that positioning is optimal to minimize progression. Bracing should be considered when the curvature (Cobb angle) exceeds 25°, if not before. When the curvature exceeds 40°, surgery is strongly recommended. In the US Natural History study, surgical instrumentation was provided in 13% of girls with definite improvement in their quality of life [102, 103].

8.7. Sleep. Abnormal sleep hygiene, that is, difficulty both with falling asleep and maintaining sleep, is very common in RTT. First, it is critical to rule out medical issues that could impact sleep including GERD, constipation, urinary tract infection, or even a missed bone fracture before considering medical management of sleep. Adequate sleep hygiene is critical for the entire family such that proper attention should be placed on both associated medical issues and sleep itself. An overnight sleep study may be helpful in identifying the specific features. Melatonin will aid sleep onset in some, although its effectiveness in maintaining sleep may be questioned. Antihistamines may be transiently effective but may lose their efficacy over time, so-called tachyphylaxis. Trazodone and clonidine are generally quite effective. Chloral hydrate has long been known to be an effective sedative, but its strong taste may make it undesirable unless it can be satisfactorily compounded. However, if a G-tube is present, it can be regarded as a suitable alternative.

8.8. Ambulation. As noted previously, 80% of girls with RTT are able to walk independently. However, 30% will lose this ability during or after the period of regression such that about 50% of girls overall remain ambulatory. Anxiety is a major problem in many aspects of RTT and will certainly lessen security in maintaining independent gait or even in navigating changes in floor coverings or uneven terrain. With assistance, in some only minor degrees of support, in others significant assistance, another 20% continue to be able to walk. Whether independent or assisted, ambulation should be encouraged as much and as long as possible. For those who do not walk, weight-bearing should be an essential part of therapy, either standing frames or gait-trainers and at least twice daily. In addition to providing effective therapy, this should assist the management of bone undermineralization. In this regard, the utilization of recommended amounts of calcium and vitamin D and the periodic assessment of vitamin D levels are essential elements for optimizing bone health.

8.9. Self-Abuse. Self-abusive behavior in the form of hair pulling, biting the fingers, hands, or other parts of the upper extremities, and head banging may be noted occasionally. Further, aggressive behavior towards others may be seen such as hitting, biting, or hair pulling. While the tendency may be to provide medication for this, medical issues such as underlying infections, gastrointestinal dysfunction (GERD,

constipation, or gallbladder dysfunction) as noted above, bone fractures, or the side effect of a medication already in use should first be considered. If such problems are excluded, these behaviors may be reduced by low dose risperidone (0.5 mg BID) or by an SSRI such as escitalopram. Behavioral management may also be considered as these girls do respond to specific modification techniques.

8.10. Quality of Life. As assessed by the Child Health Questionnaire Parent form (CHQ-PF50) in the US Natural History study, quality of life (QOL) in RTT syndrome revealed that individuals with lower motor abilities had less behavioral problems but that individuals with more preserved motor functions had greater behavioral issues [104]. These included aggressive behaviors toward others and a greater risk of potentially dangerous activities such as touching a hot pan or stove, climbing on furniture, or even wandering outside the home. As we are engaged in clinical trials, the idea of improving motor abilities while leading to functional concerns is a matter requiring vigilance.

8.11. Longevity. Previous reports had suggested markedly reduced survival in RTT [105]. However, more recent information indicates that survival into adulthood is more likely. A systematic study in the US revealed that survival was normal up to age of 10 and that median survival exceeded age of 50 years [106]. More recently, this was substantiated by review of data from the US Natural History study. These data not only represent critical information for parents and other caregivers about long-term care but also represent an important issue for the public health authorities. In the USA, the parents continue to provide care for most individuals with RTT. However, contingency plans involving a complex set of issues are required for the future when this is no longer possible.

8.12. Other Associated Features. Hypertonia and progressive dystonia, cardiac conduction QTc interval prolongation [107, 108], bruxism (teeth grinding), and vasomotor disturbances of feet and hands, the former more so than the latter, can be major concerns.

Muscle tone is generally reduced in infancy and early childhood, but this gradually increases with time leading to hypertonia and increased rigidity by teenage years or beyond. Dystonic posturing, particularly in the feet, but also occurring occasionally in the hands and the axial skeleton, is also prominent. These factors represent major therapeutic challenges for physical medicine and orthopedics. In addition, contractures in the lower extremities for those who are nonambulatory and spend most of the day seated or even at the elbows related to the constant midline hand stereotypies are often problematic. Orthotic devices are generally effective in maintaining neutral positions of the distal extremities, but the use of botulin toxin injections may be required.

Already in the early 1990s, prolongation of the QTc interval and an increase in nonspecific T-wave abnormalities were found in girls with RTT compared to healthy age-matched girls. These findings appeared to worsen with increasing age. Examination of QTc intervals in the US Natural History Study revealed that nearly 20% of girls had prolongation beyond 450 msec [107]. Although most remained asymptomatic and were not treated specifically, a few girls had marked prolongation necessitating medical management, generally with β-blockers and at least one young woman received a pacemaker. Animal model studies have suggested that treatment should involve a sodium channel blocking agent rather than the utilization of a β-blocker [107].

Bruxism tends to be the most prominent during early childhood and less problematic over time. Attempts to modify this often harsh sound have not been overly helpful. Vasomotor disturbances producing cold feet and hands appear to be associated with exaggerated sympathetic tone. Again, effective treatment is elusive.

9. Neuropathology

In keeping with the abnormal deceleration in head growth, the main neuropathologic features on gross inspection are reduced brain weight and reduced volume of frontal and temporal cortex [109–121]. Volumetric MRI confirmed reduction in cortical volume as well as noting reduction in deep gray nuclei [122]. On microscopic assessment, neurons are small and closer together (increased packing density), dendritic arborizations were reduced, and melanin deposition is markedly diminished or absent in the substantia nigra [117]. Remarkably, no evidence of any recognizable disease process is evident. The absence of any progressive neuropathologic features, namely, any evidence of neuronal loss or extensive gliosis, suggests that the fundamental neurobiologic problem in RTT is neurodevelopmental and not neurodegenerative. The brain does appear normal but is generally about 60–70% of expected weight for age. Golgi studies were highly informative revealing shortened and primitive dendritic arborizations supporting the notion of a failure in the proper development and maintenance of synaptic connections. In subsequent animal model studies, similar features were noted, namely, small neurons and deficient dendrites and dendritic spines. Although the fundamental cause is quite different, similar neuropathologic features have been observed in other neurodevelopmental disorders. Dendritic spines are deficient already by 4 months of age in Down syndrome and in Angelman syndrome. Increased packing density and decreased cell size have been noted in autistic spectrum disorder [123].

10. Genetic Basis of Rett Syndrome

As a genetic disorder predominantly affecting females with a different and generally much more aggressive phenotype in some males or even fetal demise, RTT is established definitively as an X-linked dominant disorder. It typically occurs sporadically as a *de novo* mutation in germinal cells. As a majority of individuals with RTT arise from the paternal cell line mutations, these mutations appear to occur predominantly in the more rapidly developing germinal cells, namely, the sperm. Recurrences within families are much less than 1%. Despite this observation, parents desiring additional children should obtain specific information from a genetic counselor and may wish to assess the carrier status of the mother by testing for the same mutation in her peripheral blood. Although a germline mutation is considered unlikely, such testing in either the mother or fathers blood would not exclude its presence. In fact, one instance of recurrent germline mutation in a father has been reported as the result of sperm analysis [124].

Among participants in the US Natural History Study, 8 specific point mutations account for about 60% of the total and specific deletions and insertions account for another 15–18% of mutations. However, over 200 different mutations have been defined in *MECP2* in girls or women with RTT identified to-date worldwide such that numerous mutations occur in only one or a small number of individuals. In the US study, mutations in *MECP2* have been identified in >95% of females with classic RTT. Greater than 75% of females with atypical forms of RTT also have mutations. When considered as specific groups in classic RTT, R133C, R294X, R306C, and $3'$-truncations are associated with a milder phenotype and the remaining five common point mutations as well as large deletions are associated with more severe clinical involvement. These data suggest that specific phenotype-genotype correlations exist [125–129]. However, when considering the impact of a specific mutation in a given situation, two girls with exactly the same mutation may have a quite different clinical profile. Several factors are involved in this difference, the most important determinant being variability in X-chromosome inactivation (XCI). Skewing of XCI can lead to milder or more significant clinical involvement regardless of the specific mutation. However, XCI determined in blood may not represent the same distribution in other cell populations such that other factors should be considered. These include the distribution of the mutation in brain cells as it is unlikely to be uniform and may vary significantly both within a given individual and between different individuals. MeCP2 is known to regulate the transcription of other genes. These effects may vary between different individuals. Finally, the involvement of other unknown factors including environmental influences such as activity level, different therapeutic programs, and dietary patterns could also be important contributors to outcome.

The same factors are likely responsible for the broad spectrum of clinical phenotypes associated with *MECP2* mutations. This spectrum may range from completely normal females to autistic spectrum disorder and nonsyndromic mental retardation and may affect both females and males. Thus, *MECP2* mutations have a very broad clinical impact apart from RTT. Following the identification of *MECP2* mutations, subsequent evaluations revealed a quite different process that explained previous observations of chromosomal rearrangement associated with developmental delays and other features as described above Section 6. Inasmuch as the clinical picture differs substantially from RTT, identification of males with duplications represents a much smaller number to-date. However, the increased availability of genome-wide array studies will likely result in increased identification of this disorder.

In recent years, girls with mutations in three other genes have had phenotypes resembling atypical RTT. *CDKL5*, expressing cyclin-dependent kinase-like 5, is located on X-chromosome at Xp22. It has an as yet unknown function but does appear to be a target of MeCP2 transcriptional repression. It produces significant developmental delay and epilepsy in both females and males and some females have the early-onset seizure variant of RTT [130, 131]. *FOXG1*, expressing forkhead box G1, is located at 14q12 and is a transcriptional repressor involved in early embryonic to adult telencephalon function. It has been associated with the congenital or limited development variant of RTT [132, 133]. A more recent and very rare cause of the early onset seizure variant of RTT involves the *NTNG1* gene located on chromosome 1 [134]. *NTNG1* is important for axonal guidance and NMDA receptor function. An attempt to identify additional affected individuals was not fruitful.

11. Functions of MECP2

MECP2, located at Xq28, encodes methyl-CpG-binding protein 2 (MeCP2). *MECP2*, derived from four exons, is ubiquitous in mammalian cells and is highly expressed in brain. It functions principally in the nucleus where it is important in the regulation of gene transcription. The MeCp2 protein occurs as two isoforms, MeCP2_e1 and MeCP2_e2, with the former being more highly expressed in brain. MeCP2 contains two functional domains, the methyl-binding domain (amino acids 78–162) that binds to methylated CpGs in DNA and the transcriptional regulating domain (amino acids 207–311) that recruits other proteins to mediate transcription of other genes. In addition, a nuclear localization signal (amino acids 255–271) directs MeCP2 to the cell nucleus. In the human brain, MeCP2 has a characteristic ontogeny first appearing in the brainstem during the first trimester with a subsequent caudal-to-rostral progression of expression such that, by 35 weeks of gestation, the protein is evident in forebrain and by age of 10 the protein is distributed widely throughout both the forebrain and brainstem. This ontogenetic pattern fits well with the onset of the disorder. Prior to the third trimester, MeCP2 is scarcely present in the forebrain, explaining the absence of abnormality in neuronal proliferation and migration at the cortical level. As MeCP2 expression in forebrain increases more significantly at or after the end of the third trimester, the delay in onset of clinical expression of RTT is not surprising.

MeCP2 was initially felt to be a transcriptional repressor, but more recent findings indicate that it has both activating and repressing functions, actually with more genes being activated than repressed [135]. The precise number and identification of genes affected are not known at present. However, several genes are known to be impacted including *BDNF* [136], expressing brain derived neurotrophic factor, *CRH*, expressing corticotrophic releasing hormone [137], and *FYXD1*, expressing phospholemman [138]. Whether MeCP2 is involved in the transcriptional regulation of additional genes is critical to a complete understanding of its function. Initial emphasis was placed on the role of MeCP2 in normal

TABLE 5: Rett syndrome animal models of Rett syndrome.

Mouse model type	Genetic composition	Reference
Null mutation		
Tm1.1Bird	Exon 3-4 deletion	[139]
Tml1.1Jae	Exon 3 deletion	[140]
Tm1.Pplt	Methyl-binding domain deletion	[141]
2loxB *TH-Cre*	Dopaminergic/noradrenergic neurons	[142]
2loxB *PET1-Cre*	Serotonergic neurons	[143]
2loxJ *hGFAP-CreT2*	Astrocytes	[144]
Truncated mutation		
Tm1Hzo	Nucleotide 308 truncation	[145]
Human point mutation		
Tm1.1Coyle	R168X	[146]
Tm1.1Vnar	A140V	[147]
Tm1.1Hup	R168X	[148]
Tm1.1Joez	T158A	[149]
Tm1.1IRSF	R255X	Unpublished

neuronal function as the principal pathologic changes were noted in neurons, namely, small neurons with abnormalities in dendritic size and complexity, synaptic organization, and axonal arborization. However, the importance of MeCP2 in glial development has received recent attention. Among the important roles of glial cells, the astrocytic role for controlling extracellular glutamate levels appears to be critical.

12. Animal Models

With the identification of *MECP2* mutations being responsible for RTT, the development of animal models advanced dramatically [139]. Prior attempts, before the linkage with RTT, at creating a knockout model, that is, with an absent *Mecp2* gene, were regarded as difficult due to prenatal demise of the null animals. Later efforts proved more successful such that both knockout and knock-in models are now available [139, 150, 151]. Animal models are available that restrict *Mecp2* deletion to the forebrain [140], the hypothalamus [152], and to dopaminergic/noradrenergic neurons [142], serotonergic neurons [143], or astrocytes [144] (Table 5). A key National Institutes of Health consensus conference was held in 2011 resulting in the elaboration of a comprehensive summary of animal models and their clinical phenotypes and clear standards for the design of preclinical studies to include adequate sample size, proper outcome measures, statistical methodologies, reporting of both positive and negative results, and replication of results in multiple animal models with varying genetic backgrounds and in independent laboratories [150]. The goal is to improve on the rather poor overall performance in moving from translational studies in animal models of a number of human disorders to specific clinical trials. Several aspects of this require emphasis related to RTT. Much of the animal work has occurred in male mice as male siblings tend to be quite similar in onset and character of their disease expression. Secondly, these male mutants are considerably more mature at the onset of symptoms than the corresponding time of onset in humans. Further, female mice are generally several months older with considerable variation among siblings at onset of their symptomatology. Finally, while these male mice do have a characteristic phenotype, by definition, they do not represent the genetic mosaicism seen in RTT in humans. Thus, it is critical that evidence of effective therapies in males be validated carefully in the more appropriate female heterozygotes and with animals that represent different genetic backgrounds and express a variety of *Mecp2* mutations to be certain that effectiveness is evident in the more relevant female phenotype. It has been demonstrated clearly that specific features of RTT may vary with different genetic backgrounds both in the presence or absence of particular features and in the timing of their appearance. Such background effects were noted both with respect to the timing of the appearance of impaired social behavior, prepulse inhibition, and increases in weight and the overall occurrence of stress-related reduction in corticosterone levels [153]. In addition, female mice from at least two different backgrounds did not display the increase in anxiety typically noted in individuals with RTT [153].

Critical research models have explored the role of Mecp2 in specific cell populations. Thus, removal of *Mecp2* from tyrosine hydroxylase-expressing dopaminergic and noradrenergic neurons or tryptophan hydroxylase-expressing serotonergic neurons reduced the levels of their respective metabolites, homovanillic acid (HVA), or 5-hydroxyindole acetic acid (5-HIAA) [142]. This study recapitulated the very early findings in girls with RTT and provided additional evidence for such decreases from an expanded group of individuals with RTT, particularly associated with the R168X mutation. In the HVA deficient animals, abnormalities in motor activity were evident whereas abnormalities in motor learning, anxiety, social interaction, learning, and memory or in breathing function were not noted. This differed from observations in 5-HIAA deficient animals in which motor activity was not reduced whereas increased aggression was noted. In higher functioning individuals with RTT, aggressive behaviors toward parents and siblings, teachers, and classmates are common and often problematic. Interestingly, both of these animal models had a normal life span indicating that Mecp2 function in these cells did not appear essential for determining longevity.

In a related study of serotonin function in male *Mecp2* mutant mice, use of the serotonin reuptake inhibitor, citalopram, resulted in improved carbon dioxide chemosensitivity, suggesting that elevation of serotonin levels has a beneficial effect [154]. The number of animals tested was small and, unfortunately, did not include females. Nevertheless, replication of these results in appropriate numbers and with appropriate inclusion of both sexes is warranted.

In a similar cell-type specific study, *Mecp2* was removed from GABA (γ-aminobutyric acid) neurons resulting in the occurrence of specific features of RTT including stereotypic movements, motor difficulties, compulsive behaviors,

and severe breathing abnormalities [143]. When the *Mecp2* removal was limited to forebrain nuclei, the RTT behaviors were preserved, but the abnormalities in breathing were absent, supporting the role of brainstem nuclei as critical for this particular feature of RTT. In addition, this model provided support for the notion of excitatory-inhibitory imbalance in RTT, particularly related to the concept of glutamate hyperexcitability.

More recently, a novel approach to *Mecp2* mutant mice involved the creation of a mutagenesis suppressor screen [155]. One of the five suppressors that resulted produced a stop-codon in the rate limiting enzyme for cholesterol biosynthesis, squalene epoxidase, and this suppressor resulted in a reduction of symptoms in the *Mecp2* mutant animals. Examining cholesterol metabolites in nonsuppressed mutant mice revealed significant abnormalities that were reversed in part along with motor performance abnormalities by the statin drugs, fluvastatin, and lovastatin in male animals and fluvastatin in female animals. This finding was prominent in a mouse strain that is obese and needs to be repeated in other strains as well to allay this concern.

13. Translational Research

The impetus for translational studies in RTT rests in part on the pivotal findings of reversing the abnormality in the null mutant model. Utilizing clever genetic engineering, null mice were produced that contained the *Mecp2* gene lying dormant under the control of the estrogen receptor [156]. At different time points, both male and female mutant animals were treated with the estrogen analogue, tamoxifen. Regardless of the level of disease expression in these animals, the tamoxifen-produced activation of the *Mecp2* resulted in remarkable improvement. Consideration has long been given to the necessity for early diagnosis to allow for earlier implementation of treatment. These findings underscored the notion that RTT represents a neurodevelopmental and not a neurodegenerative disorder and provided proof of principle that if effective therapies could be developed, they could be beneficial. Moreover, this study suggested that treatment could be effective even if implemented later in the course of the disease process. Thus, the long-term goal in RTT research continues to be identification and testing appropriate agents for therapeutic trials in animals or cell-based systems as a prelude to the necessary clinical trials in individuals with RTT. These therapeutic options are outlined in Table 6 and include restoration of the activity of mutant MeCP2, a variety of different symptomatic therapies, and gene replacement strategies. These approaches are already being assessed as described in the following paragraphs. However, additional points should be made. Attempts should be made to target the missense mutations in order to reactivate the full-length protein and with the effective promotion of full-length proteins in nonsense mutations to secondarily reactivate these as well. In total, that would deal effectively with about 70% of participants with known mutations in *MECP2*. Strategies for correcting deletion and insertion truncating mutations are more complicated to resolve in this manner.

TABLE 6: Rett Syndrome (therapeutic options).

MeCP2 restoration
Missense mutations: reactivate full-length protein
Nonsense (stop) mutations: promote full-length protein; may require "reactivation"
Deletions/insertions: more complicated

Symptomatic therapy
Serotonin reuptake inhibitors: ameliorate anxiety
NMDA receptor blocker: memantine reverse glutamate hyperexcitability
IGF-1: full length and tri-peptide downstream effect in BDNF cascade
BDNF-mimetics: TrkB agonists restore BDNF levels
Read-through compounds: stop mutations produce full length MeCP2

Gene therapy
Gene correction correct only abnormal allele
Stem cell transplant
X chromosome activation of normal allele activate normal allele in all cells

Symptomatic therapies are being addressed as described below. Gene therapy through provision of a normal gene or stem cell transplantation has been attempted. Theoretically, X chromosome activation of the normal allele is feasible but requires that all cells be activated to the normal allele.

While the principal research themes to-date have targeted neurons virtually exclusively, recent efforts have been extended to glia, providing yet another series of important and provocative observations. While RTT had long been considered to represent a disorder of neuronal function, very early studies had actually provided strong support for the role of MeCP2 in glia. Through the use of immunofluorescence and laser scanning cytometry, it was noted that both oligodendroglia and astrocytes express MeCP2 [157]. Certainly, the predominance of behaviors related to neuronal dysfunction was the subject of intense investigation and likely led to an active search regarding the role of neuronal cells in the disease process. However, with the notion that neuronal-glial interactions are critical, more recent attention has been directed to the glial cell population, recognizing that important pathological consequence could arise from glial dysfunction as well. Using an *in vitro* coculture system, *Mecp2* mutant astrocytes produced deleterious effects on dendritic morphology in both mutant and wild-type hippocampal neurons providing evidence for the lack of cell autonomous effects [158]. The authors suggested that these effects represented abnormalities in secretion of soluble factors. Subsequently, work from the same laboratory demonstrated that reexpression of *Mecp2* in astrocytes alone was sufficient to improve motor activity, anxiety, breathing pattern, and survival in null mutant mice and to reverse dendritic abnormalities in neurons from these animals [144]. Thus, unlike the cell autonomous effects noted with neuronal models, the impact

of altered Mecp2 function in astrocytes is clearly noncell autonomous. Not considered in this model were the potential adverse effects of excess glutamate on neuronal function. Astrocytes are known to represent an important sink for extracellular glutamate and inasmuch as both brain glutamate levels and NMDA-receptors are increased in young girls with RTT, it is likely that astrocytes, normally responsible for the clearance of extracellular glutamate, are unable to maintain normal expression of relevant proteins in the absence of normal Mecp2 [159–161]. As a result, abnormalities in control of extracellular glutamate levels adversely affect neurons in terms of synapse formation and dendritic morphology. These studies correlate well with evidence that hippocampal slices from *Mecp2* mutant mice are extremely hyperexcitable [162, 163]. While additional work is required to identify the factor or factors responsible for this abnormality in astrocytic function, it is tempting to suggest that a reduction in network hyperexcitability could be achieved by modulating glutamate levels or interfering with glutamate-related synaptic activity. In this regard, the NMDA receptor antagonist, memantine, is capable of restoring two components of short-term plasticity, posttetanic potentiation, and paired-pulse facilitation [164]. As such, the prospect of modulating glutamate levels deserves scrutiny in future preclinical trials.

BDNF (brain-derived neurotrophic factor) has also received significant attention in relation to RTT [136, 165]. BDNF expression is reduced both in autopsy-derived brain samples from individuals with RTT and in *Mecp2* mutant mice. Coupled with the finding that *Bdnf* levels were reduced in Mecp2 mutant mice, excitement has been raised regarding increasing BDNF levels in RTT. However, application of BDNF directly is limited by two factors, one being its short half-life, the other being that BDNF does not readily cross the blood-brain barrier. Thus, preclinical studies have focused on the activation of endogenous BDNF or the application of compounds that are capable of mimicking BDNF. It is known that, when *Bdnf* is overexpressed in *Mecp2* mutant mice or in neurons transfected with relevant RTT *MECP2* mutations, the behavioral phenotypes in animals and dendritic abnormalities in cultured primary neurons can be reversed [166, 167]. Similarly, application of the so-called nootropic AMPAkines, molecules known to increase BDNF expression, has reversed the synaptic impairments in the brainstem of *Mecp2* mutant models with abnormal breathing patterns [167–169]. Finally, the BDNF mimetic drugs have superior blood-brain barrier profiles and have been demonstrated to modulate function in *Mecp2* mutant models. Molecules that act like BDNF, termed "BDNF mimetics," have the capability to pass through the blood-brain barrier and bind to the TrkB receptor. The TrkB agonists, LM22A-4 and 7,8-DHF, are two agents that appear capable of reversing features of RTT in these animal models [170, 171].

Operating within the same pathway as BDNF, a tripeptide of IGF-1 was noted to produce better motor performance, to increase dendritic spine density and motility, and to correct breathing dysfunction in *Mecp2* mutant mice [172]. In a separate study using induced pleuripotential stems cells reprogrammed from skin fibroblasts of individuals with RTT, full-length IGF-1 application resulted in an increase in synaptic development in neurons derived from this technique [173]. These results led directly to on-going clinical trials in RTT as described below.

A completely different approach has been taken directed at nonsense or so-called STOP mutations. It has been known for some time that the aminoglycosides, a class of potent antibiotics, are capable of reading through the premature STOP codon to achieve a protein of full-length. Although this protein will not have the correct amino acid composition, it is posited that the full-length protein will have greater functional capabilities than its mutant precursor. Knockout mutations occur in approximately 35% of girls with RTT in the US Natural History study such that this approach could target a significant number of affected participants. Animal studies utilizing *MECP2* nonsense mutations have shown promise when exposed to gentamycin as well as to small molecule compounds with similar read through properties [148, 174, 175]. The development of gentamycin analogues lacking the toxic side effects of gentamycin or the class of small molecules is crucial as gentamycin itself is associated with significant ototoxicity and renal toxicity when used chronically. Studies are ongoing to evaluate the effects of these compounds in mutant *Mecp2* animal models with knockout mutations. Similarly, studies using the induced pleuripotential stem cell-derived neurons from an individual with RTT carrying a nonsense mutation indicated that the aminoglycoside, gentamycin, increased levels of MeCP2 although this finding was not reproduced at a higher gentamycin dosage [173].

Efforts at hematopoietic stem cell transplantation (HSCT) have been revealing but not overall successful. Presymptomatic male and female mutant mice did appear to have improved survival and motor performance, but symptomatic males were not benefited and female symptomatic mice were not tested [176]. However, the studies suggested that microglia resulting from the HSCT did have improved function over endogenous microglia from the mutant mice suggesting that pharmacologic manipulation of microglial cells could be a therapeutic target [177]. Unfortunately, efforts to reproduce these findings have not been forthcoming. Furthermore the methodology utilized in HSCT is inherently problematic in and of itself.

Systemic delivery of intact Mecp2 to female *Mecp2* mutant mice using the adenoassociated virus as a vehicle resulted in improved survival and overall motor performance but did not appear to produce resolution of breathing dysfunction [178]. The gene replacement either did not reach critical brainstem nuclei or did not have a brainstem impact. The number of animals treated was small. Further, animals treated by direct cranial injection had only modest improvement and more concerning the appearance of parkinsonian features that were attributed to the scAAV9/cre virus utilized, independent of the Mecp2.

14. Treatment

14.1. Clinical Trials. Clinical trials have been relatively few in RTT. Naltrexone was employed in the premutation era in an effort to ameliorate breathing dysfunction. While the treatment group in this double-blind, placebo-controlled trial did appear to have a reduction in breathing abnormalities, this could not be distinguished from the sedating properties of the opiate antagonist. Further, stratification of participants did not yield balanced groups such that individuals in the treatment group actually progressed more rapidly than those in the control group.

Shortly after identification of *MECP2* mutations as the cause of RTT and with knowledge that one role of MeCP2 is to bind to methylated CpG nucleotides, a double-blind, placebo-controlled trial of folate and betaine was employed. No objective evidence of improvement was noted although some parents of participants in the treated group observed subjective improvement in overall behavior.

Active clinical trials currently involve the use of either IGF-1 (NCT01777542) or a tripeptide fragment of IGF-1 (NCT01703533). The mechanisms of action of the full length IGF-1 and the tripeptide are felt to differ. The full length compound is a 70-amino acid peptide that inserts itself downstream of BDNF at the IGF-1 receptor and activates the same Akt pathway. The tripeptide is only bound weakly to the IGF-1 receptor and has other actions that are independent of the full-length molecule. Based on studies in *Mecp2* mutant mice, the IGF-1 tripeptide was shown to penetrate the blood-brain barrier and to promote increased longevity and improved motor performance as well as improve neurite outgrowth and synaptogenesis. The full-length IGF-1 is approved for use in children with short stature and an IND was obtained to utilize this compound in RTT. Due to its effect on bone growth, IGF-1 is approved for use in RTT participants less than age of 11 years. As a subcutaneous injection, the phase 2 safety trial showed that the agent had no concerns in the RTT participants. An advanced phase 2 double-blind, placebo controlled, crossover design trial is now in progress (two 20-week assessments with an intervening 10-week washout period) with outcome information expected in about one year.

A separate phase 2 trial with the modified initial tripeptide of the IGF-1 molecule is also being conducted. Inasmuch as this tripeptide is being trialed in individuals age of 15–45 years with traumatic brain injury, significant safety data already exist allowing a similar 40-day double-blind, placebo-controlled safety trial to proceed in a two-phase dose escalation protocol. This agent is provided as an oral preparation. It is anticipated that this trial will be concluded before the end of 2104 and at that time additional approval will be received to test this agent in younger participants.

A double-blind, placebo-controlled trial with secondary crossover for both groups to active agent is on-going with the serotonin reuptake inhibitor, escitalopram, to evaluate its anxiolytic properties. This agent is approved for use in children at age of 12 years and older.

An additional trial involves the use of dextromethorphan (NCT01520363). It is a three-month double blind, placebo-controlled trial involving girls, age 2–10 years with classic or atypical RTT. Dextromethorphan is an NMDA receptor antagonist and the trial proposes to evaluate its efficacy in alleviating glutamate hyperexcitability. This phase 2 safety assessment will examine improvements in cognitive function.

14.2. Clinical Therapies. Current recommendations regarding on-going treatment for individuals with RTT include aggressive physical, occupational, and speech and appropriate interventions as required for nutrition and optimal growth, orthopedic concerns, proper assessment and management of epilepsy and GI dysfunction, and other issues as they become relevant. Despite the limitations in motor performance, physical and occupational strategies should be employed daily. The establishment of optimal communication is also essential. This should take advantage of the improved social interaction and eye contact which develop by school age and involve the application of the recently available computer technologies as best as possible. Optimal growth and nutrition are especially relevant by school age and beyond. An expert in nutrition is often necessary to maintain proper guidance. The principal orthopedic concerns relate to scoliosis and limitation of joint mobility. Scoliosis should be assessed regularly and bracing or surgical intervention with stabilizing rods should be implemented based on these assessments. The presence of epilepsy should be assessed accurately, including the use of video-EEG where necessary. While antiepileptic agents may be warranted, care should be used in selecting the proper agents, being mindful to observe the potential side-effects and to remove drugs that are not effective before adding a new agent. Great care should be taken to avoid multiple drugs that may be ineffective as a group. Inasmuch as GI issues play a major role in the general well-being of those with RTT, careful attention must be paid to all aspects.

As suggested above, long-term care and planning are crucial. Proper attention to other medical and dental issues is essential in view of the potential longevity of individuals with RTT. An ECG for prolongation of the QTc interval and gynecologic assessment should be performed annually. Inasmuch as adult physicians have little experience in dealing with RTT or other neurodevelopmental disorders for that matter, their education must be accelerated to allow for the proper provision of continuity of care.

The principal caregivers must also develop a long-term care plan. When individuals with RTT reach the age of majority, certificates of guardianship must be obtained by their responsible caregivers. As formal school options end, usually by age of 22, the treatment and social programs available during the prior 21 years will cease. It is essential that planning for satisfactory replacements is made well in advance in order to maintain a stable transition to an adult program. This is a major issue from both the public health and societal perspectives. Finally, in planning for the future, a blind trust is necessary in order for individuals with RTT to preserve their resources.

In summary, women with RTT may well survive into middle age. Parents and other caregivers may require guidance and assistance both to promote the well-being of individuals with RTT including socialization and interaction with family and friends and to address the specific issues involving health care and continuing therapies specific to RTT.

15. Future Perspectives

Understanding the complexities of *MECP2* mutations, the dysregulated genes that contribute to specific symptoms of RTT, and rational approaches to effective therapy represent the major challenges for the future. The effective management of RTT will depend on finding and implementing FDA-approved and repurposed agents and investigating novel compounds through continued research. While current emphasis is focused on addressing specific symptoms related to RTT, continued emphasis must be placed on treating the underlying cause in a manner to provide an effective and lasting cure. This will rely on promoting the interaction of both basic and clinical research through major efforts in translational research and the necessary and critical collaboration with pharmaceutical enterprises and regulatory agencies.

Conflict of Interests

The author declares that there is no conflict of interests regarding the publication of this paper.

Acknowledgment

The author recognizes with deep respect and admiration the many girls and women with RTT and their families and caregivers whose support over the past thirty years made this work possible. Support is provided by Grants from the International Rett Syndrome Foundation and from the NIH, including the Angelman, Rett, and Prader-Willi syndrome consortium (U54HD61222), a part of the National Institutes of Health (NIH) Rare Disease Clinical Research Network (RDCRN), supported through collaboration between the NIH Office of Rare Diseases Research (ORDR) at the National Center for Advancing Translational Science (NCATS) and the *Eunice Kennedy Shriver* Child Health and Human Development Institute. The content is solely the responsibility of the author and does not necessarily represent the official views of the National Institutes of Health.

References

[1] A. Rett, "Uber ein eigenartiges hirnatrophisches Syndrom bei Hyperammonamie im Kindesalter," *Wiener Medizinische Wochenschrift*, vol. 116, pp. 723–726, 1966.

[2] A. Rett, *Uber ein cerebral-atrophisches Syndrom bei Hyperammonaemie*, Bruder Hollinek, Wien, Germany, 1966.

[3] A. Rett, "Cerebral atrophy associated with hyperammonemia," in *Handbook of Clinical Neurology*, P. J. Vincken and G. W. Bruyn, Eds., pp. 305–329, North-Holland Publishing, Amsterdam, The Netherlands, 1977.

[4] B. Hagberg, J. Aicardi, K. Dias, and O. Ramos, "A progressive syndrome of autism, dementia, ataxia, and loss of purposeful hand use in girls: Rett's syndrome. Report of 35 cases," *Annals of Neurology*, vol. 14, no. 4, pp. 471–479, 1983.

[5] A. Rett, "Rett syndrome: history and general overview," *American Journal of Medical Genetics*, vol. 24, no. 1, pp. 21–25, 1986.

[6] A. K. Percy, H. Zoghbi, and V. M. Riccardi, "Rett syndrome: initial experience with an emerging clinical entity," *Brain and Development*, vol. 7, no. 3, pp. 300–304, 1985.

[7] B. Hagberg, F. Goutieres, and F. Hanefeld, "Rett syndrome: criteria for inclusion and exclusion," *Brain and Development*, vol. 7, no. 3, pp. 372–373, 1985.

[8] H. Y. Zoghbi, A. K. Percy, and D. G. Glaze, "Reduction of biogenic amine levels in the Rett syndrome," *The New England Journal of Medicine*, vol. 313, no. 15, pp. 921–924, 1985.

[9] A. Lekman, I. Witt-Engerstrom, J. Gottfries, B. A. Hagberg, A. K. Percy, and L. Svennerholm, "Rett syndrome: biogenic amines and metabolites in postmortem brain," *Pediatric Neurology*, vol. 5, no. 6, pp. 357–362, 1989.

[10] C. A. Kozinetz, M. L. Skender, N. MacNaughton et al., "Epidemiology of Rett syndrome: a population-based registry," *Pediatrics*, vol. 91, no. 2, pp. 445–450, 1993.

[11] D. F. Wong, J. C. Harris, S. Naidu et al., "Dopamine transporters are markedly reduced in Lesch-Nyhan disease in vivo," *Proceedings of the National Academy of Sciences of the United States of America*, vol. 93, no. 11, pp. 5539–5543, 1996.

[12] R. J. Schultz, D. G. Glaze, K. J. Motil et al., "The pattern of growth failure in Rett syndrome," *American Journal of Diseases of Children*, vol. 147, no. 6, pp. 633–637, 1993.

[13] R. Schultz, D. Glaze, K. Motil, D. Hebert, and A. Percy, "Hand and foot growth failure in Rett syndrome," *Journal of Child Neurology*, vol. 13, no. 2, pp. 71–74, 1998.

[14] D. G. Glaze, J. D. Frost Jr., H. Y. Zoghbi, and A. K. Percy, "Rett's syndrome. Correlation of electroencephalographic characteristics with clinical staging," *Archives of Neurology*, vol. 44, no. 10, pp. 1053–1056, 1987.

[15] D. G. Glaze, R. J. Schultz, and J. D. Frost, "Rett syndrome: characterization of seizures versus non-seizures," *Electroencephalography and Clinical Neurophysiology*, vol. 106, no. 1, pp. 79–83, 1998.

[16] I. Hagne, I. Witt-Engerstrom, and B. Hagberg, "EEG development in Rett syndrome. A study of 30 cases," *Electroencephalography and Clinical Neurophysiology*, vol. 72, no. 1, pp. 1–6, 1989.

[17] E. Niedermeyer and S. Naidu, "Further EEG observations in children with the Rett syndrome," *Brain and Development*, vol. 12, no. 1, pp. 53–54, 1990.

[18] E. Niedermeyer, A. Rett, and H. Renner, "Rett syndrome and the electroencephalogram," *American Journal of Medical Genetics*, vol. 24, supplement 1, pp. 195–199, 1986.

[19] E. Lugaresi, F. Cirignotta, and P. Montagna, "Abnormal breathing in the Rett syndrome," *Brain and Development*, vol. 7, no. 3, pp. 329–333, 1985.

[20] D. Glaze, J. Frost, R. Schultz, and A. Percy, "Effect of naloxone on breathing, hand movements, electroencephalogram during wakefulness in patients in rett syndrome," *Annals of Neurology*, vol. 26, article 486, 1989.

[21] D. G. Glaze, J. D. Frost, H. Y. Zoghbi, and A. K. Percy, "Rett's syndrome: characterization of respiratory patterns and sleep," *Annals of Neurology*, vol. 21, no. 4, pp. 377–382, 1987.

[22] C. L. Laurvick, N. de Klerk, C. Bower et al., "Rett syndrome in Australia: a review of the epidemiology," *Journal of Pediatrics*, vol. 148, no. 3, pp. 347–352, 2006.

[23] B. Hagberg and P. Rasmussen, "'Forme fruste' of Rett syndrome. A case report," *American Journal of Medical Genetics*, vol. 24, supplement 1, pp. 175–181, 1986.

[24] B. A. Hagberg and O. H. Skjeldal, "Rett variants: a suggested model for inclusion criteria," *Pediatric Neurology*, vol. 11, no. 1, pp. 5–11, 1994.

[25] M. Zappella, "The Rett girls with preserved speech," *Brain and Development*, vol. 14, no. 2, pp. 98–101, 1992.

[26] O. H. Skjeldal, S. von Tetzchner, K. Jacobsen, L. Smith, and A. Heiberg, "Rett syndrome—distribution of phenotypes with special attention to the preserved speech variant," *Neuropediatrics*, vol. 26, no. 2, p. 87, 1995.

[27] F. Hanefeld, B. Hagberg, and A. Percy, "Molecular and neurobiology aspects of Rett syndrome," *Neuropediatrics*, vol. 26, no. 2, pp. 60–61, 1995.

[28] H. Y. Zoghbi, A. K. Percy, R. J. Schultz, and C. Fill, "Patterns of X chromosome inactivation in the Rett syndrome," *Brain and Development*, vol. 12, no. 1, pp. 131–135, 1990.

[29] H. Y. Zoghbi, D. H. Ledbetter, R. Schultz, A. K. Percy, and D. G. Glaze, "A de novo X;3 translocation in Rett syndrome," *American Journal of Medical Genetics*, vol. 35, no. 1, pp. 148–151, 1990.

[30] N. C. Schanen, E. J. R. Dahle, F. Capozzoli, V. A. Holm, H. Y. Zoghbi, and U. Francke, "A new Rett syndrome family consistent with X-linked inheritance expands the X chromosome exclusion map," *American Journal of Human Genetics*, vol. 61, no. 3, pp. 634–641, 1997.

[31] C. Schanen, "A severely affected male born into a Rett syndrome kindred supports X-linked inheritance and allows extension of the exclusion map," *American Journal of Human Genetics*, vol. 63, no. 1, pp. 267–269, 1998.

[32] N. C. Schanen, "Molecular approaches to the Rett syndrome gene," *Journal of Child Neurology*, vol. 14, no. 12, pp. 806–814, 1999.

[33] N. Sirianni, S. Naidu, J. Pereira, R. F. Pillotto, and E. P. Hoffman, "Rett syndrome: confirmation of X-linked dominant inheritance, and localization of the gene to Xq28," *American Journal of Human Genetics*, vol. 63, no. 5, pp. 1552–1558, 1998.

[34] K. A. Ellison, C. P. Fill, J. Terwilliger et al., "Examination of X chromosome markers in Rett syndrome: exclusion mapping with a novel variation on multilocus linkage analysis," *American Journal of Human Genetics*, vol. 50, no. 2, pp. 278–287, 1992.

[35] K. A. Ellison, E. J. Roth, E. R. B. McCabe, A. C. Chinault, and H. Y. Zoghbi, "Isolation of a yeast artificial chromosome contig spanning the X chromosomal translocation breakpoint in a patient with Rett syndrome," *American Journal of Medical Genetics*, vol. 47, no. 7, pp. 1124–1134, 1993.

[36] R. E. Amir, I. B. van den Veyver, M. Wan, C. Q. Tran, U. Francke, and H. Y. Zoghbi, "Rett syndrome is caused by mutations in X-linked *MECP2*, encoding methyl-CpG-binding protein 2," *Nature Genetics*, vol. 23, no. 2, pp. 185–188, 1999.

[37] B. R. Migeon, M. A. Dunn, G. Thomas, B. J. Schmeckpeper, and S. Naidu, "Studies of X inactivation and isodisomy in twins provide further evidence that the X chromosome is not involved in Rett syndrome," *American Journal of Human Genetics*, vol. 56, no. 3, pp. 647–653, 1995.

[38] N. Sirianni, S. Naidu, J. Pereira, R. F. Pillotto, and E. P. Hoffman, "Rett syndrome: confirmation of X-linked dominant inheritance, and localization of the gene to Xq28," *American Journal of Human Genetics*, vol. 63, no. 5, pp. 1552–1558, 1998.

[39] B. Hendrich and A. Bird, "Identification and characterization of a family of mammalian methyl-CpG binding proteins," *Molecular and Cellular Biology*, vol. 18, no. 11, pp. 6538–6547, 1998.

[40] J. Christodoulou, A. Grimm, T. Maher, and B. Bennetts, "RettBASE: the IRSA *MECP2* variation database—a new mutation database in evolution," *Human Mutation*, vol. 21, no. 5, pp. 466–472, 2003.

[41] M. J. Friez, J. R. Jones, K. Clarkson et al., "Recurrent infections, hypotonia, and mental retardation caused by duplication of *MECP2* and adjacent region in Xq28," *Pediatrics*, vol. 118, no. 6, pp. e1687–e1695, 2006.

[42] A. K. Percy, "Rett syndrome: recent research progress," *Journal of Child Neurology*, vol. 23, no. 5, pp. 543–549, 2008.

[43] A. K. Percy, "Rett syndrome: from recognition to diagnosis to intervention," *Expert Review of Endocrinology and Metabolism*, vol. 3, no. 3, pp. 327–336, 2008.

[44] E. Trevathan and H. W. Moser, "Diagnostic criteria for Rett syndrome," *Annals of Neurology*, vol. 23, no. 4, pp. 425–428, 1988.

[45] B. Hagberg, F. Hanefeld, A. Percy, and O. Skjeldal, "An update on clinically applicable diagnostic criteria in Rett syndrome: comments to Rett syndrome clinical criteria consensus panel satellite to European Paediatric Neurology Society Meeting Baden Baden, Germany, 11 September 2001," *European Journal of Paediatric Neurology*, vol. 6, no. 5, pp. 293–297, 2002.

[46] J. L. Neul, W. E. Kaufmann, D. G. Glaze et al., "Rett syndrome: revised diagnostic criteria and nomenclature," *Annals of Neurology*, vol. 68, no. 6, pp. 944–950, 2010.

[47] A. K. Percy, J. L. Neul, D. G. Glaze et al., "Rett syndrome diagnostic criteria: lessons from the Natural History study," *Annals of Neurology*, vol. 68, no. 6, pp. 951–955, 2010.

[48] G. Hagberg, Y. Stenbom, and I. Witt Engerström, "Head growth in Rett syndrome," *Acta Paediatrica, International Journal of Paediatrics*, vol. 89, no. 2, pp. 198–202, 2000.

[49] D. C. Tarquinio, K. J. Motil, W. Hou et al., "Growth failure and outcome in Rett syndrome: specific growth references," *Neurology*, vol. 79, no. 16, pp. 1653–1661, 2012.

[50] C. Philippe, L. Villard, N. de Roux et al., "Spectrum and distribution of *MECP2* mutations in 424 Rett syndrome patients: a molecular update," *European Journal of Medical Genetics*, vol. 49, no. 1, pp. 9–18, 2006.

[51] A. Quenard, S. Yilmaz, H. Fontaine et al., "eleterious mutations in exon 1 of *MECP2* in Rett syndrome," *European Journal of Medical Genetics*, vol. 49, no. 4, pp. 313–322, 2006.

[52] I. Kim, Y. Kim, B. Son et al., "Diagnostic mutational analysis of *MECP2* in Korean patients with Rett syndrome," *Experimental and Molecular Medicine*, vol. 38, no. 2, pp. 119–125, 2006.

[53] D. Zahorakova, R. Rosipal, J. Hadac et al., "Mutation analysis of the *MECP2* gene in patients of Slavic origin with Rett syndrome: novel mutations and polymorphisms," *Journal of Human Genetics*, vol. 52, no. 4, pp. 342–348, 2007.

[54] K. Sampieri, I. Meloni, E. Scala et al., "Italian Rett database and biobank," *Human Mutation*, vol. 28, no. 4, pp. 329–335, 2007.

[55] L. Abuhatzira, K. Makedonski, Y. P. Galil et al., "Splicing mutation associated with Rett syndrome and an experimental approach for genetic diagnosis," *Human Genetics*, vol. 118, no. 1, pp. 91–98, 2005.

[56] R. Khajuria, S. Sapra, M. Ghosh et al., "Rapid detection of deletions in hotspot C-terminal segment region of *MECP2* by routine PCR method: report of two classical Rett syndrome patients of Indian origin," *Genetic Testing and Molecular Biomarkers*, vol. 13, no. 2, pp. 277–280, 2009.

[57] M. Li, H. Pan, X. Bao, Y. Zhang, and X. Wu, "*MECP2* and CDKL5 gene mutation analysis in Chinese patients with Rett syndrome," *Journal of Human Genetics*, vol. 52, no. 1, pp. 38–47, 2007.

[58] K. A. Percy, B. J. Lane, J. Childers et al., "Rett syndrome: North American database," *Journal of Child Neurology*, vol. 22, no. 12, pp. 1338–1341, 2007.

[59] T. Bienvenu, L. Villard, N. de Roux et al., "Spectrum of *MECP2* mutations in Rett syndrome," *Genetic Testing*, vol. 6, no. 1, pp. 1–6, 2002.

[60] I. M. Buyse, P. Fang, K. T. Hoon, R. E. Amir, H. Y. Zoghbi, and B. B. Roa, "Diagnostic testing for Rett syndrome by DHPLC and direct sequencing analysis of the *MECP2* gene: identification of several novel mutations and polymorphisms," *American Journal of Human Genetics*, vol. 67, no. 6, pp. 1428–1436, 2000.

[61] V. Bourdon, C. Philippe, O. Labrune, D. Amsallem, C. Arnould, and P. Jonveaux, "A detailed analysis of the *MECP2* gene: prevalence of recurrent mutations and gross DNA rearrangements in Rett syndrome patients," *Human Genetics*, vol. 108, no. 1, pp. 43–50, 2001.

[62] R. C. Samaco, R. P. Nagarajan, D. Braunschweig, and J. M. LaSalle, "Multiple pathways regulate *MECP2* expression in normal brain development and exhibit defects in autism-spectrum disorders," *Human Molecular Genetics*, vol. 13, no. 6, pp. 629–639, 2004.

[63] A. Shibayama, E. H. Cook Jr., J. Feng et al., "*MECP2* structural and 3′-UTR variants in schizophrenia autism and other psychiatric diseases: a possible association with autism," *American Journal of Medical Genetics B: Neuropsychiatric Genetics*, vol. 128, no. 1, pp. 50–53, 2004.

[64] K. Augenstein, J. B. Lane, A. Horton, C. Schanen, and A. K. Percy, "Variable phenotypic expression of a *MECP2* mutation in a family," *Journal of Neurodevelopmental Disorders*, vol. 1, no. 4, article 313, 2009.

[65] J. S. Schwartzman, A. Bernardino, A. Nishimura, R. R. Gomes, and M. Zatz, "Rett syndrome in a boy with a 47,XXY karyotype confirmed by a rare mutation in the *MECP2* gene," *Neuropediatrics*, vol. 32, no. 3, pp. 162–164, 2001.

[66] J. S. Schwartzman, M. Zatz, L. dos Reis Vasquez et al., "Rett syndrome in a boy with a 47,XXY karyotype," *American Journal of Human Genetics*, vol. 64, no. 6, pp. 1781–1785, 1999.

[67] S. G. Vorsanova, Y. B. Yurov, V. Y. Ulas et al., "Cytogenetic and molecular-cytogenetic studies of Rett syndrome (RTT): a retrospective analysis of a Russian cohort of RTT patients (the investigation of 57 girls and three boys)," *Brain and Development*, vol. 23, supplement 1, pp. S196–S201, 2001.

[68] J. Clayton-Smith, P. Watson, S. Ramsden, and G. C. M. Black, "Somatic mutation in *MECP2* as a non-fatal neurodevelopmental disorder in males," *The Lancet*, vol. 356, no. 9232, pp. 830–832, 2000.

[69] L. Villard, "*MECP2* mutations in males," *Journal of Medical Genetics*, vol. 44, no. 7, pp. 417–423, 2007.

[70] P. Kankirawatana, H. Leonard, C. Ellaway et al., "Early progressive encephalopathy in boys and *MECP2* mutations," *Neurology*, vol. 67, no. 1, pp. 164–166, 2006.

[71] T. Ylisaukko-Oja, K. Rehnström, R. Vanhala et al., "*MECP2* mutation analysis in patients with mental retardation," *American Journal of Medical Genetics*, vol. 132, no. 2, pp. 121–124, 2005.

[72] D. Lugtenberg, A. P. M. de Brouwer, T. Kleefstra et al., "Chromosomal copy number changes in patients with non-syndromic X linked mental retardation detected by array CGH," *Journal of Medical Genetics*, vol. 43, no. 4, pp. 362–370, 2006.

[73] D. Lugtenberg, T. Kleefstra, A. R. Oudakker et al., "Structural variation in Xq28: *MECP2* duplications in 1% of patients with unexplained XLMR and in 2% of male patients with severe encephalopathy," *European Journal of Human Genetics*, vol. 17, no. 4, pp. 444–453, 2009.

[74] H. van Esch, M. Bauters, J. Ignatius et al., "Duplication of the *MECP2* region is a frequent cause of severe mental retardation and progressive neurological symptoms in males," *American Journal of Human Genetics*, vol. 77, no. 3, pp. 442–453, 2005.

[75] M. B. Ramocki, S. U. Peters, Y. J. Tavyev et al., "Autism and other neuropsychiatric symptoms are prevalent in individuals with *MECP2* duplication syndrome," *Annals of Neurology*, vol. 66, no. 6, pp. 771–782, 2009.

[76] M. B. Ramocki, Y. J. Tavyev, and S. U. Peters, "The *MECP2* duplication syndrome," *American Journal of Medical Genetics A*, vol. 152, no. 5, pp. 1079–1088, 2010.

[77] S. U. Peters, R. J. Hundley, A. K. Wilson et al., "The behavioral phenotype in *MECP2* duplication syndrome: a comparison with idiopathic autism," *Autism Research*, vol. 6, no. 1, pp. 42–50, 2013.

[78] B. Hagberg and I. Witt-Engerstrom, "Rett syndrome: a suggested staging system for describing impairment profile with increasing age towards adolescence," *American Journal of Medical Genetics*, vol. 24, supplement 1, pp. 47–59, 1986.

[79] C. A. Chapleau, J. Lane, J. Larrimore, W. Li, L. Pozzo-Miller, and A. Percy, "Recent progress in Rett syndrome and *MECP2* dysfunction: assessment of potwntial treatment options," *Future Neurology*, vol. 8, pp. 21–28, 2013.

[80] P. M. Baptista, M. T. Mercadante, E. C. Macedo, and J. S. Schwartzman, "Cognitive performance in Rett syndrome girls: a pilot study using eyetracking technology," *Journal of Intellectual Disability Research*, vol. 50, part 9, pp. 662–666, 2006.

[81] A. Djukic and M. V. McDermott, "Social preferences in Rett syndrome," *Pediatric Neurology*, vol. 46, no. 4, pp. 240–242, 2012.

[82] A. Djukic, M. V. McDermott, K. Mavrommatis, and C. L. Martins, "Rett syndrome: basic features of visual processing: a pilot study of eye-tracking," *Pediatric Neurology*, vol. 47, no. 1, pp. 25–29, 2012.

[83] D. G. Glaze, "Neurophysiology of Rett syndrome," *Mental Retardation and Developmental Disabilities Research Reviews*, vol. 8, no. 2, pp. 66–71, 2002.

[84] D. G. Glaze, "Neurophysiology of Rett syndrome," *Journal of Child Neurology*, vol. 20, no. 9, pp. 740–746, 2005.

[85] D. G. Glaze, A. K. Percy, S. Skinner et al., "Epilepsy and the natural history of Rett syndrome," *Neurology*, vol. 74, no. 11, pp. 909–912, 2010.

[86] E. E. J. Smeets, P. O. O. Julu, D. van Waardenburg et al., "Management of a severe forceful breather with Rett Syndrome using carbogen," *Brain and Development*, vol. 28, no. 10, pp. 625–632, 2006.

[87] A. K. Percy, "Clinical trials and treatment prospects," *Mental Retardation and Developmental Disabilities Research Reviews*, vol. 8, no. 2, pp. 106–111, 2002.

[88] A. K. Percy, D. G. Glaze, R. J. Schultz et al., "Rett syndrome: controlled study of an oral opiate antagonist, naltrexone," *Annals of Neurology*, vol. 35, no. 4, pp. 464–470, 1994.

[89] E. E. Hagebeuk, R. P. Bijlmer, J. H. Koelman, and B. T. Poll-The, "Respiratory disturbances in rett syndrome: don't forget to evaluate upper airway obstruction," *Journal of Child Neurology*, vol. 27, no. 7, pp. 888–892, 2012.

[90] K. J. Motil, R. J. Schultz, W. W. Wang, and D. G. Glaze, "Increased energy expenditure associated with repetitive involuntary movement does not contribute to growth failure in girls with Rett syndrome," *Journal of Pediatrics*, vol. 132, no. 2, pp. 228–233, 1998.

[91] K. J. Motil, R. Schultz, B. Brown, D. G. Glaze, and A. K. Percy, "Altered energy balance may account for growth failure in Rett syndrome," *Journal of Child Neurology*, vol. 9, no. 3, pp. 315–319, 1994.

[92] K. J. Motil, R. J. Schultz, K. Browning, L. Trautwein, and D. G. Glaze, "Oropharyngeal dysfunction and gastroesophageal dysmotility are present in girls and women with Rett syndrome," *Journal of Pediatric Gastroenterology and Nutrition*, vol. 29, no. 1, pp. 31–37, 1999.

[93] K. J. Motil, E. Caeg, J. O. Barrish et al., "Gastrointestinal and nutritional problems occur frequently throughout life in girls and women with rett syndrome," *Journal of Pediatric Gastroenterology and Nutrition*, vol. 55, no. 3, pp. 292–298, 2012.

[94] K. J. Motil, M. Morrissey, E. Caeg, J. O. Barrish, and D. G. Glaze, "Gastrostomy placement improves height and weight gain in girls with rett syndrome," *Journal of Pediatric Gastroenterology and Nutrition*, vol. 49, no. 2, pp. 237–242, 2009.

[95] G. S. Bassett and V. T. Tolo, "The incidence and natural history of scoliosis in Rett syndrome," *Developmental Medicine and Child Neurology*, vol. 32, no. 11, pp. 963–966, 1990.

[96] S. Ager, S. Fyfe, J. Christodoulou, P. Jacoby, L. Schmitt, and H. Leonard, "Predictors of scoliosis in Rett syndrome," *Journal of Child Neurology*, vol. 21, no. 9, pp. 809–813, 2006.

[97] E. Stokland, J. Lidstrom, and B. Hagberg, "Scoliosis in Rett Syndrome," in *Rett Syndrome—Clinical & Biological Aspects*, B. Hagberg, Ed., pp. 61–71, Mac Keith Press, London, UK, 1993.

[98] J. Lidstrom, E. Stokland, and B. Hagberg, "Scoliosis in Rett syndrome: clinical and biological aspects," *Spine*, vol. 19, no. 14, pp. 1632–1635, 1994.

[99] A. M. Kerr, P. Webb, R. J. Prescott, and Y. Milne, "Results of surgery for scoliosis in Rett syndrome," *Journal of Child Neurology*, vol. 18, no. 10, pp. 703–708, 2003.

[100] D. J. Harrison and P. J. Webb, "Scoliosis in the Rett syndrome: natural history and treatment," *Brain and Development*, vol. 12, no. 1, pp. 154–156, 1990.

[101] V. A. Holm and H. A. King, "Scoliosis in the Rett syndrome," *Brain and Development*, vol. 12, no. 1, pp. 151–153, 1990.

[102] A. K. Percy, H. Lee, J. L. Neul et al., "Profiling scoliosis in rett syndrome," *Pediatric Research*, vol. 67, no. 4, pp. 435–439, 2010.

[103] J. Downs, A. Bergman, P. Carter et al., "Guidelines for management of scoliosis in rett syndrome patients based on expert consensus and clinical evidence," *Spine*, vol. 34, no. 17, pp. E607–E617, 2009.

[104] J. B. Lane, H.-S. Lee, L. W. Smith et al., "Clinical severity and quality of life in children and adolescents with Rett syndrome," *Neurology*, vol. 77, no. 20, pp. 1812–1818, 2011.

[105] M. Freilinger, A. Bebbington, I. Lanator et al., "Survival with Rett syndrome: comparing Rett's original sample with data from the Australian Rett Syndrome Database," *Developmental Medicine and Child Neurology*, vol. 52, no. 10, pp. 962–965, 2010.

[106] R. S. Kirby, J. B. Lane, J. Childers et al., "Longevity in Rett Syndrome: analysis of the North American database," *Journal of Pediatrics*, vol. 156, no. 1, pp. 135–138, 2010.

[107] M. D. McCauley, T. Wang, E. Mike et al., "Rett syndrome: pathogenesis of lethal cardiac arrhythmias in *MECP2* mutant mice: implication for therapy in Rett syndrome," *Science Translational Medicine*, vol. 3, no. 113, Article ID 113ra125, 2011.

[108] E. A. Sekul, J. P. Moak, R. J. Schultz, D. G. Glaze, and A. K. Percy, "Electrocardiographic findings in Rett syndrome: an explanation for sudden death?" *Journal of Pediatrics*, vol. 125, no. 1, pp. 80–82, 1994.

[109] D. D. Armstrong, "Review of Rett syndrome," *Journal of Neuropathology and Experimental Neurology*, vol. 56, no. 8, pp. 843–849, 1997.

[110] D. Armstrong, "Recent developments in neuropathology—electron microscopy—brain pathology," *European Child and Adolescent Psychiatry*, vol. 6, supplement 1, pp. 69–70, 1997.

[111] D. Armstrong, J. K. Dunn, B. Antalffy, and R. Trivedi, "Selective dendritic alterations in the cortex of Rett syndrome," *Journal of Neuropathology and Experimental Neurology*, vol. 54, no. 2, pp. 195–201, 1995.

[112] D. D. Armstrong, "The neuropathology of the Rett syndrome," *Brain and Development*, vol. 14, supplement, pp. S89–S98, 1992.

[113] D. D. Armstrong, "The neuropathology of Rett syndrome—overview 1994," *Neuropediatrics*, vol. 26, no. 2, pp. 100–104, 1995.

[114] D. D. Armstrong, "Rett syndrome neuropathology review 2000," *Brain and Development*, vol. 23, supplement 1, pp. S72–S76, 2000.

[115] D. D. Armstrong, "Neuropathology of Rett syndrome," *Mental Retardation and Developmental Disabilities Research Reviews*, vol. 8, no. 2, pp. 72–76, 2002.

[116] D. D. Armstrong, "Neuropathology of Rett syndrome," *Journal of Child Neurology*, vol. 20, no. 9, pp. 747–753, 2005.

[117] D. D. Armstrong, K. Dunn, and B. Antalffy, "Decreased dendritic branching in frontal, motor and limbic cortex in Rett Syndrome compared with Trisomy 21," *Journal of Neuropathology and Experimental Neurology*, vol. 57, no. 11, pp. 1013–1017, 1998.

[118] K. Jellinger, D. Armstrong, H. Y. Zoghbi, and A. K. Percy, "Neuropathology of Rett syndrome," *Acta Neuropathologica*, vol. 76, no. 2, pp. 142–158, 1988.

[119] K. Jellinger and F. Seitelberger, "Neuropathology of Rett syndrome," *American Journal of Medical Genetics*, vol. 24, supplement 1, pp. 259–288, 1986.

[120] K. Jellinger, D. Armstrong, H. Zoghbi, and A. Percy, "The Rett Syndrome: an overview," in *Movement Disorders in Neurology and Neuropsychiatry*, A. B. Joseph and R. Young, Eds., pp. 667–678, Blackwell Scientific Publications, 1992.

[121] K. A. Jellinger, "Rett syndrome—an update: review," *Journal of Neural Transmission*, vol. 110, no. 6, pp. 681–701, 2003.

[122] A. L. Reiss, F. Faruque, S. Naidu et al., "Neuroanatomy of Rett syndrome: a volumetric imaging study," *Annals of Neurology*, vol. 34, no. 2, pp. 227–234, 1993.

[123] A. Percy, J. Dragich, and N. Schanen, "Rett Syndrome: clinical-molecular correlates," in *Genetics and Genomics of Neurobehavioral Disorders*, G. Fisch, Ed., pp. 391–418, Humana Press, Totowa, NJ, USA, 2003.

[124] J. C. Evans, H. L. Archer, S. D. Whatley, and A. Clarke, "Germline mosaicism for a *MECP2* mutation in a man with two Rett daughters," *Clinical Genetics*, vol. 70, no. 4, pp. 336–338, 2006.

[125] J. Dragich, I. Houwink-Manville, and C. Schanen, "Rett syndrome: a surprising result of mutation in *MECP2*," *Human Molecular Genetics*, vol. 9, no. 16, pp. 2365–2375, 2000.

[126] C. Schanen, E. J. F. Houwink, N. Dorrani et al., "Phenotypic manifestations of *MECP2* mutations in classical and atypical Rett Syndrome," *American Journal of Medical Genetics A*, vol. 126, no. 2, pp. 129–140, 2004.

[127] A. Bebbington, A. Anderson, D. Ravine et al., "Investigating genotype-phenotype relationships in Rett syndrome using an international data set," *Neurology*, vol. 70, no. 11, pp. 868–875, 2008.

[128] A. Bebbington, A. Percy, J. Christodoulou et al., "Updating the profile of C-terminal *MECP2* deletions in Rett syndrome," *Journal of Medical Genetics*, vol. 47, no. 4, pp. 242–248, 2010.

[129] J. L. Neul, P. Fang, J. Barrish et al., "Specific mutations in Methyl-CpG-Binding Protein 2 confer different severity in Rett syndrome," *Neurology*, vol. 70, no. 16, pp. 1313–1321, 2008.

[130] G. Pini, S. Bigoni, I. Engerström et al., "Variant of rett syndrome and CDKL5 gene: clinical and autonomic description of 10 cases," *Neuropediatrics*, vol. 43, no. 1, pp. 37–43, 2012.

[131] N. Rademacher, M. Hambrock, U. Fischer et al., "Identification of a novel CDKL5 exon and pathogenic mutations in patients with severe mental retardation, early-onset seizures and rett-like features," *Neurogenetics*, vol. 12, no. 2, pp. 165–167, 2011.

[132] F. Ariani, G. Hayek, D. Rondinella et al., "FOXG1 is responsible for the congenital variant of Rett Syndrome," *American Journal of Human Genetics*, vol. 83, no. 1, pp. 89–93, 2008.

[133] C. Philippe, D. Amsallem, C. Francannet et al., "Phenotypic variability in Rett syndrome associated with FOXG1 mutations in females," *Journal of Medical Genetics*, vol. 47, no. 1, pp. 59–65, 2010.

[134] H. L. Archer, J. C. Evans, D. S. Millar et al., "NTNG1 mutations are a rare cause of Rett syndrome," *American Journal of Medical Genetics A*, vol. 140, no. 7, pp. 691–694, 2006.

[135] M. Chahrour, Y. J. Sung, C. Shaw et al., "*MECP2*, a key contributor to neurological disease, activates and represses transcription," *Science*, vol. 320, no. 5880, pp. 1224–1229, 2008.

[136] W. Li, G. Calfa, J. Larimore, and L. Pozzo-Miller, "Activity-dependent BDNF release and TRPC signaling is impaired in hippocampal neurons of *MECP2* mutant mice," *Proceedings of the National Academy of Sciences of the United States of America*, vol. 109, no. 42, pp. 17087–17092, 2012.

[137] B. E. McGill, S. F. Bundle, M. B. Yaylaoglu, J. P. Carson, C. Thaller, and H. Y. Zoghbi, "Enhanced anxiety and stress-induced corticosterone release are associated with increased Crh expression in a mouse model of Rett syndrome," *Proceedings of the National Academy of Sciences of the United States of America*, vol. 103, no. 48, pp. 18267–18272, 2006.

[138] C. Garcia-Rudaz, V. Deng, V. Matagne et al., "FXYD1, a modulator of Na+, K+-ATPase activity, facilitates female sexual development by maintaining gonadotrophin-releasing hormone neuronal excitability," *Journal of Neuroendocrinology*, vol. 21, no. 2, pp. 108–122, 2009.

[139] J. Guy, B. Hendrich, M. Holmes, J. E. Martin, and A. Bird, "A mouse *MECP2*-null mutation causes neurological symptoms that mimic rett syndrome," *Nature Genetics*, vol. 27, no. 3, pp. 322–326, 2001.

[140] R. Z. Chen, S. Akbarian, M. Tudor, and R. Jaenisch, "Deficiency of methyl-CpG binding protein-2 in CNS neurons results in a Rett-like phenotype in mice," *Nature Genetics*, vol. 27, no. 3, pp. 327–331, 2001.

[141] G. J. Pelka, C. M. Watson, T. Radziewic et al., "*MECP2* deficiency is associated with learning and cognitive deficits and altered gene activity in the hippocampal region of mice," *Brain*, vol. 129, no. 4, pp. 887–898, 2006.

[142] R. C. Samaco, C. Mandel-Brehm, H. Chao et al., "Loss of *MECP2* in aminergic neurons causes cell-autonomous defects in neurotransmitter synthesis and specific behavioral abnormalities," *Proceedings of the National Academy of Sciences of the United States of America*, vol. 106, no. 51, pp. 21966–21971, 2009.

[143] H. Chao, H. Chen, R. C. Samaco et al., "Dysfunction in GABA signalling mediates autism-like stereotypies and Rett syndrome phenotypes," *Nature*, vol. 468, no. 7321, pp. 263–269, 2010.

[144] D. T. Lioy, S. K. Garg, C. E. Monaghan et al., "A role for glia in the progression of Rett-syndrome," *Nature*, vol. 475, no. 7357, pp. 497–500, 2011.

[145] M. D. Shahbazian, J. I. Young, L. A. Yuva-Paylor et al., "Mice with truncated *MECP2* recapitulate many Rett syndrome features and display hyperacetylation of histone H3," *Neuron*, vol. 35, no. 2, pp. 243–254, 2002.

[146] A. Lawson-Yuen, D. Liu, L. Han et al., "Ube3a mRNA and protein expression are not decreased in *MECP2*R168X mutant mice," *Brain Research*, vol. 1180, no. 1, pp. 1–6, 2007.

[147] G. M. Jentarra, S. L. Olfers, S. G. Rice et al., "Abnormalities of cell packing density and dendritic complexity in the *MECP2* A140V mouse model of Rett syndrome/X-linked mental retardation," *BMC Neuroscience*, vol. 11, article 19, 2010.

[148] C. Brendel, V. Belakhov, H. Werner et al., "Readthrough of nonsense mutations in Rett syndrome: evaluation of novel aminoglycosides and generation of a new mouse model," *Journal of Molecular Medicine*, vol. 89, no. 4, pp. 389–398, 2011.

[149] D. Goffin, M. Allen, L. Zhang et al., "Rett syndrome mutation *MECP2* T158A disrupts DNA binding, protein stability and ERP responses," *Nature Neuroscience*, vol. 15, no. 2, pp. 274–283, 2012.

[150] D. M. Katz, J. E. Berger-Sweeney, J. H. Eubanks et al., "Preclinical research in Rett syndrome: setting the foundation for translational success," *Disease Models and Mechanisms*, vol. 5, no. 6, pp. 733–745, 2012.

[151] W. Li and L. Pozzo-Miller, "Beyond widespread *MECP2* deletions to model Rett syndrome: conditional spatio-temporal knockout, single-point mutations and transgenic rescue mice," *Autism*, supplement 1, pp. 1–10, 2012.

[152] S. L. Fyffe, J. L. Neul, R. C. Samaco et al., "Deletion of *MECP2* in Sim1-expressing neurons reveals a critical role for *MECP2* in feeding behavior, aggression, and the response to stress," *Neuron*, vol. 59, no. 6, pp. 947–958, 2008.

[153] R. C. Samaco, C. M. McGraw, C. S. Ward, Y. Sun, J. L. Neul, and H. Y. Zoghbi, "Female *MECP2*(+/-) mice display robust behavioral deficits on two different genetic backgrounds providing a framework for pre-clinical studies," *Human Molecular Genetics*, vol. 22, no. 1, pp. 96–109, 2013.

[154] M. A. Toward, A. P. Abdala, S. J. Knopp, J. F. Paton, and J. M. Bissonnette, "Increasing brain serotonin corrects CO_2 chemosensitivity in methyl-CpG-binding protein 2 (*MECP2*)-deficient mice," *Experimental Physiology*, vol. 98, no. 3, pp. 842–849, 2013.

[155] C. M. Buchovecky, S. D. Turley, H. M. Brown et al., "A suppressor screen in *MECP2* mutant mice implicates cholesterol metabolism in Rett syndrome," *Nature Genetics*, vol. 45, pp. 1013–1020, 2013.

[156] J. Guy, J. Gan, J. Selfridge, S. Cobb, and A. Bird, "Reversal of neurological defects in a mouse model of Rett syndrome," *Science*, vol. 315, no. 5815, pp. 1143–1147, 2007.

[157] J. M. LaSalle, J. Goldstine, D. Balmer, and C. M. Greco, "Quantitative localization of heterogeneous methyl-CpG-binding protein 2 (*MECP2*) expression phenotypes in normal and Rett syndrome brain by laser scanning cytometry," *Human Molecular Genetics*, vol. 10, no. 17, pp. 1729–1740, 2001.

[158] N. Ballas, D. T. Lioy, C. Grunseich, and G. Mandel, "Non-cell autonomous influence of *MECP2*-deficient glia on neuronal dendritic morphology," *Nature Neuroscience*, vol. 12, no. 3, pp. 311–317, 2009.

[159] J. W. Pan, J. B. Lane, H. Hetherington, and A. K. Percy, "Rett syndrome: 1H spectroscopic imaging at 4.1 Tesla," *Journal of Child Neurology*, vol. 14, no. 8, pp. 524–528, 1999.

[160] M. E. Blue, W. E. Kaufmann, J. Bressler et al., "Temporal and regional alterations in NMDA receptor expression in *MECP2*-null mice," *Anatomical Record*, vol. 294, no. 10, pp. 1624–1634, 2011.

[161] M. V. Johnston, O. Jeon, J. Pevsner, M. E. Blue, and S. Naidu, "Neurobiology of Rett syndrome: a genetic disorder of synapse development," *Brain and Development*, vol. 23, supplement 1, pp. S206–S213, 2001.

[162] G. Calfa, J. J. Hablitz, and L. Pozzo-Miller, "Network hyperexcitability in hippocampal slices from *MECP2* mutant mice revealed by voltage-sensitive dye imaging," *Journal of Neurophysiology*, vol. 105, no. 4, pp. 1768–1784, 2011.

[163] G. Calfa, A. K. Percy, and L. Pozzo-Miller, "Experimental models of rett syndrome based on *MECP2* dysfunction," *Experimental Biology and Medicine*, vol. 236, no. 1, pp. 3–19, 2011.

[164] S.-M. Weng, F. McLeod, M. E. S. Bailey, and S. R. Cobb, "Synaptic plasticity deficits in an experimental model of rett syndrome: long-term potentiation saturation and its pharmacological reversal," *Neuroscience*, vol. 180, pp. 314–321, 2011.

[165] W. Li and L. Pozzo-Miller, "BDNF deregulation in Rett syndrome," *Neuropharmacology*, vol. 76, pp. 737–746, 2014.

[166] J. L. Larimore, C. A. Chapleau, S. Kudo, A. Theibert, A. K. Percy, and L. Pozzo-Miller, "Bdnf overexpression in hippocampal neurons prevents dendritic atrophy caused by Rett-associated *MECP2* mutations," *Neurobiology of Disease*, vol. 34, no. 2, pp. 199–211, 2009.

[167] H. Wang, S. Chan, M. Ogier et al., "Dysregulation of brain-derived neurotrophic factor expression and neurosecretory function in *MECP2* null mice," *The Journal of Neuroscience*, vol. 26, no. 42, pp. 10911–10915, 2006.

[168] M. Ogier, H. Wang, E. Hong, Q. Wang, M. E. Greenberg, and D. M. Katz, "Brain-derived neurotrophic factor expression and respiratory function improve after ampakine treatment in a mouse model of Rett syndrome," *The Journal of Neuroscience*, vol. 27, no. 40, pp. 10912–10917, 2007.

[169] D. D. Kline, M. Ogier, D. L. Kunze, and D. M. Katz, "Exogenous brain-derived neurotrophic factor rescues synaptic dysfunction in *MECP2*-null mice," *The Journal of Neuroscience*, vol. 30, no. 15, pp. 5303–5310, 2010.

[170] D. A. Schmid, T. Yang, M. Ogier et al., "A TrkB small molecule partial agonist rescues TrkB phosphorylation deficits and improves respiratory function in a mouse model of rett syndrome," *The Journal of Neuroscience*, vol. 32, no. 5, pp. 1803–1810, 2012.

[171] R. A. Johnson, M. Lam, A. M. Punzo et al., "7,8-dihydroxyflavone exhibits therapeutic efficacy in a mouse model of Rett syndrome," *Journal of Applied Physiology*, vol. 112, no. 5, pp. 704–710, 2012.

[172] D. Tropea, E. Giacometti, N. R. Wilson et al., "Partial reversal of Rett Syndrome-like symptoms in *MECP2* mutant mice," *Proceedings of the National Academy of Sciences of the United States of America*, vol. 106, no. 6, pp. 2029–2034, 2009.

[173] M. C. N. Marchetto, C. Carromeu, A. Acab et al., "A model for neural development and treatment of rett syndrome using human induced pluripotent stem cells," *Cell*, vol. 143, no. 4, pp. 527–539, 2010.

[174] C. Brendel, E. Klahold, J. Gärtner, and P. Huppke, "Suppression of nonsense mutations in Rett syndrome by aminoglycoside antibiotics," *Pediatric Research*, vol. 65, no. 5, pp. 520–523, 2009.

[175] A. C. Popescu, E. Sidorova, G. Zhang, and J. H. Eubanks, "Aminoglycoside-mediated partial suppression of *MECP2* nonsense mutations responsible for Rett syndrome in vitro," *The Journal of Neuroscience Research*, vol. 88, no. 11, pp. 2316–2324, 2010.

[176] N. C. Derecki, J. C. Cronk, Z. Lu et al., "Wild-type microglia arrest pathology in a mouse model of Rett syndrome," *Nature*, vol. 484, no. 7392, pp. 105–109, 2012.

[177] N. C. Derecki, J. C. Cronk, and J. Kipnis, "The role of microglia in brain maintenance: implications for Rett syndrome," *Trends in Immunology*, vol. 34, no. 3, pp. 144–150, 2013.

[178] S. K. Garg, D. T. Lioy, H. Cheval et al., "Systemic delivery of *MECP2* rescues behavioral and cellular deficits in female mouse models of Rett syndrome," *The Journal of Neuroscience*, vol. 33, no. 34, pp. 13612–13620, 2013.

4

Contemporary Review of the Management of Brain Metastasis with Radiation

Deepak Khuntia

Varian Medical Systems, 3100 Hansen Way, E-175, Palo Alto, CA 94340, USA

Correspondence should be addressed to Deepak Khuntia; deepak.khuntia@varian.com

Academic Editor: Aimee J. Nelson

Brain metastases are an important cause of morbidity and mortality, afflicting approximately 200,000 Americans annually. The prognosis for these patients is poor, with median survivals typically measured in months. In this review article, we present the standard treatment approaches with whole brain radiation and as well as novel approaches in the prevention of neurocognitive deficits.

1. Introduction

Brain metastases (BrM) represent an important cause of morbidity and mortality and are the most common intracranial tumors in adults, occurring in up to 30% of adult cancer patients [1, 2]. It is estimated that up to 170,000 new cases of brain metastases occur in the United States each year [3, 4]. It is speculated that the annual incidence is rising for several reasons, including an aging population, better treatment of systemic disease, and improvements in imaging, such as magnetic resonance imaging (MRI), to detect smaller metastases in asymptomatic patients [1, 5, 6].

The risk of developing BrM varies according to primary tumor type, with lung cancer accounting for approximately one-half of all brain metastases and is likely rising [7, 8]. Two large series have shown the cumulative incidence of BrM to be between 16 and 20% for lung cancer, 7–10% for renal cell carcinoma, 7% for melanoma, 5% for breast cancer, and <2% for colorectal cancer [9, 10]. One disease in particular, breast cancer, has seen increases in survival even in the metastatic setting. Patients with HER2 overexpression are particularly sensitive to developing BrM, especially those that also have a history of lung metastasis [11]. Longer survival in colorectal cancer has also contributed to the rise in BrM with this diagnosis [12].

The prognosis of patients with brain metastases is poor with the median survival time of untreated patients being approximately one month [13]. With treatment, the overall median survival time after diagnosis is typically still less than one year [14]. Brain metastases present cancer patients with significant neurologic, cognitive, and emotional difficulties and, once diagnosed, generally convey a poor outcome. In this paper, we will review standard treatment approaches with whole brain radiotherapy (WBRT) and discuss new directions in brain metastasis therapy, specifically focusing on the role of radiosurgery and chemical modifiers of the radiation effect. Since neurocognitive dysfunction following brain metastasis is a major concern, we will focus a significant portion of our discussion on this issue.

2. Diagnosis

The differential diagnosis for brain metastasis includes infection, paraneoplastic diseases, bleeding, and radiation necrosis (often from previous radiosurgery). As a result biopsies are considered when the diagnosis is uncertain. In fact, in the landmark study from Patchell in colleagues randomizing patients to surgery and whole brain versus biopsy and whole brain, approximately 10% of patients on the biopsy arm had tumors other than metastasis [15].

On MRI, brain metastases are typically found in the watershed areas of the brain (areas where blood vessels narrow and act as a trap for clumps of tumor cells). Approximately 80% of the lesions are found in the cerebral hemispheres, 15% in the cerebellum and 5% in the brain stem. This is largely

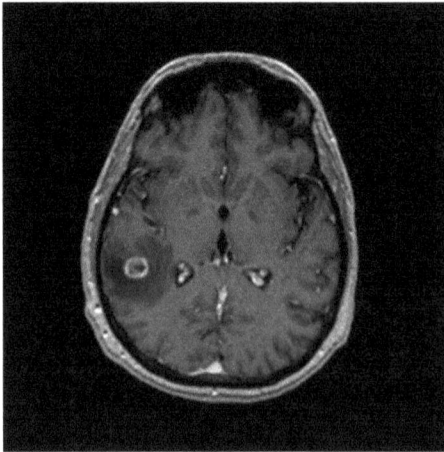

FIGURE 1: T1-weighted brain magnetic resonance imaging scans of a patient with NSCLC: contrast scan showing a 2 cm right sided parenchymal lesion (courtesy of Sam Chao, MD, Cleveland Clinic Foundation).

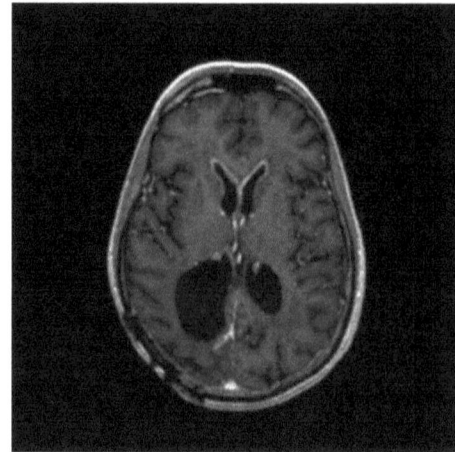

FIGURE 2: A patient with leptomeningeal enhancement (courtesy of Sam Chao, MD, Cleveland Clinic Foundation).

based on the general volume of brain in these regions. Areas that are often strategically avoided by therapies, such as the hippocampus, have low propensity for the development of brain metastasis and this has special significance, as will be discussed later [16]. Most of the lesions are intensely enhanced by gadolinium contrast as a result of disruption of the blood brain barrier (see Figure 1). Leptomeningeal metastases, also known as carcinomatous meningitis, are another less common presentation of advanced cancer that occurs when tumor breaks through the arachnoid and pia mater and spreads throughout the subarachnoid space. This is a very aggressive form of metastasis. Symptoms can be quite varied from headaches, to mass effect, to cranial nerve root dysfunction. The most common primary for this to occur is breast cancer but it can occur with other cancers such as lung, melanoma, gastrointestinal tumors, and gynecologic malignancies. MRI is the diagnosis tool of choice and typically one will see enhancement along the walls of the gyri and sulci or multiple nodular deposits throughout the subarachnoid space (see Figure 2). Due to the wide spread dissemination of tumor, WBRT is often employed as part of the treatment strategy for leptomeningeal disease.

3. Treatment Options with Radiation

Treatment has evolved over the last several decades. Dexamethasone, for example, has been used to improve symptoms by decreasing capillary permeability and subsequently reducing intracranial edema. A typical dose is 16 mg/day in 2–4 divided doses. Gastrointestinal prophylaxis with ranitidine or other drugs in its class is often recommended to combat the GI side effects of dexamethasone. For patients on the drug for extended periods of time, thrush prophylaxis is also considered. Steroids are not without side effects as patients can experience weight gain, Cushingoid appearance, proximal muscle weakness, hyperglycemia, fluid retention, and, if tapered to quickly, even adrenal insufficiency. In addition to helping alleviate symptoms, steroids were felt to prolong survival from about 1 to 2 months [17].

Traditionally, the most widely used treatment for patients with multiple brain metastases is WBRT. The 1954 article, "Roentgen-ray therapy of cerebral metastases," was one of the earliest reviews of the use of WBRT for the treatment of BrM [32]. The appropriate use of WBRT can provide rapid improvements of many neurologic symptoms, improve quality of life, and may be especially beneficial in patients whose brain metastases are surgically inaccessible or when other medical considerations remove surgery from the list of appropriate options [32–34]. The use of adjuvant WBRT, following resection or radiosurgery has been proven to be effective in terms of improving local control of brain metastases, and, furthermore, the likelihood of neurologic death is decreased based on a randomized trial [35]. The majority of patients who achieve local tumor control die from progression of disease outside of the brain, whereas the cause of death is most often due to central nervous system (CNS) disease in patients with recurrent brain metastases [36]. However, the use of whole brain has come under criticism recently due to the possibility of neurocognitive decline related to brain radiation [37].

Three areas of investigation are attempting to improve the survival of patients with unresectable brain metastases: (1) WBRT in conjunction with radiosurgery (RS), an area that is further explored in other manuscripts in this issue, (2) radiosensitizers, and (3) new chemotherapeutic agents that synergize (or are additive) with radiation. Older studies of radiosensitizers have not resulted in clinical benefit [38, 39]. Other promising developments in the treatment of brain metastases include new chemotherapy agents such as temozolomide (Temodar), which crosses the blood-brain barrier. Other tumor specific drugs, such as lapatinib (Tykerb), are also being considered for certain primaries, such as HER2 positive breast cancer [40].

3.1. Whole Brain Radiation Therapy. In patients who have brain metastases that impinge upon eloquent areas or are

TABLE 1: Dose fractionation schemes of WBRT in various tumor types*.

Study	Number of patients	Randomization Gy/# fractions	Median survival (months)
Harwood and Simpson [18]	101	30/10 versus 10/1	4.0–4.3
Kurtz et al. [19]	255	30/10 versus 50/20	3.9–4.2
Borgelt et al. [17, 20]	138	10/1 versus 30/10 versus 40/20	4.2–4.8
Borgelt et al. [17, 20]	64	12/2 versus 20/5	2.8–3.0
Chatani et al. [21]	70	30/10 versus 50/20	3.0–4.0
Haie-Meder et al. [22]	216	18/3 versus 36/6 or 43/13	4.2–5.3
Chatani et al. [23]	72	30/10 versus 50/20 or 20/5	2.4–4.3
Murray et al. [24]	445	54.4/34 versus 30/10	4.5

*Adapted from Khuntia et al. [25].

TABLE 2: (a) Median survival according to RPA class following WBRT [26]. (b) RTOG Graded Prognostic Assessment (GPA) is felt to be a more sensitive tool for predicting outcomes in BrM patients. They are assigned a score of 0, 0.5, or 1 for each of 4 characteristics. The sum of the score predicts median survival both as a whole (RTOG MS) and with therapy such as WBRT ± SRS [27]. (c) Disease Specific GPA [28].

(a)

Treatment	Patients (n)	Median survival (months) by RPA class		
		Class 1 (Primary controlled, age <65, no extracranial metastases, KPS ≥ 70)	Class 2 (primary uncontrolled OR age ≥65, OR extracranial metastases)	Class 3 (KPS < 70)
WBRT (RTOG phase III trials)	1176	7.1	4.2	2.3

(b)

Score	0	0.5	1	Sum GPA score	RTOG MS	WBRT and/or SRS MS**
Age	>60	50–59	<50	3.5–4	11.0	21.7
KPS	<70	70–80	90–100	3	6.9	17.5
Number brain mets	>3	2–3	1	1.5–2.5	3.8	5.9
ExtraCNS mets	Present	—	None	0–1	2.6	3.0

MS = median survival (months).

(c)

Primary	Median survival (Months)	95% CI
Non-small-cell lung cancer	7.00	6.53–7.50
Small cell lung cancer	4.90	4.30–6.20
Melanoma	6.74	5.90–7.57
Renal cell carcinoma	9.63	7.66–10.91
Breast cancer	11.93	9.69–12.85
Gastrointestinal cancer	5.36	4.30–6.30
Unknown	6.37	5.22–7.49

too large, numerous, or disseminated for surgery or RS or in patients that performance status does not allow for more aggressive therapy, WBRT alone remains the treatment of choice and provides effective symptom relief in the majority [34]. Response rates following WBRT vary, with complete or partial responses being documented in more than 60% of patients in randomized controlled studies conducted by the Radiation Therapy Oncology Group (RTOG). Table 1 summarizes results of different dose and fractionation schedules from 8 randomized studies in patients receiving WBRT alone, with median survival ranges from 2.4 to 4.8 months. The consensus from these studies of fractionation schedules is that differences in dose, timing, and fractionation have

not significantly altered the median survival time for WBRT treatment of BrM. The landmark RTOG recursive partitioning analysis (RPA) describes three prognostic classes, defined by age, Karnofsky performance status (KPS), and disease status [26]. RPA class 1 patients are younger (<65), have higher KPS scores (70 or greater), no other sites of metastases, and controlled extracranial disease, and have the longest median survival (Table 2(a)).

As treatments for BrM continued to evolve, it became necessary to have additional granularity into the predictive factors associated with BrM to help tailor treatments. The RTOG RPA, for example, was limited in that it did not include the number of lesions. As a result, the RTOG Graded

Prognostic Assessment (GPA) was developed (Table 2(b)) [27]. In the GPA, data from multiple RTOG studies, including patients from the RTOG 95-08 radiosurgery study, were analyzed and a more sensitive predictive tool was developed that also included number of lesions. With the GPA, primary histology was not included as in the RPA. Therefore, a subsequent disease specific GPA was developed (DS-GPA) (Table 2(c)) [28], but even this system had limitations as we know that the biology is also an important factor in predicting outcomes.

Reports indicate that response to WBRT may be related to the primary histology. Nieder and colleagues [41] studied 108 patients and assessed CT-response based on tumor type following WBRT alone. Complete response was obtained in 24% of patients and partial response in 35%. Response rates ranged from 81% for small cell lung carcinoma to 0% for malignant melanoma (although other series have shown response rates of 45 to 65% for melanoma brain metastases) [42]. Other retrospective investigations of treatment for brain metastases from various primaries suggest relatively clustered survival statistics: 6 months for female genitourinary cancers [43], 4.2 months for breast cancer [44], 2.3 months [45] for melanoma, and so forth. The RTOG RPA multivariate analysis, however, did not find histology to be an independent predictor of survival following WBRT and this was also factored in the subsequent GPA report.

Another major use of WBRT, which is declining, is as an adjuvant following surgery or radiosurgery. Magnetic resonance imaging reveals that about 80% of patients have more than 1 metastasis, and ~50% have 3 or more metastases so treating microscopic disease with WBRT is of value. Furthermore, 70% of patients with brain metastases experience relapse after resection, if WBRT is omitted [46].

It is important to recognize that there are some arguments against the use of WBRT. Many have questioned its ability to reverse neurologic symptoms [47] and its use has been putatively associated with debilitating complications in long-term survivors [37, 48]. Furthermore, many patients have short term side effects such as fatigue, alopecia, and erythema. Less common side effects include ear pain, headaches, alterations in smell and taste, and nausea. As a result, the use of WBRT has been declining in the USA.

3.2. Stereotactic Radiosurgery. Traditionally, radiosurgery (SRS) has required the use of Gamma Knife (Elekta, Stockholm, Sweden) radiosurgery system. This is a cobalt based dedicated system used to treat lesions in the brain. As technology has evolved, other manufactures have developed tools such as the Cyberknife (Accuray, Inc., Sunnyvale, CA), Novalis Tx (Varian Medical Systems, Palo Alto, CA and BrainLab, Munich, Germany), TrueBeam (Varian Medical Systems, Palo Alto, CA), and Edge Radiosurgery System (Varian Medical Systems, Palo Alto, CA). Many consider both linac based and cobalt based systems as equivalent and this has allowed for the rapid increase in both intra- and extracranial SRS [49, 50].

SRS is now standard practice for patients with 4 or fewer metastases in the brain and this has been validated

TABLE 3: RTOG 9005 [29].

Tumor diameter ≤20 mm		21–30 mm		31–40 mm	
Dose	Toxicity	Dose	Toxicity	Dose	Toxicity
18 Gy	8%	15 Gy	13%	12 Gy	10%
21 Gy	11%	**18 Gy**	20%	**15 Gy**	14%
24Gy	10%	21 Gy	38%	18 Gy	50%
		24 Gy	58%		

The MTD for tumors ≤20 mm is 24 Gy, for tumors 21–30 mm it is 18 Gy, and for tumors 31–40 mm it is 15 Gy. Doses in yellow represent the recommended MTD.

by multiple prospective trials. The controversy arises when considering its utilization with or without WBRT which is discussed later in detail. The original dose escalation study was reported by Shaw and colleagues in RTOG 9005 where 100 patients with brain metastasis underwent a dose escalation regimen based on the size of the tumor [29]. Smaller tumors were escalated to higher doses (since this could be done safer given the more favorable dosimetry for small lesions) in 3 Gy increments. The authors concluded that the maximum tolerated dose for tumors <20 mm was 24 Gy, between 21 and 30 mm was 18 Gy, and between 31 and 40 mm is 15 Gy (see Table 3).

One of the early efforts reviewing the utility of SRS involved a randomized trial comparing WBRT with or without a SRS boost was done by the University of Pittsburgh. Researchers attempted a phase III study comparing 30 Gy in 12 fractions of WBRT with a 16 Gy boost, but the study was terminated earlier as it was felt unethical to continue given the high control rate in the WBRT + SRS arm (100%) versus WBRT alone (8%) [51]. In what is considered one of the defining studies in SRS, the RTOG conducted a 333-patient randomized trial comparing WBRT alone (37.5 Gy in 15 fractions) with or without SRS (dosing per RTOG 9005) [30]. The primary endpoint to the study was overall survival with secondary endpoints of tumor response, local control, intracranial recurrence, cause of death, and performance status changes. This study included patients with up to 3 BrM. Patients with a single BrM were found to improve in overall survival. The study helped to establish a new standard of care for patients with a single BrM.

The Japanese Radiation Oncology Study Group (JROSG) also conducted a randomized study of SRS versus SRS + WBRT (JROSG 99-1) where 132 patients with up to 4 lesions were randomized [31]. They found that the use of WBRT delayed the occurrence of new brain metastases at 12 months and also reduced the likelihood of the need for salvage brain treatments. The authors concluded that WBRT should not be withheld as intracranial control is paramount (Table 5).

In a provocative study challenging the previous randomized trials mentioned above, Chang and colleagues conducted a single institution randomized trial of SRS with or without WBRT at the MD Anderson Cancer Center [52]. In this study, 58 patients with 1–3 brain metastases (RPA class I or II) were randomized and stratified by RPA class, number of lesions, and radioresistant histologies (melanoma or renal cell versus other). The primary endpoint of the study was the Hopkins Verbal Learning Test-Recall (HVLT-R) at 4 months by more than 5 points. Doses used were similar to those in RTOG 95-08 with WBRT given at 30 Gy in 12 fractions. The investigators stopped the study early due to a decreased survival in the WBRT arm (15.2 months versus 5.7 months) which challenged conventional thinking and the data from previous trials (no difference in survival in both RTOG 95-08 and JROSG 99-01). This has come under some criticism in that some argue that the arms were not well balanced as there was more visceral metastatic disease in the WBRT arm and did not take into account subsequent recovery of neurocognitive function as 4 months was the endpoint and that there was a time bias from the fact that WBRT had to be given within 3 weeks after SRS so there could be a 5-week delay in the time points of when the data was analyzed. Given the fact that there were both a reduction of neurocognitive function and also increased death in the WBRT, those that believe in SRS alone have level 1 evidence supporting that decision.

In a European effort, Kocher and colleagues conducted a randomized multi-institutional study comparing adjuvant WBRT versus observation after SRS or surgical resection in patients with 1 to 3 brain metastases [53]. This study randomized a total of 359 patients (199 underwent SRS and 160 underwent resection). After SRS or surgery, adjuvant WBRT was found to reduce intracranial relapse (59% to 27% after surgery, $P < 0.001$, and 31% to 19% after SRS, $P = 0.040$) and neurologic deaths but did not show improvements in functional independence (10 versus 9.5 months) or overall survival.

Another area of increased interest involves the use of adjuvant SRS after surgical resection. It has been previously noted that the landmark study by Patchell et al. showed the benefits of adjuvant WBRT in improving local control not only in the brain, but also in particular in the site of the resection cavity [35]. However, with the fear of the WBRT toxicities, some have argued that an SRS cavity boost be considered instead of WBRT. In a poll conducted in the 2006 Congress of Neurological Surgeons Meeting, one-third of neurosurgeons resect metastases and follow it by an SRS boost. Soltys and colleagues conducted a retrospective review of 72 patients with 76 cavities from 1998 to 2006 who underwent SRS with a median marginal dose of 18.6 Gy (range of 15–30 Gy) [54]. Actuarial local control was found to be respectable 88% and 79% at 6 and 12 months, respectively. This compared favorably to their historical control rate of 54% for observation alone and 80–90% with adjuvant WBRT. Furthermore, they recommended using a 2 mm margin with their technique on the resection cavity. Though this study showed very reasonable results with an SRS cavity boost, other authors have not been able to replicate these results with local control rates as low as 35% [55]. Part of the poor results may be related to the difficulty in identifying the areas at risk of recurrence due to the difficulty in identifying the postresection cavity. In an effort to clarify this discrepancy, a phase III study is currently under way. In this effort run by the Alliance and endorsed by NRG, NCCTG N107c is currently accruing patients. In this study, patients are randomized to adjuvant whole brain radiation to a dose of 37.5 Gy in 15

fractions versus SRS to the surgical resection bed to a dose between 12 and 20 Gy in a single fraction. Patients will be stratified based on age, duration of controlled extracranial disease, number of preoperative BrM, histology, and size of the resection cavity. The dose in the SRS arm is based on the size of the cavity with the high dose patients exhibiting targets <4.2 cc receiving 20 Gy in a single fraction and the low dose region between ≥30 cc and 5 cm max of 12 Gy. The study is expected to accrue a total of 174 eligible patients.

4. The Controversy Surrounding the Use of Whole Brain Radiotherapy

With the increased availability of radiosurgery, a new trend has been emerging in the management of patients with brain metastases. In this approach, patients with a *limited* number of brain metastatic lesions (the exact definition of *limited* is based on institutional preference and varies from 3 to 10 or more) [30, 31, 52, 53, 56] are treated with radiosurgery alone, without WBRT, and are then closely monitored, which involves regular MR imaging. Repeat radiosurgery is performed for new intracranial metastases, with the intent of avoiding or eliminating WBRT in as many patients for as long as possible. The rationale is the avoidance of neurotoxicity from WBRT. However, this approach is still considered controversial by some and definitive controlled clinical trials can support either argument. Delaying WBRT in favor of active surveillance increases the overall cost of managing these patients, with multiple and expensive imaging studies and repeat radiosurgical procedures which also need also needs to be taken into account.

Advocates of withholding WBRT suggest that WBRT may be "ineffective," patients may have "oligometastatic disease," survival is unaltered whether upfront WBRT is used or not, radiosurgery is adequate for local control, and neurologic status and quality of life of patients in whom WBRT is withheld are superior.

Historically, when steroids alone were used for the management of BrM, survival was only about 1 month. The addition of WBRT was found to increase survival by several months. The most common WBRT regimen uses 30 Gy in 2 weeks; this dose is designed to be palliative and was never intended to cure epithelial tumors but rather strikes a balance of minimizing toxicity but still helping to relieve symptoms. When reviewing data within BrM studies in the RTOG, control of disease is realized in approximately 50% of patients at 6 months. Therefore, enhancing the effect of WBRT in controlling the macroscopically visible tumor with the addition of radiosurgery makes sense and is now supported by level 1 evidence [30, 31]. For example, in the phase III RTOG 9508 trial of WBRT with or without radiosurgery boost, the actuarial 1-year local control was 82 versus 71% ($P = 0.01$), in favor of the radiosurgery boost [30] (Table 4). Furthermore, WBRT can and does add to the local control on top of the SRS treatments as based on both the RTOG and JROSG studies, which does have value.

Some may argue that BrM may be oligometastatic and therefore we only need to worry about the disease that is

TABLE 4: RTOG 9508 [30]. SRS improved survival in patients with a single BrM. Subset analysis suggested there was a potential benefit for patients with NSCLC, RPA class I, or patients that were <50 years old with 2 to 3 metastasis. Patients in the study receiving SRS also had improved KPS with decreased steroid dependence.

Med OS	All pts	Single brain met	1–3 mets, age <50	1–3 mets, NSCLC	1–3 mets, RPA class I
WBRT alone	5.7 mos	4.9 months	8.3 months	3.9 months	9.6 months
WBRT + SRS	6.5 mos	6.5 months	9.9 months	5.0 months	11.6 months
P value	0.14	**0.04**	**0.04**	**0.05**	**0.05**

TABLE 5: JROSG 99-1 [31] study comparing SRS with or without WBRT. Omission of WBRT was found to decrease intracranial control, and, as a result, the authors recommended SRS + WBRT for patients with up to 4 brain metastases.

	MS	OS @ 1 yr	Freedom from new brain mets @ 1 mos	Salvage brain tx	Neuro death
SRS	8.0 months	28.4%	46.8%	43%	19.3%
SRS + WBRT	7.5 months	38.5%	76.4%	15%	22.8%
P value	0.42	0.42	**<0.001**	**<0.001**	0.64

seen on MR. However, older autopsy and CT-imaging studies suggest that the rate of multiple brain metastases ranges from 58 to 86%, with a mean of 66%, but these have been criticized on several grounds [25]. In one MRI-based study, only 19% of the 336 patients had a single lesion; the percentage of patients with 2, 3, 4, and 5 or more lesions was 16, 13, 10, and 40%; in most trials of radiosurgery, <5 is considered the upper limit, in terms of the definition of oligometastases, and, in this trial, 50% of patients had more than 3 lesions on MR imaging [57]. Therefore, most reports suggest that only about 20% of patients have one brain met, and this is especially important, as evidence-based data suggest no survival benefit from aggressive local treatments such as surgery or radiosurgery in patients with more than 1 metastatic lesion [58].

Others have argued that survival is unaltered whether upfront WBRT is used or not. This is indeed true as there are other competing risks of death, such as systemic disease. However, the value proposition here is that of local control [59]. Many of these studies were not designed to answer an overall survival question as the true value is preventing future complications from recurrent disease and improving or maintaining quality of life [35]. That being said, caution should be used in oversimplifying this statement. For example, Pirzkall et al. reported that, for brain metastases patients without extracranial disease, (i.e., patients with a much lower likelihood of dying from systemic metastases) the median survival following radiosurgery alone with WBRT used for salvage was 8.3 months, compared to 15.4 months for patients treated up-front with radiosurgery plus WBRT [60]. Similar results were seen in a retrospective study from the Mayo Clinic where a survival benefit for adjuvant WBRT limited to patients without systemic disease was realized; 5-year survival rates of 21% for those who received adjuvant WBRT compared to 4% for those patients who did not [61]. These observations are crucial, implying that, for those patients where prolonged survival is likely, failure to control the intracranial disease by omitting or delaying WBRT may negatively impact survival.

Some have argued that SRS is good enough for local control. In the phase III study, JROSG 99-1, patients were randomized to radiosurgery alone, versus whole brain radiotherapy

and radiosurgery [31]. The actuarial 6-month freedom from new brain metastases was 48% in the SRS alone arm and 82% in the SRS plus WBRT (log rank, $P = 0.003$). Actuarial 1-year brain tumor control rate for the lesions treated with radiosurgery was 70% in the radiosurgery alone arm and 86% in the radiosurgery and whole brain radiation arm (log rank, $P = 0.019$) [31]. In another randomized trial [62] comparing SRS alone versus WBRT and SRS versus WBRT, the local brain control rate was highest in the radiosurgery plus WBRT arm. A prospective single arm, multi-institutional ECOG phase II study of radiosurgery alone for "radioresistant" histologies [63] (such as melanoma, sarcoma, and renal cell carcinoma) in patients with 1–3 brain metastases reported at 6 months, 39.2% failed within the radiosurgery volume, and 39.4% failed outside the radiosurgery volume, thereby supporting the case of limited benefit from radiosurgery alone. Clinical trial-based assessments therefore suggest high rates of intracranial failures and reduced local control rates when WBRT is omitted or delayed.

Finally, an argument has been made that neurologic status and quality of life of patients in whom WBRT is withheld is superior. In the JRSG 99-01 study, patients were randomized to radiosurgery alone or with WBRT but detailed neurocognitive assessments were not performed, and the primary assessment was by an evaluation of performance status and neurologic functional status, using RTOG criteria [31]. There were no differences in these endpoints between the two study arms, belying the claims of worse neurologic outcomes in the WBRT arm [31]. In fact, some have argued that withholding WBRT increases intracranial failure and neurologic deterioration is more directly related to disease progression in the brain [64]. In a phase III trial of WBRT with or without the radiosensitizer, motexafin gadolinium, the most significant predictor for neurologic and neurocognitive decline, as well as deterioration in quality of life was disease progression in the brain [65].

Therefore, the switch to omitting WBRT is still considered controversial and data supports both withholding and administering WBRT. In large measure, it is fair to say that this switch has been made because physicians have observed some patients experiencing neurocognitive and neurologic decline (the causes for which could in fact be multifactorial). This is supported by the Chang study showing a doubling of the rate of neurocognitive decline as a result of WBRT [52]. As a result, efforts, as described below, are underway to help mitigate the toxicities associated with WBRT. Also, multiple studies are underway in single institution phase III studies evaluating the possibility of eliminating WBRT in patients with 5 or more metastases (including UCSF [ClinicalTrials.gov identifier NCT01731704] and MDACC [ClinicalTrials.gov identifier NCT01644591 and NCT01592968]).

4.1. Mechanism of Neurocognitive Dysfunction. Toxicity from radiation can be stratified based on the timing of onset of symptoms: acute, subacute, and late [66]. Acute effects typically occur during the first few weeks of treatment and are often characterized by drowsiness, headache, nausea, vomiting, and worsening focal deficits (typically in the first 30 days). Often, cerebral edema is the cause of these symptoms and corticosteroids such as dexamethasone may improve these symptoms. Subacute symptoms related to encephalopathy (early delayed reaction) occurring at 1 to 6 months after completion of radiation may be secondary to diffuse demyelination [67, 68]. Symptoms include headache, extreme somnolence, fatigability, and deterioration of preexisting deficits that resolve within several months. Late delayed effects appear more than 6 months after radiation and can be irreversible and progressive [69]. This may be a result of white matter damage due to vascular injury, demyelination, or even necrosis. Symptoms can vary from mild lassitude to significant memory loss and even severe dementia [70]. The pathophysiology of radiation induced neurocognitive damage is complex and multifactorial. Oligodendrocytes, which are important for myelination, are likely at least partially to blame. Oligodendrocyte death can occur either as a result of direct p53 dependent radiation apoptosis or due to exposure to radiation induced tumor necrosis factor α (TNFα) [71, 72]. Postradiation injury to the vasculature damages the endothelium leading to platelet aggregation and thrombus formation, followed by abnormal endothelial proliferation and intraluminal collagen deposition [73, 74]. Another area receiving increased attention is hippocampal-dependent functions of learning, memory, and spatial information processing that seem to be preferentially affected by radiation [75]. Animal studies reveal that doses as low as 2 Gy can induce apoptosis in the proliferating cells in the hippocampus leading to decreased repopulative capacity [76].

4.2. Management and Prevention of Neurocognitive Deficits from WBRT. Treatment (or prophylaxis) of cognitive sequelae of cranial radiation has been limited until recently. In the past, methylphenidate has been used in a few small series of patients exhibiting neurobehavioral slowing with limited response [77–79]. Patients who develop psychomotor slowing, decline in executive functioning, or general apathy may benefit [78]. Though these studies suggest beneficial

effects with methylphenidate, they have significant limitations including small sample size, lack of a blinded control, high toxicity of methylphenidate (including addiction potential), and therefore the widespread use of methylphenidate should not be considered standard of care.

Erythropoietin has been used as a central nervous system protectant in a number of studies and this has generated some interest in the utilization of this agent [80, 81]. A blinded, randomized trial of erythropoietin (compared to saline) found less motor impairment in erythropoietin treated rats 2 days after 100 Gy was delivered to the right striatum; by day 10 the erythropoietin treated rats had returned to near control levels while the deficits persisted in the saline treated rats [82]. A similar study found erythropoietin delivered one hour after whole brain radiotherapy (17 Gy in one fraction) was neuroprotective in mice [83]. That being said, currently erythropoietin has not been validated in large human studies and it is not considered a routine part of the management of BrM.

There has been significant interest in using Alzheimer's therapeutic agents to treat radiation induced injury, since many aspects radiation induced injury are clinically and radiographically similar to Alzheimer's dementia. In a trial from Wake Forest University, 24 previously irradiated brain tumor patients were treated with 24 weeks of donepezil [84]. Neurocognitive tests were performed at multiple time points which included tests of verbal fluency, verbal memory, attention, and figural memory scores. Patients were significantly improved between baseline and week 24, but there was no change on global cognitive function or executive function. There was no significant worsening of performance noted on any measures. The limitations of this study include the small sample size and the potential (as well as uncontrolled) impact of practice (i.e., neurocognitive measures repeated over multiple evaluations) and the placebo effect.

Prior studies have suggested that vitamin E may benefit patients with Alzheimer's disease and potentially radiation toxicity [85]. Researchers at the Queen Elizabeth Hospital in Hong Kong treated 19 patients with temporal lobe radionecrosis with a daily megadose of vitamin E for 1 year, whereas 10 other patients with temporal lobe radionecrosis served as controls (treatment assignment was decided on a voluntary basis) [86]. Significant improvement in global cognitive ability, memory, and executive function occurred among patients in the treatment group after 1-year of vitamin E treatment. However, there are significant limitations of this study in that the patients were not randomized or blinded to treatment, and therefore the results should be considered hypothesis generating.

Although a neurocognitive conceptual framework for understanding the effects of radiotherapy on the brain is limited [87], it seems that the pathophysiology of late RT injury is dynamic and complex, and a result of inter- and intracellular interactions between the vasculature and parenchymal compartments and injury is most likely multifactorial (i.e., demyelination, proliferative and degenerative glial reactions, endothelial cell loss, and capillary occlusion) [75]. The vascular hypothesis is the most recognized and longest standing premise as the primary cause of radiation induced damage [88]. The vascular hypothesis of radiation-induced injury attributes accelerated atherosclerosis and mineralizing microangiopathy resulting in vascular insufficiency and infarction to radiation injury and inflammation. These mechanisms result in a picture similar to the small vessel disease, as is often seen with vascular dementia and Alzheimer's dementia [89]. For this reason there is interest in using pharmaceutical agents that are effective in the treatment of vascular dementia for irradiated brain tumor patients to serve as a chemoprotectant. One of these agents is memantine, a NMDA receptor antagonist induced by ischemia, which blocks excessive NMDA stimulation leading to excitotoxicity. Agents that block pathologic stimulation of NMDA receptors may protect against further damage in patients with vascular dementia [90]. Thus, NMDA receptor antagonists such as memantine are thought to be a potential neuroprotector when patients are exposed to brain radiation and these drugs will help to prevent neuronal injury associated with radiation-induced ischemia. Furthermore, the physiologic function of the remaining neurons could be restored, resulting in symptomatic improvement [91] and both preclinical in vitro and in vivo data support this hypothesis [92–95]. Phase III clinical trials of memantine in patients with vascular dementia demonstrated clinical benefit, with the subgroup of patients with small-vessel disease responding better to memantine than other types of dementia again, supporting the hypothesis that memantine may function as a neuroprotector [96, 97]. In addition, there is anecdotal experience using memantine in primary CNS lymphoma patients with cognitive dysfunction after radiation has shown dramatic clinical improvement [98]. With the beneficial findings of these studies and the limitations of treatment of cognitive decline after radiation, the Radiation Therapy Oncology Group (RTOG) has launched and completed a large phase III study comparing patients receiving WBRT to either memantine (Namenda) or placebo (RTOG 0614) [99]. In this landmark study, 508 eligible patients were randomized to the two arms. Patients receiving memantine had less decline in delayed recall at 24 weeks (primary endpoint of the study) though this was not significantly significant. However, this was thought to be partially due to significant patient loss from competing factors such as death from extracranial disease progression. There was better cognitive function over time in many domains of neurocognition, such as memory, executive function, and processing speed. Furthermore, the improved cognition was maintained over time, even when the drug was discontinued, suggesting a protective effect of memantine. Since the drug had relatively few side effects associated with it, the authors concluded that the memantine can be considered along with WBRT when used in the management of BrM. Also of interest in this study is that there are significant biospecimens available for translational research. The investigators are currently analyzing both inflammatory cytokines and biomarkers such as apolipoprotein E (apoE) as a predictor of patients that are likely to develop neurocognitive decline. Early single institution reports show that those carrying the ApoE allele are more likely to have adverse cognition from radiation [100].

Furthermore, biomarkers can be modulated by the presence of brain radiation [101].

Besides pharmaceutical interventions, others are considering modifying how WBRT is delivered to decrease the risk of neurotoxicity. As mentioned earlier, doses of 2 Gy or less can damage the hippocampus in the mouse model [76]. However, more recent data has shown that hippocampal dosimetry does indeed predict neurocognitive function impairment. Gondi and colleagues recently reported a prospective study in which 29 patients with benign or low grade brain tumors were treated with fractionated stereotactic radiotherapy. The authors measured the dose to the hippocampi and correlated the outcome to the 18 patients that completed both baseline and 18-month neurocognitive function testing. The study revealed that if that biologically equivalent dose in 2 Gy fractions exceeded 7.3 Gy, there was a higher likelihood of neurocognitive decline [102]. As a result, current investigations are underway using new technology to conformally avoid the hippocampus. With the use of intensity modulated radiotherapy, it is possible to create isodose distributions that treat the majority of the brain to full dose, while keeping the radiation dose to the hippocampus relatively low. Furthermore, it may be possible to even incorporate a simultaneous boost to the gross disease at the same time (Figure 3).

Prior to investigating the possibilities of hippocampal avoidance WBRT (HA-WBRT), it is necessary to identify the likelihood of developing BrM within the hippocampi to ensure that sparing the area would not result in an increase in recurrences. Ghia and colleagues reviewed 100 patients treated with radiation for brain metastasis and found that, of the 100 patients, only 8 had metastases within 5 mm of the hippocampus [103]. These results were further validated in a larger multi-institutional effort including over 1100 metastases in 371 patients [104]. Less than 9% of the patients had lesions within 5 mm of the hippocampus and there were no tumors seen in the hippocampus. As a result, 5 mm was selected as a safe avoidance region of the hippocampus for a prospective evaluation of HA-WBRT. Furthermore, efforts were made to standardize the technique of how to plan such cases [105].

The major study to date evaluating the effectiveness of HA-WBRT was RTOG 0933 [106]. This study was a single-arm, multi-institutional phase II study evaluating 113 brain metastases patients undergoing HA-WBRT. The study involved a battery of neurocognitive tests (similar to what was seen in RTOG 0614-WBRT with or without memantine) as well as significant credentialing before an institution was able to accrue a patient. Each physician enrolling a patient on the study was required to pass both contouring and planning of a HA-WBRT case. Furthermore, each plan for an enrolled patient underwent central review by RTOG prior to delivery of therapy. Of the 100 analyzable patients, 76% were categorized as RPA class II. All patients underwent 30 Gy in 10 fractions of HA-WBRT. The mean dose to the hippocampus was below 10 Gy in all patients with the maximum dose not exceeding 17 Gy. Patients were assessed using the HVLT-Delayed Recall, (DR) the HVLT-Recall, and the HVLT-Immediate Recognition tests. The primary endpoint of the study was HVLT-DR at 4 months. There were

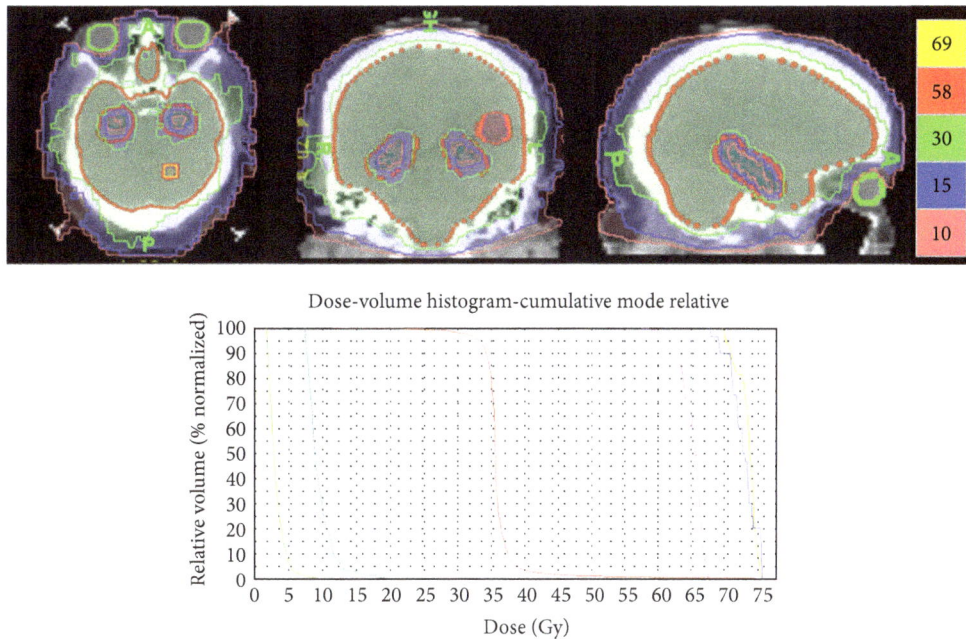

FIGURE 3: Hippocampal sparing whole brain radiotherapy plan showing treatment of the whole brain to 30 Gy while sparing the hippocampi from high doses of radiation which is receiving less than 10 Gy mean dose. Furthermore, it is also possible to dose escalate the gross disease simultaneously (courtesy of Wolfgang Tomé, Ph.D.).

42 analyzable patients that had four month post-RT data. These patients experienced only a 7% decline in HVLT-DR which was significantly lower (95% CI, −4.7% to 18.7%) of the historical control group of 30% decline at 4 months. At 6-month follow-up, the decline was even less at 2%, though only 29 patients were analyzable at this point. There were two grade 3 toxicities and no grade 4 or 5 toxicities. The median survival on the study was 6.8 months. As a result of these promising findings, a new phase III study, CC001 has been developed randomizing patients to HA-WBRT versus WBRT. Both study arms will include memantine based on the results seen in RTOG 0614. The study is expected to accrue patients in mid 2015.

5. Conclusion

In summary, WBRT continues to be a standard and efficacious treatment in the management of brain metastasis. Despite the use of whole brain radiation and radiosurgery, outcomes are poor and efforts are being made to incorporate multimodality approaches including surgery, radiosurgery, and chemotherapy to improve outcomes. Patients with brain metastasis are susceptible to deficits in neurocognition because of their disease and potentially from the treatment for their brain metastasis. As a result, the use of WBRT is declining despite ample evidence supporting the efficacy. For patients with >4 lesions, WBRT still remains the standard of care. For 4 or fewer lesions, SRS alone can be considered but active surveillance for recurrence is needed. Adjuvant SRS to the resection cavity is currently being evaluated in a randomized trial and remains a study question.

Innovative strategies for preventing and treating neurocognitive deficits are actively under investigation and include chemoprevention with drugs such as memantine, but also the use of advanced radiation delivery techniques to spare regions of the brain susceptible to radiation injury to reduce the likelihood of neurocognitive deficits. Phase II studies suggest a strong benefit for HA-WBRT. Many of the recently closed and currently open cooperative group trials have extensive translational components as part of the studies. It is the hope that biomarkers may be able to predict which patients are likely to develop neurocognitive decline and which ones will not, even in the presence of WBRT. These types of study will allow clinicians to personalize the WBRT and SRS treatment strategies for the patients they see.

Conflict of Interests

In addition to being a practicing Radiation Oncologist, Dr. Khuntia serves as the Vice-President of Medical Affairs at Varian Medical Systems, a leading manufacturer of radiation oncology hardware and software.

Acknowledgments

The author would like to offer special thanks to Minesh Mehta, MD, at the University of Maryland, Wolfgang Tomé, Ph.D., from Albert Einstein University, Vinai Gondi, MD, from Cadence Health, and Paul Brown, MD, from MD Anderson Cancer center for their years of support in the advancement of technology and delivery of radiation for the care of patients with brain metastases.

References

[1] P. Y. Wen, P. M. Black, and J. S. Loeffler, "Metastatic brain cancer," in *Cancer: Principles and Practice of Oncology*, V. DeVita, S. Hellman, and S. A. Rosenberg, Eds., pp. 2655–2670, Lippincott, WIlliams, & Wilkins, Philadelphia, Pa, USA, 6th edition, 2001.

[2] A. D. Norden, P. Y. Wen, and S. Kesari, "Brain metastases," *Current Opinion in Neurology*, vol. 18, no. 6, pp. 654–661, 2005.

[3] M. P. Mehta and I. Tremont-Lukats, "Radiosurgery for single and mutliple brain metastasis," in *Intracranial Metastases: Current Management Strategies*, R. Sawaya, Ed., pp. 139–164, Futura Division, Blackwell Publishing, Malden, Mass, USA, 2004.

[4] H. Greenberg, W. F. Chandler, and H. M. Sandler, "Brain metastases," in *Brain Tumors*, H. Greenberg, W. F. Chandler, and H. M. Sandler, Eds., pp. 299–317, Oxford University Press, New York, NY, USA, 1999.

[5] M. L. Sundermeyer, N. J. Meropol, A. Rogatko, H. Wang, and S. J. Cohen, "Changing patterns of bone and brain metastases in patients with colorectal cancer," *Clinical Colorectal Cancer*, vol. 5, no. 2, pp. 108–113, 2005.

[6] J. D. Johnson and B. Young, "Demographics of brain metastasis," *Neurosurgery Clinics of North America*, vol. 7, no. 3, pp. 337–344, 1996.

[7] B. P. Yawn, P. C. Wollan, C. Schroeder, L. Gazzuola, and M. Mehta, "Temporal and gender-related trends in brain metastases from lung and breast cancer," *Minnesota Medicine*, vol. 86, no. 12, pp. 32–37, 2003.

[8] H. J. Mamon, B. Y. Yeap, P. A. Jänne et al., "High risk of brain metastases in surgically staged IIIA non-small-cell lung cancer patients treated with surgery, chemotherapy, and radiation," *Journal of Clinical Oncology*, vol. 23, no. 7, pp. 1530–1537, 2005.

[9] J. S. Barnholtz-Sloan, A. E. Sloan, F. G. Davis, F. D. Vigneau, P. Lai, and R. E. Sawaya, "Incidence proportions of brain metastases in patients diagnosed (1973 to 2001) in the Metropolitan Detroit Cancer Surveillance System," *Journal of Clinical Oncology*, vol. 22, no. 14, pp. 2865–2872, 2004.

[10] L. J. Schouten, J. Rutten, H. A. M. Huveneers, and A. Twijnstra, "Incidence of brain metastases in a cohort of patients with carcinoma of the breast, colon, kidney, and lung and melanoma," *Cancer*, vol. 94, no. 10, pp. 2698–2705, 2002.

[11] K. Slimane, F. Andre, S. Delaloge et al., "Risk factors for brain relapse in patients with metastatic breast cancer," *Annals of Oncology*, vol. 15, no. 11, pp. 1640–1644, 2004.

[12] T. J. Kruser, S. T. Chao, P. Elson et al., "Multidisciplinary management of colorectal brain metastases: a retrospective study," *Cancer*, vol. 113, no. 1, pp. 158–165, 2008.

[13] S. Zimm, G. L. Wampler, D. Stablein, T. Hazra, and H. F. Young, "Intracerebral metastases in solid-tumor patients: natural history and results of treatment," *Cancer*, vol. 48, no. 2, pp. 384–394, 1981.

[14] J. T. Sundström, H. Minn, K. K. Lertola, and E. Nordman, "Prognosis of patients treated for intracranial metastases with whole-brain irradiation," *Annals of Medicine*, vol. 30, no. 3, pp. 296–299, 1998.

[15] R. A. Patchell, P. A. Tibbs, J. W. Walsh et al., "A randomized trial of surgery in the treatment of single metastases to the brain," *The New England Journal of Medicine*, vol. 322, no. 8, pp. 494–500, 1990.

[16] V. Gondi, W. A. Tomé, and M. P. Mehta, "Why avoid the hippocampus? A comprehensive review," *Radiotherapy and Oncology*, vol. 97, no. 3, pp. 370–376, 2010.

[17] B. Borgelt, R. Gelber, M. Larson, F. Hendrickson, T. Griffin, and R. Roth, "Ultra-rapid high dose irradiation schedules for the palliation of brain metastases: final results of the first two studies by the radiation therapy oncology group," *International Journal of Radiation Oncology, Biology, Physics*, vol. 7, no. 12, pp. 1633–1638, 1981.

[18] A. R. Harwood and W. J. Simpson, "Radiation therapy of cerebral metastases: a randomized prospective clinical trial," *International Journal of Radiation Oncology Biology Physics*, vol. 2, no. 11-12, pp. 1091–1094, 1977.

[19] J. M. Kurtz, R. Gelber, L. W. Brady, R. J. Carella, and J. S. Cooper, "The palliation of brain metastases in a favorable patient population: a randomized clinical trial by the radiation therapy oncology group," *International Journal of Radiation Oncology, Biology, Physics*, vol. 7, no. 7, pp. 891–895, 1981.

[20] B. Borgelt, R. Gelber, S. Kramer et al., "The palliation of brain metastases: final results of the first two studies by the radiation therapy oncology group," *International Journal of Radiation Oncology, Biology, Physics*, vol. 6, no. 1, pp. 1–9, 1980.

[21] M. Chatani, T. Teshima, K. Hata, and T. Inoue, "Prognostic factors in patients with brain metastases from lung carcinoma," *Strahlentherapie und Onkologie*, vol. 162, no. 3, pp. 157–161, 1986.

[22] C. Haie-Meder, B. Pellae-Cosset, A. Laplanche et al., "Results of a randomized clinical trial comparing two radiation schedules in the palliative treatment of brain metastases," *Radiotherapy and Oncology*, vol. 26, no. 2, pp. 111–116, 1993.

[23] M. Chatani, Y. Matayoshi, N. Masaki, and T. Inoue, "Radiation therapy for brain metastases from lung carcinoma. Prospective randomized trial according to the level of lactate dehydrogenase," *Strahlentherapie und Onkologie*, vol. 170, no. 3, pp. 155–161, 1994.

[24] K. J. Murray, C. Scott, H. M. Greenberg et al., "A randomized phase III study of accelerated hyperfractionation versus standard in patients with unresected brain metastases: A report of the Radiation Therapy Oncology Group (RTOG) 9104," *International Journal of Radiation, Oncology, Biology, Physics*, vol. 39, no. 3, pp. 571–574, 1997.

[25] D. Khuntia, P. Brown, J. Li, and M. P. Mehta, "Whole-brain radiotherapy in the management of brain metastasis," *Journal of Clinical Oncology*, vol. 24, no. 8, pp. 1295–1304, 2006.

[26] L. Gaspar, C. Scott, M. Rotman et al., "Recursive Partitioning Analysis (RPA) of prognostic factors in three Radiation Therapy Oncology Group (RTOG) brain metastases trials," *International Journal of Radiation Oncology Biology Physics*, vol. 37, no. 4, pp. 745–751, 1997.

[27] C. M. Sperduto, Y. Watanabe, J. Mullan et al., "A validation study of a new prognostic index for patients with brain metastases: the Graded Prognostic Assessment," *Journal of Neurosurgery*, vol. 109, pp. 87–89, 2008.

[28] P. W. Sperduto, S. T. Chao, P. K. Sneed et al., "Diagnosis-specific prognostic factors, indexes, and treatment outcomes for patients with newly diagnosed brain metastases: a multi-institutional analysis of 4,259 patients," *International Journal of Radiation Oncology Biology Physics*, vol. 77, no. 3, pp. 655–661, 2010.

[29] E. Shaw, C. Scott, L. Souhami et al., "Single dose radiosurgical treatment of recurrent previously irradiated primary brain tumors and brain metastases: final report of RTOG protocol 90-05," *International Journal of Radiation Oncology Biology Physics*, vol. 47, no. 2, pp. 291–298, 2000.

[30] D. W. Andrews, C. B. Scott, P. W. Sperduto et al., "Whole brain radiation therapy with or without stereotactic radiosurgery

boost for patients with one to three brain metastases: phase III results of the RTOG 9508 randomised trial," *The Lancet*, vol. 363, no. 9422, pp. 1665–1672, 2004.

[31] H. Aoyama, H. Shirato, M. Tago et al., "Stereotactic radiosurgery plus whole-brain radiation therapy vs stereotactic radiosurgery alone for treatment of brain metastases: a randomized controlled trial," *The Journal of the American Medical Association*, vol. 295, no. 21, pp. 2483–2491, 2006.

[32] J. H. Chao, R. Phillips, and J. J. Nickson, "Roentgen-ray therapy of cerebral metastases," *Cancer*, vol. 7, no. 4, pp. 682–689, 1954.

[33] S. E. Order, S. Hellman, C. F. von Essen, and M. M. Kligerman, "Improvement in quality of survival following whole-brain irradiation for brain metastasis," *Radiology*, vol. 91, no. 1, pp. 149–153, 1968.

[34] L. R. Coia, "The role of radiation therapy in the treatment of brain metastases," *International Journal of Radiation Oncology Biology Physics*, vol. 23, no. 1, pp. 229–238, 1992.

[35] R. A. Patchell and W. F. Regine, "The rationale for adjuvant whole brain radiation therapy with radiosurgery in the treatment of single brain metastases," *Technology in Cancer Research and Treatment*, vol. 2, no. 2, pp. 111–115, 2003.

[36] E. Arbit, M. Wroński, M. Burt, and J. H. Galicich, "The treatment of patients with recurrent brain metastases. A retrospective analysis of 109 patients with nonsmall cell lung cancer," *Cancer*, vol. 76, no. 5, pp. 765–773, 1995.

[37] M. Mehta, "The dandelion effect: treat the whole lawn or weed selectively?" *Journal of Clinical Oncology*, vol. 29, no. 2, pp. 121–124, 2011.

[38] M. D. Prados, C. B. Scott, M. Rotman et al., "Influence of bromodeoxyuridine radiosensitization on malignant glioma patient survival: a retrospective comparison of survival data from the Northern California Oncology Group (NCOG) and Radiation Therapy Oncology Group Trials (RTOG) for glioblastoma multiforme and anaplastic astrocytoma," *International Journal of Radiation Oncology Biology Physics*, vol. 40, no. 3, pp. 653–659, 1998.

[39] M. D. Prados, W. Seiferheld, H. M. Sandler et al., "Phase III randomized study of radiotherapy plus procarbazine, lomustine, and vincristine with or without BUdR for treatment of anaplastic astrocytoma: final report of RTOG 9404," *International Journal of Radiation Oncology Biology Physics*, vol. 58, no. 4, pp. 1147–1152, 2004.

[40] C. Arslan, O. Dizdar, and K. Altundag, "Chemotherapy and biological treatment options in breast cancer patients with brain metastasis: an update," *Expert Opinion on Pharmacotherapy*, vol. 15, no. 12, pp. 1643–1658, 2014.

[41] C. Nieder, W. Berberich, and K. Schnabel, "Tumor-related prognostic factors for remission of brain metastases after radiotherapy," *International Journal of Radiation Oncology Biology Physics*, vol. 39, no. 1, pp. 25–30, 1997.

[42] J. Ellerhorst, E. Strom, E. Nardone, and I. McCutcheon, "Whole brain irradiation for patients with metastatic melanoma: a review of 87 cases," *International Journal of Radiation Oncology Biology Physics*, vol. 49, no. 1, pp. 93–97, 2001.

[43] A. S. Mahmoud-Ahmed, P. A. Kupelian, C. A. Reddy, and J. H. Suh, "Brain metastases from gynecological cancers: factors that affect overall survival," *Technology in Cancer Research and Treatment*, vol. 1, no. 4, pp. 305–310, 2002.

[44] A. S. Mahmoud-Ahmed, J. H. Suh, S.-Y. Lee, R. L. Crownover, and G. H. Barnett, "Results of whole brain radiotherapy in patients with brain metastases from breast cancer: a retrospective study," *International Journal of Radiation Oncology Biology Physics*, vol. 54, no. 3, pp. 810–817, 2002.

[45] J. C. Buchsbaum, J. H. Suh, S.-Y. Lee, M. A. Chidel, J. F. Greskovich, and G. H. Barnett, "Survival by radiation therapy oncology group recursive partitioning analysis class and treatment modality in patients with brain metastases from malignant melanoma: a retrospective study," *Cancer*, vol. 94, no. 8, pp. 2265–2272, 2002.

[46] R. A. Patchell, P. A. Tibbs, W. F. Regine et al., "Postoperative radiotherapy in the treatment of single metastases to the brain: a randomized trial," *Journal of the American Medical Association*, vol. 280, no. 17, pp. 1485–1489, 1998.

[47] A. Bezjak, J. Adam, R. Barton et al., "Symptom response after palliative radiotherapy for patients with brain metastases," *European Journal of Cancer*, vol. 38, no. 4, pp. 487–496, 2002.

[48] L. M. DeAngelis, J.-Y. Delattre, and J. B. Posner, "Radiation-induced dementia in patients cured of brain metastases," *Neurology*, vol. 39, no. 6, pp. 789–796, 1989.

[49] V. W. Stieber, J. D. Bourland, W. A. Tomé, and M. P. Mehta, "Gentlemen (and ladies), choose your weapons: gamma Knife vs. linear accelerator radiosurgery," *Technology in Cancer Research and Treatment*, vol. 2, no. 2, pp. 79–85, 2003.

[50] E. M. Thomas, R. A. Popple, X. Wu et al., "Comparison of plan quality and delivery time between volumetric arc therapy (rapidarc) and gamma knife radiosurgery for multiple cranial metastases," *Neurosurgery*, vol. 75, no. 4, pp. 409–418, 2014.

[51] D. Kondziolka, A. Patel, L. D. Lunsford, A. Kassam, and J. C. Flickinger, "Stereotactic radiosurgery plus whole brain radiotherapy versus radiotherapy alone for patients with multiple brain metastases," *International Journal of Radiation Oncology Biology Physics*, vol. 45, no. 2, pp. 427–434, 1999.

[52] E. L. Chang, J. S. Wefel, K. R. Hess et al., "Neurocognition in patients with brain metastases treated with radiosurgery or radiosurgery plus whole-brain irradiation: a randomised controlled trial," *The Lancet Oncology*, vol. 10, no. 11, pp. 1037–1044, 2009.

[53] M. Kocher, R. Soffietti, U. Abacioglu et al., "Adjuvant whole-brain radiotherapy versus observation after radiosurgery or surgical resection of one to three cerebral metastases: results of the EORTC 22952-26001 study," *Journal of Clinical Oncology*, vol. 29, no. 2, pp. 134–141, 2011.

[54] S. G. Soltys, J. R. Adler, J. D. Lipani et al., "Stereotactic radiosurgery of the postoperative resection cavity for brain metastases," *International Journal of Radiation Oncology Biology Physics*, vol. 70, no. 1, pp. 187–193, 2008.

[55] A. Narayana and K. Chan, "A phase II trial of stereotactic radiosurgery boost following surgical resection for solitary brain metastases," *Journal of Clinical Oncology*, vol. 24, p. 71S, 2006, ASCO Abstract.

[56] W. S. Chang, H. Y. Kim, J. W. Chang, Y. G. Park, and J. H. Chang, "Analysis of radiosurgical results in patients with brain metastases according to the number of brain lesions: is stereotactic radiosurgery effective for multiple brain metastases?" *Journal of Neurosurgery*, vol. 113, supplement, pp. 73–78, 2010.

[57] G. Sze, M. Mehta, C. J. Schultz et al., *Radiologic Response Evaluation of Brain Metastases: Uni-Dimensional (1D) W.H.O. Recist vs. Bi-Dimensional (2D) Or 3-Dimensional (3D) Criteria*, American Society of Clinical Oncology, 2001.

[58] M. P. Mehta, M. N. Tsao, T. J. Whelan et al., "The American Society for Therapeutic Radiology and Oncology (ASTRO)

evidence-based review of the role of radiosurgery for brain metastases," *International Journal of Radiation Oncology Biology Physics*, vol. 63, no. 1, pp. 37–46, 2005.

[59] C. J. Langer and M. P. Mehta, "Current management of brain metastases, with a focus on systemic options," *Journal of Clinical Oncology*, vol. 23, no. 25, pp. 6207–6219, 2005.

[60] A. Pirzkall, J. Debus, F. Lohr et al., "Radiosurgery alone or in combination with whole-brain radiotherapy for brain metastases," *Journal of Clinical Oncology*, vol. 16, no. 11, pp. 3563–3569, 1998.

[61] S. R. Smalley, E. R. Laws Jr., J. R. O'Fallon, E. G. Shaw, and M. F. Schray, "Resection for solitary brain metastasis. Role of adjuvant radiation and prognostic variables in 229 patients," *Journal of Neurosurgery*, vol. 77, no. 4, pp. 531–540, 1992.

[62] P. B. Chougule, M. Burton-Williams, S. Saris et al., "Randomized treatment of brain metastasis with gamma knife radiosurgery, whole brain radiotherapy or both," *International Journal of Radiation Oncology, Biology, Physics*, vol. 48, no. 3, supplement 1, p. 114, 2000.

[63] R. Manon, A. O'Neill, J. Knisely et al., "Phase II trial of radiosurgery for one to three newly diagnosed brain metastases from renal cell carcinoma, melanoma, and sarcoma: an eastern cooperative oncology group study (E 6397)," *Journal of Clinical Oncology*, vol. 23, no. 34, pp. 8870–8876, 2005.

[64] W. F. Regine, J. L. Huhn, R. A. Patchell et al., "Risk of symptomatic brain tumor recurrence and neurologic deficit after radiosurgery alone in patients with newly diagnosed brain metastases: results and implications," *International Journal of Radiation Oncology, Biology, Physics*, vol. 52, no. 2, pp. 333–338, 2002.

[65] C. A. Meyers, J. A. Smith, A. Bezjak et al., "Neurocognitive function and progression in patients with brain metastases treated with whole-brain radiation and motexafin gadolinium: results of a randomized phase III trial," *Journal of Clinical Oncology*, vol. 22, no. 1, pp. 157–165, 2004.

[66] G. E. Sheline, W. M. Wara, and V. Smith, "Therapeutic irradiation and brain injury," *International Journal of Radiation Oncology Biology Physics*, vol. 6, no. 9, pp. 1215–1228, 1980.

[67] A. J. van der Kogel, "Radiation-induced damage in the central nervous system: an interpretation of target cell responses," *British Journal of Cancer*, vol. 53, no. 7, pp. 207–217, 1986.

[68] E. Boldrey and G. Sheline, "Delayed transitory clinical manifestations after radiation treatment of intracranial tumors," *Acta Radiologica: Therapy, Physics, Biology*, vol. 5, pp. 5–10, 1966.

[69] S. Kramer, "The hazards of therapeutic irradiation of the central nervous system," *Clinical neurosurgery*, vol. 15, pp. 301–318, 1968.

[70] T. E. Schultheiss, L. E. Kun, K. K. Ang, and L. C. Stephens, "Radiation response of the central nervous system," *International Journal of Radiation Oncology, Biology, Physics*, vol. 31, no. 5, pp. 1093–1112, 1995.

[71] B. M. Chow, Y. Q. Li, and C. S. Wong, "Radiation-induced apoptosis in the adult central nervous system is p53-dependent," *Cell Death and Differentiation*, vol. 7, no. 8, pp. 712–720, 2000.

[72] W. Cammer, "Effects of TNFα on immature and mature oligodendrocytes and their progenitors in vitro," *Brain Research*, vol. 864, no. 2, pp. 213–219, 2000.

[73] J. R. Crossen, D. Garwood, E. Glatstein, and E. A. Neuwelt, "Neurobehavioral sequelae of cranial irradiation in adults: a review of radiation-induced encephalopathy," *Journal of Clinical Oncology*, vol. 12, no. 3, pp. 627–642, 1994.

[74] P. C. Burger, M. S. Mahaley Jr., L. Dudka, and F. S. Vogel, "The morphologic effects of radiation administered therapeutically for intracranial gliomas. A postmortem study of 25 cases," *Cancer*, vol. 44, no. 4, pp. 1256–1272, 1979.

[75] M. L. Monje and T. Palmer, "Radiation injury and neurogenesis," *Current Opinion in Neurology*, vol. 16, no. 2, pp. 129–134, 2003.

[76] W. Peißner, M. Kocher, H. Treuer, and F. Gillardon, "Ionizing radiation-induced apoptosis of proliferating stem cells in the dentate gyrus of the adult rat hippocampus," *Molecular Brain Research*, vol. 71, no. 1, pp. 61–68, 1999.

[77] R. DeLong, H. Friedman, N. Friedman, K. Gustafson, and J. Oakes, "Methylphenidate in neuropsychological sequelae of radiotherapy and chemotherapy of childhood brain tumors and leukemia," *Journal of Child Neurology*, vol. 7, no. 4, pp. 462–463, 1992.

[78] M. A. Weitzner, C. A. Meyers, and A. D. Valentine, "Methylphenidate in the treatment of neurobehavioral slowing associated with cancer and cancer treatment," *Journal of Neuropsychiatry and Clinical Neurosciences*, vol. 7, no. 3, pp. 347–350, 1995.

[79] C. A. Meyers, M. A. Weitzner, A. D. Valentine, and V. A. Levin, "Methylphenidate therapy improves cognition, mood, and function of brain tumor patients," *Journal of Clinical Oncology*, vol. 16, no. 7, pp. 2522–2527, 1998.

[80] S. A. Lipton, "Erythropoietin for neurologic protection and diabetic neuropathy," *The New England Journal of Medicine*, vol. 350, no. 24, pp. 2516–2517, 2004.

[81] H. Ehrenreich, M. Hasselblatt, C. Dembowski et al., "Erythropoietin therapy for acute stroke is both safe and beneficial," *Molecular Medicine*, vol. 8, no. 8, pp. 495–505, 2002.

[82] J. P. Knisely, A. C. de Lotbiniere, N. C. de Lanerolle, and M. L. Brines, "Randomized trial of erythropoietin as a central nervous system radioprotectant," *International Journal of Radiation Oncology, Biology, Physics*, vol. 60, no. 1, supplement, pp. S343–S344, 2004.

[83] M. Hossain and C. S. Wong, "Abstract 3125: erythropoietin improves learning and memory impairment after whole brain irradiation," *Cancer Research*, vol. 64, p. 724, 2004.

[84] S. R. Rapp, R. Rosdhal, R. D'Agostino et al., "Phase II study of *Ginkgo biloba* in irradiated brain tumor patients: effect on cognitive function, quality of life, and mood," *Journal of Neuro-Oncology*, vol. 109, no. 2, pp. 357–363, 2012.

[85] M. Sano, C. Ernesto, R. G. Thomas et al., "A controlled trial of selegiline, alpha-tocopherol, or both as treatment for Alzheimer's disease," *The New England Journal of Medicine*, vol. 336, no. 17, pp. 1216–1222, 1997.

[86] A. S. Chan, M.-C. Cheung, S. C. Law, and J. H. Chan, "Phase II study of alpha-tocopherol in improving the cognitive function of patients with temporal lobe radionecrosis," *Cancer*, vol. 100, no. 2, pp. 398–404, 2004.

[87] C. L. Armstrong, K. Gyato, A. W. Awadalla, R. Lustig, and Z. A. Tochner, "A critical review of the clinical effects of therapeutic irradiation damage to the brain: the roots of controversy," *Neuropsychology Review*, vol. 14, no. 1, pp. 65–86, 2004.

[88] S. B. Wolbach, "The pathologic history of chronic X-ray dermatitis & early X-ray carcinoma," *The Journal of Medical Research*, vol. 21, pp. 415–449, 1909.

[89] C. Belka, W. Budach, R. D. Kortmann, and M. Bamberg, "Radiation induced CNS toxicity—molecular and cellular mechanisms," *British Journal of Cancer*, vol. 85, no. 9, pp. 1233–1239, 2001.

[90] E. Lancelot and M. F. Beal, "Glutamate toxicity in chronic neurodegenerative disease," *Progress in Brain Research*, vol. 116, pp. 331–347, 1998.

[91] J. Kornhuber, M. Weller, K. Schoppmeyer, and P. Riederer, "Amantadine and memantine are NMDA receptor antagonists with neuroprotective properties," *Journal of Neural Transmission Supplementum*, no. 43, pp. 91–104, 1994.

[92] J. W. Pellegrini and S. A. Lipton, "Delayed administration of memantine prevents N-methyl-D-aspartate receptor-mediated neurotoxicity," *Annals of Neurology*, vol. 33, no. 4, pp. 403–407, 1993.

[93] H. S. V. Chen, J. W. Pellegrini, S. K. Aggarwal et al., "Open-channel block of N-methyl-D-aspartate (NMDA) responses by memantine: therapeutic advantage against NMDA receptor-mediated neurotoxicity," *The Journal of Neuroscience*, vol. 12, no. 11, pp. 4427–4436, 1992.

[94] H.-S. V. Chen and S. A. Lipton, "Mechanism of memantine block of NMDA-activated channels in rat retinal ganglion cells: uncompetitive antagonism," *The Journal of Physiology*, vol. 499, no. 1, pp. 27–46, 1997.

[95] H.-S. V. Chen, Y. F. Wang, P. V. Rayudu et al., "Neuroprotective concentrations of the N-methyl-D-aspartate open-channel blocker memantine are effective without cytoplasmic vacuolation following post-ischemic administration and do not block maze learning or long-term potentiation," *Neuroscience*, vol. 86, no. 4, pp. 1121–1132, 1998.

[96] J.-M. Orgogozo, A.-S. Rigaud, A. Stöffler, H.-J. Möbius, and F. Forette, "Efficacy and safety of memantine in patients with mild to moderate vascular dementia: a randomized, placebo-controlled trial (MMM 300)," *Stroke*, vol. 33, no. 7, pp. 1834–1839, 2002.

[97] G. Wilcock, H. J. Möbius, and A. Stöffler, "A double-blind, placebo-controlled multicentre study of memantine in mild to moderate vascular dementia (MMM500)," *International Clinical Psychopharmacology*, vol. 17, no. 6, pp. 297–305, 2002.

[98] M. P. Mehta and I. Robbins, "Improvement in cognitive function with memantine in patient with PCNSL and cognitive impairment after therapy," *Personal Communication*. In press.

[99] P. D. Brown, S. Pugh, N. N. Laack et al., "Memantine for the prevention of cognitive dysfunction in patients receiving whole-brain radiotherapy: a randomized, double-blind, placebo-controlled trial," *Neuro-Oncology*, vol. 15, no. 10, pp. 1429–1437, 2013.

[100] D. D. Correa, J. Satagopan, R. E. Baser et al., "APOE polymorphisms and cognitive functions in patients with brain tumors," *Neurology*, vol. 83, no. 4, pp. 320–327, 2014.

[101] M. Kalm, E. Abel, P. Wasling et al., "Neurochemical evidence of potential neurotoxicity after prophylactic cranial irradiation," *International Journal of Radiation Oncology, Biology, Physics*, vol. 89, no. 3, pp. 607–614, 2014.

[102] V. Gondi, B. P. Hermann, M. P. Mehta, and W. A. Tomé, "Hippocampal dosimetry predicts neurocognitive function impairment after fractionated stereotactic radiotherapy for benign or low-grade adult brain tumors," *International Journal of Radiation Oncology, Biology, Physics*, vol. 85, no. 2, pp. 348–354, 2013.

[103] A. Ghia, W. A. Tomé, S. Thomas et al., "Distribution of brain metastases in relation to the hippocampus: implications for neurocognitive functional preservation," *International Journal of Radiation Oncology Biology Physics*, vol. 68, no. 4, pp. 971–977, 2007.

[104] V. Gondi, W. A. Tome, J. Marsh et al., "Estimated risk of perihippocampal disease progression after hippocampal avoidance during whole-brain radiotherapy: safety profile for RTOG 0933," *Radiotherapy and Oncology*, vol. 95, no. 3, pp. 327–331, 2010.

[105] V. Gondi, R. Tolakanahalli, M. P. Mehta et al., "Hippocampal-sparing whole-brain radiotherapy: a 'how-to' technique using helical tomotherapy and linear accelerator-based intensity-modulated radiotherapy," *International Journal of Radiation Oncology Biology Physics*, vol. 78, no. 4, pp. 1244–1252, 2010.

[106] V. Gondi, S. L. Pugh, W. A. Tome et al., "Preservation of memory with conformal avoidance of the hippocampal neural stem-cell compartment during whole-brain radiotherapy for brain metastases (RTOG 0933): a phase II multi-institutional trial," *Journal of Clinical Oncology*, vol. 32, no. 34, pp. 3810–3816, 2014.

5

Developing Attention: Behavioral and Brain Mechanisms

Michael I. Posner,[1] **Mary K. Rothbart,**[1] **Brad E. Sheese,**[2] **and Pascale Voelker**[1]

[1] *University of Oregon, Eugene, OR 97403, USA*
[2] *Illinois Wesleyan University, Bloomington, IL 61701, USA*

Correspondence should be addressed to Michael I. Posner; mposner@uoregon.edu and Mary K. Rothbart; maryroth@uoregon.edu

Academic Editor: Jan Gläscher

Brain networks underlying attention are present even during infancy and are critical for the developing ability of children to control their emotions and thoughts. For adults, individual differences in the efficiency of attentional networks have been related to neuromodulators and to genetic variations. We have examined the development of attentional networks and child temperament in a longitudinal study from infancy (7 months) to middle childhood (7 years). Early temperamental differences among infants, including smiling and laughter and vocal reactivity, are related to self-regulation abilities at 7 years. However, genetic variations related to adult executive attention, while present in childhood, are poor predictors of later control, in part because individual genetic variation may have many small effects and in part because their influence occurs in interaction with caregiver behavior and other environmental influences. While brain areas involved in attention are present during infancy, their connectivity changes and leads to improvement in control of behavior. It is also possible to influence control mechanisms through training later in life. The relation between maturation and learning may allow advances in our understanding of human brain development.

1. Introduction

Few life changes are as dramatic as the development that occurs between infancy and elementary school, with locomotion, language, and voluntary control as the most obvious behavior changes. We also know that the brain changes in size, connectivity, and synaptic density during this period. What is least explored is exactly how these brain changes support behavioral change. Our research traces the development of attention networks that support the mechanisms of self-regulation, allowing children to control their emotions and behavior. In this paper, we first outline the connection between attention and self-regulation. In the next section, we examine measurement of individual differences in attention in adults. The heart of the paper summarizes the relation of early temperament (7 months) to later temperament and attention (age: 7 years). We show how changes in mechanisms of control over this period relate to genes and to the environment provided by the caregiver. Finally, we examine training studies that influence some of the same brain connections that change during development.

During infancy, the caregiver provides much of the child's regulation. Soothing by holding and rocking or by orienting of attention is a common practice for control of distress. Holding supports the child's focus on the external physical environment, and the social world of interaction with the caregiver provides a means of raising and lowering sensory stimulation [1]. This process allows the caregiver to accommodate the child to controls appropriate for a given culture and environment. External controls on arousal, distress, and sensory input eventually become internalized as toddlers come to control their own emotional and cognitive levels through self-regulation. Success in the development of self-regulation has many advantages for the child's future.

2. Attention and Self-Regulation

Starting at about the age of 3 years, parents can answer questions about their children's ability to control their own emotions and behavior. For example, caregivers answer questions such as when playing alone, how often is your child distracted? How often does your child look immediately when you point? The answers are aggregated to form scales measuring attention focusing, inhibitory control, low intensity pleasure, and perceptual sensitivity. These are summarized in a higher order scale called effortful control (EC) [1]. Effortful control has been studied in relation to many important achievements of childhood. For example, empathy is strongly related to EC, with children high in EC showing greater empathy [1].

Imaging the human brain has revealed brain networks related to specific aspects of attention, including obtaining and maintaining the alert state, orienting to sensory stimuli, and resolving conflict among competing responses [2, 3].

The alerting network is modulated by the brain's norepinephrine system and involves major nodes in frontal and parietal cortex. The alert state is critical to high level performance. Phasic changes in alertness can be produced by the presentation of a signal warning of an impending target. This leads to a rapid change from a resting state to one of increased receptivity to the target. The orienting network interacts with sensory systems to improve the priority of information relevant to task performance. The orienting network exerts much of the control over other brain networks during infancy and early childhood [4, 5].

The executive network is involved in resolving competing actions in tasks where there is conflict. The executive network includes the anterior cingulate cortex, anterior insula, areas of the midprefrontal cortex, and the underlying striatum [2, 3]. Regulation occurs by enhancing activity in networks related to our goals and inhibiting activity in conflicting networks. These controls operate through long connections between the nodes of the executive network and cognitive and emotional areas of the frontal and posterior brain. In this way, the executive network is important for voluntary control and self-regulation [6, 7]. As mentioned previously, effortful control is a higher order temperamental factor assessing self-regulation that is obtained from parent report questionnaires [1]. In childhood, performance on conflict related cognitive tasks is positively related to measures of children's effortful control [1]. During childhood and in adulthood, effortful control and self-regulation are correlated with school performance and with indices of life success, including health, income, and successful human relationships [8, 9]. In Figure 1 we illustrate our hypothesis about the relative influence of the attention networks on self control in early development.

3. Measuring Individual Differences in Executive Attention

There are individual differences in the efficiency of each of the three attentional networks. The attention network test (ANT) was devised as a means of measuring these differences [10]. The task requires the person to press one key if a central arrow points to the left and another if it points to the right. Conflict is introduced by having surrounding flanker arrows point in either the same (congruent) or the opposite (incongruent) direction. Cues presented prior to the target provide information on where or when the target

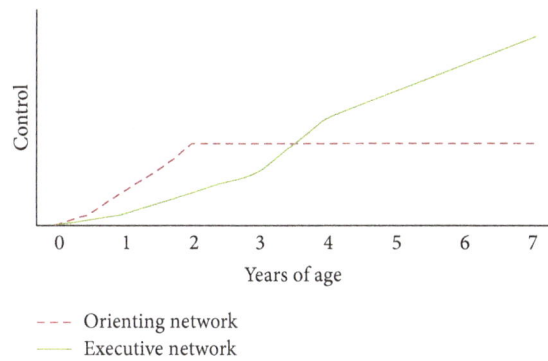

FIGURE 1: Hypothesized relation between brain attention networks and dominance of control between birth and adulthood.

will occur. Three scores are computed that are related to the performance of each individual in alerting, orienting, and executive control. In our work, we have used the ANT to examine the efficiency of brain networks underlying attention [10]. A children's version of this test is very similar to the adult test but replaces the arrows with animal figures [11].

Studies have shown moderate reliability of conflict scores and lower reliability for the orienting and alerting scores [12], but recent revisions of the ANT provide better measures of orienting and alerting that may improve these results [13]. The attentional networks involve different cortical brain areas [14], and scores on the ANT are related to distinct white matter pathways [15] as well as structural differences in cortical thickness [16]. Thus, the attentional networks show independent anatomy and connectivity. However, the ANT and its various revisions show significant interaction among networks [13, 17]. The networks communicate and work together in many situations, even though their anatomy is mostly distinct. The dorsal part of the anterior cingulate cortex (ACC) is involved in the regulation of conflict in cognitive tasks, while the more ventral part of the cingulate is involved in regulation of emotion [6, 18]. One way to examine regulation is to image the structural connections of different parts of the cingulate using diffusion tensor imaging (DTI). This form of imaging traces diffusion of water molecules in long myelinated fibers and provides a means of examining the physical connections present in the brain. DTI studies have shown that the dorsal (cognitive) part of the ACC is connected primarily to parietal and frontal lobes, while the ventral (emotional) part of the ACC has strong connections to subcortical limbic areas [19].

The executive attention network also includes the underlying striatum and adjacent areas of the midprefrontal cortex. There is evidence that the anterior insula is involved particularly in switching between tasks [20], while adjacent midprefrontal cortex is important during complex decision making [21]. Comparative anatomical studies point to important differences in the evolution of cingulate connectivity between nonhuman primates and humans. Anatomical studies show the great expansion of white matter, which has increased more in recent evolution than has the neocortex itself [22]. One type of projection cell called the von Economo neuron is found only in the anterior cingulate and a related area of the anterior insula, two brain areas that are active together even when the person is resting and not performing a task [23, 24]. It is thought that von Economo neurons are important in communication between the cingulate and other brain areas. This neuron is not present at all in monkeys and there are many more such neurons present in adult humans than in great apes. Moreover, there is some evidence that the frequency of the neuron increases in development between infancy and later childhood [23].

4. Principles of Development of Self-Regulation

4.1. Control Systems. Some individuals have stronger activations and connectivity in brain areas related to self-regulation than others and are thus better able to exercise the various functions of self-regulation. Moreover, childhood assessments of self-regulation as measured by the ability to delay rewards [25] and by observer reports of the child's self-control predict performance as adults [9]. How do these individual differences arise?

To investigate this question, we have run a longitudinal study of the development of attentional networks starting in infancy (7 months), and now the children are 7 years of age. In our longitudinal study, we have found evidence of both behavioral and neural mechanisms of self-regulation. The earliest form of regulation appeared to come from the orienting rather than the executive network (see Figure 1). This conclusion was based on several findings. First, parent reports of their child's orienting to the environment were correlated with reports of their positive and negative affect [5, 26]. Moreover, direct tests were done on the role of orienting to novel objects in soothing. Distressed infants, while orienting was maintained showed a reduction in overt signs of distress, but the distress returned when orienting was broken [27].

Second, in our longitudinal study, we observed that children of 7 months showed evidence of behavior related to self-regulation. When confronted with novel objects, some infants oriented for a long period before reaching towards them. This tendency for a cautious reach was positively correlated with the number of anticipations infants made in orienting to a repetitive sequence of visual events [26]. This striking observation showed that infants fast in orienting to repetitive visual sequences, often in anticipation of the object, exercised stronger controls over whether and when they reached for an object by moving toward it slowly. At the time, we did not know if rapid orienting to repetitive locations was controlled by the executive or the orienting network, but because ours was a longitudinal study, we later found that anticipations at 7 months were more closely related to orienting at 4 years than to the executive network [4]. We have confirmed this idea in our examination of the children at 7 years. The time that infants examined a novel toy before starting to reach for it, their overall latency to reach, and the total time they examined the toy were all significantly correlated with the orienting network at the age of 7.

Lewkowicz and Hansen-Tift [29] provided dramatic evidence that orienting can demonstrate a high level of discrimination in attending environmental events. Infants prior to 6 months and after one year oriented primarily to the eyes of pictures of faces, just as adults do, but between 6 and 12 months when language learning was prominent they were more likely to orient to the mouth. This shows direction of attention by orienting, but it does not let us know whether this control also involves the executive network.

Resting state brain imaging data have also indicated that the orienting system shows greater connectivity during infancy than do brain areas associated with the executive network [30]. In the first week of life, resting state data show an important hub in infants in the ACC/SMA area. Although this hub shows the largest number of connections in infancy, [31]; it is much less strongly activated than hubs found in adults. Fransson et al. also report a hub area in the left parietal lobe during infancy. Menon [32] indicates a substantial increase in connectivity between core areas of what he calls the salience network, but we term the executive network (ACC and insula) between childhood (7–9 years) and adulthood (20 years). He finds no significant developmental change in connections between lateral parietal and frontal areas (orienting network). This imaging data provides further support for the slow development of control from the ACC and the early dominance of the orienting network (see Figure 1). In addition, most hubs for information processing in the infant brain are closely related to sensory and motor brain areas [31, 32] that would be targets of the orienting network. While there is evidence that some of these resting state studies may be confounded by greater movement that can occur in younger subjects [33], in our view it seems unlikely that this artifact will change the conclusions discussed above. However, the problems that occur with any one imaging method support the approach of relating different imaging methods [34] and establishing their connections to behavior as we have sought to do in this paper.

We think the relatively slow development of long-term connections to distant brain areas allows the executive network to provide more control at later ages. Indeed direct evidence on this point came from a study of 7-month-old infants viewing visual displays [35]. They oriented longer when the display was in error [36] and this behavior was associated with a set of scalp electrodes at the frontal midline which localized to the anterior cingulate, an important node of the executive network. However, the lack of connections of the cingulate to remote areas was shown in an inability to use error to control behavior. The most frequent adult response to a self-made error is to slow down during the next trial [37]. We traced the evidence for this kind of control and found that it emerged around three years of age and was not found at the age of 2 [38].

The growing behavioral influence of executive control is shown in an MRI study of the resolution of conflict in the flanker task [39] by 725 children from 4 to 21 years [40]. From 4 to 8 years, ability to resolve conflict was positively related to the size of the anterior cingulate. Beyond the age of 8, the connectivity of the anterior cingulate was correlated with the speed of response. The brain and behavior correlation in early childhood was similar to our finding that flanker task performance showed a specific improvement in children of 6–8 years, but reaction time in the task continued to improve until adulthood [11]. A different study [41] used emotional responses to a fear face during a rewarded go/no-go task to explore the role of brain connectivity in regulation of the amygdala from the ventral anterior cingulate. They found a significant correlation between age and the efficiency of connectivity between the ventral ACC and amygdala during the presentation of fear faces.

The major change in connectivity took place between ages 5 and 7. These studies show substantial overlap in age between development of purely cognitive and emotional self-regulation. We do not believe that the flanker task and emotional go/no-go tasks index the full development of control mechanisms, since more complex tasks may show longer periods of development, but these studies do provide strong confirmation of growing executive system control during early childhood and the close correspondence of brain connectivity to behavioral performance.

In summary, we have discovered a transition between the brain networks responsible for control at 7 months and those at 4 years and later. At 7 months, control involves the orienting network, but by 4 years the executive network dominates. Behaviorally, the orienting network involves sensory stimulation and we believe this is a major reason why infants show control by external stimulation provided by caregivers and sensory events. We also do not believe that control through orienting ends with the preschool transition. We view adults as having dual control. Looking away from disturbing or highly arousing events is clearly a major coping strategy in adults. However, the growing influence of executive control allows the person's internally controlled goals to become generally dominant.

4.2. Control of Emotion and Cognition. The structural connectivity of the anterior cingulate reflects its control functions [6, 18]. The ventral portion of the ACC and adjacent orbital frontal cortex connects mainly to limbic regions and its function is thought to be related to control of emotions [6, 42]. The more dorsal part of the cingulate connects more strongly to cortical areas in the frontal and parietal lobes. This is reflected in evidence of increased connectivity between the dorsal ACC and auditory areas when attending to speech, while a switch to visual input is reflected in increased connectivity between the ACC and occipital lobe [43]. The developmental data cited in the last section [40, 41] support separate functions for the ventral and dorsal ACC and show they both develop strongly between 5 and 8 years of age.

We want to understand the origins of cognitive and emotional controls in the developing infant and child. As mentioned previously, one important function of the anterior cingulate is to play a role in the detection of error [44]. Error detection found at 7 months may reflect either the cognitive or emotional aspects related to the violation of expectation. However, studies using high density scalp EEG at 4–6 years suggest that the resolution of conflict at 4

TABLE 1: Correlations between temperament measures at 7 months and ANT scores at 7 years.

| IBQ | ANT at age 7 | | | | | |
| | Alerting | | Orienting | | Conflict | |
	r	P	r	P	r	P
Perceptual sensitivity	.56*	.02	.18	.51	−.07	.79
Duration of orienting	.55*	.03	.01	.96	.03	.91
Approach	.29	.27	.76*	.001	−.28	.29
Soothability	.13	.63	.56*	.024	−.24	.37
Smiling and laughter	.17	.53	.06	.84	−.60*	.015
Vocal reactivity	.24	.37	.20	.47	−.64*	.007
Cuddliness	−.04	.88	.08	.77	−.64*	.008
Positive Affect (higher order)	.43	.10	.38	.15	−.58*	.019

*denotes $P < .05$.

years involves primarily ventral areas of the cingulate [45, 46]; later more dorsal areas become involved. In addition, studies of resting state MRI in infancy suggest a node in the midprefrontal cortex adjacent to emotional parts of the ACC [30]. This evidence fits with the idea that emotional control develops more quickly than cognitive control during early life, although there is strong overlap in their later development. While the data are not completely clear on this point, it is of obvious importance to parents in fostering the development of these controls.

5. Early Temperament Predicts Later Control

By temperament, we mean constitutionally based individual differences in reactivity and self-regulation [47]. At 7 months, we used a parent report scale, the Infant Behavior Questionnaire (IBQ), which heavily weighs reactive responses of the infant, although it does provide a measure of orienting that involves an early control network.

5.1. Predicting Attention Networks. We found surprisingly high and significant correlations between temperament measures at 7 months and performance on the attention network test at 7 years. Our surprise reflects the fact that these correlations are found over an extended time course during which there is considerable neural maturation and they also involve parent report during infancy and behavior in a cognitive reaction time task (ANT) during childhood. These correlations must be regarded as tentative, however, since they involve only sixteen of the seventy infants who remained in the study when the ANT was measured at 7 years of age. The small remaining sample is partly self-selected (some loss resulting from moving away may have been involuntary) from the larger number of infants involved at 7 months.

Separate aspects of temperament were related to each of the attention networks. For a correlation matrix, see Table 1, and in what follows we report significant correlations. Infants' perceptual sensitivity to the environment (.56) and duration of orienting (.55) were correlated with ANT scores of the alerting network at the age of 7 years. While we did not predict that parent ratings of orienting would be related to the alerting network rather than the orienting network, this may reflect dependence of orienting on alertness during infancy when sleep occupies so much of the day.

Infant approach behavior (.76) and soothability (.56) as rated by parents were correlated with ANT scores for the orienting network at the age of 7. As we have seen previously, orienting as reported by parents and measured in the laboratory can be used to control emotional reactivity in infancy, and this aspect seems to predict the skill of taking in sensory information later in life. Soothability as reported by the parent may reflect both the child's propensity and the parent's skill. This could mean that the parents' ability to provide emotional soothing to the child is an important determinant of cognition via the orienting network.

The scales of infant smiling and laughter (−.60), vocal reactivity (−.64), and cuddliness (−.64) were negatively correlated with the ability to resolve conflict and, in addition, the higher order factor of positive affect that contains these scales was also negatively correlated with ANT conflict at 7 years. Multiple regression indicates that these factors could account for about 50 percent of the variance in the difference between reaction time in incongruent and congruent flankers.

In addition, negative affect measured in infancy is correlated with the total errors found in the ANT at the age of 7. It is interesting that positive affect was related to the speed of the children's response, which may largely reflect the efficiency of white matter connections [40], while negative affect predicted the errors that arise due to competition from the incompatible flankers.

Many older ideas of temperament are based on stability between childhood and adults traits. However, Rothbart and Derryberry [47] suggested that we should expect temperament to change as new neural systems come on line. They recognize that there is stability, but change is be expected as neural systems and connections are established. A number of the temperament correlations between infancy and childhood in the previous literature support the ability to predict control in children from infant emotion. Putnam et al. [48] found that positive emotion in infancy is related to later parent reports of their child's effortful control and that infant surgery (smiling and laughter and approach) predicted high effortful control in toddlers. Komsi et al. [49] also found that infant smiling and laughter predicted effortful control in children when they were 5 years old. In addition, the overall orienting measure in infancy predicted 7-year-old soothability, effortful control, and interest. Thus, both ANT cognitive tests and parent reported effortful control support the relation of early reactive emotion in infancy to control systems of childhood.

The correlations found between parent reported temperament at 7 months and ANT performance at 7 years were as high or higher than those found between temperament at the two ages. It is possible these high correlations are due to the unique nature of the 16 families who persisted from 7 months to 7 years. Comparison of those infants who remained in the study until the age of 7 with those who dropped out did not reveal any striking differences, although there was some evidence that the parents continuing with the study were more committed to timely submission of questionnaires

TABLE 2: Relating attention networks to dominant modulators and relevant genes.

Network	Modulator	Genes
Alerting	Norepinephrine	ADRA2A
		NET
Orienting	Acetylcholine	CHRNA4 APOE
Executive	Dopamine	DRD4, DAT1, and COMT
		MAOA, DBH
	Serotonin	TPH2, 5HTT

This table is adapted from Green et al., 2008 [28].

than those who dropped out. Moreover, we found neither significant demographic nor behavioral differences between the 16 persistent families and those who were involved at 7 years but not at 7 months.

However, the 16 children who had participated at 7 months were faster in ANT performance than the new recruits. Since faster speed of responding is frequently related to better overall performance, this finding suggests that the 16 children who persisted from time 1 were relatively high performing children. This effect was probably not due to practice, since a direct comparison of performance on the ANT at the age of 7 of children who had also taken the test at the age of 6 and those who had not practiced it previously showed no differences in speed. The speed differences may have reflected recruitment of lower SES families at the age of 7 years than we had previously recruited or other unknown characteristics of the persistent families. A more interesting possibility is that early positive emotional reactivity reflects a particularly predictive feature of child behavior. One possible mechanism for the strong influence of early positive emotion on later control is that more reactive children in infancy come to control their positive emotions more strongly and that this transfers to cognitive control as measured by the ANT.

5.2. Role of Genetic Variation. We have pursued two strategies to help understand how genes are related to the individual efficiency of attention networks. One approach involves adults and uses the association of attentional networks with particular neuromodulators. These associations have led to identification of candidate genes that relate to each network. The results were summarized by Green et al. [28] and are shown in Table 2. A number of other results have qualified the view of Green et al. somewhat. It seems clear that serotonin as well as dopamine can influence the executive attention network [50] and that there are interactions between dopaminergic and cholinergic genes at the molecular level that modify the degree of independence between them [51]. Nonetheless, the scheme in Table 2 provides a degree of organization and prediction that is often lacking in studies of genetic influences on cognition and behavior.

In our longitudinal study, we examined genetic variation in twelve genes that had been related to attention in adult studies (see Table 2 and [52]). The children had been evaluated when they were 7 months old, and genotyping took place when they returned to the laboratory at 18–20 months. We also genotyped all of the children at 7 years. We compared the results at two ages to be sure of high replication of our classifications. We found supportive evidence for some of the genes discussed in Table 2. The COMT gene was related to number of anticipatory looks at 7 and 18 months [53]. The DRD4 7 repeat allele was not related to our attention measures in infancy or among toddlers but did relate to effortful control at the age of 4 [54]; [55]. This discontinuity likely reflected the change in networks of control from orienting to executive control that we found between 2 and 4 years of age.

In addition, parenting quality at 18–20 months was examined through observation of caregiver-child interactions in which the children played with toys in the presence of one of their caregivers. Raters reviewed videotapes of the caregiver-child interaction and rated the parent on five dimensions of parenting quality according to a schedule developed by NICHD [56]: support, autonomy, stimulation, lack of hostility, and confidence in the child. According to their scores, parents were divided at the median into two groups: one showing a higher quality of parenting and the other a lower quality.

We reported previously [57] that variations in COMT, SNAP25, CHRNA4, and DRD4 were related to elements of emotion during infancy (age of 7 months) and during the toddler period (18–20 months). COMT was related to positive affect including smiling and laughter and high intensity pleasure at 7 months. SNAP 25 was related to negative affect, mainly distress at 7 and 18 months. CHRNA 4 was related to effortful control at 18 months and DRD4 was related to sensation seeking at 18 months.

However, unlike the temperament measure of emotion to which the genetic variations were often related, there was little evidence that the genetic variations by themselves predicted behavior at 7 years on the ANT. A recent meta-analysis of studies of twins indicates that genetic factors that influence cognition at one point are largely different from those at later times (see, [58], p. 19). Our studies suggest that shifts in control networks and gene X environment interactions may be among the reasons for this lack of prediction in early life.

6. Simulating Development through Training

Development in the title of this paper refers both to changes in attention through the natural maturation of the brain and to our efforts to develop attention through training. Below we discuss similarities between the development of white matter pathways between infancy and childhood with the influence of meditation training on adult white matter. It is our hope that efforts to train attention may help us to better understand the process of infant and child development. As we have seen, parenting influences this development, and we hope to better inform parents about what can be done to improve this process.

The developmental process through which attention networks and self-regulation mature is very complex. There are many changes in brain structure and function that may be related to the multiple changes in voluntary behavior in early development. As discussed previously, an increasingly popular way of tracing brain changes is to use resting state MRI to characterize how the brain changes in development [30, 59]. In our recent work, we have tried to relate behavior changes to changes in functional connectivity [4].

The changes in connectivity during development reported in resting state MRI studies involve functional connectivity based upon correlations between BOLD activity in separated brain areas. There is also evidence of actual physical changes in the white matter thought to underlie these correlations [34]. Our recent training work with adults using diffusion tensor imaging (DTI) has uncovered white matter changes that have some similarities to those found in development. Changes in connectivity surrounding the ACC have been shown to be critical to improved reaction time in the flanker task during development [40]. Training adults might thus allow us to uncover how connections developing during childhood support the changes in self- control between infancy and adulthood.

During development, there is a large change in the physical connections between brain areas. The density of axons in pathways connecting brain areas increases, followed by an increase in the myelin sheath that surrounds the axons and provides insulation. Together, these changes result in more efficient connections [60]. Fractional anisotropy (FA) is the main index for measuring the integrity of white matter fibers when using DTI.

In our work, we studied FA in college students before and after a form of mindfulness meditation called integrated body mind training (IBMT) in comparison to a control group given the same amount of relaxation training. We found clear improvement in the executive attention network after only five days of training [61]. After two to four weeks of training, we found significantly greater change in FA following meditation training than following the relaxation training control. This change was found in all white matter tracts surrounding the ACC, but not in other brain areas [62]. This was particularly striking because one of these pathways, the anterior corona radiata, has previously been reported to be correlated with individual differences in the ability to resolve conflict using the ANT [15].

These alterations in FA could originate from several factors, such as changes in myelination, axon density, axonal membrane integrity, axon diameter, intravoxel coherence of fiber orientation, and others. Several DTI studies have examined axial diffusivity (AD) and radial diffusivity (RD), the most important indices associated with FA, to understand the mechanisms of FA change [63, 64]. Changes in AD are associated with axon morphological changes, with lower AD value indicating higher axonal density. In contrast, RD relates to the myelin insulation surrounding the axons. Decreases in RD imply increased myelination, while increases represent demyelination.

In our study [65], we investigated AD and RD where FA indicated that integrity of white matter fibers was enhanced in the IBMT group more than control group. We found that after two weeks of training, there were changes in axonal density but not in myelination. In some areas, these changes in axonal density were correlated with improved mood and affect as measured by self-report. After 4 weeks of training, we found evidence of myelination changes. Our studies also found that reaction time in the attention network test and specifically the executive network was improved more by IBMT training than by the control. Since the developmental changes in childhood first involve changes in axonal density and only later myelination, our training may provide changes that are somewhat similar to those found in development. If so, it might be possible to use training to study how physical changes in connectivity alter aspects of control, including reaction time, control of affect, stress reduction, and other changes found with training.

7. Future Directions

The work described here has barely begun to open up a window on the dramatic changes in control between infancy and childhood. Some changes in the size and connectivity of brain areas related to cognitive and emotional control have been documented by resting state and task related MRI methods. More work needs to be done in these areas.

Moreover, we are at the very beginning of understanding the joint role of caregivers and genetic endowment in creating the brain networks of control. We have clear evidence that parents can rate in infancy critical aspects of their child's emotions and behavior that seem to exert influence on the development of control and in some cases we know that specific genes are important, but confirmation and extension of these ideas are critical to understand what environments and experiences will foster self-regulation. Research is starting to provide ideas as to the epigenetic basis of environmental influence [66, 67], and these need to be expanded and applied to the development of self-regulation.

It is important that specific interventions can influence connectivity even into adulthood. More studies are needed to connect brain changes fostered by learning with specific behavioral gains and then to determine if there are more than superficial similarities between adult development through specific interventions and the changes that take place in early child development. We think the small scale and tentative steps outlined in this report point the way to the types of studies that can lead to improved understanding of how specific brain changes support the child's developing abilities for self-regulation.

Conflict of Interests

The authors declare that there is no conflict of interests regarding the publication of this paper.

Acknowledgment

This research was supported in part by NIH Grant HD 060563 to the Georgia State University.

References

[1] M. K. Rothbart, *Becoming Who We Are: Temperament, Personality and Development*, Guilford Press, New York, NY, USA, 2011.

[2] M. I. Posner and S. E. Petersen, "The attention system of the human brain," *Annual Review of Neuroscience*, vol. 13, pp. 25–42, 1990.

[3] S. E. Petersen and M. I. Posner, "The attention system of the human brain: 20 years after," *Annual Review of Neuroscience*, vol. 35, pp. 73–89, 2012.

[4] M. I. Posner, M. K. Rothbart, B. E. Sheese, and P. Voelker, "Control networks and neuromodulators of early development," *Developmental Psychology*, vol. 48, no. 3, pp. 827–835, 2012.

[5] M. K. Rothbart, B. E. Sheese, M. R. Rueda, and M. I. Posner, "Developing mechanisms of self-regulation in early life," *Emotion Review*, vol. 3, no. 2, pp. 207–213, 2011.

[6] G. Bush, P. Luu, and M. I. Posner, "Cognitive and emotional influences in anterior cingulate cortex," *Trends in Cognitive Sciences*, vol. 4, no. 6, pp. 215–222, 2000.

[7] S. A. Sheth, M. K. Mian, S. R. Patel et al., "Human dorsal anterior cingulate cortex neurons mediate ongoing behavioural adapation," *Nature*, vol. 488, no. 7410, pp. 218–221, 2012.

[8] P. Checa and M. R. Rueda, "Behavioral and brain measures of executive attention and school competence in late childhood," *Developmental Neuropsychology*, vol. 36, no. 8, pp. 1018–1032, 2011.

[9] T. E. Moffitt, L. Arseneault, D. Belsky et al., "A gradient of childhood self-control predicts health, wealth, and public safety," *Proceedings of the National Academy of Sciences of the United States of America*, vol. 108, no. 7, pp. 2693–2698, 2011.

[10] J. Fan, B. D. McCandliss, T. Sommer, A. Raz, and M. I. Posner, "Testing the efficiency and independence of attentional networks," *Journal of Cognitive Neuroscience*, vol. 14, no. 3, pp. 340–347, 2002.

[11] M. R. Rueda, J. Fan, B. D. McCandliss et al., "Development of attentional networks in childhood," *Neuropsychologia*, vol. 42, no. 8, pp. 1029–1040, 2004.

[12] J. W. MacLeod, M. A. Lawrence, M. M. McConnell, G. A. Eskes, R. M. Klein, and D. I. Shore, "Appraising the ANT: psychometric and theoretical considerations of the Attention Network Test," *Neuropsychology*, vol. 24, no. 5, pp. 637–651, 2010.

[13] J. Fan, X. Gu, K. G. Guise et al., "Testing the behavioral interaction and integration of attentional networks," *Brain and Cognition*, vol. 70, no. 2, pp. 209–220, 2009.

[14] J. Fan, B. D. McCandliss, J. Fossella, J. I. Flombaum, and M. I. Posner, "The activation of attentional networks," *NeuroImage*, vol. 26, no. 2, pp. 471–479, 2005.

[15] S. Niogi, P. Mukherjee, J. Ghajar, and B. D. McCandliss, "Individual differences in distinct components of attention are linked to anatomical variations in distinct white matter tracts," *Frontiers in Neuroanatomy*, vol. 4, article 2, 2010.

[16] L. T. Westlye, H. Grydeland, K. B. Walhovd, and A. M. Fjell, "Associations between regional cortical thickness and attentional networks as measured by the attention network test," *Cerebral Cortex*, vol. 21, no. 2, pp. 345–356, 2011.

[17] A. Callejas, J. Lupiáñez, and P. Tudela, "The three attentional networks: on their independence and interactions," *Brain and Cognition*, vol. 54, no. 3, pp. 225–227, 2004.

[18] M. Beckmann, H. Johansen-Berg, and M. F. S. Rushworth, "Connectivity-based parcellation of human cingulate cortex and its relation to functional specialization," *The Journal of Neuroscience*, vol. 29, no. 4, pp. 1175–1190, 2009.

[19] M. I. Posner, B. E. Sheese, Y. Odludaş, and Y. Tang, "Analyzing and shaping human attentional networks," *Neural Networks*, vol. 19, no. 9, pp. 1422–1429, 2006.

[20] K. Supekar and V. Menon, "Developmental maturation of a dynamic causal control signals in higher-order cognition: a neurocognitive network model," *PLOS Computational Biology*, vol. 8, no. 2, Article ID e1002374, 2012.

[21] T. E. Behrens, "Neural mechanisms underlying human choice in frontal cortex," in *Neurosciences and the Human Person: New on Human Activities*, W. Singer S, Dehaene, and A. Batro, Eds., Pontifical Academy of Sciences, Vatican, 2014.

[22] K. Zilles, "Evolution of the human brain and comparative syto and receptor architecture," in *From Monkey Brain to Human Brain*, S. Dehaene, J. R. Duhamel, M. D. Rizzolatti, and G. Rizzolatti, Eds., pp. 41–56, MIT Press, Cambridge Mass, 2005.

[23] J. M. Allman, K. K. Watson, N. A. Tetreault, and A. Y. Hakeem, "Intuition and autism: a possible role for Von Economo neurons," *Trends in Cognitive Sciences*, vol. 9, no. 8, pp. 367–373, 2005.

[24] N. U. F. Dosenbach, D. A. Fair, F. M. Miezin et al., "Distinct brain networks for adaptive and stable task control in humans," *Proceedings of the National Academy of Sciences of the United States of America*, vol. 104, no. 26, pp. 11073–11078, 2007.

[25] B. J. Casey, L. H. Somerville, I. H. Gotlib et al., "Behavioral and neural correlates of delay of gratification 40 years later," *Proceedings of the National Academy of Sciences of the United States of America*, vol. 108, no. 36, pp. 14998–15003, 2011.

[26] B. E. Sheese, M. K. Rothbart, M. I. Posner, L. K. White, and S. H. Fraundorf, "Executive attention and self-regulation in infancy," *Infant Behavior and Development*, vol. 31, no. 3, pp. 501–510, 2008.

[27] C. Harman, M. K. Rothbart, and M. I. Posner, "Distress and attention interactions in early infancy," *Motivation and Emotion*, vol. 21, no. 1, pp. 27–43, 1997.

[28] A. E. Green, M. R. Munafò, C. G. DeYoung, J. A. Fossella, J. Fan, and J. R. Gray, "Using genetic data in cognitive neuroscience: from growing pains to genuine insights," *Nature Reviews Neuroscience*, vol. 9, no. 9, pp. 710–720, 2008.

[29] D. J. Lewkowicz and A. M. Hansen-Tift, "Infants deploy selective attention to the mouth of a talking face when learning speech," *Proceedings of the National Academy of Sciences of the United States of America*, vol. 109, no. 5, pp. 1431–1436, 2012.

[30] W. Gao, H. Zhu, K. S. Giovanello et al., "Evidence on the emergence of the brain's default network from 2-week-old to 2-year-old healthy pediatric subjects," *Proceedings of the National Academy of Sciences of the United States of America*, vol. 106, no. 16, pp. 6790–6795, 2009.

[31] P. Fransson, U. Åden, M. Blennow, and H. Lagercrantz, "The functional architecture of the infant brain as revealed by resting-state fMRI," *Cerebral Cortex*, vol. 21, no. 1, pp. 145–154, 2011.

[32] V. Menon, "Developmental pathways to function brain networks: emerging principles," *Trends in Cognitive Science*, vol. 17, no. 12, pp. 627–639, 2013.

[33] J. D. Power, K. A. Barnes, A. Z. Snyder, B. L. Schlaggar, and S. E. Petersen, "Spurious but systematic correlations in functional connectivity MRI networks arise from subject motion," *NeuroImage*, vol. 59, no. 3, pp. 2142–2154, 2012.

[34] L. Q. Uddin, K. S. Supekar, S. Ryali, and V. Menon, "Dynamic reconfiguration of structural and functional connectivity across core neurocognitive brain networks with development," *The Journal of Neuroscience*, vol. 31, no. 50, pp. 18578–18589, 2011.

[35] A. Berger, G. Tzur, and M. I. Posner, "Infant brains detect arithmetic errors," *Proceedings of the National Academy of Sciences of the United States of America*, vol. 103, no. 33, pp. 12649–12653, 2006.

[36] K. Wynn, "Addition and subtraction by human infants," *Nature*, vol. 358, no. 6389, pp. 749–750, 1992.

[37] P. M. A. Rabbitt, "Three kinds of error-signalling responses in a serial choice task," *Quarterly Journal of Experimental Psychology*, vol. 20, no. 2, pp. 179–188, 1968.

[38] L. B. Jones, M. K. Rothbart, and M. I. Posner, "Development of executive attention in preschool children," *Developmental Science*, vol. 6, no. 5, pp. 498–504, 2003.

[39] B. A. Eriksen and C. W. Eriksen, "Effects of noise letters upon the identification of a target letter in a nonsearch task," *Perception & Psychophysics*, vol. 16, no. 1, pp. 143–149, 1974.

[40] A. M. Fjell, K. B. Walhovd, T. T. Brown et al., "Multi modal imaging of the self-regulating brain," *Proceedings of the National Academy of Sciences of the United States of America*, vol. 109, no. 48, pp. 19620–19625, 2012.

[41] S. B. Perlman and K. A. Pelphrey, "Developing connections for affective regulation: age-related changes in emotional brain connectivity," *Journal of Experimental Child Psychology*, vol. 108, no. 3, pp. 607–620, 2011.

[42] A. Etkin, T. Egner, D. M. Peraza, E. R. Kandel, and J. Hirsch, "Resolving emotional conflict: a role for the rostral anterior cingulate cortex in modulating activity in the amygdala," *Neuron*, vol. 51, no. 6, pp. 871–882, 2006.

[43] S. Crottaz-Herbette and V. Menon, "Where and when the anterior cingulate cortex modulates attentional response: combined fMRI and ERP evidence," *Journal of Cognitive Neuroscience*, vol. 18, no. 5, pp. 766–780, 2006.

[44] S. Dehaene, M. I. Posner, and D. M. Tucker, "Localization of a neural system for error detection and compensation," *Psychological Science*, vol. 5, no. 5, pp. 303–305, 1994.

[45] M. R. Rueda, M. K. Rothbart, B. D. McCandliss, L. Saccomanno, and M. I. Posner, "Training, maturation, and genetic influences on the development of executive attention," *Proceedings of the National Academy of Sciences of the United States of America*, vol. 102, no. 41, pp. 14931–14936, 2005.

[46] M. R. Rueda, P. Checa, and L. M. Cómbita, "Enhanced efficiency of the executive attention network after training in preschool children: immediate changes and effects after two months," *Developmental Cognitive Neuroscience*, vol. 2, supplement 1, pp. S192–S204, 2012.

[47] M. K. Rothbart and D. Derryberry, "Development of individual differences in temperament," in *Advances in Developmental Psychology*, M. E. Lamb and A. L. Brown, Eds., pp. 37–86, Erlbaum, Hillsdale, NJ, USA, 1981.

[48] S. P. Putnam, M. K. Rothbart, and M. A. Gartstein, "Homotypic and heterotypic continuity of fine-grained temperament during infancy, toddlerhood, and early childhood," *Infant and Child Development*, vol. 17, no. 4, pp. 387–405, 2008.

[49] N. Komsi, K. Räikkönen, A.-K. Pesonen et al., "Continuity of temperament from infancy to middle childhood," *Infant Behavior and Development*, vol. 29, no. 4, pp. 494–508, 2006.

[50] M. Reuter, U. Ott, D. Vaitl, and J. Hennig, "Impaired executive control is associated with a variation in the promoter region of the tryptophan hydroxylase 2 gene," *Journal of Cognitive Neuroscience*, vol. 19, no. 3, pp. 401–408, 2007.

[51] S. A. Markett, C. Montag, and M. Reuter, "The association between dopamine DRD2 polymorphisms and working memory capacity is modulated by a functional polymorphism on

the nicotinic receptor gene CHRNA4," *Journal of Cognitive Neuroscience*, vol. 22, no. 9, pp. 1944–1954, 2010.

[52] B. E. Sheese, P. M. Voelker, M. K. Rothbart, and M. I. Posner, "Parenting quality interacts with genetic variation in dopamine receptor D4 to influence temperament in early childhood," *Development and Psychopathology*, vol. 19, no. 4, pp. 1039–1046, 2007.

[53] P. Voelker, B. E. Sheese, M. K. Rothbart, and M. I. Posner, "Variations in catechol-*O*-methyltransferase gene interact with parenting to influence attention in early development," *Neuroscience*, vol. 164, no. 1, pp. 121–130, 2009.

[54] B. E. Sheese, M. K. Rothbart, P. Voelker, and M. I. Posner, "The dopamine receptor D4 gene 7 repeat allele interacts with parenting quality to predict Effortful Control in four-year-old children," *Child Development Research*, vol. 2012, Article ID 863242, 6 pages, 2012.

[55] H. J. Smith, H. I. Sheikh, M. W. Dyson et al., "Parenting and child *DRD4* genotype interact to predict children's early emerging Effortful Control," *Child Development*, vol. 83, no. 6, pp. 1932–1944, 2012.

[56] NICHD Early Child Care Research Network, "The NICHD Study of Early Child Care: a comprehensive longitudinal study of young children's lives," ERIC Document Reproduction Service ED3530870, 1993.

[57] B. E. Sheese, P. Voelker, M. I. Posner, and M. K. Rothbart, "Genetic variation influences on the early development of reactive emotions and their regulation by attention," *Cognitive Neuropsychiatry*, vol. 14, no. 4-5, pp. 332–355, 2009.

[58] E. M. Tucker-Drob and D. A. Briley, "Continuity of genetic and environmental influences on cognition across the life span: a meta analysis of longitudinal twin and adoption studies," *Psychological Bulletin*, 2014.

[59] D. A. Fair, A. L. Cohen, J. D. Power et al., "Functional brain networks develop from a "local to distributed" organization," *PLoS Computational Biology*, vol. 5, no. 5, Article ID e1000381, 2009.

[60] C. Lebel, M. Gee, R. Camicioli, M. Wieler, W. Martin, and C. Beaulieu, "Diffusion tensor imaging of white matter tract evolution over the lifespan," *NeuroImage*, vol. 60, no. 1, pp. 340–352, 2012.

[61] Y.-Y. Tang, Y. Ma, J. Wang et al., "Short-term meditation training improves attention and self-regulation," *Proceedings of the National Academy of Sciences of the United States of America*, vol. 104, no. 43, pp. 17152–17156, 2007.

[62] Y.-Y. Tang, Q. Lu, X. Geng, E. A. Stein, Y. Yang, and M. I. Posner, "Short-term meditation induces white matter changes in the anterior cingulate," *Proceedings of the National Academy of Sciences of the United States of America*, vol. 107, no. 35, pp. 15649–15652, 2010.

[63] I. J. Bennett, D. J. Madden, C. J. Vaidya, D. V. Howard, and J. H. Howard Jr., "Age-related differences in multiple measures of white matter integrity: a diffusion tensor imaging study of healthy aging," *Human Brain Mapping*, vol. 31, no. 3, pp. 378–390, 2010.

[64] A. Z. Burzynska, C. Preuschhof, L. Bäckman et al., "Age-related differences in white matter microstructure: region-specific patterns of diffusivity," *NeuroImage*, vol. 49, no. 3, pp. 2104–2112, 2010.

[65] Y.-Y. Tang, Q. Lu, M. Fan, Y. Yang, and M. I. Posner, "Mechanisms of white matter changes induced by meditation," *Proceedings of the National Academy of Sciences of the United States of America*, vol. 109, no. 26, pp. 10570–10574, 2012.

[66] N. Provencal, M. J. Suderman, C. Guillemin et al., "The signature of maternal rearing in the methylome in rhesus macaque prefrontal cortex and T cells," *The Journal of Neuroscience*, vol. 32, no. 44, pp. 15626–15642, 2012.

[67] N. Provençal, M. J. Suderman, F. Vitaro, M. Szyf, and R. E. Tremblay, "Childhood chronic physical aggression associates with adult cytokine levels in plasma," *PLos ONE*, vol. 8, no. 7, Article ID e69481, 2013.

6

Structure-Function Relationships behind the Phenomenon of Cognitive Resilience in Neurology: Insights for Neuroscience and Medicine

David Rudrauf

Laboratory of Functional Imaging (LIF), INSERM U678S, 91 Boulevard de l'Hôpital, 75013 Paris, France

Correspondence should be addressed to David Rudrauf; david.rudrauf@gmail.com

Academic Editor: Jan Gläscher

The phenomenon of cognitive resilience, that is, the dynamical preservation of normal functions despite neurological disorders, demonstrates that cognition can be highly robust to devastating brain injury. Here, cognitive resilience is considered across a range of neurological conditions. Simple computational models of structure-function relationships are used to discuss hypotheses about the neural mechanisms of resilience. Resilience expresses functional redundancies in brain networks and suggests a process of dynamic rerouting of brain signals. This process is underlined by a global renormalization of effective connectivity, capable of restoring information transfer between spared brain structures via alternate pathways. Local mechanisms of synaptic plasticity mediate the renormalization at the lowest level of implementation, but it is also driven by top-down cognition, with a key role of self-awareness in fostering resilience. The presence of abstraction layers in brain computation and networking is hypothesized to account for the renormalization process. Future research directions and challenges are discussed regarding the understanding and control of resilience based on multimodal neuroimaging and computational neuroscience. The study of resilience will illuminate ways by which the brain can overcome adversity and help inform prevention and treatment strategies. It is relevant to combating the negative neuropsychological impact of aging and fostering cognitive enhancement.

1. Introduction

In neurology, one is often faced with a relative disconnect between the clinical presentation and the underlying neuropathology or amount of brain damage [1–10]. One observes cognitive functions that appear to be relatively preserved in spite of damage to brain systems that one would expect to be normally implicated in these functions. Patients with similar brain damage or neurological disorder often show quite different neuropsychological profiles, with different evolutions, and cliniconeuropathological relationships are characterized by a strong between-subject variability [2, 9].

Part of this between-subject variability is underlined by static intrinsic differences in structure-function relationships in different subjects, for example, the lateralization of language, which makes certain patients less susceptible than others to certain impairments for similar brain damage, for example, damage to the left hemisphere, in which many critical functions for language are most often implemented in humans. Part of the variability is related to processes of recovery that are more or less efficient across individuals following similar initial impairments due to similar brain damage. But more generally, as reviewed below, quite often patients with severe, extensive, irreversible bilateral brain damage show preserved functions or eventually recover in full or in part over time in a dynamic manner from brain damage causing initial cognitive impairments, sometimes very rapidly, often after a long and painful struggle. Thus, in cases in which brain structures cannot be rebuilt through structural plasticity, there are within-subject changes in structure-function relationships manifested in the recovery of cognition.

In other words, there is a phenomenon of "cognitive resilience" to brain damage. Resilience, generally speaking, is the ability of a system to resist dynamically a perturbation or adverse condition that challenges the integrity of its normal operation and to preserve function as a result in reference to some initial design or normative functional standards. The concept of resiliency is relevant to and employed in many scientific domains, including material science, biology, ecology, economy, computer and network science, psychiatry, and neurology. In computer networking, which is relevant here: "resilience is the ability of the network to provide and maintain an acceptable level of service in the face of various faults and challenges to normal operation" (see ResiliNets initiative: https://wiki.ittc.ku.edu/resilinets). It features disruption tolerance; that is, "the ability of a system to tolerate disruptions in connectivity among its components", and fault tolerance against failure, that is, "the occurrence of an event in which an entity does not meet its in-service functional and performance requirements or expectations" (see https://wiki.ittc.ku.edu/resilinets_wiki). According to this model (see ResiliNets Architecture), which has broad applications, resilient systems will integrate expectations about the inevitability of fault, understand (or possess a model of) normal operations, expect adverse events and respond to adverse events and conditions. Resilience can build upon a strategy involving detection, defense, remediation and recovery mechanisms, based on a control loop.

In the context of the present paper, I am discussing the resilience of cognition despite brain damage that results in extensive and irreversible destruction and disconnection of the structural backbone of the brain. In neurological resilience, the overall architecture of information processing and control that underlies normal cognition appears to resist the structural perturbations that challenge its integrity. There is an apparent decoupling between structure and function, in relation to normative anatomical expectations or previous structure-function relationships, which allows the brain to recover function in a manner that is compatible with normal functional or cognitive standards.

The phenomenon of cognitive resiliency is pervasive and observed across a large spectrum of neurological disorders. It is present in cases of focal and stable brain damage—even in dramatic cases of very extensive lesions (e.g., [2, 3]). Cognitive resilience is also found in cases of diffuse brain damage, both with stable lesions, for example, following traumatic brain injury [4], as well as progressive lesions, for example, neurodegenerative processes such as Alzheimer's disease [11]. Likewise it is found in dramatic developmental cases [10]. It is difficult to quantify, and the interindividual variability it introduces in neurological populations complicates our ability to understand and model neurological conditions with specificity (and thus approach treatments). It challenges the central aim of maximizing sensitivity and specificity in diagnostics, prognostics, treatment planning, treatment outcome monitoring, and more generally neurological research.

Theoretical rationale and empirical evidence [2, 3, 8, 12–15] suggest that cognitive resilience may, in part, take advantage of the existence of processing resources that are distributed across large portions of the brain and which are highly redundant. It builds upon the possibility of exploiting alternative pathways, which can be direct or indirect, for restoring information transfer and maintain cognitive functions (e.g., [13]). The notion of resilience is related to that of

"cognitive reserve" [8], an innate and acquired "reserve" of compensatory mechanisms, which can support resilience as a phenomenon and which notably appears to be correlated with premorbid, higher-order cognitive skills.

Resilience notably concerns "higher-order cognition," which entails an ensemble of psychological mechanisms and phenomena including executive functions, attention, general intelligence, and self-awareness. These form, together, a coherent functional whole that normally constitutes the core of a wakeful and willful mind in the process of conscious perception, imagination, decision-making, and action planning [12, 16, 17]. "Higher-order cognition" itself appears to be generally more resilient to damage than more specialized, modal forms of cognition, such as basic vision and audition [1, 12, 18, 19].

In this paper, I argue that beyond reflecting sheer redundancies in the brain, the phenomenon of resilience manifests degrees of freedom in anatomofunctional relationships, which in turn challenge to some extent the standard anatomofunctional framework as it traditionally supposes a strong and direct relationship between structure and function. It therefore represents a methodological challenge for functional neuroanatomy and research on biomarkers from multimodal neuroimaging.

I argue that resilience manifests mechanisms of dynamic rerouting of information streams in the brain that are necessary to maintain functional integrity in face of network structural failure. I propose a framework for understanding, modeling, and quantifying resilience in this perspective. I also argue that resilience can provide a paradigm for approaching fundamental questions about mind-brain relationships. It suggests provocative hypotheses about the mechanisms and principles underlying brain computation, including the possibility that some integrative aspects of cognition relate to the brain according to principles that are analogous to those underlying virtualization in computer and network science. It thus reopens the question of the neural code.

In the following, I first consider the phenomenon of cognitive resilience in the context of various neurological disorders, from stable focal brain damage—with an example of preserved higher-order cognition following extensive bilateral damage—to stable diffuse brain damage, using the example of disorders of consciousness, and progressive diffuse brain damage, exemplified by Alzheimer's disease. I briefly consider resilience to developmental aberrations such as hydrocephaly. I then discuss hypotheses regarding the relationships between resilience, distributed processing, and anatomofunctional dissociations. I also discuss the corollary hypothesis that the mind might relate to the brain through a pile of layers of abstraction and a process of virtualization (in the sense that these phrases have in computer and network science). I consider possible research directions and highlights challenges for understanding and controlling resilience based on multimodal neuroimaging and computational neuroscience. I conclude that resilience offers new venues for clinical and basic research, in particular with regard to preventive and clinical medicine, but also for the mitigation of aging and cognitive enhancement.

2. The Phenomenon of Cognitive Resilience to Neurological Disorders

2.1. Resilience to Developmental Aberrations: Setting the Stage. One of the most striking illustrations of the resilience of normal cognition to the presence of severely abnormal brain structures can be found in the literature on abnormal development (see [10]), which I will only briefly mention here. This literature challenges how one thinks about anatomical-functional relationships and illustrates how extreme resilience can be in certain rare developmental cases.

While genetic and environmental factors can result in extremely aberrant brain development (with dramatic morphological and structural alterations), in many cases, there is often a relative preservation of core mental abilities [10]. In a rather extreme example, a 44-year-old civil servant and father of two with relatively low intelligence, but normal social functioning, was found to have preserved mental abilities despite significant ventricular enlargement and a very thin cortical mantle due to a history of hydrocephaly [20] (Figure 1(a)). While the processes underlying neuroanatomical reorganization and recovery after brain damage remain unclear, developmental cases suggest that extremely different brains across individuals can support normal cognition. Furthermore, it is textbook knowledge and common clinical observation that age plays a critical role in resilience, since early in development when the potential for brain plasticity is highest resilience can be greater.

2.2. Resilience to Stable Focal Brain Damage. Stable, focal brain damage, which is damage encompassed by a continuous and unique lesion which can nevertheless be extensive and bilateral, can be caused by a variety of etiologies and mechanisms, ranging from ischemic or hemorrhagic strokes to surgery of tumors or epileptic foci and certain types of encephalitis, such as herpes simplex virus encephalitis. These sources of brain damage constitute the most common basis for the human lesion method ([21]; see [22, 23]).

It is well established that many higher cognitive functions do not appear to be completely and systematically disrupted by focal brain damage to the cerebral cortex [1, 2, 15, 19, 24]. In contrast, such damage can cause systematic and durable impairments in more specialized aspects of cognition, in particular in sensorimotor processing, for example, vision and audition. Impairments can also affect speech and language, for example, aphasia, or memory-laden functions, for example, the case of anterograde amnesia, which is quite a systematic syndrome following bilateral damage to the medial temporal lobe. These disorders are also susceptible to relatively systematic and sometimes permanent impairments. Working memory, decision-making, attention, and other executive functions, for example, the frontal syndromes of perseveration, may also be impaired and may engender a loss of autonomy to various degrees, more or less systematically and persistently, in particular when damage is bilateral [19, 25]. Such impairments are thought to be caused either by the disruption of modular processing in functionally specialized, cortical, and subcortical regions, or by the dissection of fiber tracts, causing disconnection syndromes (see [23, 26]). But

overall: "one sided removal of, or injury to, any area of the cerebral cortex does not abolish conscious thinking. It may change the content of awareness, interfere with voluntary acts, render less effective planned action, and deprive the patient of word symbols—but he still thinks and weeps, perhaps, at his own pitiful incapacity" [18]. Moreover, except in specific cases, higher-order cognition in its core remains generally quite robust even to extensive and bilateral focal brain damage, or recovers sometimes quite fast after the acute phase following damage onset. A striking illustration of resilience of higher-order cognition to extensive bilateral brain damage can be found in neurological cases that challenge contemporary knowledge and hypotheses about the neural substrate of self-awareness (SA).

Over the past decade, an ever-growing body of functional neuroimaging research has explored the neural basis of SA. For instance, largely based on such findings, it has recently been proposed that the anterior insula (AI) represents one of the most critical and essential substrates underlying SA in humans [27–30]. In addition, the medial prefrontal cortex (mPFC) has been proposed to be essential for self-related processing [31–34]. These hypotheses predict that damage to these regions should disrupt, or perhaps even abolish essential aspects of SA. However, an emerging body of work in a rare patient with extensive bilateral damage encompassing both the AI and mPFC directly contradicts this prediction [3, 13, 35].

The patient, Roger, is a male in his late 50s with a college education whose brain was severely damaged in 1980 as a result of herpes simplex encephalitis (Figure 1(b)). His brain damage is bilateral, more extensive on the right, and encompasses the insular cortex, the anterior cingulate cortex (ACC), and the mPFC. Moreover the damage extends to the basal forebrain and the entire medial temporal lobe, including the amygdala and hippocampus bilaterally. In addition, the white matter is extensively damaged, in particular on the right, extending from the frontal and temporal poles to the anterior inferior parietal lobule. The damage spares the brainstem, cerebellum, thalamus, hypothalamus, basal ganglia, and most posterior cortical structures in the occipital and parietal lobes.

Studies from our group have demonstrated that Roger has largely intact cognitive abilities with normal intelligence, language, and even executive functioning [35]. Roger exhibits an overall normal neuropsychological profile except for a profound anterograde amnesia and a temporally graded retrograde amnesia that is most apparent during the 10 years preceding the onset of his brain damage.

Moreover, Roger has preserved interoceptive awareness of cardiac sensations [13]. We used a double-blind, randomized, pharmacological protocol involving the infusion of Isoproterenol—a Beta-adrenergic agonist, which provokes well-titrated, transient increases in heart rate and heart contraction. The results supported the hypothesis that interoceptive awareness is an integrative and synthetic phenomenon that relies on multiple pathways, including somatosensory pathways. The latter are traditionally conceived as transducing and carrying exteroceptive signals. The study suggested that these pathways constitute a sufficient channel to carry

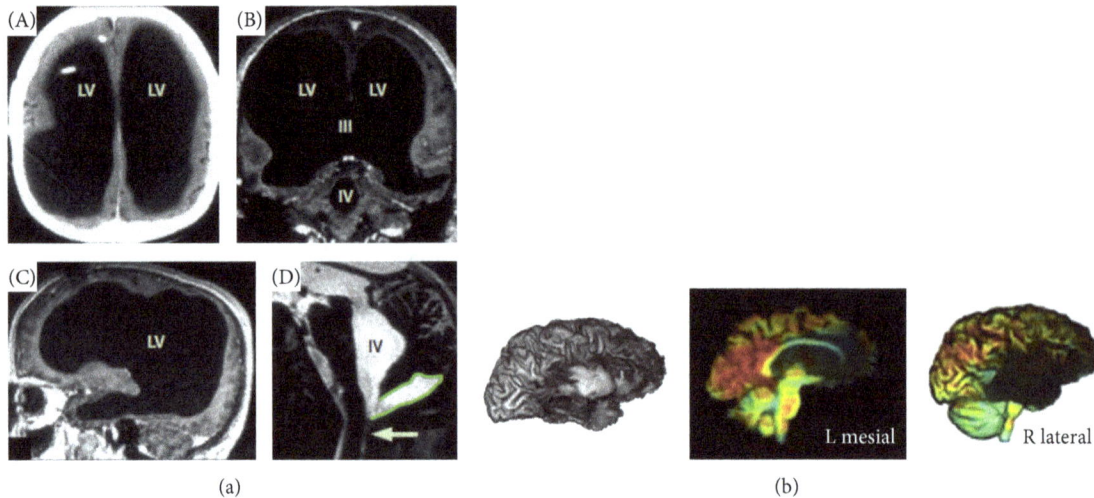

FIGURE 1: Examples of resilience to brain damage. (a) A 44-year-old civil servant and father of two with relatively low intelligence, but normal social functioning, was found to have preserved mental abilities despite significant ventricular enlargement and a very thin cortical mantle due to a history of hydrocephaly [20]. (b) Roger: patient with bilateral destruction of the limbic system following herpes simplex virus encephalitis. Contrary to all expectations, the patient presents largely preserved cognition and self-awareness (adapted from [3]).

peripheral visceral information to the brain for an integration that cannot be performed at the level of the insula in this patient.

We also demonstrated that Roger's SA was largely preserved, at all levels of its functional hierarchy, from core, to extended and reflective SA (see [3, 12]), using a battery of tests targeting SA at multiple levels (mirror test, self-recognition from pictures, self-agency tasks, personality ratings, and self-awareness questionnaire). Furthermore, functional connectivity analyses from resting state fMRI collected in Roger suggested that the dynamics of interaction among preserved sectors of his brain, including preserved medial parietal regions of the so-called default mode network (see [36]), could contribute to support Roger's preserved functions with regard to SA (Figure 1(b)).

In conclusion, Roger is a conscious, self-aware, and sentient human being despite the destruction of nearly one-third of his brain, including cortical centers presumed to play a critical role in SA according to some prominent hypotheses in the literature. His general appreciation of his memory deficit indicates that he has some awareness of his cognitive limitations. However due to Roger's pervasive amnesia, his autobiographical SA, especially with regard to his autobiographical self [19], that is, his own representations and narratives of himself built upon autobiographical memory, appears to be largely limited to the repositories of stored episodic and semantic knowledge consolidated during his childhood and young adult life.

This is not a completely isolated case. Other herpes simplex encephalitis patients, with brain damage almost identical to Roger's, and even more extensive, have been described [37] but had never been presented as showing any evidence for defective SA ([19], p. 117–121). A retrospective report following up on Philippi et al. [3], with a focus on emotion and sentience, found indications of similarly preserved functions in such herpes simplex encephalitis patients [38]. In such patients, emotions, from basic to social emotions, from experience to recognition, also appear more preserved than what could be expected from their damage to regions of the brain supposed to be critical for emotions, including the amygdala, anterior cingulate cortex (ACC), and insular cortex [38–40].

SA also appears to remain largely preserved in neuropsychological cases of patients with profound retrograde and anterograde amnesia [19], including patients with extreme amnesia such as Clive Wearing [41]. Interestingly, the patient demonstrated intact Core Consciousness ([19]; see also [12]), that is, the core, preattentive private experience and feeling of being a willful agent owner of his own thoughts and at least minimally aware of himself as such. The patient also had remaining controlled, self-reflective abilities pertaining to SA. They were expressed in distressful statements like: "I'm alive for the very first time." He could remember much of his previous self and had in recent years shown an ability to integrate an awareness of his memory deficit.

2.3. Resilience to Stable Diffuse Brain Damage: The Case of Disorders of Consciousness. Recent research in patients with disorders of consciousness (DOC), such as persistent vegetative states (PVS) or minimally conscious state (MCS) patients, can further provide some surprising support for the notion that many higher-order cognitive functions are highly resilient to neuropathological insults. This is expressed clinically through a within-subject process of recovery of function, often accompanied with daily fluctuations in mental status and marked by an important between-subject variability in capacity for resilience [4, 5, 42, 43].

Contrary to coma, which generally arises from damage to the upper brainstem's Ascending Reticular Activating System (ARAS), in PVS and MCS there is sufficient diencephalic and upper brainstem preservation of function for supporting basic sleep-wake cycles, primitive orienting responses, and basic brainstem and spinal reflexes. In PVS, cognitive functions, sensory modalities, speech, and movement are dramatically interrupted, and the patients are entirely noncommunicative. In MCS, there can be rare and intermittent signs of following simple commands, occasional yes/no responses and verbalizations, and congruent basic affective responses. From a pathological standpoint, PVS generally results from very diffuse necrosis of the cerebral cortex and/or diffuse shear injury of axons in the thalamocortical system, and/or damage to the thalamic intralaminar nuclei. PVS can occur following traumatic brain injury (TBI), metabolic failure (e.g., anoxia), and poisoning, as well as massive or diffuse strokes. MCS is caused by a similar etiology and pathology, with damage however often less diffuse topographically. Overall, the metabolic rate of glucose in PVS and MCS ranges between 40% and 50% of a normal wakeful brain, and it is comparable with that of coma and general anesthesia (see [44]).

Apart from cases of focal brain damage that affect subcortical regions of the thalamus, basal ganglia, or brainstem, many PVS cases suggest that consciousness may only disappear whenever extensive, diffuse, bilateral damage disrupts much of the thalamocortical system and large-scale functional interactions between brain regions [45, 46]. Nevertheless, even in such circumstances, evidence suggests that residual consciousness can be present in some PVS patients [4–6, 44].

In a series of studies [5, 6], several PVS patients were able to perform mental imagery of playing tennis or walking through different rooms, following verbal cues. Playing tennis is reliably associated with activation of the supplementary motor area (SMA) and navigating rooms is reliably associated with activation of the parahippocampal gyrus, posterior parietal lobe, and premotor cortex. While instructed to perform the task, the patient activated the exact same regions as predicted based on data collected in normal participants, in accordance with the instructions. Furthermore, in a follow-up experiment, one of the patients was asked a few biographical questions [6]. The patient was instructed to perform one or the other type of mental imagery depending on whether the answer to the questions was "yes" or "no." As measured by the activation of the target regions, the "answers" were 100% correct. Further neuroanatomical investigations will be essential to establish whether the integrity of certain regions of the thalamocortical system (e.g., regions of the default mode network (DMN) that are discussed below), is more critical than that of other regions for PVS cases to demonstrate such preserved covert consciousness.

More generally, resilience is also manifested in the impressive capacity of many patients to recover from coma, PVS, and MCS [47], and this may depend on the details of the anatomy of the damage. In Giacino and Kalmar's study [48], up to seventy-three percent of PVS patients showing early signs of intact visual pursuit were able to recover other clear-cut signs of consciousness by 12 months. Fifty percent of MCS patients and three percent of PVS patients had "no disability" to "moderate disability" at 1-year post injury.

2.4. Resilience to Progressive Diffuse Brain Damage: The Case of Alzheimer's Disease. In addition to the aforementioned neurological cases of DOC, neurodegenerative diseases, such as Alzheimer's disease (AD) and frontotemporal dementia (FTD), represent further examples of the clinical manifestation of within-subject cognitive resilience, with pronounced fluctuations in mental status and a strong between-subject variability, following this time a progressively aggravating, irreversible distributed neuropathology affecting both structure and function [8].

Understanding the specific mechanisms associated with resilience to AD is an important clinical, financial, and societal challenge for public health, because AD is turning into an epidemic among the aging population. This issue strongly affects AD care-burden management, prognosis, the development of strategies of rehabilitation, treatment planning and management, and more generally behavioral neurology. There is currently no known treatment for AD. According to the 2010 World Alzheimer report, about 35.6 million people in the world struggle with dementia, representing an annual cost of more than US $600 billion. The prospect is to see the incidence of the disease double over the next 20 years.

AD is a "dual clinicopathological entity" (see [9]) that is characterized by a neurodegenerative process [49]. It presents a typical pattern of progression [50], including the following.

(1) A clinical phenotype, which entails progressive dementia following a prodromal phase, often developing over decades, with quite variable rates of decline across individuals. Typically, symptomatic phase starts with episodic memory impairments and is followed by anomia, disorders of controlled and executive process, appearance of prevalent spatial cognition impairments, and emotional disorders (e.g., apathy, panic attacks), personality changes, and impaired judgment and consciousness, progressing into a complete breakdown of the mind. Anosognosia, a reduced self-awareness regarding one's own deficits [51], is also a prevalent symptom in AD [52] that can lead to unsafe behaviors [53], neuropsychiatric comorbidities, including apathy and panic attacks [54, 55]. Moreover, it represents a strong burden for caregivers and has deleterious effects on quality of the patient's life [56].

(2) A progressive pattern of neuropathological alterations [57], which seemingly propagates along neural pathways [58, 59]. Senile plaques (often presymptomatic and weakly correlated with clinical expression) are associated with extracellular β-amyloid (Aβ) aggregates. Neurofibrillary tangles (more strongly correlated with clinical expression) are associated with intracellular tau-amyloid fibril aggregates. A progressive pattern of diffuse atrophy [57] and abnormal resting metabolism [60] develops consecutively with collateral oxidative and inflammatory stress, synaptic loss and neuronal loss, especially in association cortices. Damage starts with mesial-temporal lobe structures (medial temporal atrophy is one of

the biomarkers most associated with cognitive decline [57]) and progresses with temporal, parietal, and frontal atrophy, while also affecting many subcortical structures [61, 62].

Several variants of the disease exist, and its etiology can be idiopathic or genetic, in particular in rare cases of early-onset manifestations of the disease. Multiple demographic and functional factors contribute either to mitigate or aggravate the risk of disease. (http://www.alz.co.uk/research/world-report).

There is a growing consensus [63–68], on both clinical and neuropathological grounds, that AD is a disconnection syndrome [26], with clinical expression in impaired cross-modal integration. A progressive breakdown of communication between brain systems at the large scale is observed and is reflected in both structural and functional connectivity (see Definitions). It affects both interhemispheric and intrahemispheric interactions, notably in frontoparietal, parietotemporal, and temporofrontal networks that are all affected by AD pathology. Fiber tracts such as the cingulum, the superior longitudinal fasciculus, uncinate fasciculus, corpus callosum, and most association tracts [69] are affected. Beyond the sheer loss of neurons, the global organization and hierarchy of normal brain networks break down, and random patterns of connectivity replace the so-called "small-world" organization of normal brain networks, in which specialized subnetworks with dense intrinsic connections are well connected together at the large scale but at low wiring cost. The central "hubs" of the networks appear to undergo reorganization, that is, the regions characterized by the highest degree or bandwidth of connectivity with the rest of the network, from both a structural and functional standpoint. These hubs typically include midline structures such as the precuneus and medial prefrontal cortex. Global and local processing efficiency cannot be maintained in the context of shrinking processing resources and routes to connect them. As a result integrative and specialized functional processes cannot carry on the task of supporting normal cognition, and the mind as an integrated functional whole collapses.

Within this overall pathological process, the neuropsychological dependence of manifestations of cognitive impairments on the amount of brain alterations appears to be marked by a substantial interindividual variability [8, 49]. Full pathologic criteria for AD have been observed *post mortem* in 25% to 67% of the brains of elderly individuals with no indication of cognitive impairment prior to death [9, 70–72]. Certain AD patients show increased functional connectivity within frontal sectors as well as between frontal, thalamic, and striatal regions, which in turn suggests the presence of compensatory mechanisms aimed at coping with large-scale disconnection [67]. Generally speaking, in AD, variability across individuals in cerebral metabolic patterns is at least partly related to strategies of compensations aiming at optimizing the efficacy of key processes in a context of progressive decimation of resources [66].

Intriguingly, resilience in AD appears to be partly mediated by variables such as general intelligence, degree of literacy, educational attainment, occupational complexity, interpersonal skills, integration in social networks, personality variables, and leisure activity. These are all aspects of what has been referred to as "cognitive reserve" (CR) (see [8]). In other words, higher-order cognition and behaviors interact with the capacity for resilience. Given a comparable amount of brain damage, individuals who score higher in such variables tend to present with better cognitive performance and social adjustment, and also tend to be more easily managed by healthcare professionals, than individuals with lower CR. Furthermore, individuals with lower CR demonstrated a relative risk of developing dementia that was between 2.2 and 2.85 higher than individuals with higher CR [73]. In a meta-analysis, higher CR was associated with a lowered risk for incident dementia with summary odds ratio of 0.54, and increased complex mental activity in late life was associated with lower dementia rates independent of other predictors [74].

Likewise, individuals with AD pathology and higher CR tend to present a point of inflexion in the progression of the disease, which marks the transition from a prodromal phase to dementia, which occurs at a more advanced stage of brain pathology [75] than individuals with low CR. Biomarkers of AD pathology, such as the uptake of ^{11}CPiB in positron emission tomography (PET) interacts with the number of years of education in predicting cognitive performance on scales such as the Clinical Dementia Rating sum of boxes, Mini-Mental State Examination, and Short Blessed Test [76]. Evidence also suggests that the relation between senile plaques and level of cognitive function differs by years of formal education [77]. Moreover, it has been shown that there is a relationship between higher CR and lower incidence or severity of anosognosia in dementia [78]. In other words, individuals with higher CR tend to be more resilient.

3. Hypotheses about the Mechanisms of Cognitive Resilience

As reviewed above, a wealth of clinical facts demonstrates that brains can preserve core aspects of the functional architecture of information processing that sustains higher-order cognition in spite of substantial structural damage causing irreversible losses of neuronal ensembles and systems of wires at multiple scales. Here I discuss a set of coherent hypotheses, often reasoning based on postulates, in order to explore possible explanations. Alternative explanations not envisioned in this paper probably exist. I am only proposing one possible conceptual approach, which I believe offers at this point the best overall explanatory power. As it will be apparent, some of those ideas are mainstream and others are more idiosyncratic and speculative, but I believe warrant attention. I frame the rationale and discussion by adopting a perspective on neural computation aimed at neural engineering.

3.1. Limits of Structural Plasticity for Recovery of Function. The brain is constituted by populations of neurons and glial cells distributed over many different anatomical locations. They are locally connected through intrinsic networks and at the large-scale through the white matter via neuronal bundles of fibers containing axons. At all scales, synapses mediate the functional interactions between connected neurons via fast electrochemical signaling. The integrity of structural connections, for example, long-range fiber bundles, is critical for many aspects of normal cognition. Our group has shown for instance that sectors of the white matter which contain large association fiber bundles connecting fronto-parietal systems play a causal role in general intelligence [79].

However, with resilience, functions are preserved or recover in spite of structural damage to gray matter regions and/or fiber tracts normally implicated in these functions. This process implies some form of anatomofunctional "plasticity."

Structural plasticity, for example, axonal regeneration, and synaptic and dendritic sprouting, can contribute to such plasticity [80]. However, lesions observed in the neurological cases considered here are too extended and severe for being compensated by a direct, large-scale physical rewiring of the entire system based on structural plasticity that would rebuild the original anatomical structures.

Thus structural plasticity alone cannot account for the anatomofunctional adaptations that appear necessary to support and account for the phenomenon of resilience.

Central tendencies in the relationships between structure and function, for example, anatomical location and task-related responses, which are observed in normal brains may appear integral to how the brain implements cognition. But these central tendencies are to some degree contingent, and their regularity often masks a strong interindividual variability in actual structure-function relationships. Such regularities should not be confused with an actual, strong, and rigid dependency between specific structures and specific functions [2]. The brain may have many alternative solutions to cognition built-in, which are revealed and manifested via neurological cases of resilience.

If large-scale structural plasticity alone cannot account for cognitive resilience, then anatomofunctional relationships, or more generally structure-function relationships, must undergo transformations in the process of resilience. Damage to the physical integrity of neural systems is present, but functions normally relying on these damaged resources appear preserved. It is reasonable as a first approximation to hypothesize that resilience is related to compensatory mechanisms that will be reflected in dissociations between normal structure-function relationships and pathological structure-function relationships for equivalent performance [34].

3.2. Evidence from Neuroimaging and Computational Modeling for Dissociations in Structure-Function Relationships and Renormalization of Function.

Recent methodological advances in neuroimaging acquisition and data analysis have enabled the estimation in vivo of large-scale interactions in the brain, in normal and pathological contexts. Tractography in diffusion weighted imaging (DWI) can be used to quantify structural connectivity, and analyses of covariance in resting state functional MRI (rsfMRI) can be used to quantify functional connectivity. Advanced statistical analyses often based on graph theory can further be applied in order to characterize topological properties of structural and functional connectivity [36, 67, 81–84]. Studying the relationships between structural and functional connectivity is a suitable paradigm to investigate large-scale structure-function relationships in the brain in connection to resilience.

Analyses of functional connectivity have shown that the brain is organized in functionally coherent large-scale networks at baseline (e.g., during wakeful rest and inactivity), the so-called "resting state networks" (RSNs)—that is, intrinsic networks constituted by sets of brain regions whose activity appears reliably correlated at rest [85]. Some of these so-called "resting state networks" (RSNs), such as the default mode network (DMN), have been associated with higher-order cognitive functions, including consciousness [86, 87], autobiographical memory [36], executive control [88], and language [89, 90].

Abnormal resting state functional connectivity has been implicated in multiple neurological disorders [91]. RSNs, including the DMN, were altered in patients diagnosed with AD [92–94] or at risk of AD [95], and in patients with traumatic brain injury [96, 97]. Functional connectivity alterations appeared partially correlated with AD neuropathology [98]. DMN activity was correlated longitudinally with the course of AD [66, 94]. Also, studies of RSNs in normal aging have shown age-related RSN changes [99, 100].

These networks appear to depend on complex mechanisms and can show flexible relationships to the underlying structural connectivity. Stationary neurodynamical models of physiological functions can predict, taking structural connectivity as an input, the topological and topographical organization of some of the main RSNs [101–103]. However, a large amount of prediction error variance between simulated and empirical functional connectivity remains and cannot be reduced based on the manipulation of structural parameters [102]. Nonstationary dynamics are likely to contribute to this variance. The relationship between functional connectivity and structural connectivity is complex and indirect (Figure 3).

Nevertheless, some systems of structural connections are predicted by a range of generative models to play a particularly critical role in shaping the overall topographical organization of RSNs across the brain. According to the models, the commissural system of homotopic fibers that passes through the corpus callosum and connects functionally homologous regions of the cerebral cortex across the two hemispheres plays a critical role in the emergence of bilateral symmetrical RSNs across the two hemispheres [102] (Figure 2).

However, a few studies of patients with corpus callosum abnormalities, including complete commissurotomy [104] and congenital callosal agenesis [105], have found RSNs to be remarkably normal and symmetrical in these patients. This challenges the idea that interhemispheric symmetries in major RSNs are necessarily mediated by callosal fibers and shows that functional networks can survive major changes in structural connectivity (Figure 3(a)).

Moreover, resting state fluctuations are large in magnitude and normally consistent across participants and

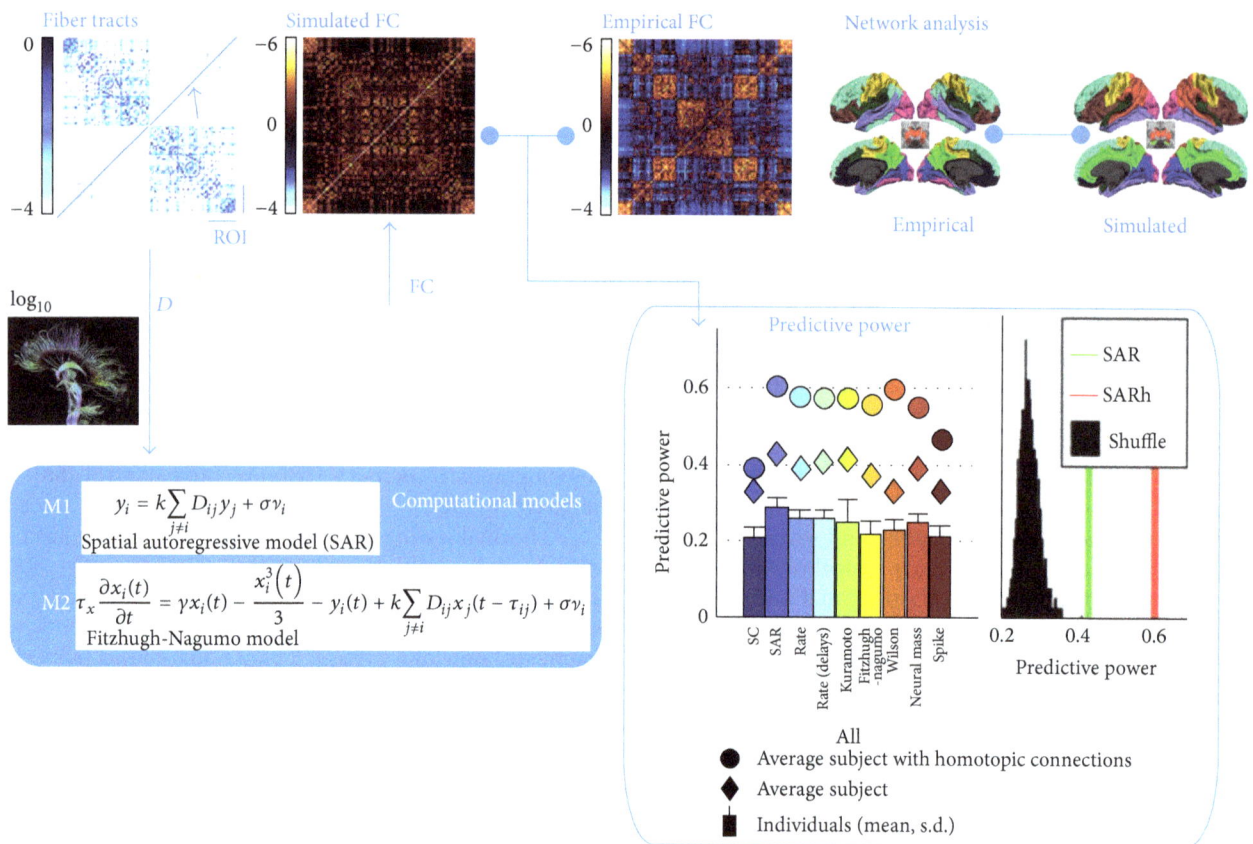

FIGURE 2: Modeling structure-function relationships. Left. *Upper-tier*: matrices of (anatomical, simulated-functional, and empirical-functional) average connectivity, between a set of 160 regions of interest derived from automated segmentations of the human cerebral cortex. Network analysis: connectivity information is also represented as cluster of similarly connected regions over the cerebral cortex for empirical and simulated functional connectivity (SAR model, i.e., spatial autoregressive model). *Lower-tier*: matrices of anatomical connectivity (from DWI-based tractography) are used as inputs to computational models of neurophysiology, with increasing complexity and realism (from SAR to Spike models), from which simulated matrices of functional connectivity are derived. Predictive power: the correlation between simulated and empirical data (predictive power) is highly increased (circle color dots) when missing interhemispheric and homotopic connections are added (the effect is specific to this fiber tract system and robust to permutation schemes [histogram chart]). (Adapted from [102]).

across time [106–109]. Part of these fluctuations might have functional significance and might be related to fluctuations in cognitive and behavioral performance. Fluctuations in functional connectivity following brain damage could be an important functional marker of the process of compensation and rescue of function, useful for the development of strategies of rehabilitation [110–112].

RSNs have a tendency to shift towards a more random structure of connectivity in patients with nonfocal brain pathology, for example, in brain tumors [113, 114], AD [93], epilepsy [115], and severe TBI [96]. A study of patients with multiple sclerosis showed that some RSNs were altered and others were reorganized [116]. There are a few studies in patients with more focal disorders. Carter et al. [82] studied 23 acute stroke patients and found that the dorsal attention network and arm somatomotor networks were altered. Moreover, the loss of coherence among different RSNs predicted behavioral deficits. Wang et al. [112] studied 10 patients with subcortical infarctions. They investigated RSNs across 5 consecutive time points within a single year

and observed gradual changes in networks and associated functions. In particular, they found a tendency for the motor executive network to gradually transits through a random mode during the recovery process. Vanhaudenhuyse et al. [46] found that DMN connectivity was decreased in 14 severely brain damaged patients, in proportion to the patients' degree of impairment in consciousness (e.g., locked-in syndrome, coma, and vegetative state). Recent research on patients with disorders of consciousness, such as patients in a persistent vegetative state (PVS) or a minimally conscious state (MCS), also suggested the importance of RSNs' functional connectivity in functional preservation or recovery [4, 5, 42]. Nakamura et al. [96] demonstrated evidence of rapid renormalization of functional connectivity (3–6 months) in the process of recovery from trauma after an initial phase of high perturbation of the normal pattern of functional connectivity (Figure 3(b)).

In the framework of these large-scale structural and functional parameters, the problem of understanding and controlling the mechanisms of resilience in neurology is

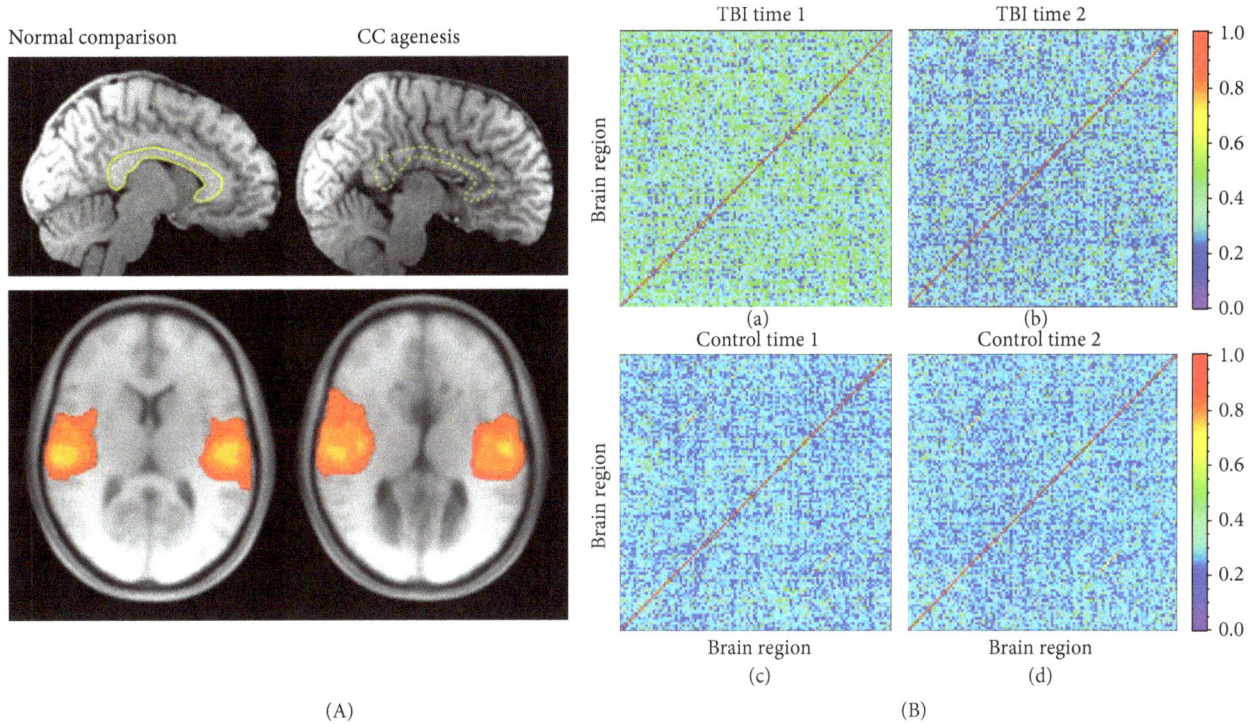

FIGURE 3: Dissociations between functional and structural connectivity and renormalization of function. (a) Preserved bilateral, symmetrical functional connectivity from resting fMRI in patients with agenesis of the corpus callosum (from [105]). *Top-tier*: sagittal slices of T1-weighted MRI data from a normal comparison participant (left) and an agenesis patient (right). The normal location of the corpus callosum (CC) is indicated with dashed yellow lines. *Bottom-tier*: axial slices showing similar bilateral functional connectivity from resting fMRI in both patients and normal comparison participants. (b) Evidence for rapid renormalization of functional connectivity (3–6 months) in the process of recovery from traumatic brain injury (TBI) (from [96]). Charts represent matrices of functional connectivity derived from resting fMRI for the patients (upper-tier) and the comparison participants (lower-tier), at two time points after TBI onset (left versus right tiers). Functional connectivity in the patients progressively renormalizes in conjunction with behavioral recovery after an initial phase of perturbation.

a problem of modeling how normal functional connectivity can be preserved in the context of abnormal structural connectivity. Models can be modified to incorporate *ad hoc* neuropharmacological or electrophysiological mechanisms (e.g., additional norepinephrine-related neurotransmission; new inhibitory receptors-conductances; electrical potentiation of connectivity along alternate, indirect pathways) (Figure 4).

3.3. Setting and Operationalizing Resilience: Brain Computation and Mutual Information. In order to better understand possible underlying mechanisms for resilience, it is useful to start from a simple operationalization of brain computation. Let us define the normal brain as a structural network S_N of n regions/nodes, associated with a generative model G of the dynamics (generally a set of differential equations), yielding a functional network M_N, such that

$$M_N = G\left(S_N\right). \qquad (1)$$

Both networks S_N and M_N can be described as weighted graphs associated with corresponding adjacency $n \times n$ matrices $S(i, j)$ and $M(i, j)$. An adjacency matrix is simply a square matrix informing the level of (structural or functional) connectivity between each pair of nodes.

Let us now assume that the brain performs some form of computation, executing processes $\{A, B, \ldots, Z\}$ which implement functions and operate over partially encapsulated (i.e., specialized) subsets of the brain network. One can conceive of such subsets or subnetworks as RSNs or task based networks (TBNs), that is, networks of brain regions that are reliably activated (e.g., in fMRI) during specific tasks [122]. Though they interact, such networks, which are related to different cognitive functions, can operate in a relatively independent manner (which is why they can be revealed with techniques such as independent component analysis for RSNs, and statistical contrasts between conditions for TBNs).

Within each of these subnetworks, network nodes interact through structural wiring to implement a function. The computation involves exchanges of information between the nodes. Here by node, we do not necessarily mean individual neurons, but also entire neuronal ensembles, which are partially specialized (e.g., cortical area V4 in the visual system) acting as a unit, depending on the scale considered (see Figure 5(a)).

We can further operationalize this model by describing the direct or indirect exchange of information between nodes using Information Theory and the concept of mutual information [123]. Mutual information is a quantity derived

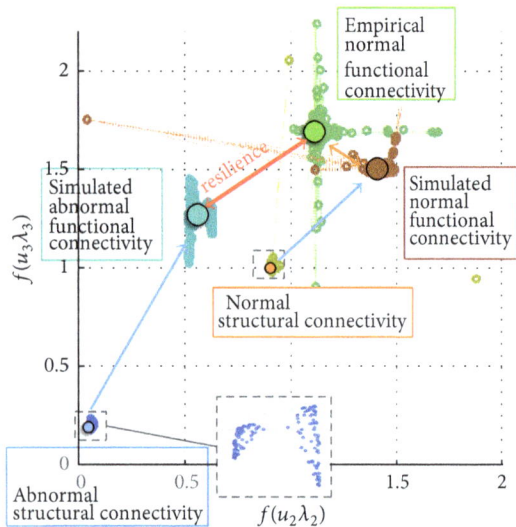

FIGURE 4: Research on resilience and modeling of structure-function relationships. Example of Laplacian matrices of anatomical and functional connectivity, for empirical and simulated, normal and pathological instances represented in a vector space over two components following singular value decomposition and additional transformations providing an optimal layout and metrics for comparing topological properties of networks. A simple SAR model (see [102]) is used to predict matrices of functional connectivity from matrices of structural connectivity. Normal anatomical connectivity predicts a simulated-functional connectivity that is close to empirical-functional connectivity, whereas abnormal anatomical connectivity (simulated callosectomy) predicts abnormal functional connectivity, farther away from empirical-functional connectivity. The distance between simulated and empirical functional connectivity, given anatomical connectivity, provides the parameter of control to drive research on mechanisms of renormalization of function and resilience.

from Shannon's entropy [124], which characterizes the degree of statistical dependence between two variables X and Y. It is minimal when two systems do not exchange information and maximum when they share the exact same information.

Let us now consider the case of a pathological brain with a damaged structural network S_P and an abnormal functional network M_P. Let us say that two of the network nodes (i, j) are now disconnected. This means that their effective connectivity $w(i, j)$, which is an indicator of presence of anatomical connectivity weighted by a transmission or synaptic gain (see Definitions), is equal to 0. The nodes cannot directly interact and thus cannot exchange information. As a result their mutual information $m(i, j)$ is also equal to 0.

However, if there are alternative, indirect pathways that structurally connect the nodes i and j with sufficient effective connectivity to provide bandwidth then the two nodes can interact and exchange information, and their mutual information $m(i, j)$ is not equal to 0.

From the standpoint of resilience, it is also important to exploit alternative pathways that do not imply prohibitive transmission delays for the integrity of the cognitive process. It is customary to observe a slowing down of processing in

brain damaged patients reflected in behavioral performance (e.g., [13]).

Likewise, if nodes or pathways become shared by different processes—for example, to compensate for lost resources pertaining to one of the processes by using alternative, indirect pathways associated with other processes—then access conflicts, cross-talks and interferences may arise between the processes, depending on how the transmission channels and effective connectivity are set. Phenomena such as tinnitus and pathologies such as epilepsy are pathological testimonies of such interferences.

Figure 5 presents simple illustrations of such an overall operational model from which we can analyze the implications of resilience for neuroscience.

3.4. Redundancy: Structural, Topological, and Combinatorial Bases of Resilience in the Brain. Redundancy is intrinsic to the brain's anatomofunctional architecture, and plays a natural role in its capacity for resilience. Redundancy may provide the brain with the ability to switch to alternate processing resources when others become unavailable or untrustworthy (Figure 5). From a combinatorial standpoint, the brain appears well equipped for functional resilience to structural challenges.

It has been proposed that the structural balance between segregation (functional specialization of subnetworks) and integration (their degree of interconnectedness), in the overall anatomofunctional organization of the brain presents a so-called small-world topology (see [125]). Such topology maximizes the number of short pathways between any two nodes in the entire network, while reducing wiring cost (overall number of necessary structural connections) and make the network's short connectedness resilient to disconnection. This hypothesis has recently been challenged (see [126]) to favor instead a bow tie architecture, in which dense peripheral subnetworks are highly pluripotent and not specialized. In both cases the architectures have properties of resilience.

More basically, structural parameters such as premorbid neuronal count and its volumetric proxies, the so-called "passive brain reserve" (see [8]), are highly relevant. The high number of neurons in the brain and between-subject differences in overall neuronal resources represents a strong source of redundancy and variability in redundancy. In principle, larger brains can sustain more insult up to a certain threshold.

However, redundancy in the brain is intimately related to functional parameters. It is expressed in at least two complementary ways (Figure 5(d)) [2, 14, 127]. There can be a relative "degeneracy" among processing units/nodes: different nodes are capable of handling the same function or output, it is a many-to-one mapping (e.g., parallel array of identical specialized processors). There can also be a relative "pluripotency" in processing units: individual nodes are capable of handling multiple functions contextually; it is a one-to-many mapping (e.g., processor individually executing different tasks sequentially by switching between them). Examples of possible anatomical substrates for such processes would include, with unilateral lesions, contralateral homologue regions taking over; the direct penumbra of the lesion,

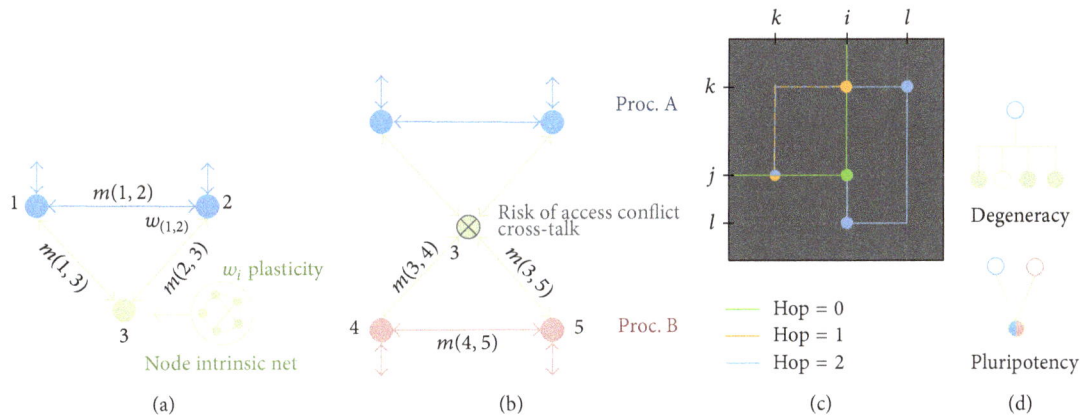

FIGURE 5: Redundancy and resilience. (a) Simple model of network with 3 nodes (1, 2, and 3). Nodes 1 and 2 interact to perform process A (blue), implementing a function, with inputs and outputs from and to other unrepresented nodes (little blue arrows). Node 3 is structurally connected with nodes 1 and 2 but is assumed to present little effective connectivity $w(i, j)$ and thus not to interact much with nodes 1 and 2. Each node, which can be a region of the brain, can contain multiple intrinsic processing units (subregions or neurons), working together and capable of plasticity, that is, of modification of their effective connectivity via synaptic tuning. One can define a quantity of mutual information $m(i, j)$ between any two nodes (i, j) in the network (see text). If the effective connectivity of node 3 with nodes 1 and 2 increases, node 3 will relay information between nodes 1 and 2, and the chaining of $m(1, 3)$ and $m(2, 3)$ will contribute to $m(1, 2)$: node 3 and its wires can become an indirect, parallel, alternate carrier of signal for nodes 1 and 2. This represents a form of redundancy. (b) Extended model from (a) with two additional nodes, 4 and 5, assumed to support a process B, irrelatively independent from process A, through their interactions. A quantity of mutual information can also be defined between nodes 4 and 5, and any other nodes in the network. In this case, node 3 is placed in a position of "hub"; that is, it is highly connected structurally with the other nodes of the network ("degree" = 4 versus 2 connections). If its effective connectivity with all its neighbors (i.e., directly connected nodes) is increased, it will start indirectly relaying signals not only among nodes of the same process (A or B), but also between nodes subserving the different processes (A and B). Without further filtering to separate and channel sources of signals, there is thus a risk of cross-talk and interferences between the processes A and B. If for functional reasons, the processing capacity of node 3 becomes shared by processes A and B, and plasticity within the node manages to reduce cross-talk between them, for example, by serializing the access, and to handle the source separation and channeling problem, there is nevertheless a risk of "access conflict" for the resource represented by node 3. (c) Theoretical matrix of structural connectivity (i.e., adjacency matrix) informing the existence of structural connections between each pair of nodes in a network. The analysis of such matrix can identify all direct and indirect, alternate structural pathways between any two nodes (i, j), and sort them according to their "hop" distance, that is, the number of intermediary nodes along the pathway connecting i and j (which is 0 when the connection is direct, 1 when it has one relay, 2 when 2, and so on). (d) Two types of functionally relevant redundancy: degeneracy and pluripotency (see text). Assuming that it is functional, node 3 in (b) can potentially represent a pluripotent resource for both processes A and B.

that is, tissues around the lesion, being sufficient to compensate; or entirely different structures and circuits, not already pluripotent, being recruited to compensate. More generally, individual neurons are capable of switching between different information processing modes in a pluripotent and highly contextual manner, notably in the prefrontal cortex (see [128]).

Further mechanisms have been discussed in the field, often in the context of the notion of "cognitive reserve" [8, 11, 72, 129]. Resilience can build upon preexisting cognitive skills and thereby facilitate problem-solving in cognitively challenging environments. It can use resources within brain networks that normally support these specific cognitive skills, or alternate resources that do not normally support such skills. It can optimize the balance between two main categories of parameters. The first parameter is "efficiency," minimizing the number of operations and energy expenditure. The second is "capacity," that is, the maximal processing power or capacity of integration per neuronal unit, based on which a stronger processing demand can be placed on preserved neurons by making them operate at fuller capacity.

It is generally the case that brain damaged patients demonstrate slower cognition and behavior, often accompanied with decreased cerebral metabolism such as in AD. This suggests that both capacity and efficiency in their brain reach a limit. In AD (see above), patterns of higher metabolic activity in certain regions of the brain have been hypothesized to reflect compensatory mechanisms [66]. This could be an illustration of a case of increased processing capacity per unit time for neuronal units in these regions. Activation studies using fMRI can study efficiency and capacity in brain processing using event-related designs in which cognitive load during task is manipulated [8].

Alternatively, the brain can build upon a flexible use of cognitive strategies and brain systems that are not normally involved in the skills (e.g., mnemonic strategies to compensate impaired recall, and interhemispheric transfer of psycholinguistic functions after a stroke). Partial evidence suggests both an enhancement of the processing in neural networks that are specifically related to the task demand, and the participation of more general "cognitive reserve networks," involving frontal sectors, which have been otherwise associated with controlled processes, task switching, and working memory [66, 72, 79]. Emotional and motivational factors may also contribute to fueling resilience [130], notably via the noradrenergic tone [131].

Thus cognitive resilience can rely on the combinatorial power of redundancy (degeneracy and pluripotency) in the anatomofunctional architecture of the brain, including on the presence of multiple alternate indirect pathways [2, 13, 22]. It can build upon a plastic capacity for adaptively switching between alternate resources, as well as upon mechanisms optimizing efficiency of processing within networks.

3.5. Renormalization of Function, Dynamic ReRouting, and Plasticity: A Complex Inverse Problem over the Structural Backbone for the Brain. Under the models described above, resilience corresponds to a general "renormalization" of the core functional/processing architecture supporting cognition (e.g., as suggested in [96, 105], in the context of analyses of functional connectivity from fMRI; see Figure 3). Such renormalization occurs in the context of a severely modified processing and wiring structure. By "renormalization" I explicitly mean a relative preservation of—or return to—the "normal," overall core computational scheme characterizing normal cognition. This process must be achieved in a manner that is compatible with available structural and metabolic resources, given a structurally modified brain network and a corresponding loss of previously dedicated processing power. This does not imply that the overall computational scheme of cognition is not substantially modified in its details. Multiple strategies may arise for specific cognitive processes.

For such renormalization, the brain must solve a routing problem. It must be capable of managing and recombining resource allocation adaptively via the dynamic "rerouting" and addressing of distributed signal streams along alternate neural pathways at multiple scales. It must dynamically identify, address, and allocate redundant, functionally compatible residual resources by a two-pronged approach: bringing alternate neural resources online, while coping with other neural resources that are dysfunctional and thus untrustworthy (e.g., noise in sensorimotor systems related to disease processes), for instance by setting them offline in order to minimize perturbation (e.g., progressive inhibition). The frequent observation in many conditions [1], as it was also the case for the patient Roger [3], of strikingly rapid recovery from extensive damage that had initially caused profound cognitive deficits (e.g., stupor, delirium, neglect, and anosognosia), emphasizing the dynamic and massive nature of such reboot and general reorganization.

As damage becomes more extended (e.g., in the course of AD), the brain must face increasing difficulties in finding resources available for compensation, in order to preserve core, critical cognitive functions. Solving the allocation and routing problem underlying resilience must become increasingly difficult. It is predictable that the brain will encounter more and more access conflicts for resources (Figure 5) and will have to rely on the pluripotency of residual resources. Such an increasing reliance on pluripotency can only result in slower, noisier, and ultimately dedifferentiated processing, with a lower capacity for information processing. This implies

subsequently placing more stress on available resources, as a condition for maintaining relative efficiency and specificity in a manner that is compatible with the timing and energetics of core adaptation. Such suboptimal processing can eventually become incompatible with the throughput required for adaptation and functional coherence. To some extent, this process is somewhat reflected in resilient AD patients who generally reach an inflexion point in their mental status. At this point, the cognitive apparatus that had been, until then, relatively resilient (generally at the expenditure of a high metabolic pressure over remaining functional tissues) collapses dramatically, plunging the patients into a rapidly progressing dementia. Such inflection point is observed at stages that are closer to organ failure in resilient patients than in nonresilient patients [8].

The overall guiding principles of the execution of such renormalization and the control of this global reweighting of effective connectivity in the brain remain mysterious.

The capacity for renormalization of function must at least in part be self-contained in the brain and robust: it operates and deploys in a rather systematic manner, at the cost of much energy expenditure, since all living individuals are more or less resilient, in a more or less efficient and powerful manner, as it is obvious in the psychological struggle of humanity [17]. It must itself be one of the most resilient general features of brain computation: a process in charge of controlling overall resilience in the brain must be itself resilient to fulfill its function.

The brain can functionally reconnect itself after damage via alternate, indirect pathways, based on local mechanisms of plasticity related to learning and adaptation, such as the modulation of synaptic plasticity [80]. Modulating synaptic efficacy, that is, synaptic transmission gain, which is equivalent to modulating effective connectivity in the network, will control information transfer and can be used to restore it (Figure 5). Figure 6 illustrates these concepts using the simple model of brain processing introduced above (see Figure 5), by showing how structural connectivity, effective connectivity and mutual information interact in a small network undergoing disconnection and synaptic plasticity over pluripotent resources. After disconnection of two nodes performing a coordinated process in the model, information flow is disrupted. The process fails. It can be partially restored, as reflected in their mutual information, thanks to a reweighting of the effective connectivity matrix, enabling indirect pathways to carry signals between the two disconnected nodes.

Yet, this process of synaptic plasticity must operate over massively distributed local nodes. Deciphering how such rerouting scheme can be coded and deployed in the brain is key to understanding fundamental relationships between structure and function in neuroscience.

As a first approximation and in all generality, the problem can be formulated as an inverse problem (see [132]). In our reduced model, the forward problem corresponds to that of defining a generative model G, taking a matrix of effective connectivity W as an input and outputting a matrix of mutual information: $M = G(W, S)$, with S the associated binary matrix of structural connections. The inverse problem

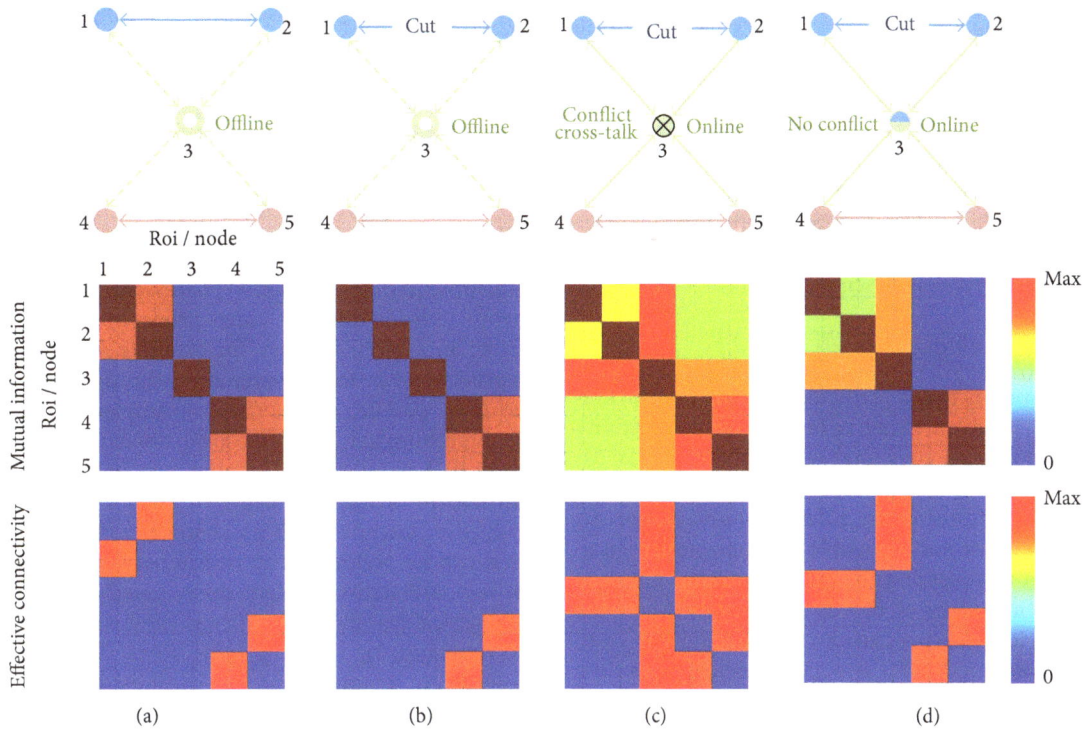

FIGURE 6: Information transfer and functional resilience in a model of small network subjected to disconnection. The principles, basic nodes, and (two-way) connections of the model are the same as in Figure 5(b). *Upper-tier.* Graphs of different states of the basic model. Two processes A and B implement some functions within, respectively, nodes (1, 2) and nodes (4, 5). It is assumed that the processes rely on an exchange of information between their respective nodes to compute the output of the functions. Disruption of information flow between nodes after structural disconnection (b, c, d) implies a failure of the process. A central node 3 or "hub" is connected to all the other nodes. Node 3 can be "offline" (a, b); that is, its effective connectivity with the other nodes is very low, and thus signals cannot flow through it even in the presence of structural connections. Alternatively it can be "online" (c, d); that is, its effective connectivity with the other nodes is high, and thus signals can directly flow through it. When node 3 is online, cross-talks and interferences between processes will arise (c), except if the node internal structure fully supports pluripotency (d), in case that information flow between nodes 1 and 2 is restored indirectly via node 3 without interference. *Lower-Tier.* Adjacency matrices of effective connectivity (bottom row) and associated mutual information (top row) for the different states of the network in (a, b, c, and d). Each square within the matrix represents the strength of the corresponding parameter between two nodes (i, j) among the 5 nodes of the network. The color bars on the right indicate the relative strength of the parameters. *Model specification and simulations.* In order to demonstrate the property illustrated in (a, b, c, and d), we used a simple generative model. Binary matrices of structural connectivity were first defined to implement the structure of connectivity. Matrices of effective connectivity were defined by reweighting the matrix of structural connectivity in order to implement the different states of effective connectivity in the network in (a), (b), (c), and (d) (e.g., high versus low connectivity; disconnection). Effective connectivity matrices were used as an input to a spatial autoregressive model (SAR), which demonstrates the best predictive power among many other more complex and realistic models in predicting empirical functional connectivity (from fRMI), based on empirical structural connectivity (from DWI) (see [102]). The SAR model assumes a stationary, multivariate, independently, and identically distributed Gaussian process with covariance matrix F. It corresponds to the equilibrium solution of a simple linear dynamical system of n nodes interacting through a set of structural connections, with effective connectivity matrix W. The covariance matrix has a closed form solution with the SAR model and can be computed based on the matrix of effective connectivity W: $F = s^2(I-kW)^{-1}(I-kW)^{-1T}$, with "$s^2$" being the variance of the process, "I" being the identity matrix, $(\cdot)^{-1}$ and $(\cdot)^{T}$, respectively, being the inverse and transpose of the matrices within the parenthesis, and k being a parameter of overall connectivity within the network (here k was set to .8). The covariance F corresponds to what is measured as functional connectivity in functional neuroimaging: functional connectivity is generally defined as the covariance between measured signals. A correlation matrix R can be derived from the covariance matrix F, and there is a simple relation between the correlation $r(i, j)$ in the dynamics of two nodes i and j and their mutual information (expressed in bits of information) because of the statistical properties of the SAR model. Thus $m(i, j) = \ln(1/\mathrm{sqrt}(1 - r(i, j)^2))$, with $\ln(\cdot)$ being the natural logarithm and $\mathrm{sqrt}(\cdot)$ being the square root functions. (a) Information flows between nodes 1 and 2, thanks to their high effective connectivity; mutual information is high between them. (b) Nodes 1 and 2 have been structurally disconnected, information does not flow, and their mutual information is zero. (c) Nodes 1 and 2 have been structurally disconnected, information does not flow directly, but node 3 has been brought online and information can flow through it indirectly. Mutual information between nodes 1 and 2 is partially restored, but there are also interfering cross-talks between nodes (1, 2) and (4, 5) through node 3 (see green squares in the corresponding matrix). (d) Nodes 1 and 2 have been structurally disconnected, information does not flow directly, and node 3 has been brought online but in a pluripotent manner that filters out cross-talks, resulting in no mutual information between nodes (1, 2) and (4, 5). Mutual information between nodes 1 and 2 is partially restored, as signals can flow through node 3. Information processing has been partially renormalized by playing on effective connectivity over redundancies in the model.

consists in finding an inverse generative model or inverse map G^{-1} to infer W from M and S: $W = G^{-1}(M, S)$. G^{-1} must select the set of W_i that are compatible with S and the topology of its embedded pathways. The problem of the brain then becomes a problem of optimization, which can be formulated as a process of minimization of the difference between a target, internal model M_N of normal information processing, and an internal measure of pathological information processing M_P, such that the renormalized matrix of effective connectivity W_R is chosen as

$$W_R = \mathrm{argmin}\left\{\left|M_N - M\left(W, S_P\right)\right|\right\}. \qquad (2)$$

$M(W, S_P)$ corresponds to the predicted measure of information processing M, given a matrix of effective connectivity W and the pathological structural connectivity matrix S_P, assuming an internal forward model: $M = G(W, S)$. W_R is the matrix W that minimizes the difference between normal information processing and a possible alternate implementation of information processing given the constraints imposed by S_P. Internal measures of the discrepancy between the current pathological matrix of effective connectivity W_P and the normal internal model W_N associated with M_N can then provide signals to control local synaptic plasticity in order to renormalize function.

In this framework, in order to be resilient, a brain must therefore embed fairly abstract, innate or acquired, internal, normative models of itself and of processing strategies serving as a compass for adaptive cognition and renormalization. It must also embed an algorithm that can perform such minimization, in a manner that is energetically and functionally viable and robust. One option that could be envisioned as a possible solution to the global renormalization problem would be to implement processes similar to simulated annealing and random walk search. They might account for the between-subject variability observed for similar cases of damage in recovery of function, both in terms of timing and performance. It is likely that what matters is to optimize the output function of processes, that is, optimize functions in a task-oriented manner based on desired goals that are internally modeled and a signal of reinforcement. This is compatible with textbook knowledge about operant learning in the brain.

3.6. Local Synaptic Plasticity and Resolution of Conflict in Pluripotent Nodes.

The hypothesis is that, at the lowest level of implementation, all local computational principles and corresponding biophysical and biochemical mechanisms involved in synaptic plasticity and learning, that is, one of the key interface between structure and function, are exploited by such an overall algorithm of renormalization to tune the routing of signals and transfer functions between and within neural ensembles, that is, in this framework, effective connectivity.

One of the problems that local synaptic plasticity will have to resolve is the mutualisation of a limited pool of neural resources to reconnect disconnected systems and replace damaged ones. It will have to create well-tuned properties of pluripotency in neural resources as they become shared between different processes, for example, for providing an alternate, indirect channel of information transfer between disconnected nodes associated with the different processes (Figures 5 and 6). Cross-talks between processes can occur during renormalization as access-demand by the different processes for the shared bandwidth of the pluripotent node increases the risk of conflicts and interferences (Figures 5 and 6).

In principle, synaptic plasticity can drive intrinsic units in pluripotent nodes to channel processes by dividing their total bandwidth for different client processes. This may be done either in a serial manner, for example, by enabling switching between processes over time through cross-inhibition, or in a parallel manner, for example, by frequency filtering/multiplexing or the local rewiring of resource into dedicated, parallel physical pipelines. In all case, it generally involves resolving a problem of blind-source separation [118]. Figure 7 illustrates such mechanisms. Blind-source separation can be performed by neural network implementations of standard statistical algorithms, based on various versions of classical leaning rules such as the famous Hebb rule (see [119]; Figure 7), which possess some degree of biological plausibility, supported by empirical evidence (e.g., NMDA-receptor-mediated long term potentiation).

But, even though, the implementation of such algorithms in artificial neural networks is relatively straightforward [121], there are many customary issues concerning the normalization and stabilization of the underlying process of reweighting of effective connectivity/synaptic gain over the ensembles of units in the network [133]. For many neural network implementations of these algorithms, it is necessary, in order to avoid divergence and enable convergence, to perform for each iteration of the learning process a normalization of the local synaptic weights in the network, that is, of effective connectivity. This must be done based on a measure of the overall weight of connection in the entire network. Such constraint somewhat defeats the purpose of providing implementations of learning algorithms based on purely local plasticity and principles. In such cases, individual synapses must still "know" the states of all the other synapses to renormalize their own weight. This comes down to expecting neurons to encode routing tables of the entire network or to broadcast information about their own effective connectivity to others or to have access to a central repository or hub capable of informing the entire network about its own state by broadcasting global parameters (see [134]). Evidence indicates that sleep and dreaming may be key periods during which brain processing enters a special mode in order to perform memory encoding and globally normalize local synaptic weights after a day of overall synaptic potentiation related to active, wakeful learning [135].

3.7. Resilience: The Manifestation of Layers of Abstraction at the Core of Structure-Function Relationships in the Brain.

In resilience, the renormalization process involves something global, and the relationships between the "global" level (general routing scheme and strategy) and the "local" levels (synaptic plasticity) appear and remain quite mysterious (see

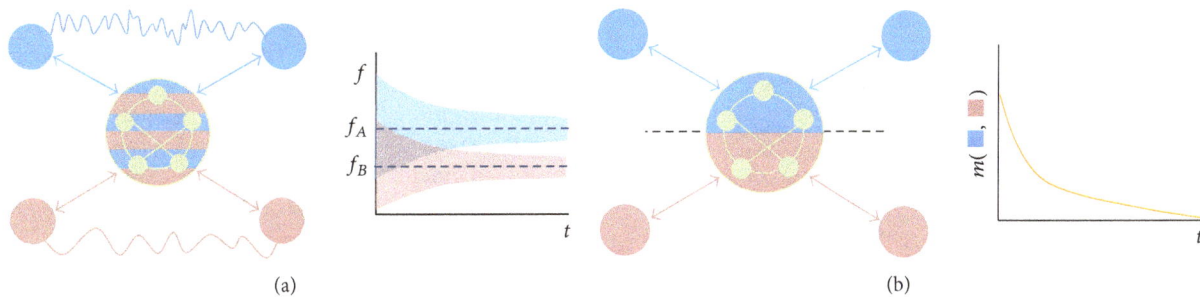

FIGURE 7: Plasticity and pluripotency. Pluripotent nodes can be recruited to provide a common alternate relay between groups of nodes subserving different, independent processes (Figure 5). As the different processes compete for the pluripotent node's bandwidth, the pluripotent node's intrinsic subnetwork of processing units must learn to carry and output the signals from the different competing processes in a manner that is ultimately unadulterated. One option is to multiplex signals from different processes over the subnetwork, for instance based on their frequency content (a). If two processes A and B (blue and red) generate nonoverlapping, narrow-band signals with different central frequencies f_A and f_B, the subnetwork can learn to tune its output nodes' transfer functions so that they separately filter the two frequency bands, and relay adequately the signals (see little chart on the right). Oscillations and the emission of power from multiple frequency bands over the same regions of the brain are reliably observed in electrophysiological signals (see [117]). Another option is to keep the signals from the different processes separated within the subnetwork over different, potentially cross-inhibiting subpipelines. Many other options can be envisioned. In all cases, somewhat, the pluripotent node must learn, as it is recruited for renormalization of information transfer, to separate independent sources of signals (b). Blind source separation can be performed by unsupervised algorithms such as principal component analyses (PCA), for uncorrelated sources of Gaussian signals, and by independent component analysis (ICA), for statistically independent sources of signals (see [118]). In both cases, source separation enables the absence of cross-talks and interference between processes. This is expressed in a mutual information $m(i, j)$ between the nodes of different processes that becomes null (see (b) little chart). These algorithms can easily be implemented in small neural networks. PCA is formally equivalent to neural network implementations based on classical learning rules from connectionism such as Hebb's rule for unsupervised learning (see [119]). Hebb's rule increases synaptic weight $w(i, j)$, that is, local effective connectivity, between a presynaptic neuron i and a postsynaptic neuron j based on the presence of sustained correlations in their activity (see [120]). In this framework, synaptic weights behave just like the loadings of principal components along directions of maximal covariance. ICA can be implemented with modifications and generalizations of Hebb's rule in a manner that minimizes mutual information between processes while maximizing their own intrinsic quantity of information (e.g., infomax algorithm, [121]).

[136]). In order to approach this issue, we must first wonder what processes are the main targets for renormalization in resilience.

The brain is a highly complex biological machine that resolves extremely difficult problems of coordination, learning, inference, anticipation, modeling, integration of information, constitution, and storage of knowledge, as well as sequencing and execution of commands and actions. It does so through a unified framework or "global workspace," for perception, imagination, learning, inference, decision, and action that we call our minds when we are awake (see [127, 137–140]). At the core of this framework there is what I have called "higher-order cognition," which encompasses and unites together in the subjective frame, executive functions, attention, general intelligence, and self-awareness; which are all functionally related. For instance, in healthy individuals, higher metacognitive skills are associated with greater intelligence [141]. Dementia corresponds to a dramatic and radical dissolution of such integrative cognition.

As will be explained in detail in future reports I hold that such a cognitive framework of the human mind is characterized by two main components, for which we recently gained indirect empirical evidence [122]. On the one hand, there is a central process of ongoing computation of inferences in frontotemporal cortices on the physical and social causes of sense data, based on internal models of the world and self, and heavily relying on language and symbolic logic (following principles similar to a hierarchical Bayesian scheme). This process heavily relies on long-term memory and operates over time to satisfy a core utility function related to innate or vital goals and needs, which is expressed through emotion and feeling. On the other hand, there is the real-time multisensory computation and rendering in posterior cortices of a specific type of projective spaces (in a technical sense of that term in projective geometry; see [142]), which frames our three-dimensional experience of the world and self, in perception and imagination, and more generally in spatial cognition. Such internal projective space also serves for the programming of actions in connection with the real space to which it is coupled via sensorimotor interfaces. These two central components of cognition are functionally coupled, just like thought and perception or emotion and action are in the vocabulary of classical philosophy. Their anatomical substrate may be reflected in major anatomofunctional subdivisions in the brain recently uncovered by our group [122].

Irrespective of the details of the mind's cognitive framework, one can safely postulate that such framework exists and directly depends on the overall functional scheme of information processing in the brain. From a neurological standpoint, this functional scheme thus appears most important to preserve for overall cognitive resilience. It is first and foremost at the level of this "functional brain," so to speak, that the brain as a whole must be resilient to preserve cognition.

Neuropsychiatric conditions such as schizophrenia, and their wealth of distress and anxiety for the patients, which is notably related to their frequent self-awareness of global cognitive dysfunction, or autism are a striking demonstration of the importance of preserving the overall cognitive framework, as a condition for autonomy and adaptation to the world's demands [17].

A key fact to integrate is that part of the process underlying resilience is driven by top-down cognition. Often, in the process of recovery, patients painstakingly struggle to rebuild awareness of their deficit, as a first necessary step for learning solutions to cope with it. Awakening and recovering from coma, vegetative states and minimally conscious states to regain full-fledged consciousness are striking examples of such struggle. They are cruel evidence that rebooting a general state of consciousness is the first critical step in cognitive resilience, before any other recovery process pertaining to more specialized skills can be engaged willfully to regain autonomy (see [43]). Then becoming self-aware of deficit, as disorienting and distressing as it may be, is, in and of itself, a root principle for reorganization: one must become aware of malfunctioning to be able to willfully act upon any malfunction. Anosognosia, the lack of self-awareness of one's own deficits, is negatively correlated with resilience [78]. There is clinical evidence that in many cases, higher-order cognition, for example, self-awareness, plays a key role in enabling and driving cognitive resilience itself. The concept of CR discussed previously brings forth the importance for resilience of neuropsychological variables such as general intelligence, degree of literacy, educational attainment, occupational complexity, interpersonal skills, integration in social networks, personality variables, and leisure activity.

More generally, self-representations, self-awareness of deficits, executive functions for self-control, goal-directed cognition, and intelligence, all, are enabling conditions and motivating factors for engaging in a process of frustrating, often painful and uncertain, sometimes lifelong rehabilitation.

In such context, if resilience implies a global reweighting of local synaptic plasticity, then there is a top-down control mechanism based on seeds of preserved higher-order cognition that is capable of acting upon local plasticity to support resilience.

Moreover, it is impossible to overlook the importance of social cognition and support in such process [143]. A supportive social environment of clinicians, friends, and family, providing social feedback signals can be key for resilience. It is a source of normative models of cognition and behavior, which can potentially be used by the patient in order to define cognitive and behavioral references or standards and better supervise the renormalization process as he struggles to find the pathways of resilience. This principle is at the center of most rehabilitation strategies.

At a slightly lower level of cognitive integration, phenomena such as sensory substitution (see [144]) demonstrate that, at an intermediate level, basic perceptual experiences are synthetized based on flexible relations to the brain hardware. In sensory substitution, a category of experience (e.g., visual) is induced in a functional manner, based on the stimulation of sensory systems normally associated with other categories of experience (e.g., touch). The stimulation is designed to reproduce sensorimotor contingencies that are intrinsic to the first category of experience (e.g., telemetry versus direct contact), based on intermediary devices augmenting the sensory channel associated with the second category of experience. The ability of the brain to sense the same sources of information and to build the same overall qualitative experience in multiple indirect ways is also illustrated by patients without insula who can nevertheless continue feeling interoceptive information via alternate pathways normally associated with exteroception [13].

Therefore, a hierarchy of top-down processes contributes to controlling resilience and renormalization of effective connectivity in a robust manner, from higher-order self-awareness and perceptual gestalt synthesis to basic operant learning.

In order to understand in an operational manner what exactly must be renormalized in resilience, it is important to identify specific levels of expression of cognitive processing that are as close as possible to observable physical levels of implementation. Information processing in the brain must ultimately embed cognition, even when considered at a level of observation close to hardware implementation (see the illustrative models presented in Figures 5–7).

At such level of implementation, information processing, for example, mutual information, at first appears to entertain a close relationship with the structural network, for example, matrices of structural and functional connectivity resemble each other and there are generative rules between them. However, as reviewed above, evidence suggests that the renormalization of functional connectivity correlates more with recovery of function than the rigid structure of processing units and wires that remains largely invariant at the large-scale, following extensive brain damage.

The effective, in-use, functional wiring diagram of information processing supporting ongoing core cognition in the brain is to some extent different from the structural implementations that may be expected to serve as a preset, somewhat rigid, specialized set of pipelines to support it. As reviewed in this paper, the robustness of higher-order cognitive functions and their striking ability for resilience demonstrate that central aspects of higher-order cognition may rely on information processing mechanisms that are unlikely to rigidly depend upon a static, fixed set of specialized brain regions and anatomical connections. They are more likely to operate by dynamically exploiting available neural resources and possible routes between them, based on the resilient use of flexible, degenerate, and pluripotent brain systems. If higher-order cognition is so transferable and capable of dynamic reinstantiation and reinitialization, then, in principle, higher-order cognition might have multiple solutions of implementation with respect to the brain substrate [2]. More generally, in normal conditions, neural networks show collective behaviors that are manifested in higher-order parameters controlling highly contextual information processing modes, notably in the prefrontal cortex (see [128]).

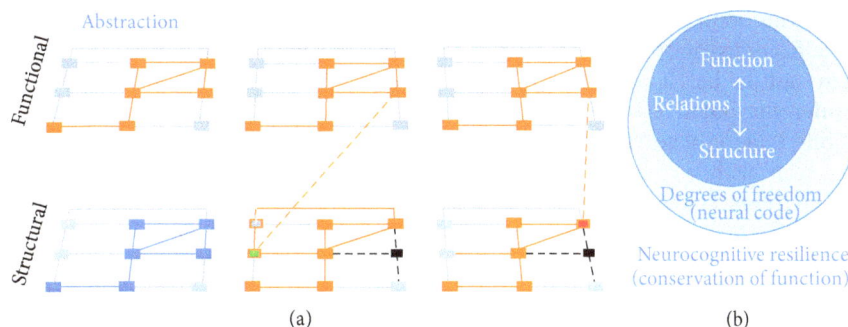

FIGURE 8: Abstraction of function from structure. (a) The relationships of connectivity among the nodes of a network can reside at, at least, two levels, structural and functional levels. Modifications at the structural level (black squares and lines representing damage) can be compensated by reassigning nodes and nodes' relationships to keep invariant (or similar) the map of the process of information transfer at the level of the functional map. *Left.* The structural and functional map over the network are identical. *Center.* After damage, the structural map is modified. Degeneracy in the structure is used to compensate for the lost node (black) and another available node in the structure is allocated (green). Topologically, the functional network is equivalent to the original structural network. *Right.* Pluripotency is used to compensate for the lost node, while another node, but already used in the structure is allocated (red). This nevertheless maximally preserves network's topology. (b) Illustration of the notion of degrees of freedom in structure-function relationships in the brain, and of their role in resilience.

Such capacity for relative decoupling between structure and function in the brain appears quite adaptive vis-à-vis evolution. It implements a somewhat universal resilient functional architecture capable of rerouting and sustaining itself, in a manner that is partially independent from the fixed structure of connectivity that is most directly susceptible to irreversible damage. In summary, it suggests the hypothesis that

(i) core higher-order cognition behaves like a general algorithm that relates to the brain qua a hierarchy of layers of abstraction, and participates in driving its own resilience in a top-down manner (qua self-awareness);

(ii) interfaces between layers exploit combinatorial principles, just as with code execution in computers, in order to handle resource allocation and dynamic routing,

(iii) the process ultimately does so by dynamically controlling local biophysical and biochemical parameters involved in synaptic plasticity.

In other words, under such hypothesis, the relation between higher-order cognition, the brain, and the principles driving resilience appears to be of a relatively abstract or algorithmic nature. In this framework the neural correlates of the mind has to be understood via layers of abstractions (Figures 8 and 9). Resilience would reflect the presence of intrinsic degrees of freedom in structure-function relationships. It would be linked to combinatory rules implemented in the brain for flexible allocation of resources, operating at the interface between structure and function. The rules and mechanisms of these flexible relationships, which are nothing but the neural "code" itself, need to be studied, understood, modeled, and exploited in medicine and neuroengineering. I would even argue that there is no definitive reason at this point to reject the hypothesis that such code may exist and

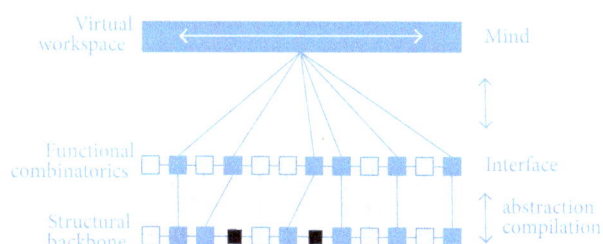

FIGURE 9: Structure-function relationships, abstraction layers and resilience. Beyond the notion of redundancy in distributed brain systems, hypothesis of the existence of abstraction layers, that is, a neural code, contributing to resilience, involving a partial virtualization of the functional architecture underlying cognition (see text).

even perhaps present features as universal as the genetic code but for biological cognition. It remains an open question.

Standard anatomofunctional explanations—in which a strong and rigid relationship between structure and function is generally expected—will miss essential aspects of the neural correlate of the mind. Understanding the nature of such "computation" and how it relates to the brain will present many theoretical and methodological challenges to cognitive neuroscience. If true, to some extent, such a framework will automatically raise potential concerns regarding the validity, in this context, of neuroanatomical hypotheses involving specific critical regions, either localized or distributed over several locations. Indeed in such a framework, the link between the brain substrate and the most integrative aspects of the mind might have to be reconceived on the model of the flexible relationships existing between hardware and software in computer science. As just mentioned, this would reopen profound questions about neural coding and suggest an approach to neuroscience returning to models inspired from system engineering and computer design, which have become often considered as inappropriate to understand biological systems such as the brain as a whole [16, 145]. No matter what the specifications of such computational relationships would turn out to be, it would seem like an impossible task to infer the putative "coding scheme" from empirical observations, looking at correlations between structure and function, even with a perfect spatial and temporal resolution. In this respect it would be analogous to the impossible task of inferring the "operating system" running through a CPU by measuring the temperature of the CPU at multiple locations (which is not that much different from what we do when we use functional imaging or macroscopic electrophysiology in cognitive neuroscience). Nevertheless this is a task that neuroscience might eventually have to take on again, perhaps with the help of new theoretical breakthrough and computational resources. Models that are driven by first principles (such as Friston's free-energy driven Bayesian scheme for the brain; see [139, 140]) might help to resolve this issue, and there is a strong need for progress in theoretical neuroscience and psychology.

3.8. Is the Mind a Virtual Machine Running on a Distributed Computer? We have envisioned in the previous section a series of arguments in support of the hypothesis that the mind relates to the brain through layers of abstraction, similar to what is implemented in computer science. We argued for the existence of low-level interfaces that govern the relationships between the rigid structural organization of the brain and information processing in neural networks, based on abstract combinatorial rules. The existence of such interfaces is suggested by the process of renormalization of information processing patterns that is observed in cognitive resilience to neurological insult, and unfolds while structural connectivity remains invariant. Such process and its top-down driving demonstrate the existence of degrees of freedom and of a relative independence between structure and function in the brain.

Similar features are found in virtual machines, or more generally in virtualization of distributed computer resources [146, 147]. "Virtualization" is a strategy aimed at simplifying and rendering more resilient interactions between systems, applications, or end users and complex distributed computing resources and devices, operating with rigidly set rules. It involves a set of operations that are precisely and explicitly aimed at hiding the physical characteristics or complicated details of an underlying hardware implementation, and at mapping function over structure flexibly, so that higher-order processes to which they are transparent can continue to operate independently of changes in the underlying hardware. The functional environment that is thereby created facilitates a resilient interfacing with other resources, by reducing dependency with the lower-layers of implementation down to the microdesign of the hardware. It allows the system to transfer entire processes from one physical environment to the other. It is used to facilitate multiplexed access, to combine resources at different physical locations under one virtual interface, and more generally to simplify the control of a complex device (in our case, the brain and the body in interaction with their environment). It generally takes many more cycles of computation to simulate resources and run a virtual machine than it would with a direct hardware implementation, so a virtualized environment can be slower, for equivalent amounts of nominal resources. For sure, controlled cognition and more generally higher-order cognition are slow (e.g., in the second range), as compared to electrochemical signaling (e.g., in the millisecond range). Virtualization is capable of providing maximum resilience to processes operating over networks of distributed computing resources. A form of virtualization of computation in the brain would thus appear to be a sound solution to resilience from an evolutionary standpoint.

Such a hypothesis entails conceptualizing the "mind" itself as a virtual entity (Figure 9) and the brain as a code interpreter. Without entering in the details of other reports in preparation, there is undeniable evidence that the brain is a code and command interpreter. The mere existence and the properties of language are proofs that this is the case at some level. Language, with its ability to address semantic memory and evoke mental imagery, is both one of the core components of higher-order cognition and a sparse, sequential code with specific combinatory rules. It is governed by universal syntactic principles and multiple layers of abstraction and parsing rules that are hierarchically nested (e.g., phonemes, morphemes, words, phrases, propositions, and so on). It can be dematerialized and carried via multiple media (e.g., speech and writing). In parsing, interpreting and understanding words, we are the living proof and we manifest that the brain is a code interpreter.

3.9. Resilience: Between Abstraction and Resistance. In this framework, irrespective of what the principles and details of the mind-brain interfacing may ultimately turn out to be, the mind is conceived as a functional entity. Through the phenomenon of cognitive resilience, this functional entity therefore behaves as an assaulted "fortress" which attempts to defend itself against desiccation and loss of autonomy. It struggles to rebuild its functional environment, even as its shrinking neural environment forces it to take adaptive measures. This is implicit and pervasive throughout the struggle and utmost distress of patients affected by AD as the night of dementia takes over and consciousness shrinks on a background of apathy and confusion. More generally, over its lifetime, the mind struggles with and resists insults and multiple normal and/or pathological perturbations arising from its neural, psychological, and social environments. The experience of effortful cognition, emotion regulation, willpower, and resilience to life events and disease is direct evidence of this existential fact.

Searching in brain mechanisms for the expression of this self-same resistance to destruction which is embedded at the core of cognition can be a strategy for isolating key aspects of the neural correlates of the mind. Given the core role of higher-order cognition itself, for example, self-awareness, in enabling and driving cognitive resilience and functional renormalization (see above), and more generally adaptive behaviors, it is intriguing to realize that it is possible to conceive of the very function of consciousness as being, in and of itself, a form of fundamental algorithm for resilience selected by evolution.

At the core of this resilience, there is also a dimension of "resistance." The concept of resistance here is to be interpreted as a bridge-concept between phenomenology and physics. Brain computation and resilience encounter inertia in biological systems [16], including the inertia of synaptic plasticity, which slow down functional processes and render them as energetically costly. My hypothesis is that this plays a central role in shaping the phenomenology of the mind. This inner resistance of the mind against inertia that resilience manifests suggests that the mind also features a behavior of perturbed dynamical system: it drains energy to maintain its dynamics in a timely manner within certain boundaries of its state space based on an adaptive tuning of its control parameters (see [12, 16, 17, 136]). As far as the mind is concerned, abstract computation thus seems to be intimately coupled with the physics of out-of-equilibrium systems.

For the longest, schools in the cognitive science opposed two views. On the one hand, there was the computational view on mind-brain relationships, sometimes construed as "ancient" with its software-hardware analogy and its emphasis on symbolic processing; what we could call the Von Neumann's brain. On the other hand, there was a more "modern" biophysical view on mindbrain relationships, which brings forth self-organization, complexity, and dynamical system theories, and relies implicitly or explicitly on the generic model of coupled differential equations and the notion of emergence, what we could call the Varela's brain (see [136, 148, 149]). This academic antinomy was not in the mind of von Neumann when he developed his famous architecture at the core of all modern computers [150], as he based his reflections upon the architecture of the brain and the abstract model of neuron by McCulloch and Pitts [151], and derived the principles of implementation of universal arithmetical operations based on simple accumulators functioning as logical gates, by reasoning about small networks of interconnected formal neurons.

A network of computers—such as the Internet—is in turn certainly a complex, distributed dynamical system, embedding much self-organization (we need only consider all the various "bots" and autonomous agents trawling the web today), myriads of coupled oscillators at numerous scales, all while being run ultimately through the combinatory principles of a Von Neumann architecture. The possibility that the brain embeds similar principles should (re-)open many directions of research and therefore should be an opportunity to bring together several scientific communities that may have lost the habit of working together, or at the very least, that of cross-pollinating their research findings in ways that would ultimately prove mutually beneficial.

In summary, according to such a view, our mind is mediated by an algorithm that mimics a virtual machine and that governs the execution of an adaptive program in the brain, following inchoate and abstract combinatorial rules. The algorithm is characterized by principles that make the execution of such program resilient to structural damage, and more generally capable of coping, within the boundaries of energetic and chronometric constraints, with the inertia of its own biophysical implementation to produce adaptive cognition and behaviors. Behind a resilient mind there is

a computation depending on a capacity to control routing and information transfer among distributed resources by building new paths of least resistance in the brain substrate. This requires both abstract principles and energy.

It is intriguing to consider that if evolution implies selecting resilient systems, in such framework, the ability to relate function and structure via layers of abstraction, or more generally abstraction, might paradoxically appear as a summit of biological evolution. It is further intriguing to consider that if functionally, consciousness itself is a form of higher-order, universal algorithm for resiliency, consciousness might itself appear to be the pinnacle of biological evolution qua abstraction. It is relevant to reemphasize here that basic consciousness appears to be one of the most resilient feature of cognition (see first part of the paper), as would be predicted based on the rationale that a mechanism optimized for the resiliency of cognitive and control systems should itself be maximally resilient (see also [12]).

4. Studying the Mechanisms of Resilience: A Challenge for Neuroscience and Neuroimaging Methods

One important venue for research on cognitive resilience is the study of structure-function relationships and their degrees of freedom at the large scale level. Several methodological challenges can be distinguished regarding this endeavor.

The Challenge of Multimodality. The disease processes and neurological disorders that manifest and call for cognitive resilience in patients struggling with their condition are diverse and complex. Their physiopathology often affects the brain at multiple scales and in multiple ways. The relative disconnect, extensively discussed above, between clinical expression and gross structural neuropathology that exists in resilient patients suggests the importance of specifically studying (1) functional parameters related to large-scale interactions and metabolism, in reference to (2) structural parameters, related to structural connectivity and morphometry (e.g., neuronal count). In order to (1) increase specificity, (2) adequately map this uncharted territory of compensatory anatomofunctional reorganizations, and (3) test hypotheses in a well-controlled, meaningful and conclusive way, we should endeavor to take into account the various levels of structural and metabolic brain alterations affecting the patients.

It is particularly important to find powerful and reliable solutions to analyze multimodal neuroimaging data together, as well as multiple dependent parameters. Thereby we can open multiple windows on one underlying brain. Contemporary medical imaging and multicentric projects foster the simultaneous use of complementary imaging modalities over a large number of patients at multiple time points. However solutions for proper data integration still need to be discovered and implemented in order to reduce the risk of data cemeteries, with an enormous amount of data that might not be exploited to their full potential.

Multimodality can increase sensitivity and specificity, and it can offer better inferential power and better potential for pathophysiological interpretation [57]. It is particularly relevant for studying large-scale, higher-order, neurodynamical phenomena with specificity [67]. For instance, matching brains based on gray matter atrophy and accounting for structural disconnection and baseline metabolism are essential if one is to study which aspects of residual functional connectivity could account for CR specifically (see [8]). For example, significant differences in residual functional connectivity in fMRI between AD patients and healthy controls remained after accounting for structural damage such as cortical atrophy [152]. This suggests that it is important to extract information that is specific to each modality by taking into account the shared variance with the others. Yet studies combining structural and functional connectivity analyses are still in their infancy [66].

Multimodality is also important for understanding the relationships between different levels of observation in the brain, as well as making causal inferences about them. For instance, hippocampal atrophy in AD has been shown to be related to cingulum bundle atrophy, itself correlated with hypometabolism of the posterior cingulate cortex [153]. This suggested that the observed hypometabolism was related to the impact of hippocampal atrophy and mediated by the cingulum.

The Challenge of Integrating Longitudinal Information and Dynamics. Beyond multimodality, it is important to integrate a longitudinal perspective. Resilience is by definition a dynamical process that unfolds over time and at time scales that can vary greatly among disease processes and individuals. It can manifest through very rapid compensations over a matter of hours or days following certain strokes (e.g., the resolution of several acute-phase deficits like certain forms of anosognosia and aphasia) as well as through decades of struggle in the case of neurodegenerative processes such as AD.

Thus within its course, AD presents fluctuations that could contain critical information about nonlinear transitions between stages of disease progression [154], reflecting critical neuropathological processes, mechanisms of vulnerability, and resilience. Therefore, it is important to study such processes using longitudinal paradigms, which can also yield an increase in sensitivity, specificity, and physiopathological interpretability, as well as enhance the translational impact of research on individual patients.

Integration of longitudinal data in discriminant analyses has proven to ameliorate early estimates of conversion from MCI to AD up to 6 months before conversion [155]. Given the high interindividual variability in clinical response to neuropathological processes, being able to model and account for within-subject variability can substantially improve the heuristic value of studies and signal detection. This view of the importance of longitudinal analyses is largely shared by the research community [8, 78]. Many research groups from around the world are implementing large-scale multimodal longitudinal studies, for example, the Alzheimer's disease neuroimaging initiative (ADNI) [57], which includes more than 800 healthy elderly participants, MCI and AD patients. A further important one is the French MEMENTO project. Nevertheless few longitudinal studies in functional connectivity have been conducted in AD [66, 67]. Some longitudinal studies suggest an accelerated aging, a central role of the DMN and a driving role of the posterior cingulate cortex connectivity pattern in disease progression (see [94, 156]).

Of course, the ideal rate of longitudinal acquisition should be adjusted to the "natural" rate of evolution that is specific to the neurological disorder or process under consideration. For instance, in awakening from coma, the ability to acquire data several times a week over the relatively short period during which there is a maximum expectation of change in mental status in the patients, would bring new fundamental insights about the mechanisms of recovery from the disorder, and have an impactful and lasting translational value. Of course, there are major practical issues of feasibility in such projects, due to safety concerns and clinical constraints, such as problems with titration as well as a lack of adequate infrastructures.

Several other important challenges face research about the dynamics of structure-function relationships. It is paramount to have well-controlled, basic research on the impact of experimental lesions of specific systems of fiber tracts and cortical regions on structural and functional connectivity over time. We must also look at the potential of electrical stimulation and pharmacology to renormalize functional connectivity, cognition and behavior following lesions. For these reasons, it is very important to support the development of valid, imageable, well-documented animal models, (e.g., macaque fascicularis and rat). A multitude of questions remains unanswered that only animal experiments on the topic will be able to address. A solid ground of basic research is necessary for interpreting the mass of multicentric, exploratory, observational human neuroimaging studies that are acquired everywhere in the world at great cost. Likewise, it is important to develop a sound computational framework in order to handle the different levels of observations involved, and quantify and model large-scale structure-function relationships (Figures 2, 4, and 10). New multimodal multidimenional metrics will have to be developed, based on well-conceived models, in order to provide new biomarkers of disease processes and compensatory mechanisms with maximum sensitivity and specificity. Last but not least, there is the challenge of defining and implementing a heuristic framework to develop new strategies of treatments and solutions of renormalization of function. Such framework should be based on sound physiopathological and resilience-related mechanisms, derived from observation and modeling, and aimed at cognitive/behavioral rehabilitation strategies, electromagnetic stimulations, surgery and/or pharmacology.

5. Perspectives for Medicine

The relative disconnect between the clinical and neuropathological aspects of various neurological disorders, both within individuals across time and between individuals, has puzzled the research and clinical communities. Resilience is a central, positive contributor to such disconnect. By remaining

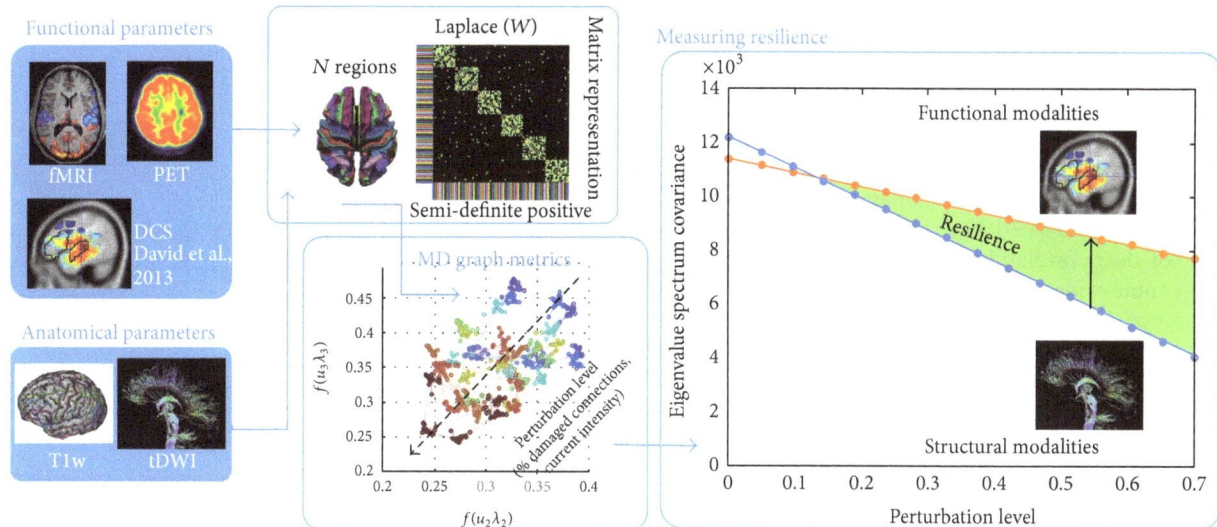

FIGURE 10: Addressing the challenges of quantifying resilience. Schema of a multimodal framework that distinguishes functional and anatomical parameters for key neuroimaging and electrical modalities. One approach is to compute matrices of connectivity based on neuroimaging signals, and then compute their Laplacian in order to obtain matrices that are semi-definite positive. Eigenvector decompositions of the matrices enable the analysis of their topological properties within multidimensional (MD) vector spaces with well-defined bases. Relations between modalities as well as the effect of structural perturbations can be measured in these spaces (see also Figure 4). Resilience can then be studied, modeled, and measured by computing parameters over these spaces and by comparing structural and functional modalities. In the framework discussed in this paper, one working hypothesis would be that resilient patients will demonstrate functional parameters that better resist damage (perturbation), in reference to normative atlases, than corresponding structural parameters.

unmodeled, it challenges the aim of achieving specificity and sensitivity in the estimation of risk of conversion to disease, differential diagnostic, prognostic, outcome of interventions, biomarker identification, the design of inclusion criteria for clinical trials aiming at reducing sample size, and that of prospective studies in which early detection of disease and testing disease-modifying treatments are central [8, 9].

The study and modeling of the mechanisms underlying resilience will thus contribute to increase specificity and sensitivity in the characterization of clinical and neuropathological relationships, by better modeling within-individual and interindividual variability. It will be a basis for defining new biomarkers, derived based on neurophysiologically sound hypotheses and well-behaved metrics over multimodal parameters, for better diagnostic, prognostic, and treatment outcome monitoring. Likewise, a better understanding of resilience will help to improve predictions regarding the clinical evolution of cognition and behavior based on multimodal neuroimaging. It will also offer a paradigm for the search for treatments and solutions in functional rehabilitation, and more generally interventional neurology, based on an understanding of the mechanisms enabling and fostering resilience.

Moreover the mechanisms supporting resilience might in certain cases directly alter the disease processes themselves, and not just compensate for them by providing a sheer buffer against the negative impact of the pathology on cognition. This disease-modifying effect might in part be mediated by neuromodulatory factors with anti-inflammatory and antiamyloid burden effects [131]. Exercise and cognitively stimulating experiences, notably the experience of novelty,

directly impact the brain by increasing local brain volume, neurogenesis, synaptogenesis, the release of the brain derived neurotrophic factor (BDNF), and resistance to apoptosis. This ensemble of neuroprotective mechanisms might be fostered by increasing the noradrenergic tone, which according to recent theories could play a central role in CR [131]. Likewise, environmental enrichment has been suggested in animal models to prevent or slow AD beta amyloid pathology, suggesting a disease-modifying effect of factors related to CR [157]. Moreover, a relationship between higher CR and lower incidence or severity of anosognosia has been shown in dementia [78], which in turn suggests that fostering CR and self-awareness might help to contribute to reduce the risk of developing AD.

In such a framework, research on the mechanisms of resilience and on possible treatments and interventions should strategically place some emphasis on computational modeling, building upon the potential for structure-function dissociations in the brain, and exploiting multimodal imaging to estimate relevant parameters and compare results to empirical observations. The question then can become that of the molecular and/or electrical mechanisms that could be introduced in the system as modeled (e.g., with a particular set of pathological biomarkers), in order to renormalize functional integration and cognition. A Big Data approach can help to derive priors about key features of target resilient versus nonresilient systems, which can in turn inform analyses and inferences, taking advantage for instance of web APIs. For example, one can perform automated meta-analyses of fMRI activation studies, based on text-mining and automated activation peak coordinate extraction from thousands of relevant references, in order to inform the characterization of the functional role of target systems (see http://neurosynth.org/; http://www.linkrbrain.org/; see also [14, 158]). One can also analyze data of genetic expression from microarrays sampled over the brain in order to identify molecular footprints characteristic of target systems (e.g., Allen Brain Atlas: http://human.brain-map.org). For instance, Goel et al. [159] have recently demonstrated the existence of clear correlations between structural connectivity and genome-wide genetic expression data. Such a model-driven approach will contribute to inform pharmacological research for treatments as well as possible solutions of surgery and electrostimulations. Likewise, better understanding the connections between cognition and the brain in such a framework will help to conceive functional rehabilitation strategies promoting resilience, based on cognitive stimulations and principles of computational psychology.

Finally, and importantly, adequate understanding and modeling of the mechanisms of resilience will also constitute an important basis for a reflection on preventive medicine in the domain of public health. This will help to identify factors and mechanisms for reducing the risk of disease onset or progression and for mitigating the functional impact of damage. Approaching brain disorders from the angle of resilience is developing a positive approach to medicine in the face of what cannot yet be cured.

Figure 11 summarizes the different scientific problems concerning the study of cognitive resilience to neurological insults and their organic relationships.

6. Conclusion

The present review and discussion support the hypothesis that higher-order cognition can be a highly robust, resilient, and flexible phenomenon in the face of extensive brain damage. A global process of renormalization of effective connectivity following a major disruption of structural connectivity can account for the rerouting of brain signal and for the effective preservation of the scheme of information processing subtending cognition. Bottom-up and top-down mechanisms, as well as local and global principles, are at play in the process. Self-awareness itself and more generally consciousness appear to be central in enabling top-down processes that are key for recovering impaired cognitive functions. We hypothesized that consciousness itself can be interpreted as a general algorithm for resilience selected by evolution. Progress in cognitive neuroscience of higher-order cognition might require considering computational hypotheses about brain-mind relationships and structure-function relationships in the brain, in which the standard anatomofunctional framework would need to be complemented by an understanding of the putative layers of abstraction and principles of virtualization that may be at work in neurocognitive computation. These layers would not directly and simply be reflected in the brain hardware. Their nature remains mysterious, but the place of abstraction in nature might be greater than one thought.

The study and modeling of the mechanisms of resilience are important in order to increase specificity in diagnostic,

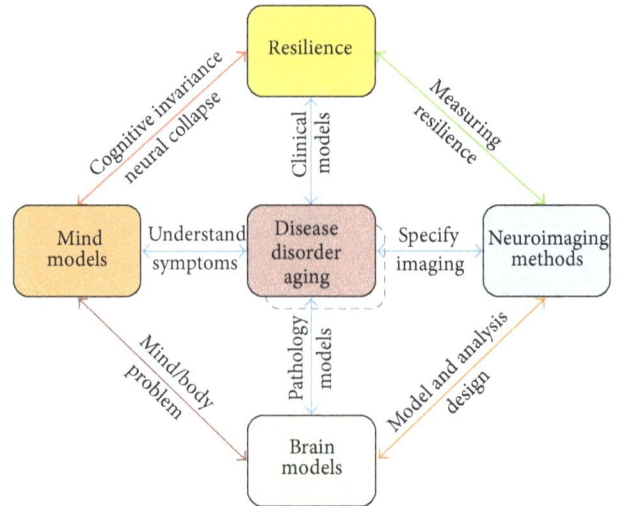

FIGURE 11: Relationships between levels of knowledge and scientific issues in the study and control of resilience. Roadmap for research on resilience. This diagram shows different scientific problems that are central to the study of cognitive resilience to neurological insults and their organic relationships.

prognostic, and treatment outcome monitoring in medicine. They also have a strong potential for informing prevention and treatment strategy, as well as technologies aimed at mitigating the functional impact of damage based on the renormalization of functions. More generally they could inform solutions to foster cognitive resilience against aging, as well as cognitive enhancement. They also open important perspectives for neuroengineering and artificial intelligence.

Definitions

Resilience. The ability for a system to resist dynamically a perturbation or adverse condition that challenges the integrity of its normal operation and to preserve function as a result in reference to some initial design or normative functional standards.

Structural Connectivity. Informs the physical connections (e.g., fiber tracts or axons) existing between pair of nodes (e.g., brain regions or neurons) in a network, at a given scale. For the brain, it is often estimated in vivo based on tractography over diffusion weighted imaging (DWI). The analysis of a matrix of structural connectivity can identify direct and indirect, alternate structural pathways between regions.

Effective Connectivity. An indicator of presence of structural connectivity weighted by a transmission or synaptic gain. This parameter regulates signal propagation and interactions between network nodes (neurons or brain regions, depending on the scale considered). It is equivalent to the concept of synaptic weight at the synaptic scale but can be used more generally to characterize the gain of transmission between network nodes at any scale. It is an essential level of modeling of functional plasticity in the brain.

Functional Connectivity. A measure of the correlations between brain signals, often empirically derived from resting state functional magnetic resonance imaging (rsfMRI) data. It reflects both direct and indirect interactions between network nodes (e.g., brain regions). It is formally similar to analyses of coherence performed on electrophysiological signals. Functional connectivity relates to structural and effective connectivity through a generative process or model of brain dynamics based on physiological mechanisms.

Mutual Information. A quantity derived from Shannon's entropy, which characterizes the degree of statistical dependence between two variables X and Y. It is minimal when two systems do not exchange information and maximum when they share the exact same information. It reflects both direct and indirect information transfer (e.g., via indirect pathways) between network nodes (e.g., brain regions). Mutual information relates to structural and effective connectivity through a generative process or model of brain dynamics based on physiological mechanisms.

Degeneracy. Form of redundancy in networks. Multiple alternate available processing units/nodes are capable of handling the same function (e.g., parallel array of identical specialized processors).

Pluripotency. Form of redundancy in networks. Processing units/nodes are individually capable of handling multiple functions contextually (e.g., processor individually executing different tasks sequentially by switching between them).

Disconnection. A disconnection of pathways in the matrix of structural connectivity following brain damage. Disconnection disrupts communication and interactions between network nodes (e.g., brain regions) normally connected and interacting via these pathways.

Routing. The mechanism regulating the transfer of information between network nodes along existing structural connections to preserve the timely execution of functional processes that critically depend on the interaction between these nodes. Dynamic routing in the brain can be controlled by modulating effective connectivity between network nodes (e.g., brain regions) along structural pathways.

Renormalization of Function. Relative preservation of or return to the "normal," overall functional scheme underlying normal cognition, following brain damage, in a manner that is compatible with residual structural and metabolic resources. It is the problem that a resilient brain must resolve after brain damage.

Conflict of Interests

The author declares that there is no conflict of interests regarding the publication of this paper.

Acknowledgments

The author would like to particularly thank Ralph Adolphs, Justin Feinstein, Katharina Orhnberger, Guillaume Marrelec, Kenneth Williford, and ZZ Packer for their invaluable feedbacks during the completion of this paper. He also thanks Dirk Neumann, Alain Giron, and Mélanie Pélégrini for their insights. Additionally the author would like to thank for their direct or indirect influence on these ideas over the years: F. Varela, A. Damasio, Th. Grabowski, D. Tranel, S. Metha, S. Khalsa, C. Philippi, H. Benali, G. Landini, Y. Burnod, D. Bennequin, and M. Le Van Quyen.

References

[1] A. Luria, *The Man with a Shattered World: The History of a Brain Wound*, Harvard University Press, Cambridge, Mass, USA, 1987.

[2] U. Noppeney, K. J. Friston, and C. J. Price, "Degenerate neuronal systems sustaining cognitive functions," *Journal of Anatomy*, vol. 205, no. 6, pp. 433–442, 2004.

[3] C. L. Philippi, J. S. Feinstein, S. S. Khalsa et al., "Preserved self-awareness following extensive bilateral brain damage to the insula, anterior cingulate, and medial prefrontal cortices," *PLoS ONE*, vol. 7, no. 8, Article ID e38413, 2012.

[4] S. Laureys, M. Boly, and P. Maquet, "Tracking the recovery of consciousness from coma," *Journal of Clinical Investigation*, vol. 116, no. 7, pp. 1823–1825, 2006.

[5] A. M. Owen, M. R. Coleman, M. Boly, M. H. Davis, S. Laureys, and J. D. Pickard, "Detecting awareness in the vegetative state," *Science*, vol. 313, no. 5792, p. 1402, 2006.

[6] M. M. Monti, A. Vanhaudenhuyse, M. R. Coleman et al., "Willful modulation of brain activity in disorders of consciousness," *The New England Journal of Medicine*, vol. 362, no. 7, pp. 579–589, 2010.

[7] O. Sacks, *Awakenings*, Pelican Books, Harmondsworth, UK, 1976.

[8] Y. Stern, "Cognitive reserve," *Neuropsychologia*, vol. 47, no. 10, pp. 2015–2028, 2009.

[9] B. Dubois, H. H. Feldman, C. Jacova et al., "Revising the definition of Alzheimer's disease: a new lexicon," *The Lancet Neurology*, vol. 9, no. 11, pp. 1118–1127, 2010.

[10] M. F. de Oliveira, F. C. G. Pinto, K. Nishikuni, R. V. Botelho, A. M. Lima, and J. M. Rotta, "Revisiting hydrocephalus as a model to study brain resilience," *Frontiers in Human Neuroscience*, vol. 5, article 181, 2012.

[11] Y. Stern, "Cognitive reserve and Alzheimer disease," *Alzheimer Disease and Associated Disorders*, vol. 20, no. 2, pp. 112–117, 2006.

[12] K. Williford, D. Rudrauf, and C. L. Philippi, "Self-consciousness," in *Encyclopedia of the Mind*, Sage, Thousand Oaks, Calif, USA, 2011.

[13] S. S. Khalsa, D. Rudrauf, J. S. Feinstein, and D. Tranel, "The pathways of interoceptive awareness," *Nature Neuroscience*, vol. 12, no. 12, pp. 1494–1496, 2009.

[14] G. M. Edelman and J. A. Gally, "Degeneracy and complexity in biological systems," *Proceedings of the National Academy of Sciences of the United States of America*, vol. 98, no. 24, pp. 13763–13768, 2001.

[15] R. G. Lee and P. van Donkelaar, "Mechanisms underlying functional recovery following stroke," *Canadian Journal of Neurological Sciences*, vol. 22, no. 4, pp. 257–263, 1995.

[16] D. Rudrauf and A. Damasio, "A conjecture regarding the biological mechanism of subjectivity and feeling," *Journal of Consciousness Studies*, vol. 12, no. 8–10, pp. 236–262, 2005.

[17] S. Paradiso and D. Rudrauf, "Struggle for life, struggle for love and recognition: the neglected self in social cognitive neuroscience," *Dialogues in Clinical Neuroscience*, vol. 14, no. 1, pp. 65–75, 2012.

[18] W. Penfield, "Neurophysiological basis of the higher functions of the nervous system," in *Handbook of Physiology; A Critical, Comprehensive Presentation of Physiological Knowledge and Concepts*, L. S. Jefferson, A. D. Cherrington, and H. M. Goodman, Eds., vol. 6, p. 1254, Oxford University Press, New York, NY, USA, 1960.

[19] A. Damasio, *The Feeling of What Happens: Body and Emotion in the Making of Consciousness*, Harvest Books, 1999.

[20] L. Feuillet, H. Dufour, and J. Pelletier, "Brain of a white-collar worker," *The Lancet*, vol. 370, no. 9583, p. 262, 2007.

[21] H. Damasio and A. Damasio, *Lesion Analysis in Neuropsychology*, Oxford University Press, New York, NY, USA, 1989.

[22] D. Rudrauf, S. Mehta,. J. Bruss, D. Tranel, H. Damasio, and T. J. Grabowski, "Thresholding lesion overlap difference maps: application to category-related naming and recognition deficits," *NeuroImage*, vol. 41, no. 3, pp. 970–984, 2008.

[23] D. Rudrauf, S. Mehta, and T. J. Grabowski, "Disconnection's renaissance takes shape: formal incorporation in group-level lesion studies," *Cortex*, vol. 44, no. 8, pp. 1084–1096, 2008.

[24] M. C. Cirstea and M. F. Levin, "Compensatory strategies for reaching in stroke," *Brain*, vol. 123, part 5, pp. 940–953, 2000.

[25] A. R. Damasio, *Descartes' Error: Emotion, Reason and the Human Brain*, Grosset/Putnam, New York, NY, USA, 1994.

[26] M. Catani and D. H. Ffytche, "The rises and falls of disconnection syndromes," *Brain*, vol. 128, no. 10, pp. 2224–2239, 2005.

[27] A. D. Craig, "Human feelings: why are some more aware than others?" *Trends in Cognitive Sciences*, vol. 8, no. 6, pp. 239–241, 2004.

[28] A. D. Craig, "How do you feel—now? The anterior insula and human awareness," *Nature Reviews Neuroscience*, vol. 10, no. 1, pp. 59–70, 2009.

[29] R. Z. Goldstein, A. D. Craig, A. Bechara et al., "The neurocircuitry of impaired insight in drug addiction," *Trends in Cognitive Sciences*, vol. 13, no. 9, pp. 372–380, 2009.

[30] T. Singer, H. D. Critchley, and K. Preuschoff, "A common role of insula in feelings, empathy and uncertainty," *Trends in Cognitive Sciences*, vol. 13, no. 8, pp. 334–340, 2009.

[31] D. A. Gusnard, E. Akbudak, G. L. Shulman, and M. E. Raichle, "Medial prefrontal cortex and self-referential mental activity: relation to a default mode of brain function," *Proceedings of the National Academy of Sciences of the United States of America*, vol. 98, no. 7, pp. 4259–4264, 2001.

[32] A. W. M. Kelley, C. N. Macrae, C. L. Wyland, S. Caglar, S. Inati, and T. F. Heatherton, "Finding the self? An event-related fMRI study," *Journal of Cognitive Neuroscience*, vol. 14, no. 5, pp. 785–794, 2002.

[33] D. M. Amodio and C. D. Frith, "Meeting of minds: the medial frontal cortex and social cognition," *Nature Reviews Neuroscience*, vol. 7, no. 4, pp. 268–277, 2006.

[34] C. L. Philippi, M. C. Duff, N. L. Denburg, D. Tranel, and D. Rudrauf, "Medial PFC damage abolishes the self-reference effect," *Journal of Cognitive Neuroscience*, vol. 24, no. 2, pp. 475–481, 2012.

[35] J. S. Feinstein, D. Rudrauf, S. S. Khalsa et al., "Bilateral limbic system destruction in man," *Journal of Clinical and Experimental Neuropsychology*, vol. 32, no. 1, pp. 88–106, 2010.

[36] R. L. Buckner, J. R. Andrews-Hanna, and D. L. Schacter, "The brain's default network: anatomy, function, and relevance to disease," *Annals of the New York Academy of Sciences*, vol. 1124, pp. 1–38, 2008.

[37] A. Damasio, *Self Comes to Mind*, Constructing the Conscious Brain, Random House, 2011.

[38] A. Damasio, H. Damasio, and D. Tranel, "Persistence of feelings and sentience after bilateral damage of the insula," *Cerebral Cortex*, vol. 23, no. 4, pp. 833–846, 2013.

[39] J. S. Feinstein, "Lesion studies of human emotion and feeling," *Current Opinion in Neurobiology*, vol. 23, no. 3, pp. 304–309, 2013.

[40] J. S. Feinstein, C. Buzza, R. Hurlemann et al., "Fear and panic in humans with bilateral amygdala damage," *Nature Neuroscience*, vol. 16, no. 3, pp. 270–272, 2013.

[41] B. A. Wilson, M. Kopelman, and N. Kapur, "Prominent and persistent loss of past awareness in amnesia: delusion, impaired consciousness or coping strategy?" *Neuropsychological Rehabilitation*, vol. 18, no. 5-6, pp. 527–540, 2008.

[42] S. Laureys, J. T. Giacino, N. D. Schiff, M. Schabus, and A. M. Owen, "How should functional imaging of patients with disorders of consciousness contribute to their clinical rehabilitation needs?" *Current Opinion in Neurology*, vol. 19, no. 6, pp. 520–527, 2006.

[43] S. Laureys and G. Tononi, *The Neurology of Consciousness*, Academic Press, London, UK, 2009.

[44] A. Owen, N. Schiff, and S. Laureys, "The assessment of conscious awareness in the vegetative state," in *The Neurology of Consciousness*, S. Laureys and G. Tononi, Eds., pp. 163–172, Academic Press, London, UK, 2009.

[45] M. Boly, L. Tshibanda, A. Vanhaudenhuyse et al., "Functional connectivity in the default network during resting state is preserved in a vegetative but not in a brain dead patient," *Human Brain Mapping*, vol. 30, no. 8, pp. 2393–2400, 2009.

[46] A. Vanhaudenhuyse, Q. Noirhomme, L. J.-F. Tshibanda et al., "Default network connectivity reflects the level of consciousness in non-communicative brain-damaged patients," *Brain*, vol. 133, no. 1, pp. 161–171, 2010.

[47] J. Giacino and N. Schiff, "The minimally conscious state: clinical features, pathophysiology and therapeutic implications," in *The Neurology of Consciousness*, S. Laureys and G. Tononi, Eds., pp. 173–190, Academic Press, London, UK, 2009.

[48] J. T. Giacino and K. Kalmar, "The vegetative and minimally conscious states: a comparison of clinical features and functional outcome," *Journal of Head Trauma Rehabilitation*, vol. 12, no. 4, pp. 36–51, 1997.

[49] B. T. Hyman, H. Damasio, A. R. Damasio, and G. W. van Hoesen, "Alzheimer's disease," *Annual Review of Public Health*, vol. 10, pp. 115–140, 1989.

[50] C. R. Jack Jr., D. S. Knopman, W. J. Jagust et al., "Hypothetical model of dynamic biomarkers of the Alzheimer's pathological cascade," *The Lancet Neurology*, vol. 9, no. 1, pp. 119–128, 2010.

[51] J. Babinski, "Anosognosia," *The Journal of Nervous and Mental Disease*, vol. 51, article 70, 1920.

[52] S. Banks and S. Weintraub, "Self-awareness and self-monitoring of cognitive and behavioral deficits in behavioral variant frontotemporal dementia, primary progressive aphasia and probable Alzheimer's disease," *Brain and Cognition*, vol. 67, no. 1, pp. 58–68, 2008.

[53] S. E. Starkstein, R. Jorge, R. Mizrahi, J. Adrian, and R. G. Robinson, "Insight and danger in Alzheimer's disease," *European Journal of Neurology*, vol. 14, no. 4, pp. 455–460, 2007.

[54] S. E. Starkstein, S. Brockman, D. Bruce, and G. Petracca, "Anosognosia is a significant predictor of apathy in Alzheimer's disease," *Journal of Neuropsychiatry and Clinical Neurosciences*, vol. 22, no. 4, pp. 378–383, 2010.

[55] G. Spalletta, P. Girardi, C. Caltagirone, and M. D. Orfei, "Anosognosia and neuropsychiatric symptoms and disorders in mild alzheimer disease and mild cognitive impairment," *Journal of Alzheimer's Disease*, vol. 29, no. 4, pp. 761–772, 2012.

[56] M. J. Al-Aloucy, R. Cotteret, P. Thomas, M. Volteau, I. Benmaou, and G. Dalla Barba, "Unawareness of memory impairment and behavioral abnormalities in patients with Alzheimer's disease: relation to professional health care burden," *Journal of Nutrition, Health and Aging*, vol. 15, no. 5, pp. 356–360, 2011.

[57] M. W. Weiner, D. P. Veitch, P. S. Aisen et al., "The Alzheimer's disease neuroimaging initiative: a review of papers published since its inception," *Alzheimer's and Dementia*, vol. 8, supplement 1, pp. S1–S68, 2012.

[58] S. E. Arnold, B. T. Hyman, J. Flory, A. R. Damasio, and G. W. van Hoesen, "The topographical and neuroanatomical distribution of neurofibrillary tangles and neuritic plaques in the cerebral cortex of patients with alzheimer's disease," *Cerebral Cortex*, vol. 1, no. 1, pp. 103–116, 1991.

[59] M.-C. de Lacoste and C. L. White III, "The role of cortical connectivity in Alzheimer's disease pathogenesis: a review and model system," *Neurobiology of Aging*, vol. 14, no. 1, pp. 1–16, 1993.

[60] S. M. Landau, D. Harvey, C. M. Madison et al., "Associations between cognitive, functional, and FDG-PET measures of decline in AD and MCI," *Neurobiology of Aging*, vol. 32, no. 7, pp. 1207–1218, 2011.

[61] J. Parvizi, G. W. van Hoesen, and A. Damasio, "Severe pathological changes of parabrachial nucleus in Alzheimer's disease," *NeuroReport*, vol. 9, no. 18, pp. 4151–154, 1998.

[62] J. Parvizi, G. W. van Hoesen, and A. Damasio, "Selective pathological changes of the periaqueductal gray matter in Alzheimer's disease," *Annals of Neurology*, vol. 48, no. 3, pp. 344–353, 2000.

[63] X. Delbeuck, M. van der Linden, and F. Collette, "Alzheimer's disease as a disconnection syndrome?" *Neuropsychology Review*, vol. 13, no. 2, pp. 79–92, 2003.

[64] X. Delbeuck, F. Collette, and M. van der Linden, "Is Alzheimer's disease a disconnection syndrome?. Evidence from a cross-modal audio-visual illusory experiment," *Neuropsychologia*, vol. 45, no. 14, pp. 3315–3323, 2007.

[65] Y. He, Z. Chen, G. Gong, and A. Evans, "Neuronal networks in Alzheimer's disease," *Neuroscientist*, vol. 15, no. 4, pp. 333–350, 2009.

[66] M. Filippi and F. Agosta, "Structural and functional network connectivity breakdown in Alzheimer's disease studied with magnetic resonance imaging techniques," *Journal of Alzheimer's Disease*, vol. 24, no. 3, pp. 455–474, 2011.

[67] T. Xie and Y. He, "Mapping the Alzheimer's brain with connectomics," *Frontiers in Psychiatry*, vol. 2, article 77, 2012.

[68] S. Neufang, A. Akhrif, V. Riedl et al., "Disconnection of frontal and parietal areas contributes to impaired attention in very early Alzheimer's disease," *Journal of Alzheimer's*, vol. 25, no. 2, pp. 309–321, 2011.

[69] M. Pievani, F. Agosta, E. Pagani et al., "Assessment of white matter tract damage in mild cognitive impairment and Alzheimer's disease," *Human Brain Mapping*, vol. 31, no. 12, pp. 1862–1875, 2010.

[70] J. L. Price and J. C. Morris, "Tangles and plaques in nondemented aging and "preclinical" Alzheimer's disease," *Annals of Neurology*, vol. 45, no. 3, pp. 358–368, 1999.

[71] Neuropathology Group of the Medical Research Council Cognitive Function and Ageing Study (MRC CFAS), "Pathological correlates of late-onset dementia in a multicentre, community-based population in England and Wales," *The Lancet*, vol. 357, no. 9251, pp. 169–175, 2001.

[72] J. Steffener and Y. Stern, "Exploring the neural basis of cognitive reserve in aging," *Biochimica et Biophysica Acta: Molecular Basis of Disease*, vol. 1822, no. 3, pp. 467–473, 2012.

[73] Y. Stern, B. Gurland, T. K. Tatemichi, M. X. Tang, D. Wilder, and R. Mayeux, "Influence of education and occupation on the incidence of Alzheimer's disease," *Journal of the American Medical Association*, vol. 271, no. 13, pp. 1004–1010, 1994.

[74] M. J. Valenzuela and P. Sachdev, "Brain reserve and dementia: a systematic review," *Psychological Medicine*, vol. 36, no. 4, pp. 441–454, 2006.

[75] H. Braak and E. Braak, "Neuropathological stageing of Alzheimer-related changes," *Acta Neuropathologica*, vol. 82, no. 4, pp. 239–259, 1991.

[76] C. M. Roe, M. A. Mintun, G. D'Angelo, C. Xiong, E. A. Grant, and J. C. Morris, "Alzheimer disease and cognitive reserve: variation of education effect with carbon 11-labeled pittsburgh compound B uptake," *Archives of Neurology*, vol. 65, no. 11, pp. 1467–1471, 2008.

[77] D. A. Bennett, R. S. Wilson, J. A. Schneider et al., "Education modifies the relation of AD pathology to level of cognitive function in older persons," *Neurology*, vol. 60, no. 12, pp. 1909–1915, 2003.

[78] M. B. Spitznagel and G. Tremont, "Cognitive reserve and anosognosia in questionable and mild dementia," *Archives of Clinical Neuropsychology*, vol. 20, no. 4, pp. 505–515, 2005.

[79] J. Gläscher, D. Rudrauf, R. Colom et al., "Distributed neural system for general intelligence revealed by lesion mapping," *Proceedings of the National Academy of Sciences of the United States of America*, vol. 107, no. 10, pp. 4705–4709, 2010.

[80] R. Chen, L. G. Cohen, and M. Hallett, "Nervous system reorganization following injury," *Neuroscience*, vol. 111, no. 4, pp. 761–773, 2002.

[81] G. Marrelec, A. Krainik, H. Duffau et al., "Partial correlation for functional brain interactivity investigation in functional MRI," *NeuroImage*, vol. 32, no. 1, pp. 228–237, 2006.

[82] A. R. Carter, S. V. Astafiev, C. E. Lang et al., "Resting interhemispheric functional magnetic resonance imaging connectivity predicts performance after stroke," *Annals of Neurology*, vol. 67, no. 3, pp. 365–375, 2010.

[83] E. M. Nomura, C. Gratton, R. M. Visser, A. Kayser, F. Perez, and M. D'Esposito, "Double dissociation of two cognitive control networks in patients with focal brain lesions," *Proceedings of the National Academy of Sciences of the United States of America*, vol. 107, no. 26, pp. 12017–12022, 2010.

[84] M. Boly, V. Perlbarg, G. Marrelec et al., "Hierarchical clustering of brain activity during human nonrapid eye movement sleep," *Proceedings of the National Academy of Sciences of the United States of America*, vol. 109, no. 15, pp. 5856–5861, 2012.

[85] M. D. Fox, A. Z. Snyder, J. L. Vincent, M. Corbetta, D. C. van Essen, and M. E. Raichle, "The human brain is intrinsically organized into dynamic, anticorrelated functional networks," *Proceedings of the National Academy of Sciences of the United States of America*, vol. 102, no. 27, pp. 9673–9678, 2005.

[86] M. Boly, C. Phillips, E. Balteau et al., "Consciousness and cerebral baseline activity fluctuations," *Human Brain Mapping*, vol. 29, no. 7, pp. 868–874, 2008.

[87] F. Cauda, B. M. Micon, K. Sacco et al., "Disrupted intrinsic functional connectivity in the vegetative state," *Journal of Neurology, Neurosurgery and Psychiatry*, vol. 80, no. 4, pp. 429–431, 2009.

[88] W. W. Seeley, V. Menon, A. F. Schatzberg et al., "Dissociable intrinsic connectivity networks for salience processing and executive control," *Journal of Neuroscience*, vol. 27, no. 9, pp. 2349–2356, 2007.

[89] V. L. Morgan, A. Mishra, A. T. Newton, J. C. Gore, and Z. Ding, "Integrating functional and diffusion magnetic resonance imaging for analysis of structure-function relationship in the human language network," *PLoS ONE*, vol. 4, no. 8, Article ID e6660, 2009.

[90] G. Lohmann, S. Hoehl, J. Brauer et al., "Setting the frame: the human brain activates a basic low-frequency network for language processing," *Cerebral Cortex*, vol. 20, no. 6, pp. 1286–1292, 2010.

[91] D. Zhang and M. E. Raichle, "Disease and the brain's dark energy," *Nature Reviews Neurology*, vol. 6, no. 1, pp. 15–28, 2010.

[92] F. Agosta, M. Pievani, C. Geroldi, M. Copetti, G. B. Frisoni, and M. Filippi, "Resting state fMRI in Alzheimer's disease: beyond the default mode network," *Neurobiology of Aging*, vol. 33, no. 8, pp. 1564–1578, 2012.

[93] C. J. Stam, W. de Haan, A. Daffertshofer et al., "Graph theoretical analysis of magnetoencephalographic functional connectivity in Alzheimer's disease," *Brain*, vol. 132, no. 1, pp. 213–224, 2009.

[94] H.-Y. Zhang, S.-J. Wang, B. Liu et al., "Resting brain connectivity: changes during the progress of Alzheimer disease," *Radiology*, vol. 256, no. 2, pp. 598–606, 2010.

[95] C. Sorg, V. Riedl, M. Mühlau et al., "Selective changes of resting-state networks in individuals at risk for Alzheimer's disease," *Proceedings of the National Academy of Sciences of the United States of America*, vol. 104, no. 47, pp. 18760–18765, 2007.

[96] T. Nakamura, F. G. Hillary, and B. B. Biswal, "Resting network plasticity following brain injury," *PLoS ONE*, vol. 4, no. 12, Article ID e8220, 2009.

[97] D. J. Sharp, C. F. Beckmann, R. Greenwood et al., "Default mode network functional and structural connectivity after traumatic brain injury," *Brain*, vol. 134, no. 8, pp. 2233–2247, 2011.

[98] R. L. Buckner, J. Sepulcre, T. Talukdar et al., "Cortical hubs revealed by intrinsic functional connectivity: mapping, assessment of stability, and relation to Alzheimer's disease," *Journal of Neuroscience*, vol. 29, no. 6, pp. 1860–1873, 2009.

[99] J. S. Damoiseaux, C. F. Beckmann, E. J. S. Arigita et al., "Reduced resting-state brain activity in the "default network" in normal aging," *Cerebral Cortex*, vol. 18, no. 8, pp. 1856–1864, 2008.

[100] M. Ystad, E. Hodneland, S. Adolfsdottir et al., "Cortico-striatal connectivity and cognition in normal aging: a combined DTI and resting state fMRI study," *NeuroImage*, vol. 55, no. 1, pp. 24–31, 2011.

[101] C. J. Honey, J.-P. Thivierge, and O. Sporns, "Can structure predict function in the human brain?" *NeuroImage*, vol. 52, no. 3, pp. 766–776, 2010.

[102] A. Messé, D. Rudrauf, H. Benali, and G. Marrelec, "Relating structure and function in the human brain: relative contributions of anatomy, stationary dynamics, and non-stationarities," *PLoS Computational Biology*, vol. 10, no. 3, Article ID e1003530, 2014.

[103] J. S. Damoiseaux and M. D. Greicius, "Greater than the sum of its parts: a review of studies combining structural connectivity and resting-state functional connectivity," *Brain Structure & Function*, vol. 213, no. 6, pp. 525–533, 2009.

[104] L. Q. Uddin, E. Mooshagian, E. Zaidel et al., "Residual functional connectivity in the split-brain revealed with resting-state functional MRI," *NeuroReport*, vol. 19, no. 7, pp. 703–709, 2008.

[105] J. Michael Tyszka, D. P. Kennedy, R. Adolphs, and L. K. Paul, "Intact bilateral resting-state networks in the absence of the corpus callosum," *Journal of Neuroscience*, vol. 31, no. 42, pp. 15154–15162, 2011.

[106] M. J. Lowe, B. J. Mock, and J. A. Sorenson, "Functional connectivity in single and multislice echoplanar imaging using resting-state fluctuations," *NeuroImage*, vol. 7, no. 2, pp. 119–132, 1998.

[107] J. S. Damoiseaux, S. A. R. B. Rombouts, F. Barkhof et al., "Consistent resting-state networks across healthy subjects," *Proceedings of the National Academy of Sciences of the United States of America*, vol. 103, no. 37, pp. 13848–13853, 2006.

[108] Y. Nir, U. Hasson, I. Levy, Y. Yeshurun, and R. Malach, "Widespread functional connectivity and fMRI fluctuations in human visual cortex in the absence of visual stimulation," *NeuroImage*, vol. 30, no. 4, pp. 1313–1324, 2006.

[109] S. Chen, T. J. Ross, W. Zhan et al., "Group independent component analysis reveals consistent resting-state networks across multiple sessions," *Brain Research*, vol. 1239, pp. 141–151, 2008.

[110] B. J. He, A. Z. Snyder, J. L. Vincent, A. Epstein, G. L. Shulman, and M. Corbetta, "Breakdown of functional connectivity in frontoparietal networks underlies behavioral deficits in spatial neglect," *Neuron*, vol. 53, no. 6, pp. 905–918, 2007.

[111] A. del Cul, S. Dehaene, P. Reyes, E. Bravo, and A. Slachevsky, "Causal role of prefrontal cortex in the threshold for access to consciousness," *Brain*, vol. 132, no. 9, pp. 2531–2540, 2009.

[112] J. Wang, X. Zuo, and Y. He, "Graph-based network analysis of resting-state functional MRI," *Frontiers in Systems Neuroscience*, vol. 4, article 16, 2010.

[113] F. Bartolomei, I. Bosma, M. Klein et al., "Disturbed functional connectivity in brain tumour patients: evaluation by graph analysis of synchronization matrices," *Clinical Neurophysiology*, vol. 117, no. 9, pp. 2039–2049, 2006.

[114] F. Bartolomei, I. Bosma, M. Klein et al., "How do brain tumors alter functional connectivity? A magnetoencephalography study," *Annals of Neurology*, vol. 59, no. 1, pp. 128–138, 2006.

[115] S. C. Ponten, F. Bartolomei, and C. J. Stam, "Small-world networks and epilepsy: graph theoretical analysis of intracerebrally recorded mesial temporal lobe seizures," *Clinical Neurophysiology*, vol. 118, no. 4, pp. 918–927, 2007.

[116] S. D. Roosendaal, M. M. Schoonheim, H. E. Hulst et al., "Resting state networks change in clinically isolated syndrome," *Brain*, vol. 133, no. 6, pp. 1612–1621, 2010.

[117] D. Rudrauf, A. Douiri, C. Kovach et al., "Frequency flows and the time-frequency dynamics of multivariate phase synchronization in brain signals," *NeuroImage*, vol. 31, no. 1, pp. 209–227, 2006.

[118] P. Comon and C. Jutten, *Handbook of Blind Source Separation, Independent Component Analysis and Applications*, Academic Press, Oxford, UK, 2010.

[119] D. O. Hebb, "Distinctive features of learning in the higher animal," in *Brain Mechanisms and Learning*, J. F. Delafresnaye, Ed., Oxford University Press, London, UK, 1961.

[120] K. I. Diamantras and S. Y. Kung, *Principal Component Neural Networks*, John Wiley & Sons, New York, NY, USA, 1996.

[121] A. J. Bell and T. J. Sejnowski, "An information-maximization approach to blind separation and blind deconvolution," *Neural Computation*, vol. 7, no. 6, pp. 1129–1159, 1995.

[122] S. Mesmoudi, V. Perlbarg, D. Rudrauf et al., "Resting state networks' corticotopy: the dual intertwined rings architecture," *PLoS ONE*, vol. 8, no. 7, Article ID e67444, 2013.

[123] T. Cover and J. Thomas, *Elements of Information Theory*, John Wiley & Sons, New York, NY, USA edition, 1991.

[124] C. E. Shannon, "A mathematical theory of communication," *Bell System Technical Journal*, vol. 27, no. 3, pp. 379–423, 1948.

[125] O. Sporns, "The human connectome: a complex network," *Annals of the New York Academy of Sciences*, vol. 1224, no. 1, pp. 109–125, 2011.

[126] N. T. Markov, M. Ercsey-Ravasz, D. C. van Essen, K. Knoblauch, Z. Toroczkai, and H. Kennedy, "Cortical high-density counterstream architectures," *Science*, vol. 342, no. 6158, Article ID 1238406, 2013.

[127] G. Tononi, "An information integration theory of consciousness," *BMC Neuroscience*, vol. 5, article 42, 2004.

[128] V. Mante, D. Sussillo, K. V. Shenoy, and W. T. Newsome, "Context-dependent computation by recurrent dynamics in prefrontal cortex," *Nature*, vol. 503, no. 7474, pp. 78–84, 2013.

[129] R. Cabeza, "Hemispheric asymmetry reduction in older adults: the HAROLD model," *Psychology and Aging*, vol. 17, no. 1, pp. 85–100, 2002.

[130] J. Domínguez-Borràs, J. L. Armony, A. Maravita, J. Driver, and P. Vuilleumier, "Partial recovery of visual extinction by pavlovian conditioning in a patient with hemispatial neglect," *Cortex*, vol. 49, no. 3, pp. 891–898, 2013.

[131] I. H. Robertson, "A noradrenergic theory of cognitive reserve: implications for Alzheimer's disease," *Neurobiology of Aging*, vol. 34, no. 1, pp. 298–308, 2013.

[132] R. C. Aster, B. Borchers, and C. H. Thurber, *Parameter Estimation and Inverse Problems*, Elsevier, 2nd edition, 2012.

[133] G. J. Goodhill and H. G. Barrow, "The role of weight normalization in competitive learning," *Neural Computation*, vol. 6, no. 2, pp. 255–269, 1994.

[134] D. Neumann, *Connectivity of the brain from magnetic resonance imaging [Ph.D. dissertation]*, California Institute of Technology, 2010, http://resolver.caltech.edu/CaltechTHESIS:04282010-153942989.

[135] G. Tononi and C. Cirelli, "Sleep function and synaptic homeostasis," *Sleep Medicine Reviews*, vol. 10, no. 1, pp. 49–62, 2006.

[136] D. Rudrauf, A. Lutz, D. Cosmelli, J.-P. Lachaux, and M. Le Van Quyen, "From autopoiesis to neurophenomenology: Francisco Varela's exploration of the biophysics of being," *Biological Research*, vol. 36, no. 1, pp. 27–65, 2003.

[137] S. Dehaene, M. Kerszberg, and J.-P. Changeux, "A neuronal model of a global workspace in effortful cognitive tasks," *Proceedings of the National Academy of Sciences of the United States of America*, vol. 95, no. 24, pp. 14529–14534, 1998.

[138] F. Varela, J.-P. Lachaux, E. Rodriguez, and J. Martinerie, "The brainweb: phase synchronization and large-scale integration," *Nature Reviews Neuroscience*, vol. 2, no. 4, pp. 229–239, 2001.

[139] K. Friston, "The free-energy principle: a rough guide to the brain?" *Trends in Cognitive Sciences*, vol. 13, no. 7, pp. 293–301, 2009.

[140] K. Friston, "The free-energy principle: a unified brain theory?" *Nature Reviews Neuroscience*, vol. 11, no. 2, pp. 127–138, 2010.

[141] M. V. J. Veenman, *Intellectual Ability and Metacognitive Skill: Determinants of Discovery Learning in Computerized Learning Environments*, University of Amsterdam, 1993.

[142] K. Williford, D. Rudrauf, and G. Landini, "The paradoxes of subjectivity and the projective structure of consciousness," in *Consciousness and Subjectivity*, S. Miguens and G. Preyer, Eds., Ontos, Frankfurt, Germany, 2012.

[143] D. A. Stanley and R. Adolphs, "Toward a neural basis for social behavior," *Neuron*, vol. 80, no. 3, pp. 816–826, 2013.

[144] J. K. O'Regan and A. Noë, "A sensorimotor account of vision and visual consciousness," *Behavioral and Brain Sciences*, vol. 24, no. 5, pp. 939–1031, 2001.

[145] D. Rudrauf, A. Lutz, D. Cosmelli, J.-P. Lachaux, and M. Le Van Quyen, "From autopoiesis to neurophenomenology: Francisco Varela's exploration of the biophysics of being," *Biological Research*, vol. 36, no. 1, pp. 27–65, 2003.

[146] R. Goldberg, "Survey of virtual machine research," *IEEE Computer*, vol. 7, no. 6, pp. 34–45, 1974.

[147] D. C. Dennett, *Consciousness Explained*, Little, Brown and Company, Boston, Mass, USA, 1991.

[148] T. J. Sejnowski, C. Koch, and P. S. Churchland, "Computational neuroscience," *Science*, vol. 241, no. 4871, pp. 1299–1306, 1988.

[149] P. S. Churchland and T. J. Sejnowski, *The Computational Brain*, MIT Press, Cambridge, Mass, USA, 1992.

[150] J. von Neumann, *First Draft of a Report on the EDVAC*, United States Army Ordnance Department, University of Pennsylvania, 1945.

[151] W. S. McCulloch and W. Pitts, "A logical calculus of the ideas immanent in nervous activity," *The Bulletin of Mathematical Biophysics*, vol. 5, no. 4, pp. 115–133, 1943.

[152] Y. He, L. Wang, Y. Zang et al., "Regional coherence changes in the early stages of Alzheimer's disease: a combined structural and resting-state functional MRI study," *NeuroImage*, vol. 35, no. 2, pp. 488–500, 2007.

[153] N. Villain, B. Desgranges, F. Viader et al., "Relationships between hippocampal atrophy, white matter disruption, and gray matter hypometabolism in Alzheimer's disease," *Journal of Neuroscience*, vol. 28, no. 24, pp. 6174–6181, 2008.

[154] L. A. Beckett, D. J. Harvey, A. Gamst et al., "The Alzheimer's Disease Neuroimaging Initiative: annual change in biomarkers and clinical outcomes," *Alzheimer's and Dementia*, vol. 6, no. 3, pp. 257–264, 2010.

[155] Y. Li, Y. Wang, G. Wu et al., "Discriminant analysis of longitudinal cortical thickness changes in Alzheimer's disease using dynamic and network features," *Neurobiology of Aging*, vol. 33, no. 2, pp. 427.e15–427.e30, 2012.

[156] D. T. Jones, M. M. MacHulda, P. Vemuri et al., "Age-related changes in the default mode network are more advanced in Alzheimer disease," *Neurology*, vol. 77, no. 16, pp. 1524–1531, 2011.

[157] O. Lazarov, J. Robinson, Y.-P. Tang et al., "Environmental enrichment reduces Aβ levels and amyloid deposition in transgenic mice," *Cell*, vol. 120, no. 5, pp. 701–713, 2005.

[158] S. M. Smith, P. T. Fox, K. L. Miller et al., "Correspondence of the brain's functional architecture during activation and rest," *Proceedings of the National Academy of Sciences of the United States of America*, vol. 106, no. 31, pp. 13040–13045, 2009.

[159] P. Goel, A. Kuceyeski, E. Locastro, and A. Raj, "Spatial patterns of genome-wide expression profiles reflect anatomic and fiber connectivity architecture of healthy human brain," *Human Brain Mapping*, 2014.

7

The Effect of Simple Melodic Lines on Aesthetic Experience: Brain Response to Structural Manipulations

Stefania Ferri,[1] **Cristina Meini,**[2] **Giorgio Guiot,**[3] **Daniela Tagliafico,**[4]
Gabriella Gilli,[5] **and Cinzia Di Dio**[1,5]

[1]*Department of Neuroscience, Università di Parma, Via Volturno 39/E, 43100 Parma, Italy*
[2]*Department of Humanistic Studies, Università del Piemonte Orientale, Via Manzoni 8, 13100 Vercelli, Italy*
[3]*Associazione Cantabile, Via Campana 2, 10125 Turin, Italy*
[4]*Department of Philosophy, Università Degli Studi di Torino, Via Sant'Ottavio 20, 10125 Turin, Italy*
[5]*Department of Psychology, Università Cattolica del Sacro Cuore, 20123 Milan, Italy*

Correspondence should be addressed to Cinzia Di Dio; cinzia.didio@unipr.it

Academic Editor: Notger G. Mueller

This fMRI study investigates the effect of melody on aesthetic experience in listeners naïve to formal musical knowledge. Using simple melodic lines, whose syntactic structure was manipulated, we created systematic acoustic dissonance. Two stimulus categories were created: canonical (syntactically "correct," in the Western culture) and modified (made of an altered version of the canonical melodies). The stimuli were presented under two tasks: listening and aesthetic judgment. Data were analyzed as a function of stimulus structure (canonical and modified) and stimulus aesthetics, as appraised by each participant during scanning. The critical contrast modified versus canonical stimuli produced enhanced activation of deep temporal regions, including the parahippocampus, suggesting that melody manipulation induced feelings of unpleasantness in the listeners. This was supported by our behavioral data indicating decreased aesthetic preference for the modified melodies. Medial temporal activation could also have been evoked by stimulus structural novelty determining increased memory load for the modified stimuli. The analysis of melodies judged as beautiful revealed that aesthetic judgment of simple melodies relied on a fine-structural analysis of the stimuli subserved by a left frontal activation and, possibly, on meaning attribution at the charge of right superior temporal sulcus for increasingly pleasurable stimuli.

1. Introduction

Music is simultaneously art and science: it allows the artist to express his/her inner world through sounds, which are linked one to another by stringent rules that are strongly influenced by culture. These rules represent hallmarks that, on one side, constrain the composer's freedom to choose associations and successions of sounds and, on the other, offer a context, within which all elements gain a meaning. Traditionally, there has been a strong tendency to emphasize the dominance of compositional structures in outlining the aesthetic character of a musical piece. In the present study, we investigated this relationship by exploring the aesthetics of melody, that is, the capacity of simple musical structures to evoke an aesthetic experience in listeners naïve to formal musical knowledge.

Music is made of rules that govern the relation between notes and of a dynamic dimension that defines its tempo and rhythm. As far as the succession of sounds is concerned, the founding rules of a musical piece are also referred to as syntactic rules (this denomination implicitly underlines the similarities between music and language). Music syntax is basically constituted by melody (horizontal syntax) and harmony (vertical syntax). Melody consists of a distribution of notes on scales that are organized into "modes" (e.g., minor and major) by our musical tradition. Harmony, on the other hand, establishes the criteria upon which chords are built and associated in time. The syntactic rules of music are not absolute; contrarily, they vary in relation to the different musical styles. For example, the rules forming the base of classic music are different from those characterizing soul music or blues. Still, dodecaphonic music arises in opposition to the norms of classical music, which are paradigmatically expressed by traditional "mozartian" music.

Recently, the growing interest of neuroscience for music has dealt with the way our brain processes the temporal and syntactic structure of music. Some evidence suggests that the neural processing of music syntax involves the activation of areas that are also involved in language processing and in motor planning [1–6]. Tillmann and colleagues [6], for example, showed that the processing of a chord unrelated to musical context modulates the activity of the inferior frontal gyrus (IFG). Similarly, Levitin and Menon [7] found enhanced activation of IFG (BA47) in the contrast between musical pieces and their scrambled versions, showing that this brain area may be involved in the coding of fine stimulus structure. A more recent study showed that even in newborn children altered music structures cause perceived dissonance, which involves the activation of the inferior frontal cortex [8].

Another aspect of music that has been investigated concerns the neural correlates of aesthetic experience evoked by music and, specifically, to its emotional dimension. A PET study by Blood and Zatorre [9] showed that the intensity of emotional experience elicited by familiar musical pieces positively correlated with signal change in subcortical structures, including ventral striatum, and in limbic structures, including insular cortex, orbitofrontal cortex, and anterior cingulated cortex. In their fMRI study, Koelsch et al. [10] reported the bilateral activation of the primary auditory cortex, IFG, and anterior insula while listening to pleasant music with respect to unpleasant music (see also [11]). Altogether, these studies emphasize the role of emotional centres during the aesthetic experience of music.

In the present study, we aimed at breaking down music in one of its building structural dimensions, namely, melody, and at clarifying whether aesthetic experience can be evoked by this single component alone in naïve listeners (nonmusic experts or players). Differently from the above studies that used complex music excerpts characterized by a rich harmonic and rhythmic structure as experimental stimuli, in the present study we used simple melodic lines. The effect of melody on aesthetic experience was investigated by systematically manipulating the syntactic structure of the stimuli. In fact, violation of the syntactic rules building a musical system creates acoustic dissonance that, phenomenically, could translate into an unpleasant emotion feeling.

For this purpose, two categories of melodies were presented: canonical, that is, syntactically "correct," and modified, that is, made of an altered version of the canonical melodies. In order to evaluate whether the structural alteration of the melodies modulates aesthetic experience, canonical and modified stimuli were presented in two experimental tasks, listening and aesthetic judgment. During listening task, participants had to merely listen to the presented melodies; during aesthetic judgment task, participants were required to overtly express a pleasantness evaluation of the same stimuli.

2. Methods

2.1. Participants. Nineteen healthy right-handed Italian native speakers (9 males and 8 females; mean age 24.3) participated in the fMRI study. They were undergraduate and graduate students naïve to music expertise: they did not play any musical instruments nor were they able to read piano score. They were unfamiliar with the presented melodies. After receiving an explanation of the experimental procedures, they gave their written informed consent. This study was approved by the Local Ethics Committee of Parma, Italy.

2.2. Stimuli. Simple tonal melodies played with piano were used in this study. The stimuli were presented in a canonical, syntactically "correct," version (CAN) and in a modified, syntactically "incorrect," version (MOD) of the canonical stimuli. In total, 10 stimuli (5 CAN and 5 MOD melodies) were selected on the basis of a preliminary behavioral study, in which a sample of 20 listeners naïve to formal musical knowledge (10 males, mean age = 28.8 yrs; 10 females, mean age = 28.2 yrs), different from the sample undergoing fMRI, were asked to evaluate a set of stimuli composed by 12 CAN and 12 MOD melodies. For each stimulus, participants were required to rate aesthetic preference and syntactic accuracy. The CAN and MOD versions that showed the highest discrepancy in aesthetic ratings were chosen; moreover, the syntactic alterations of the selected MOD melodies had to be clearly perceived.

Four CAN and 4 MOD stimuli were created by extracting pure melodic lines from unfamiliar excerpts written by illustrious classical composers (F. Chopin: preludio number 20; Gershwin: Oh, I can't sit down (Porgy and Bess); I wonder as I wander (American folk song); N. Morali: Notturno). In some instances, variations to the original excerpts were made to adapt the melodies to a piano composition and to equalize all melodies in terms of duration. The fifth CAN stimulus and MOD version were created from scratch (G. Guiot: Melodia). During postscanning debriefing, we ascertained that participants were unfamiliar with the presented melodies.

The melodies were created through an electronic musical program "NUENDO" using a piano timbre and keeping a low reverberation to avoid a superimposition of adjoining notes that could create a harmonic dimension. The modified versions of the canonical stimuli were created through ascending alterations of the fifth note of the musical scale, as exemplified in Figure 1. This type of alteration involves an increase in one semitone of the fifth degree of the musical scale. The fifth degree of a musical scale, named "dominant," is the most frequent note in a melody line and represents a keynote determining the stability of the composition. Therefore, this alteration represents the most disruptive intervention that can alter the perception of a melody (see Supplementary Material for the melodies score used in this study, available online at http://dx.doi.org/10.1155/2014/482126).

Each melody was presented to the participants for 12 s and contained, on average, 5 alterations.

Canonical melody (Gershwin—Oh, I can't sit down)   Modified melody (Gershwin—Oh, I can't sit down)

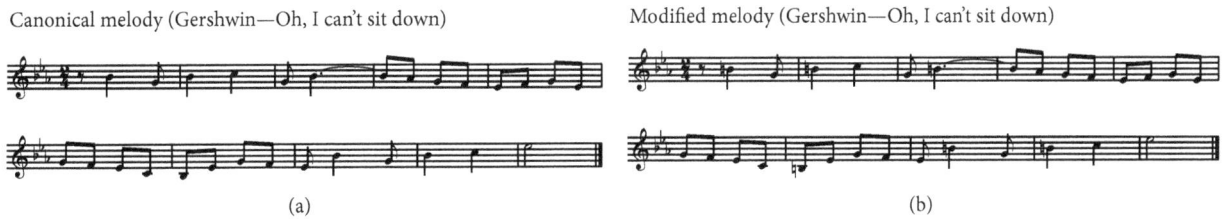

(a)   (b)

FIGURE 1: Example of melody used in this study (canonical version, upper part; modified version, bottom part). The modified version was created by alteration of the fifth note of the musical scale, which involves an increase in one semitone of the fifth degree of the musical scale.

2.3. Procedure.

During scanning, participants were provided with digital visors (VisuaSTIM, 500,000 px × 0.25-square-inch resolution, horizontal eye field of 30°) that were applied directly on the volunteers' face. The visors displayed the instructions, a fixation cross, and the question mark (see below). The participants were also provided with earphones delivering musical stimuli and a response box placed under their right hand.

The stimuli were presented in two experimental tasks: listening (L) and aesthetic judgment (AJ). The tasks were presented in separated fMRI runs; each run/task lasted about 8 minutes. The task order was maintained fixed across participants, with listening task first and aesthetic judgment last. By keeping listening task first, we aimed at measuring unbiased brain responses to the type of stimuli. Each melody was presented twice within each task, totaling 10 stimulus presentations for each category (10 CAN and 10 MOD) for each task.

At the beginning of each run, a 20 s visual instruction informed the volunteers about the upcoming task. Each experimental trial began with the musical stimulus that lasted 12 s, followed by a 6 s white noise (WN) used as explicit baseline and by a question mark that instructed the participants to respond to the music stimulus using the response box placed inside the scanner. The trials were separated by a jittered intertrial interval (ITI mean duration 3.5 s; range 2.5–4.5).

During music stimulation and white noise presentation, the volunteers were instructed to fixate on a cross randomly displaced on the visors screen across the various trials. The fixation point was placed in order to reduce eye movement; the changing spatial location of the fixation point across trials aimed at maintaining a certain attention level and to avoid eyestrain. After the white noise presentation, a question mark instructed the participants to respond to the stimulus. During listening task (L), the participants were instructed to press one of 4 buttons of the response box in a random fashion. During aesthetic judgment task (AJ), they had to express a judgment about each musical stimulus using a 4-point scale. Therefore both tasks (L and AJ) required a motor response from the participants. The scale ranged from "aesthetically pleasant" to "aesthetically unpleasant." For half of the participants, "pleasant" corresponded to 1 and "unpleasant" to 4. More specifically, they had to respond to the following question: "how much do you find it is pleasant?" (1 = very pleasant; 2 = pleasant; 3 = moderately pleasant; 4 = not pleasant at all). For the other half of

the participants, the scale was set in the opposite order ("pleasant" corresponded to 4 and "unpleasant" to 1). Each finger corresponded to one specific response: the thumb, index, medium, and ring finger produced responses 1, 2, 3, and 4, respectively. The distribution of scores ascribed to each melody is summarized the in response frequency Table S1 in Supplementary Material.

2.4. fMRI Data Acquisition and Statistical Analysis.

Functional images were acquired with a General Electric scanner operating at 3T using an 8-channel head coil. Blood oxygenation level dependent (BOLD) contrasts were obtained using echo-planar T2* weighted imaging (EPI). Each of the 185 volumes acquired was composed of 40 transverse slices, which provided coverage of the whole cerebral cortex with the exception of the primary visual cortex and the posterior part of cerebellum (TR = 2500, TE = 30 ms, flip angle = 85 degrees, FOV = 240 mm × 240, interslice gap = 0.5 mm, slice thickness = 4 mm, and plane resolution = 3 * 3). Immediately after the functional scanning, a high-resolution T1 weighted anatomical scan (150 slices, TR = 600 ms; TE = 20 ms, slice thickness = 1 mm, and in-plane resolution = 1 × 1 mm) was acquired for each participant.

Image preprocessing and statistical analysis were performed using SPM8 (Wellcome Department of Cognitive Neurology, http://www.fil.ion.ucl.ac.uk/spm/), implemented in Matlab v7.6 (Mathworks, Inc., Sherborn, MA [12]). The first four images volumes of each run were discarded to allow for stabilization of longitudinal magnetization. For each participant, the volumes were spatially realigned [13] to the first volume of the first session to correct for between-scan motion and unwarped [14]. A mean image from the realigned volumes was created. Acquisition time was then corrected using the middle slice as reference. To allow intersubject analysis, images were normalized to Montreal Neurological Institute (MNI) standard space [15], using the mean of the functional images. All images were smoothed using an isotropic Gaussian kernel (6 mm).

Two types of fMRI data analyses were performed. The "structure" analysis accounted for the effect evoked by the canonical (CAN) and modified (MOD) melodic structures on the listeners' brain, independently of the participants' explicit aesthetic response to them. The second analysis ("aesthetic" analysis) categorized each excerpt as pleasant or unpleasant according to the behavioral responses measured during AJ runs, independently of melodies modification (CAN, MOD). Statistical inference was based on a random effect approach [13] that comprised two steps: a subject-level analysis (first level analysis) and an intersubject analysis (group analysis).

With respect to the structure analysis, at the first level fMRI data were best fitted (least square fit) at every voxel using a linear combination of the effects of interest. The effects of interests were modelled as a function of the following: stimulus category (CAN, MOD), the question mark that cued overt responses, and the white noise, considered as explicit baseline, plus six regressors obtained from motion correction during the realignment process. All event types were convolved with the SPM8 standard hemodynamic function (HRF). By making linear contrasts, activation associated with WN presentation was subtracted to the activation associated with the two stimulus categories in each task (CAN-WN and MOD-WN in both L and AJ tasks). These contrasts were produced in order to isolate the specific effects of the musical stimuli partialling out the mere effect of sound.

The second step of statistical analysis comprised one flexible factorial model that included the contrast images created for each subject in the first step (CAN-WN and MOD-WN in both L and AJ tasks). This model considered the pattern of activation specific for each stimulus category in the listening and aesthetic judgment tasks. The following contrasts were tested: first, CAN versus white noise and MOD versus white noise in order to evaluate the positive effects of music on brain activation; second, CAN versus MOD within each condition to highlight specific effects of stimulus structure on brain activation.

The aesthetic analysis, carried out on data from AJ task only, examined the regional modulation of signal change induced by different levels of aesthetic judgment. As described above, judgments were recorded on a scale ranging from 1 to 4 (see Table S1 for details regarding score frequencies). Like the structure analysis, the aesthetic analysis included two different steps. At the first level of analysis, the fMRI data were best fitted (least square fit) at every voxel using a linear combination of the effects of interest. The effects of interest, modelled for each participant, were as follows: the presentation time of question mark that cued overt responses, the presentation time of the white noise, and the presentation times of the music stimuli (regardless of the type of melodic structure, CAN or MOD), plus six regressors obtained from motion correction during the realignment process. All event types were convolved with the SPM8 standard hemodynamic function (HRF). At the intersubject level, a one-sample t-test was carried out to define the brain areas modulated by increased aesthetic rating to the music stimuli regardless of stimulus type.

For all these analyses, SPM maps were thresholded at P-corrected = 0.05 at the cluster level (cluster size estimated with a voxel level threshold of P-uncorrected = 0.001). Because of acquisition plane that cut off the posterior portion of brain, it was not possible to define whether activation at its proximity constituted independent clusters or belonged to more extended activation. For this reason, the activation found in the occipitotemporal visual regions and in the cerebellum is not discussed.

TABLE 1: Activation reflecting the effect of canonical stimuli (versus white noise).

Area	Sphere	Local maxima	Z score	P-corrected (cluster)
Insula	Left	−46 −18 −2	Inf.	0.000
Middle temporal gyrus		−52 −18 4	Inf.	
Superior temporal gyrus		−58 −8 2	Inf.	
Temporal pole		−34 4 −28	6.16	
BA6 (PMd)		−54 −6 50	5.58	
BA 17		−4 −78 18	5.52	
Superior occipital lobe		−18 −76 26	5.14	0.006
Fusiform gyrus		−22 −54 −4	5.09	0.003
Temporal pole	Right	58 2 −6	Inf.	
BA6 (PMd)		56 −2 50	6.46	

3. Results

3.1. Response-Based Results. To assess aesthetic ratings provided by each participant during fMRI scanning as a function of the type of melody (CAN or MOD), a repeated measures GLM analysis, with two levels of stimulus category (CAN, MOD) and two levels of stimulus repetition (R1, R2), was carried out on responses recorded during AJ task. The data file containing the participants' responses to the stimuli is in Supplementary Material (see SDataFile.xls for the participants responses to the stimuli). The results showed that canonical stimuli were rated as more pleasant than their modified counterparts ($F_{1,18} = 8.5$, $P < 0.01$; partial-$\eta^2 = .31$; $\delta = .79$), whereas there was no effect of stimulus repetition on aesthetic appraisal ($P > 0.05$). These results indicate that acoustic dissonance created by atypical musical syntax characterizing the modified stimuli negatively affected aesthetic preference.

3.2. fMRI Results

3.2.1. Structure Analysis

Overall Effect of Melody Listening. MRI analysis was carried out by first assessing the overall activation elicited by melody, contrasting, separately, CAN and MOD (minus WN) versus baseline across listening (L) and aesthetic judgment (AJ) tasks. The contrast CAN (minus WN) versus baseline produced activation in superior occipital area, in superior temporal gyrus (STG), and in dorsal premotor cortex (dPM). Temporal activation included the primary auditory cortex and its neighbouring associative auditory regions, including BA 22, BA 21, and the superior part of BA 38. All activation was bilateral (Figure 2(a), Table 1).

As shown in Figure 2(b) (Table 2), the contrast MOD (minus WN) versus baseline revealed similar activation as that observed for the contrast CAN (minus WN) versus baseline.

Canonical versus Modified Melodies. The direct contrast CAN versus MOD was carried out for each task (L and AJ) separately to evaluate whether the structure of melodies is

(a) CAN versus WN

(b) MOD versus WN

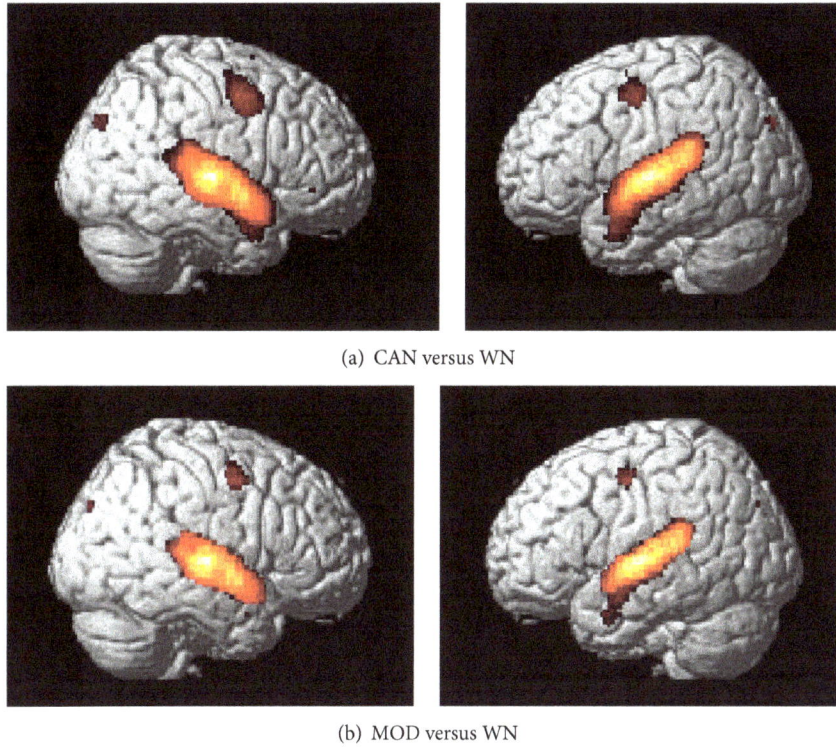

FIGURE 2: Activation observed in (a) the contrast CAN versus WN and (b) the contrast MOD versus WN averaging activation across the two experimental tasks (listening and aesthetic judgment). Group-averaged statistical parametric maps are rendered onto the MNI brain template (*P*-corr. < 0.05).

TABLE 2: Activation reflecting effect of modified stimuli (versus white noise).

Area	Sphere	Local maxima	Z score	P-corrected (cluster)
Insula	Left	−46 −18 −2	Inf.	0.000
Middle temporal gyrus		−52 −18 4	Inf.	
Superior temporal gyrus		−58 −8 2	Inf.	
Temporal pole		−34 4 −28	6.19	
BA 17		−6 −78 16	5.76	
Fusiform gyrus		−20 −52 −10	5.21	
Superior occipital lobe		−18 −76 28	5.30	
BA 6 (PMd)		−52 −8 50	5.05	0.008
Superior temporal gyrus	Right	60 −18 2	Inf.	0.000
Temporal pole		50 4 −12	7.38	
BA 6 (PMd)		56 −2 50	6.50	
BA 17		22 −82 34	5.15	0.01
Precuneus		18 −74 20	4.98	0.005
Temporal pole		40 2 −26	5.17	0.001

TABLE 3: Activation reflecting the contrast MOD versus CAN during listening (L) and aesthetic judgment (AJ) tasks.

Area	Sphere	Local maxima	Z score	P-corrected (cluster)
(a) MOD-CAN (L)				
Post central gyrus	Right	28 −36 58	4.78	0.000
Dorsal premotor cortex		32 −4 70	4.40	
(b) MOD-CAN (AJ)				
Fusiform gyrus	Left	−34 −32 −20	5.37	0.000
Middle occipital lobe		−42 −74 18	3.92	0.01
Precuneus		−6 −56 10	3.91	
Middle temporal gyrus	Right	38 −60 −4	4.69	0.000
Cerebellum		32 −40 −28	4.67	
Parahippocampal gyrus		26 −40 −4	3.96	
Precuneus		8 −46 8	3.82	

an element affecting the listeners' aesthetic experience. The results revealed no significant activation evoked by canonical stimuli with respect to the modified ones in either listening or aesthetic judgment tasks.

The opposite contrast, MOD versus CAN, assessed the neural effects of unpleasantness due to syntax alteration on brain activation within each experimental task (L and AJ). During L, the contrast MOD versus CAN showed differential activation in right dorsal premotor cortex and postcentral gyrus (Table 3(a)). With respect to AJ, differential activation between modified and canonical stimuli was observed in right middle temporal gyrus, right parahippocampus,

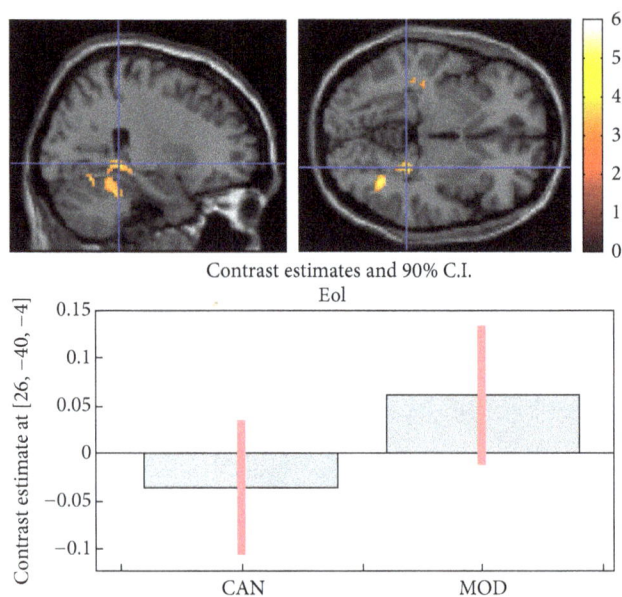

Figure 3: Activation observed in the contrast MOD versus CAN stimuli during aesthetic judgment task (AJ). Group-averaged statistical parametric maps are rendered onto the MNI brain template (*P*-corr. < 0.05). The bars show the activity profile within right parahippocampal gyrus in the contrast MOD versus CAN during AJ task in arbitrary units (a.u.).

and precuneus bilaterally, whereas, in the left hemisphere, enhanced activation was observed in middle occipital lobe and fusiform gyrus (Figure 3, Table 3(b)).

3.2.2. Aesthetic Analysis: Parametric Effect of Aesthetic Judgment. To test whether explicit aesthetic judgment modulated brain activation, independently of melody structure, we carried out a parametric analysis based on the participants' responses given during AJ task independently of stimulus type (CAN, MOD). Increasing aesthetic rating was associated with greater activation in right superior temporal sulcus (STS, maxima: 62, −26, 0; *P*-corr. < 0.05) and left IFG pars triangularis corresponding to BA 44/45 (maxima: −44, 34, 4; *P*-uncorr. = 0.02) (Figure 4). Decreasing aesthetic rating, on the other hand, was associated with greater activation in the right precuneus (maxima: 6, −78, 30).

4. Discussion

The neuroscience of music has mostly dealt with the way our brain processes and responds to the temporal and syntactic structure of music. The aim of the present study was to isolate one of the syntactic forms of music, namely, melody, to explore its independent effect on aesthetic experience in listeners naïve to formal musical knowledge. For this purpose, we used simple melodic lines whose syntactic structure was systematically manipulated to create acoustic dissonance. Two categories of melodies were presented to participants: canonical (syntactically "correct") and modified, that is, made of an altered version of the canonical melodies. In what we termed structure analysis, we evaluated the

effect on brain activation exerted by syntactic structural alterations of the melodies by comparing canonical and modified stimuli in two experimental tasks: listening and aesthetic judgment. Moreover, an aesthetic analysis, based on the listeners' responses recorded during AJ task, was carried out to evaluate the brain regions involved in aesthetic judgment, independently of structural modifications.

Our results highlighted some important aspects of neural processing underling melody listening. First, contrast analysis comparing canonical and modified stimuli with white noise showed that processing melody, regardless of structural modification and experimental task, involves activation of dorsal premotor cortex (dPM) and superior temporal gyrus (STG) bilaterally.

The activation of dorsal premotor cortex is in line with findings showing its implication in rhythm processing (e.g., [2]). In a melody, this is given by its temporal structure and phrasing, which are characterized by the pitch relationship of one note to the next [16]. In fact, melodic processing incorporates intervals between individual notes and the overall contour of the sequence, as shown by studies investigating melody or pitch perception and discrimination ([17, 18]; for a review, see [19]).

The posterior part of STG, including Heschl's gyrus (HG) and temporal planum (PT), is involved in acoustic-stimulus processing. While HG represents the first cortical step of auditory analysis, it was proposed that PT elaborates an auditory scene analysis [20] that allows one to segregate different sounds heard simultaneously and to match these with stored patterns. The output of this high level processing should inform about the acoustic environment, information that is not available from stimulus analyses elaborated at previous levels [21]. This region has been also found to be crucial for music processing. In a work including epileptic patients that underwent a unilateral temporoctomy and healthy controls, Liégeois-Chauvel and colleagues [22] found that pSTG is involved in the extraction of both contour and temporal information of melodies. The functional data of Patterson and colleagues' study [23] further clarified that cortical processing of pitch is hierarchic: this recruits not only the posterior but also the anterior part of this region (polar planum, PP) as interval information of the acoustic stimulus becomes more complex.

Coherently with these data, the bilateral activation of STG found in the present study for both CAN versus WN and MOD versus WN contrasts may represent the hierarchic neural processing of melodies. The temporal cluster expanded into the third posterior of insular cortex. This is a granular region and, as shown by several anatomical studies (e.g., [24, 25]), is connected with the medial geniculate nucleus of the thalamus, with Heschl's gyrus and superior temporal sulcus. It was shown that posterior insula might preprocess the auditory stimulus before the primary auditory cortex [25] and some neuropsychological works indicate that lesions of the posterior part of the insula are associated with auditory deficits, such as agnosia. The posterior insula might then mediate the precortical phase of auditory analysis.

Direct comparisons between stimulus types (canonical and modified) highlighted the areas specifically involved

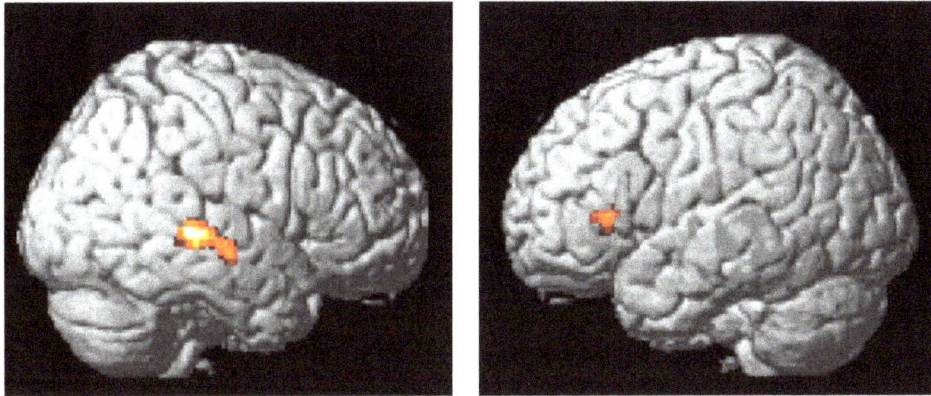

FIGURE 4: Activation observed as a function of increasing aesthetic rating on brain activation (parametric analysis) in right superior temporal sulcus and left IFG pars triangularis. Activation is rendered onto the MNI brain template.

in the syntactic processing of melodies. Direct contrasts between CAN versus MOD melodies did not produce any differential activation, suggesting that there was no specific processing associated with canonical compared to modified structures. The opposite contrast, namely, modified versus canonical stimuli, revealed on the other hand signal increase in deep temporal regions and particularly the right parahippocampal cortex. The critical role of the parahippocampal cortex in processing the emotional valence of dissonance has been shown in several works. A PET study by Blood et al. [26] showed that the increasing dissonance of the stimuli (and the relative judgments of unpleasantness) correlated with activation of right parahippocampal gyrus and precuneus, also found activated in the present study. Koelsch and colleagues [10] found activation of parahippocampal gyrus, hippocampus, amygdala, and temporal pole by contrasting dissonant stimuli judged as unpleasant with consonant classical excerpts judged as pleasant. Gosselin and coworkers [27] clarified the role of mediotemporal structures in the processing of emotional response to dissonance by studying aesthetic judgments to classical and dissonant music excerpts in both patients with lesion to medial temporal lobe and healthy subjects. While both groups gave positive aesthetic judgments to classical excerpts, the patients judged the dissonant music as slightly pleasant, opposite to healthy subjects. It was concluded that the parahippocampal cortex is specific for processing judgments of unpleasantness due to dissonance because the volume of this region, and not of other surrounding structures (like the amygdala or hippocampus), correlated with the values of judgments given by patients to the dissonant stimuli. Since the behavioral analysis of the present study showed a link between negative aesthetic judgment and modified melodies, the activation of the parahippocampal cortex found in the contrast MOD versus CAN melodies suggests a role of this region in processing the negative/emotional value of melodies driven by structural dissonance.

An alternative interpretation for parahippocampal activation favors the idea that it could have been evoked by stimulus structural novelty. The role of the hippocampus and surrounding areas in memory encoding and processing is

well known (for reviews, see e.g., [28, 29]). In this light, it is plausible to suggest that the activation of the parahippocampal cortex was determined by a stronger brain effort to decode and retain the new structures intrinsic to the MOD melodies compared to the CAN ones (increased memory load for the MOD stimuli). This interpretation of the data does not automatically discount the former emotion-related explanation for parahippocampal activation and it can serve as a suggestion for future investigations.

On the whole, the lack of enhanced brain activation for the canonical stimuli with respect to the modified ones and the presence of signal increase for the opposite contrast suggests that modified melodic structures exert a stronger effect on brain processing (in terms of either negative emotional valence and/or mnemonic-related processing), compared to melodies that respect a structural canon, at least within the Western culture.

Aesthetic preference for music, although related to a certain extent to melody structure as shown by our behavioral data, may also be guided by idiosyncratic criteria. In the present study, we attempted to capture this aspect carrying out an aesthetic analysis based on the responses from each participant during AJ task, independently of stimulus structure. This analysis revealed activation of right STS and inferior frontal gyrus (IFG) associated with increasing pleasantness expressed for the melodies, independently of structure modification (CAN, MOD).

STS cluster included BA22 that represents the homologue of Wernicke area in the right hemisphere. Recent findings suggest that the frontotemporal regions of the right hemisphere play an important role in the semantic processing of language, opposite to the traditional view that highlights the role of only the left hemisphere. Additionally, it was shown that the Wernicke homologue in the right hemisphere is involved in metaphors understanding [30, 31]. In a TMS study, Harpaz and colleagues [32] showed a crucial implication of right BA 22 in associating words with their remote meaning. In accordance with this evidence, a complex model for semantic language processing was advanced, which considers the different contribution of left and right frontotemporal regions in semantic processing. In this model, semantic processing is described as highly distributed in both hemispheres but the right regions are described to be crucial for coarser semantic coding compared with that of the left ones [33]. As language does, music conveys meaningful information. Using N400 as marker of processing meaning, it was shown that long or short music excerpts are able to prime the processing of subsequent target words [34–37]. Moreover, in an EEG-fMRI study, Steinbeis and Koelsch [37] found that right posterior STS has a key role in processing of meaning of music, as it occurs for coarse aspects of language. Although melody meaningfulness was not directly assessed in the present study, a tentative explanation for our results is that there may be a link between aesthetic preference and the coding of music meaning, in the fact that aesthetic preference was accorded to melodies that were somehow more meaningful to the listeners or, alternatively, to which the listener was able to ascribe a meaning.

Of course, other interpretations for STS activation may account for the observed data. For example, some intrinsic properties of the pleasurable stimuli may have enhanced the participants' attention, therefore modulating the activity within the STS cluster. In fact, as discussed in Himmelbach et al. [38], STG/STS seem to be involved in the attentional orienting towards potentially relevant events or stimuli [39]. Additionally, the superior temporal cortex has been shown to be a site for multimodal sensory convergence and neuronal populations in STS encode object-properties as well as spatial positions [40], orienting attention towards salient stimuli.

The results from the parametric analysis further revealed a modulation effect of the expressed aesthetic pleasure on right inferior frontal gyrus pars orbitalis corresponding to BA47 and on left IFG pars triangularis corresponding to BA44/45. With respect to activation of Broca area, several works found that Broca (left IFG) is important for both harmonic and syntactic errors processing [5, 6] and, likewise, in the present work it may be involved in syntax coding. In this study, Broca activation was associated with listening to pleasant melodies, suggesting that syntactic coding of the canonical stimuli facilitated the ascription of an aesthetic judgment as requested by the task (AJ). Since no emotional activation was found in association with aesthetic pleasurable melodies, it is possible that aesthetic judgment of the presented melodies was based on the more formal aspect of stimulus processing, namely, its syntactic analysis.

In general, in contrast with other studies that found a neural correlation between aesthetic pleasure for music and activation of emotion-related structures (see, e.g., [9–11, 41–43]), our results suggest that aesthetic preference for simple melodic pieces is mediated by a structural-syntactic and, possibly, semantic analysis of the stimuli. We suggest that the main difference across diverging findings may rest on the type of stimuli used and on the specific alterations introduced that, in our study, were different from the integer, rich stimuli (painting and sculpture images or famous musical excerpts) used in other studies. In fact, we produced a single, highly significant syntactic error, without altering in a gross and overwhelming way the original melody. Additionally, we isolated melody from a harmonic context, whose violation would have intensified melodic dissonances. Likewise, we

did not alter any other extramelodic parameter, such as rhythm, timbre, or intensity, with the aim of producing results reflecting the capability of melody alone to evoke an aesthetic experience in the listeners.

Conflict of Interests

The authors declare that there is no conflict of interests regarding the publication of this paper.

Acknowledgments

The authors wish to thank Dr. Rachel Wood, Diego Lisfera, and Edoardo Acotto for help in stimulus preparation and Professor Giacomo Rizzolatti and Professor Vittorio Gallese for theoretical and methodological suggestions; finally, they are grateful to Fondazione Cassa di Risparmio di Parma (CARIPARMA) for providing the infrastructures that made it possible to conduct this study.

References

[1] J. L. Chen, R. J. Zatorre, and V. B. Penhune, "Interactions between auditory and dorsal premotor cortex during synchronization to musical rhythms," *NeuroImage*, vol. 32, no. 4, pp. 1771–1781, 2006.

[2] J. L. Chen, V. B. Penhune, and R. J. Zatorre, "Listening to musical rhythms recruits motor regions of the brain," *Cerebral Cortex*, vol. 18, no. 12, pp. 2844–2854, 2008.

[3] P. Janata and S. T. Grafton, "Swinging in the brain: shared neural substrates for behaviors related to sequencing and music," *Nature Neuroscience*, vol. 6, no. 7, pp. 682–687, 2003.

[4] B. Maess, S. Koelsch, T. C. Gunter, and A. D. Friederici, "Musical syntax is processed in Broca's area: an MEG study," *Nature Neuroscience*, vol. 4, no. 5, pp. 540–545, 2001.

[5] B. Tillmann, S. Koelsch, N. Escoffier et al., "Cognitive priming in sung and instrumental music: activation of inferior frontal cortex," *NeuroImage*, vol. 31, no. 4, pp. 1771–1782, 2006.

[6] B. Tillmann, S. Koelsch, N. Escoffier et al., "Cognitive priming in sung and instrumental music: activation of inferior frontal cortex," *NeuroImage*, vol. 31, no. 4, pp. 1771–1782, 2006.

[7] D. J. Levitin and V. Menon, "The neural locus of temporal structure and expectancies in music: evidence from functional neuroimaging at 3 tesla," *Music Perception*, vol. 22, no. 3, pp. 563–575, 2005.

[8] D. Perani, M. C. Saccuman, P. Scifo et al., "Functional specializations for music processing in the human newborn brain," *Proceedings of the National Academy of Sciences of the United States of America*, vol. 107, no. 10, pp. 4758–4763, 2010.

[9] A. J. Blood and R. J. Zatorre, "Intensely pleasurable responses to music correlate with activity in brain regions implicated in reward and emotion," *Proceedings of the National Academy of Sciences of the United States of America*, vol. 98, no. 20, pp. 11818–11823, 2001.

[10] S. Koelsch, T. Fritz, D. Y. V. Cramon, K. Müller, and A. D. Friederici, "Investigating emotion with music: an fMRI study," *Human Brain Mapping*, vol. 27, no. 3, pp. 239–250, 2006.

[11] S. Koelsch, S. Skouras, T. Fritz et al., "The roles of superficial amygdala and auditory cortex in music-evoked fear and joy," *NeuroImage*, vol. 31, pp. 1771–1782, 2013.

[12] K. J. Worsley and K. J. Friston, "Analysis of fMRI time-series revisited—again," *NeuroImage*, vol. 2, no. 3, pp. 173–181, 1995.

[13] K. J. Friston, "Bayesian estimation of dynamical systems: an application to fMRI," *NeuroImage*, vol. 16, no. 2, pp. 513–530, 2002.

[14] J. L. R. Andersson, C. Hutton, J. Ashburner, R. Turner, and K. Friston, "Modeling geometric deformations in EPI time series," *NeuroImage*, vol. 13, no. 5, pp. 903–919, 2001.

[15] D. L. Collins, P. Neelin, T. M. Peters, and A. C. Evans, "Automatic 3D intersubject registration of MR volumetric data in standardized Talairach space," *Journal of Computer Assisted Tomography*, vol. 18, no. 2, pp. 192–205, 1994.

[16] C. J. Limb, "Structural and functional neural correlates of music perception," *Anatomical Record Part A: Discoveries in Molecular, Cellular, and Evolutionary Biology*, vol. 288, no. 4, pp. 435–446, 2006.

[17] R. J. Zatorre, A. C. Evans, and E. Meyer, "Neural mechanisms underlying melodic perception and memory for pitch," *Journal of Neuroscience*, vol. 14, no. 4, pp. 1908–1919, 1994.

[18] A. R. Halpern and R. J. Zatorre, "When that tune runs through your head: a PET investigation of auditory imagery for familiar melodies," *Cerebral Cortex*, vol. 9, no. 7, pp. 697–704, 1999.

[19] I. Peretz and R. J. Zatorre, "Brain organization for music processing," *Annual Review of Psychology*, vol. 56, pp. 89–114, 2005.

[20] A. S. Bregman, *Auditory Scene Analysis: The Perceptual Organization of Sound*, The MIT Press, Cambridge, Mass, USA, 1990.

[21] T. D. Griffiths and J. D. Warren, "The planum temporale as a computational hub," *Trends in Neurosciences*, vol. 25, no. 7, pp. 348–353, 2002.

[22] C. Liégeois-Chauvel, I. Peretz, M. Babaï, V. Laguitton, and P. Chauvel, "Contribution of different cortical areas in the temporal lobes to music processing," *Brain*, vol. 121, no. 10, pp. 1853–1867, 1998.

[23] R. D. Patterson, S. Uppenkamp, I. S. Johnsrude, and T. D. Griffiths, "The processing of temporal pitch and melody information in auditory cortex," *Neuron*, vol. 36, no. 4, pp. 767–776, 2002.

[24] J. R. Augustine, "Circuitry and functional aspects of the insular lobe in primates including humans," *Brain Research Reviews*, vol. 22, no. 3, pp. 229–244, 1996.

[25] D.-E. Bamiou, F. E. Musiek, and L. M. Luxon, "The insula (Island of Reil) and its role in auditory processing: literature review," *Brain Research Reviews*, vol. 42, no. 2, pp. 143–154, 2003.

[26] A. J. Blood, R. J. Zatorre, P. Bermudez, and A. C. Evans, "Emotional responses to pleasant and unpleasant music correlate with activity in paralimbic brain regions," *Nature Neuroscience*, vol. 2, no. 4, pp. 382–387, 1999.

[27] N. Gosselin, S. Samson, R. Adolphs et al., "Emotional responses to unpleasant music correlates with damage to the parahippocampal cortex," *Brain*, vol. 129, no. 10, pp. 2585–2592, 2006.

[28] S.-H. Wang and R. G. M. Morris, "Hippocampal-neocortical interactions in memory formation, consolidation, and reconsolidation," *Annual Review of Psychology*, vol. 61, pp. 49–79, 2010.

[29] N. M. van Strien, N. L. M. Cappaert, and M. P. Witter, "The anatomy of memory: an interactive overview of the parahippocampal- hippocampal network," *Nature Reviews Neuroscience*, vol. 10, no. 4, pp. 272–282, 2009.

[30] G. Bottini, R. Corcoran, R. Sterzi et al., "The role of the right hemisphere in the interpretation of figurative aspects of language: a positron emission tomography activation study," *Brain*, vol. 117, no. 6, pp. 1241–1253, 1994.

[31] M. Sotillo, L. Carretié, J. A. Hinojosa et al., "Neural activity associated with metaphor comprehension: spatial analysis," *Neuroscience Letters*, vol. 373, no. 1, pp. 5–9, 2005.

[32] Y. Harpaz, Y. Levkovitz, and M. Lavidor, "Lexical ambiguity resolution in Wernicke's area and its right homologue," *Cortex*, vol. 45, no. 9, pp. 1097–1103, 2009.

[33] M. Jung-Beeman, "Bilateral brain processes for comprehending natural language," *Trends in Cognitive Sciences*, vol. 9, no. 11, pp. 512–518, 2005.

[34] S. Koelsch, E. Kasper, D. Sammler, K. Schulze, T. Gunter, and A. D. Friederici, "Music, language and meaning: brain signatures of semantic processing," *Nature Neuroscience*, vol. 7, no. 3, pp. 302–307, 2004.

[35] S. Koelsch, T. Fritz, K. Schulze, D. Alsop, and G. Schlaug, "Adults and children processing music: an fMRI study," *NeuroImage*, vol. 25, no. 4, pp. 1068–1076, 2005.

[36] J. Daltrozzo and D. Schön, "Is conceptual processing in music automatic? An electrophysiological approach," *Brain Research*, vol. 1270, pp. 88–94, 2009.

[37] N. Steinbeis and S. Koelsch, "Shared neural resources between music and language indicate semantic processing of musical tension-resolution patterns," *Cerebral Cortex*, vol. 18, no. 5, pp. 1169–1178, 2008.

[38] M. Himmelbach, M. Erb, and H.-O. Karnath, "Exploring the visual world: the neural substrate of spatial orienting," *NeuroImage*, vol. 32, no. 4, pp. 1747–1759, 2006.

[39] J. Downar, A. P. Crawley, D. J. Mikulis, and K. D. Davis, "A cortical network sensitive to stimulus salience in a neutral behavioral context across multiple sensory modalities," *Journal of Neurophysiology*, vol. 87, no. 1, pp. 615–620, 2002.

[40] H.-O. Karnath, "New insights into the functions of the superior temporal cortex," *Nature Reviews Neuroscience*, vol. 2, no. 8, pp. 568–576, 2001.

[41] S. Koelsch, "Towards a neural basis of music-evoked emotions," *Trends in Cognitive Sciences*, vol. 14, no. 3, pp. 131–137, 2010.

[42] D. D. Cinzia and G. Vittorio, "Neuroaesthetics: a review," *Current Opinion in Neurobiology*, vol. 19, no. 6, pp. 682–687, 2009.

[43] D. Sammler, M. Grigutsch, T. Fritz, and S. Koelsch, "Music and emotion: electrophysiological correlates of the processing of pleasant and unpleasant music," *Psychophysiology*, vol. 44, no. 2, pp. 293–304, 2007.

8

Effect of Resveratrol as Caloric Restriction Mimetic and Environmental Enrichment on Neurobehavioural Responses in Young Healthy Mice

Mustapha Shehu Muhammad,[1] **Rabiu Abdussalam Magaji,**[2] **Aliyu Mohammed,**[2] **Ahmed-Sherif Isa,**[2] **and Mohammed Garba Magaji**[3]

[1] Department of Human Physiology, College of Medical Sciences, Gombe State University, Gombe 760214, Nigeria
[2] Department of Human Physiology, Faculty of Medicine, Ahmadu Bello University, Zaria 810001, Nigeria
[3] Department of Pharmacology and Therapeutics, Faculty of Pharmaceutical Sciences, Ahmadu Bello University, Zaria 810001, Nigeria

Correspondence should be addressed to Mustapha Shehu Muhammad; msmuhammad@gsu.edu.ng

Academic Editor: Valerio Magnaghi

Caloric restriction and environmental enrichment have been separately reported to possess health benefits such as improvement in motor and cognitive functions. Resveratrol, a natural polyphenolic compound, has been reported to be caloric restriction mimetic. This study therefore aims to investigate the potential benefit of the combination of resveratrol as CR and EE on learning and memory, motor coordination, and motor endurance in young healthy mice. Fifty mice of both sexes were randomly divided into five groups of 10 animals each: group I animals received carboxymethylcellulose (CMC) orally per kg/day (control), group II animals were maintained on every other day feeding, group III animals received resveratrol 50 mg/kg, suspended in 10 g/L of (CMC) orally per kg/day, group IV animals received CMC and were kept in an enriched environment, and group V animals received resveratrol 50 mg/kg and were kept in EE. The treatment lasted for four weeks. On days 26, 27, and 28 of the study period, the animals were subjected to neurobehavioural evaluation. The results obtained showed that there was no significant change ($P > 0.05$) in neurobehavioural responses in all the groups when compared to the control which indicates that 50 mg/kg of resveratrol administration and EE have no significant effects on neurobehavioural responses in young healthy mice over a period of four weeks.

1. Introduction

Dietary restriction (DR), otherwise known as caloric restriction (CR), has been generally defined as consumption of nutritious diet that is 30% to 40% less in calories compared to *ad libitum* diet [1]. In other words, CR can be defined as a simple reduction in caloric intake in the absence of malnutrition [2]. Caloric restriction has been demonstrated to possess many health benefits. It provides protection against numerous deadly diseases such as cancer, neurological disorders, and obesity and is found to be the only reliable treatment that extends lifespan or causes healthy aging consistently in a multitude of organisms ranging from bacteria to monkeys [3–5].

The most frequently mentioned effect of CR has been its influence on creating a mild stress in the organism and a typical upregulation of adaptive mechanisms involving stress proteins accompanied by elevated defence or survival molecules [6]. Caloric restriction (CR) has also been found to retard several aspects of the aging process in mammals, including age-related mortality, tumorigenesis, physiological decline [7], and the establishment of age-related transcriptional profiles [8].

Resveratrol (3,5′,4-trihydroxystilbene), a natural polyphenolic compound found mainly in the skin of grapes and red wine, has previously been shown to extend lifespan in yeast (*Saccharomyces cerevisiae*), nematode worm (*Caenorhabditis elegans*), fruit fly (*Drosophila melanogaster*), and short-lived fish (*Nothobranchius furzeri*) through a sirtuins 1 dependent mechanism [9–13]. Studies have shown that mice fed with a high fat diet supplemented with high levels of resveratrol were shown to have extended lifespan compared to the control animals and several metabolic alterations similar to what is observed with CR; thus, resveratrol is said to have caloric restriction-like properties [2, 14].

Environmental enrichment (EE) is defined as a sustained and progressive increase in cognitive and sensorimotor stimuli with aggregated voluntary physical activity and complex social interactions [15]. Abundant experimental evidence shows that EE is beneficial in various animal models of neurodegenerative disorders such as stroke and Alzheimer's disease [16, 17]. Environmental enrichment also induces neuroprotection against 1-methyl-4-phenyl-1,2,3,6-tetrahydropyridine (MPTP) toxicity to mice [18, 19] and improves motor function after unilateral 6-OHDA injection in rats [20]. Numerous data suggest that synthesis and release of trophic factors (TFs) may play a crucial role in mediating the neuroprotective effect of EE [16]. Environmental enrichment alters the expression of TFs and their receptors in several brain areas [21, 22] and induces astrogliogenesis [23]. In the nigrostriatal system, EE-housed animals show increased brain-derived neurotrophic factor (BDNF) expression in the striatum [18] and glia cell-line derived neurotrophic factor (GDNF) mRNA in the substantia nigra (SN) [19].

Studies have shown that CR and its mimetics such as resveratrol improve motor coordination and increase longevity in mice which may be related to the improvement in endurance and strength [2, 14, 24]. Resveratrol has also been shown to prevent cognitive decline in a number of disease models and to reduce neurodegeneration *in vivo* [25]. However, numerous works have been done on EE, CR, and its mimetics such as resveratrol and sulforaphane [1, 24], and much attention has been lavished on the effect of resveratrol, CR, and EE on aging and age related disorders but the possible beneficial role in young healthy animals has not been investigated. The beneficial role of CR in the nervous system has been extensively studied in aged animals [26]. Moreover, several reports showed the physiological, neurological, and behavioural effects of CR and EE in rodents, but the majority of efforts have been focused on the beneficial effects of CR and EE on aging and lifespan in the past decades, and little attention has been paid to the physiological effects of CR and EE especially in young healthy animals. Furthermore, there are controversial reports on the effects of CR and EE on cognition in young animals. Some investigators demonstrated that CR enhances learning and memory [27], while others have reported that CR had negative effects on cognitive functions [28]. Environmental enrichment has also been reported to improve spatial memory in aged mice with no significant effect in young and middle-aged mice [29]. Collectively, the available data suggest that both CR and EE exert similar beneficial effects on neurons in the brain and share a mechanism involving increased neurotrophic factor production [30]. Hence this study evaluates the effects of resveratrol as CR mimetic and EE on motor coordination, motor endurance, memory, and learning in young healthy Wistar albino mice over a period of four weeks.

2. Materials and Methods

2.1. Chemicals/Reagents. Resveratrol (60 g) of analytical grade was purchased from Candlewood Stars Incorporated, Danbury, USA (batch number: MR120718). Carboxymethylcellulose CMC (10 g) (product number: 27929, BDH Chemicals Ltd., Poole, UK) was obtained from Department of Pharmacology and Therapeutics, Ahmadu Bello University, Zaria. *trans*-Resveratrol, due to its low solubility in water, was suspended in 10 g/L CMC [31].

2.2. Animals. Fifty (50) Wistar albino mice of both sexes, 4 weeks of age and weighing 15–22 g, were used for this study. The animals were obtained from the Institute of Veterinary Research, Vom, Jos Plateau State. The animals were housed in standard polypropylene cages in groups of five in a temperature and humidity controlled environment subject to a 12 h light/dark cycle and fed with standard laboratory animal feed and water *ad libitum*. Dietary delivery groups were given controlled access to food; water was available *ad libitum*. The mice were allowed to acclimatize to the environment of the behavioural laboratory for the period of one week before commencement of the experiment. All experimental protocols were in accordance with the Ahmadu Bello University research policy and ethic and regulations governing the care and use of experimental animals (NIH publication number 85-23, revised 1996). The experiments were conducted in a quiet laboratory between hours of 900 h and 1600 h.

2.3. Animal Housing and Management. The enriched cage (66 cm long × 46 cm wide × 38 cm high) as described by Harburger et al. [29] was used in the study. The cage contained tubes, ramps, stairs, and different "toys" (hard plastic balls, cubes, cones, and sticks). The toys were changed twice a week to continuously encourage exploration of the environment. The complexity (number of objects) of the housing facility was increased progressively: every 2 days, two to four objects were added to the environment. Ten days after housing animals in the EE, the complexity of the cage is expected to be maximal, but the positions of the objects were changed continuously after every 2 days [15]. Five (5) mice were housed together to allow social interactions. The impoverished condition consisted of normal cages (45 cm long × 30 cm wide × 18 cm high) made without objects or running wheels, housing five (5) animals per cage.

Animals were kept in EE housing for four weeks while receiving the appropriate treatment, as described by Steiner et al. [23]. The control animals were given carboxymethylcellulose (CMC) and kept under good housing condition. Neurobehavioural study was carried out for the period of three (3) days during the last phase of the experiment.

2.3.1. Animal Groupings. The animals were divided into five (5) groups each comprising ten (10) animals of both sexes per group, that is, five (5) males and five (5) females mice kept in separate cages to prevent mating. Group I animals received carboxymethylcellulose (control group) 50 mg/kg per body weight, group II animals were maintained on every other day feeding (EODF) with standard laboratory animals diet, group III animals received resveratrol 50 mg/kg orally for four weeks as described by Blanchet et al. [32], group IV animals received CMC and were kept in an enriched housing (EE) for four weeks, and group V animals received resveratrol 50 mg/kg orally and were kept in EE housing (for 4 weeks).

2.4. Neurobehavioural Assessments. The following neurobehavioural studies were carried out for three days on days 26, 27, and 28 of the experimental period.

2.4.1. Beam Walk Test. The beam walk test was used to test motor coordination. Briefly, the beam walk apparatus consists of a beam, ruler, goal box, and an elevated wooden stand. The beam is made of wood, 8 mm in diameter, 80 cm long, and elevated 30 cm above the bench by a wooden support. Mice were allowed to walk from a start platform along a ruler (80 cm long and 3 cm wide) elevated 30 cm above the bench by a wooden support to the goal box (enclosed hamster house). Several trials were performed for each mouse and it was designed such that the mice tested were aware that there is a goal box that should be reached. A ruler was used to train the mice and once the mice find it easy to cross, they were moved immediately to the beam [33]. The mice were placed on the beam at one end and allowed to walk to the goal box. Mice that fall from the beam were returned to the position they fell from with a maximum time of 60 seconds allowed on the beam. The measurements that were taken were time on the beam, the number of foot slips (one or both hind limbs slipped from the beam), and the number of falls. After each trial, the maze was wiped with a cotton wool dipped in 70% ethyl alcohol and allowed to dry to remove any olfactory clue or odour.

2.4.2. Hang Test. The hang test was used to assess muscular endurance in mice as described by Mohanasundari et al. [34]. Briefly, the apparatus consists of a horizontal grid (grid 12 cm^2, opening 0.5 cm^2). The grid was mounted 20 cm above a hard surface, to discourage falling or injury in case of falling. The apparatus was equipped with a 3-inch wall to prevent animals from traversing to the upper side of the grid. The mice were placed on the horizontal grid and supported until they held the grid. The grid was then inverted so that the mice were allowed to hang upside down. The mice were allowed to stay on the grid for 30 s and 10 chances were given with 1 min interval and the best maximum hanging time was recorded. The percentage of success was recorded as maximum time hanging/30 s × 100 [35].

2.4.3. Elevated Plus Maze. The elevated plus maze was used to evaluate short-term spatial memory [36]. Briefly, the elevated plus maze for mice consists of two perpendicular open arms (21.5 × 7.5 cm) and two closed arms (21.5 × 7.5 × 20 cm) which extends from a central 7.5 × 7.5 cm platform. The platform and floor were made from wood, and the lateral walls of the closed arms were made of wood painted black. The maze was elevated 38 cm above the floor. On the first day (training), each animal was placed at the end of one

TABLE 1: Effect of resveratrol as CR mimetic and EE on motor coordination of mice.

Groups	Number of foot slips	Time taken to complete task (seconds)
Control (CMC)	1.13 ± 0.44	9.63 ± 1.32
EODF	1.30 ± 0.42	9.10 ± 1.39
Resveratrol only	1.20 ± 0.42	8.80 ± 1.46
EE only	0.88 ± 0.44	8.13 ± 1.30
Resveratrol + EE	0.30 ± 0.21	8.40 ± 1.94

Results were presented as mean ± SEM; CMC: carboxymethylcellulose; EODF: every other day feeding; EE: environmental enrichment; $n = 10$.

open arm, facing away from the central platform. The transfer latency of the mouse to move from the open to the enclosed arms was recorded within 90 s. Following entry into the arm, the animals were allowed to explore the apparatus for 30 s. Twenty-four hours later, the second trial (retention test) was performed and the animals were observed for 90 s. After each trial, the maze was wiped with a cotton wool dipped in 70% ethyl alcohol and allowed to dry to remove any olfactory clue or odour.

2.5. Statistical Analysis. Data obtained were expressed as mean ± SEM. Statistical analysis was carried out using SPSS version 17 and all the analysis was done using one way ANOVA followed by Tukey's post hoc test for multiple comparisons. Values of $P < 0.05$ were considered significant.

3. Results

3.1. Beam Walk Test. Table 1 represents the results observed in the beam walk test. A slight decrease in the number of foot slips was observed in the EE and RESV + EE groups, when compared to the control, though no statistical significance was recorded. On the other hand, an increase in number of foot slips was observed in EODF group when compared to the control; this also was not statistically significant (Table 1). There was no significant change in transfer latency on the beam among the groups, but lower values were recorded for the RESV, EE, and RESV + EE groups, respectively, when compared to the control group.

3.2. Hang Test. Figure 1 shows the changes in motor strength in the hang test. The percentage of hanging time was slightly lower in all the groups than the control, although it was not statistically significant.

3.3. Elevated Plus Maze. Table 2 shows the results obtained on the effect of resveratrol induced CR and EE on memory of mice. Result obtained showed no significant statistical difference in the various treatment groups when compared to the control, although there was slight decrease in transfer latency (retention) in the EODF, RESV, EE, and RESV + EE groups compared to the control group.

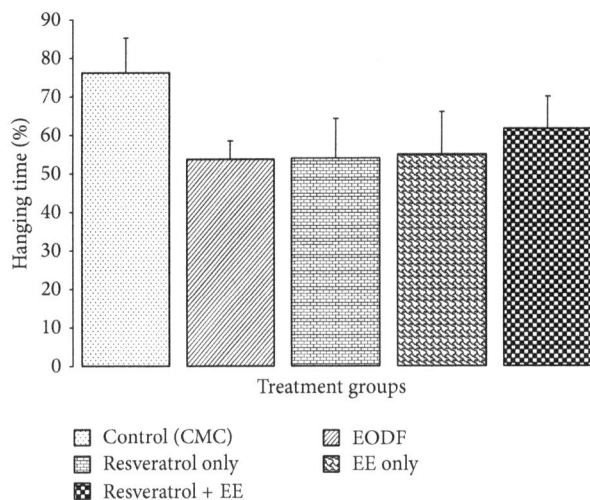

FIGURE 1: Effect of resveratrol as CR mimetic and EE on muscular endurance of mice. Results presented as mean ± SEM; $n = 10$.

TABLE 2: Effect of resveratrol as CR mimetic and EE on memory of mice.

Groups	Transfer latency (acquisition)	Transfer latency (retention)
Control (CMC)	39.75 ± 6.62	23.38 ± 9.64
EODF	53.70 ± 7.56	17.20 ± 4.18
Resveratrol only	44.60 ± 9.57	14.80 ± 3.04
EE only	25.25 ± 6.43	10.25 ± 1.32
Resveratrol + EE	25.70 ± 7.90	20.40 ± 8.01

Results were presented as mean ± SEM; CMC: carboxymethylcellulose; EODF: every other day feeding; EE: environmental enrichment; $n = 10$.

4. Discussion

The results obtained from this study demonstrated a trend towards improvement in motor coordination in the environmental enrichment and resveratrol treated group in an enriched environment using beam walk test, although the decrease in number of foot slips and latency were not statistically different when compared to the control group. The results of muscular endurance using hang test were also not significantly different between the groups. This is contrary to the findings of Anandhan et al. [37] who reported that resveratrol improves motor endurance using hang test in MPTP challenged mice. Both resveratrol and environmental enrichment have also been reported to extend lifespan and improve motor function in drosophila and rat models of Parkinson's disease, respectively, by activating sirtuins gene [15, 38].

Caloric restriction and EE have been found to attenuate age-related deficits in learning and memory [15, 39] and increase resistance of neurons to excitotoxic, oxidative, and metabolic insults and improve behavioural outcomes in experimental models of Alzheimer's and Huntington's disease [40]. The result obtained from this study using the elevated plus maze for memory, though not statistically significant,

showed a slight decrease ($P > 0.05$) in the transfer latency (retention) across the groups when compared to the control with the least mean value obtained in the EE group. This is in agreement with the findings of Harburger et al. [29] who found no significant change in spatial memory of young male mice when compared to the control after exposing them to enriched environment for a period of one month. This difference was, however, attributed to the age as well as the duration of exposure of the animals to enriched environment [29].

Although, in this study, resveratrol was used as a caloric restriction mimetic to stimulate caloric restriction, the results obtained on the effect of resveratrol as CR mimetic on memory of mice were in corroboration with the findings of Deng et al. [26] who reported no significant change in short-term memory of mice using the passive avoidance test for memory after subjecting mice to a 20% caloric restriction for one month. However, no uniform conclusion has been reached on the effect of caloric restriction or caloric restriction-like effects on cognitive functions in young animals. Nevertheless, some investigators have suggested that caloric restriction enhanced learning and memory in young animals [27, 41, 42], while others reported the contrary [28, 43]. This discrepancy was attributed to several factors including differences in caloric restriction treatment, duration of caloric restriction, species or strain of animal, and type of behavioural test [26].

There is little evidence that resveratrol enhances cognition in healthy individuals in the absence of pathological or age-related cognitive decline which indicates that resveratrol confers some protection on the brain from the effects of aging and oxidative, physical, and chemical damage to the brain without measurably improving cognition in the short term [44]; this could possibly be an explanation for the absence of an observed effect of resveratrol as CR mimetic in our study. If resveratrol can only protect the brain against damage (as opposed to being able to enhance its function), it would not be expected to produce a measurable effect on cognition in young healthy animals, such as the mice in our study, and one logical explanation for the results of these studies is that resveratrol prevented the neurological pathology that is known to increase with age [45–48] but did not enhance cognition when the animals were young. The sensitivity of the neurobehavioural test used to assess memory in young healthy animals in our study could also be considered as a factor that hinders any feasible change in memory between the treatment groups and the control.

Another possible explanation for the lack of an observed effect of resveratrol as CR mimetic in our study was the short duration of treatment. The mice received resveratrol for only four weeks before testing began, while in previous studies, where resveratrol was shown to improve cognitive functions, the subjects were given resveratrol for at least one-third of their lifespan [13, 49]. Short periods of resveratrol treatment in rats have been shown to produce positive effects on cognition, but the animals used in those studies had been subjected to neurological trauma or treatment with a neurotoxic substance [50, 51]. The failure to observe an effect after short-term treatment is a logical outcome if resveratrol's effect on cognitive function is mediated through protecting the brain against damage [44]. In previous studies where cognitive function was assessed in healthy animals, a significant effect of resveratrol was only observed in middle-aged or aged animals [13, 49].

The failure to observe an effect of resveratrol as CR mimetic may also have been due to the combined effects of both EE and resveratrol in our procedures. Results obtained in resveratrol and EE treated groups showed decrease in transfer latency though not statistically significant compared to the control group and resveratrol treated group kept in an enriched environment. A possible and logical explanation for this may be that EE alters the magnitude of improvement in spatial tasks imparted by the estrogen-like effect of resveratrol [52–55]. Studies comparing mice exposed to enriched and nonenriched environments have shown that, in certain tests of cognitive function, estrogen appeared to only improve performance in nonenriched mice [53, 54]. In some of the tests, mice that both received estrogen and were kept in an enriched environment performed worse than those that received either estrogen or enrichment alone [54], which is similar to our findings. In our studies, resveratrol failed to further enhance the performance of the enriched mice beyond an improvement ($P > 0.05$) caused by EE and resveratrol treated mice alone even though both the enriched treated mice and resveratrol treated mice did not differ significantly in cognitive performance when compared to the control but did perform better than the control group and the combined treated groups. Other studies revealed similar findings when rats were exposed to mild handling stress, where estradiol failed to enhance the cognitive performance of rats beyond the improvement caused by the increased handling in radial arm maze trial [55]. This seems to indicate the occurrence of a masking or ceiling effect by enrichment; hence, if cognitive performance is improved by EE, resveratrol probably due to estrogen-like effect may not be able to further improve the cognitive performance of mice kept in an enriched environment.

Furthermore, a more convincing explanation for our findings may be that EE and histone deacetylases (HDACs) inhibitors such as trichostatin A and sodium butyrate have been identified as being capable of improving memory function in rodent experiments [56, 57]. Some investigators reported that EE improves spatial memory capacity in mice through elevating histone acetylation in the hippocampus and further observed that the improvement in spatial memory was mimicked by HDAC inhibitors [58]. They further reported that HDAC inhibitors not only improve the capacity to form new memories but also restore the capacity to form memories in a mouse model of neurodegenerative disorders [58]. This leads to the postulation by some researchers that HDAC inhibitors could serve as a potential new therapeutic approach to human cognitive disorders and aging-related memory dysfunction arising from neurodegeneration [59].

Resveratrol which targets the sirtuin class of nicotinamide adenine dinucleotide- (NAD-) dependent deacetylases (class III histone deacetylases) mediates its beneficial effects on health and longevity in mammals through *SIRT-1* NAD-HDACs dependent activity [60]. This further explains the failure to observe an improvement in cognitive function in resveratrol treated group kept in an enriched environment beyond the trend towards improvement caused by individual treatment of EE and resveratrol, respectively, in our procedures. While EE was acting through elevating histone acetylation via the activity of histone acetyl transferases (HATs) in the hippocampus as mentioned earlier, resveratrol was probably masking this effect through HDACs dependent activity thereby catalyzing the removal of acetyl groups from lysine residues through a Zn^{2+}-dependent charge-relay system [61, 62]. Thus, if acetylation of histones is functionally significant for consolidation of memory, then disruption of HAT activity would be predicted to interfere with memory formation [63].

5. Conclusion

In conclusion, 50 mg/kg of resveratrol administered as a caloric restriction mimetic and environmental enrichment have no significant effect on neurobehavioural responses in young healthy Swiss albino mice over a period of four weeks, although slight changes that were not statistically significant were observed in both cognitive function and motor coordination and motor endurance tests; hence, extending this study period a little longer could probably produce significant changes in neurobehavioural responses.

Conflict of Interests

The authors declare that there is no conflict of interests regarding the publication of this paper.

Acknowledgments

The authors thank Malam Mu'azu in the Department of Pharmacology and Therapeutics, Ahmadu Bello University, Zaria, Nigeria, for his assistance in training and handling of the animals. They appreciate Gombe State University, Nigeria, for providing financial assistance for the success of the work through Tertiary Education Trust Fund.

References

[1] T. S. Anekonda, "The benefits of caloric restriction and caloric restriction mimetics as related to the eye," *Open Longevity Science*, vol. 3, pp. 28–37, 2009.

[2] J. A. Baur, K. J. Pearson, N. L. Price et al., "Resveratrol improves health and survival of mice on a high-calorie diet," *Nature*, vol. 444, no. 7117, pp. 337–342, 2006.

[3] M. Obin, A. Pike, M. Halbleib, R. Lipman, A. Taylor, and R. Bronson, "Calorie restriction modulates age-dependent changes in the retinas of Brown Norway rats," *Mechanisms of Ageing and Development*, vol. 114, no. 2, pp. 133–147, 2000.

[4] S. Lin, E. Ford, M. Haigis, G. Liszt, and L. Guarente, "Calorie restriction extends yeast life span by lowering the level of NADH," *Genes and Development*, vol. 18, no. 1, pp. 12–16, 2004.

[5] G. Wolf, "Calorie restriction increases life span: a molecular mechanism," *Nutrition Reviews*, vol. 64, no. 2, pp. 89–92, 2006.

[6] D. A. Sinclair, "Toward a unified theory of caloric restriction and longevity regulation," *Mechanisms of Ageing and Development*, vol. 126, no. 9, pp. 987–1002, 2005.

[7] R. Weindruch and R. L. Walford, *The Retardation of Aging and Disease by Dietary Restriction*, Charles C. Thomas, Springfield, Ill, USA, 1988.

[8] C.-K. Lee, R. G. Klopp, R. Weindruch, and T. A. Prolla, "Gene expression profile of aging and its retardation by caloric restriction," *Science*, vol. 285, no. 5432, pp. 1390–1393, 1999.

[9] K. T. Howitz, K. J. Bitterman, H. Y. Cohen et al., "Small molecule activators of sirtuins extend Saccharomyces cerevisiae lifespan," *Nature*, vol. 425, no. 6954, pp. 191–196, 2003.

[10] J. H. Bauer, S. Goupil, G. B. Garber, and S. L. Helfand, "An accelerated assay for the identification of lifespan-extending interventions in *Drosophila melanogaster*," *Proceedings of the National Academy of Sciences of the United States of America*, vol. 101, no. 35, pp. 12980–12985, 2004.

[11] J. G. Wood, B. Rogina, S. Lavu et al., "Sirtuin activators mimic caloric restriction and delay ageing in metazoans," *Nature*, vol. 430, no. 7000, pp. 686–689, 2004.

[12] M. Viswanathan, S. K. Kim, A. Berdichevsky, and L. Guarente, "A role for SIR-2.1 regulation of ER stress response genes in determining *C. elegans* life span," *Developmental Cell*, vol. 9, no. 5, pp. 605–615, 2005.

[13] D. R. Valenzano, E. Terzibasi, T. Genade, A. Cattaneo, L. Domenici, and A. Cellerino, "Resveratrol prolongs lifespan and retards the onset of age-related markers in a short-lived vertebrate," *Current Biology*, vol. 16, no. 3, pp. 296–300, 2006.

[14] M. Lagouge, C. Argmann, Z. Gerhart-Hines et al., "Resveratrol improves mitochondrial function and protects against metabolic disease by activating SIRT1 and PGC-1alpha," *Cell*, vol. 127, no. 6, pp. 1109–1122, 2006.

[15] A. Anastasía, L. Torre, G. A. de Erausquin, and D. H. Mascó, "Enriched environment protects the nigrostriatal dopaminergic system and induces astroglial reaction in the 6-OHDA rat model of Parkinson's disease," *Journal of Neurochemistry*, vol. 109, no. 3, pp. 755–765, 2009.

[16] J. Nithianantharajah and A. J. Hannan, "Enriched environments, experience-dependent plasticity and disorders of the nervous system," *Nature Reviews Neuroscience*, vol. 7, no. 9, pp. 697–709, 2006.

[17] G. Laviola, A. J. Hannan, S. Macrì, M. Solinas, and M. Jaber, "Effects of enriched environment on animal models of neurodegenerative diseases and psychiatric disorders," *Neurobiology of Disease*, vol. 31, no. 2, pp. 159–168, 2008.

[18] E. Bezard, S. Dovero, D. Belin et al., "Enriched environment confers resistance to 1-methyl-4-phenyl-1,2,3,6-tetrahydropyridine and cocaine: involvement of dopamine transporter and trophic factors," *Journal of Neuroscience*, vol. 23, no. 35, pp. 10999–11007, 2003.

[19] C. J. Faherty, K. R. Shepherd, A. Herasimtschuk, and R. J. Smeyne, "Environmental enrichment in adulthood eliminates neuronal death in experimental Parkinsonism," *Molecular Brain Research*, vol. 134, no. 1, pp. 170–179, 2005.

[20] N. M. Jadavji, B. Kolb, and G. A. Metz, "Enriched environment improves motor function in intact and unilateral dopamine-depleted rats," *Neuroscience*, vol. 140, no. 4, pp. 1127–1138, 2006.

[21] B. R. Ickes, T. M. Pham, L. A. Sanders, D. S. Albeck, A. H. Mohammed, and A. Granholm, "Long-term environmental enrichment leads to regional increases in neurotrophin levels in rat brain," *Experimental Neurology*, vol. 164, no. 1, pp. 45–52, 2000.

[22] T. L. Spires, H. E. Grote, N. K. Varshney et al., "Environmental enrichment rescues protein deficits in a mouse model of Huntington's disease, indicating a possible disease mechanism," *Journal of Neuroscience*, vol. 24, no. 9, pp. 2270–2276, 2004.

[23] B. Steiner, C. Winter, K. Hosman et al., "Enriched environment induces cellular plasticity in the adult substantia nigra and improves motor behavior function in the 6-OHDA rat model of Parkinson's disease," *Experimental Neurology*, vol. 199, no. 2, pp. 291–300, 2006.

[24] J. A. Baur, "Resveratrol, sirtuins, and the promise of a DR mimetic," *Mechanisms of Ageing and Development*, vol. 131, no. 4, pp. 261–269, 2010.

[25] D. Kim, M. D. Nguyen, M. M. Dobbin et al., "SIRT1 deacetylase protects against neurodegeneration in models for Alzheimer's disease and amyotrophic lateral sclerosis," *The EMBO Journal*, vol. 26, no. 13, pp. 3169–3179, 2007.

[26] L. Deng, Z.-N. Wu, and P.-Z. Han, "Effects of different levels of food restriction on passive-avoidance memory and the expression of synapsin I in young mice," *International Journal of Neuroscience*, vol. 119, no. 2, pp. 291–304, 2009.

[27] T. Hashimoto and S. Watanabe, "Chronic food restriction enhances memory in mice-analysis with matched drive levels," *NeuroReport*, vol. 16, no. 10, pp. 1129–1133, 2005.

[28] S. Yanai, Y. Okaichi, and H. Okaichi, "Long-term dietary restriction causes negative effects on cognitive functions in rats," *Neurobiology of Aging*, vol. 25, no. 3, pp. 325–332, 2004.

[29] L. L. Harburger, T. J. Lambert, and K. M. Frick, "Age-dependent effects of environmental enrichment on spatial reference memory in male mice," *Behavioural Brain Research*, vol. 185, no. 1, pp. 43–48, 2007.

[30] M. P. Mattson, W. Duan, J. Lee, and Z. Guo, "Suppression of brain aging and neurodegenerative disorders by dietary restriction and environmental enrichment: molecular mechanisms," *Mechanisms of Ageing and Development*, vol. 122, no. 7, pp. 757–778, 2001.

[31] M. E., lia Juan, M. Pilar Vinardell, and J. M. Planas, "The daily oral administration of high doses of trans-resveratrol to rats for 28 days is not harmful," *Journal of Nutrition*, vol. 132, no. 2, pp. 257–260, 2002.

[32] J. Blanchet, F. Longpré, G. Bureau et al., "Resveratrol, a red wine polyphenol, protects dopaminergic neurons in MPTP-treated mice," *Progress in Neuro-Psychopharmacology and Biological Psychiatry*, vol. 32, no. 5, pp. 1243–1250, 2008.

[33] J. L. Stanley, R. J. Lincoln, T. A. Brown, L. M. McDonald, G. R. Dawson, and D. S. Reynolds, "The mouse beam walking assay offers improved sensitivity over the mouse rotarod in determining motor coordination deficits induced by benzodiazepines," *Journal of Psychopharmacology*, vol. 19, no. 3, pp. 221–227, 2005.

[34] M. Mohanasundari, M. S. Srinivasan, S. Sethupathy, and M. Sabesan, "Enhanced neuroprotective effect by combination of bromocriptine and *Hypericum perforatum* extract against MPTP-induced neurotoxicity in mice," *Journal of the Neurological Sciences*, vol. 249, no. 2, pp. 140–144, 2006.

[35] J. L. Tillerson, W. M. Caudle, M. E. Reverón, and G. W. Miller, "Detection of behavioral impairments correlated to neurochemical deficits in mice treated with moderate doses of 1-methyl-4-phenyl-1,2,3,6-tetrahydropyridine," *Experimental Neurology*, vol. 178, no. 1, pp. 80–90, 2002.

[36] J. Itoh, T. Nabeshima, and T. Kameyama, "Utility of an elevated plus-maze for the evaluation of memory in mice: effects of nootropics, scopolamine and electroconvulsive shock," *Psychopharmacology*, vol. 101, no. 1, pp. 27–33, 1990.

[37] A. Anandhan, K. Tamilselvam, D. Vijayranjah, N. Ashokkumar, S. Rajasankar, and T. Manivasagam, "Resveratrol attenuate oxidative stress and improves behaviour in 1-methyl-4-phenyl-1, 2, 3, 6-tetrahydropyridine (MPTP) challenged mice," *Annals of Neuroscience*, vol. 17, no. 3, pp. 113–119, 2010.

[38] J. Long, H. Gao, L. Sun, J. Liu, and X. Zhao-Wilson, "Grape extract protects mitochondria from oxidative damage and improves locomotor dysfunction and extends lifespan in a drosophila parkinson's disease model," *Rejuvenation Research*, vol. 12, no. 5, pp. 321–331, 2009.

[39] R. Takahashi, Y. Komiya, and S. Goto, "Effect of dietary restriction on learning and memory impairment and histologic alterations of brain stem in senescence-accelerated mouse (SAM) P8 strain," *Annals of the New York Academy of Sciences*, vol. 1067, no. 1, pp. 388–393, 2006.

[40] W. Duan, Z. Guo, and M. P. Mattson, "Brain-derived neurotrophic factor mediates an excitoprotective effect of dietary restriction in mice," *Journal of Neurochemistry*, vol. 76, no. 2, pp. 619–626, 2001.

[41] A. Wu, X. Sun, and Y. Liu, "Effects of caloric restriction on cognition and behavior in developing mice," *Neuroscience Letters*, vol. 339, no. 2, pp. 166–168, 2003.

[42] M. C. Roberge, J. Hotte-Bernard, C. Messier, and H. Plamondon, "Food restriction attenuates ischemia-induced spatial learning and memory deficits despite extensive CA1 ischemic injury," *Behavioural Brain Research*, vol. 187, no. 1, pp. 123–132, 2008.

[43] V. Tucci, A. Hardy, and P. M. Nolan, "A comparison of physiological and behavioural parameters in C57BL/6J mice undergoing food or water restriction regimes," *Behavioural Brain Research*, vol. 173, no. 1, pp. 22–29, 2006.

[44] M. M. Story, J. S. Rand, M. Shyan-Norwalt, R. Mesch, J. M. Morton, and E. A. Flickinger, "Effect of resveratrol supplementation on the performance of dogs in an eight-arm radial maze," *The Open Nutrition Journal*, vol. 6, pp. 80–88, 2012.

[45] M. K. Shigenaga, T. M. Hagen, and B. N. Ames, "Oxidative damage and mitochondrial decay in aging," *Proceedings of the National Academy of Sciences of the United States of America*, vol. 91, no. 23, pp. 10771–10778, 1994.

[46] E. Head, J. Liu, T. M. Hagen et al., "Oxidative damage increases with age in a canine model of human brain aging," *Journal of Neurochemistry*, vol. 82, no. 2, pp. 375–381, 2002.

[47] P. D. Tapp, C. T. Siwak, F. Q. Gao et al., "Frontal lobe volume, function, and β-amyloid pathology in a canine model of aging," *The Journal of Neuroscience*, vol. 24, no. 38, pp. 8205–8213, 2004.

[48] C. T. Siwak-Tapp, E. Head, B. A. Muggenburg, N. W. Milgram, and C. W. Cotman, "Region specific neuron loss in the aged canine hippocampus is reduced by enrichment," *Neurobiology of Aging*, vol. 29, no. 1, pp. 39–50, 2008.

[49] K. J. Pearson, J. A. Baur, K. N. Lewis et al., "Resveratrol delays age-related deterioration and mimics transcriptional aspects of dietary restriction without extending life span," *Cell Metabolism*, vol. 8, no. 2, pp. 157–168, 2008.

[50] M. Sharma and Y. K. Gupta, "Chronic treatment with trans resveratrol prevents intracerebroventricular streptozotocin induced cognitive impairment and oxidative stress in rats," *Life Sciences*, vol. 71, no. 21, pp. 2489–2498, 2002.

[51] Ü. Sönmez, A. Sönmez, G. Erbil, I. Tekmen, and B. Baykara, "Neuroprotective effects of resveratrol against traumatic brain injury in immature rats," *Neuroscience Letters*, vol. 420, no. 2, pp. 133–137, 2007.

[52] J. L. Bowers, V. V. Tyulmenkov, S. C. Jernigan, and C. M. Klinge, "Resveratrol acts as a mixed agonist/antagonist for estrogen receptors α and β," *Endocrinology*, vol. 141, no. 10, pp. 3657–3667, 2000.

[53] J. E. Gresack and K. M. Frick, "Environmental enrichment reduces the mnemonic and neural benefits of estrogen," *Neuroscience*, vol. 128, no. 3, pp. 459–471, 2004.

[54] J. E. Gresack, K. M. Kerr, and K. M. Frick, "Short-term environmental enrichment decreases the mnemonic response to estrogen in young, but not aged, female mice," *Brain Research*, vol. 1160, no. 1, pp. 91–101, 2007.

[55] J. Bohacek and J. M. Daniel, "Increased daily handling of ovariectomized rats enhances performance on a radial-maze task and obscures effects of estradiol replacement," *Hormones and Behavior*, vol. 52, no. 2, pp. 237–243, 2007.

[56] J. M. Levenson, K. J. O'Riordan, K. D. Brown, M. A. Trinh, D. L. Molfese, and J. D. Sweatt, "Regulation of histone acetylation during memory formation in the hippocampus," *The Journal of Biological Chemistry*, vol. 279, no. 39, pp. 40545–40559, 2004.

[57] W. B. Chwang, J. S. Arthur, A. Schumacher, and J. D. Sweatt, "The nuclear kinase mitogen- and stress-activated protein kinase 1 regulates hippocampal chromatin remodeling in memory formation," *The Journal of Neuroscience*, vol. 27, no. 46, pp. 12732–12742, 2007.

[58] A. Fischer, F. Sananbenesi, X. Wang, M. Dobbin, and L. Tsai, "Recovery of learning and memory is associated with chromatin remodelling," *Nature*, vol. 447, no. 7141, pp. 178–182, 2007.

[59] T. Abel and R. S. Zukin, "Epigenetic targets of HDAC inhibition in neurodegenerative and psychiatric disorders," *Current Opinion in Pharmacology*, vol. 8, no. 1, pp. 57–64, 2008.

[60] L. Guarente and F. Picard, "Calorie restriction—the SIR2 connection," *Cell*, vol. 120, no. 4, pp. 473–482, 2005.

[61] M. S. Finnin, J. R. Donigian, A. Cohen et al., "Structures of a histone deacetylase homologue bound to the TSA and SAHA inhibitors," *Nature*, vol. 401, no. 6749, pp. 188–193, 1999.

[62] J. J. Buggy, M. L. Sideris, P. Mak, D. D. Lorimer, B. McIntosh, and J. M. Clark, "Cloning and characterization of a novel human histone deacetylase, HDAC8," *Biochemical Journal*, vol. 350, no. 1, pp. 199–205, 2000.

[63] J. D. Sweatt, "Experience-dependent epigenetic modifications in the central nervous system," *Biological Psychiatry*, vol. 65, no. 3, pp. 191–197, 2009.

9

Treatments for Neurological Gait and Balance Disturbance: The Use of Noninvasive Electrical Brain Stimulation

Diego Kaski and Adolfo M. Bronstein

Division of Brain Sciences, Imperial College London, Charing Cross Hospital, London W6 8RF, UK

Correspondence should be addressed to Diego Kaski; d.kaski@imperial.ac.uk

Academic Editor: Paul Sauseng

Neurological gait disorders are a common cause of falls, morbidity, and mortality, particularly amongst the elderly. Neurological gait and balance impairment has, however, proved notoriously difficult to treat. The following review discusses some of the first experiments to modulate gait and balance in healthy adults using anodal transcranial direct current stimulation (tDCS) by stimulating both cerebral hemispheres simultaneously. We review and discuss published data using this novel tDCS approach, in combination with physical therapy, to treat locomotor and balance disorders in patients with small vessel disease (leukoaraiosis) and Parkinson's disease. Finally, we review the use of bihemispheric anodal tDCS to treat gait impairment in patients with stroke in the subacute phase. The findings of these studies suggest that noninvasive electrical stimulation techniques may be a useful adjunct to physical therapy in patients with neurological gait disorders, but further mutlicentre randomized sham-controlled studies are needed to evaluate whether experimental tDCS use can translate into mainstream clinical practice for the treatment of neurological gait disorders.

1. Introduction

Disorders of gait are a common presentation in neurological practice and general medical settings, particularly amongst the elderly population. In addition, impairment of postural and righting reactions commonly causes falls when turning or bending over [1] leading to insecure walking and the development of a fear of falling [2]. The following review discusses some of the first ever experiments to modulate gait and balance in healthy adults using anodal transcranial direct current stimulation (tDCS) by stimulating both hemispheres simultaneously (Figure 1) and to treat locomotor and balance disorders in patients with neurological gait disturbance.

We show in a series of previously published work that bihemispheric electrical stimulation with a novel montage can increase cortical excitability of lower limb muscles and increases locomotor learning in healthy subjects. The same electrode montage increases gait speed and improves balance in patients with Parkinson's disease and gait disturbance associated with small vessel disease, when combined with physical therapy (Figure 3). Lastly, by increasing excitability in the affected hemisphere and inhibiting the unaffected

one, we were able to improve walking time in patients with stroke in the subacute phase, where the potential to modulate cortical excitability is maximal.

2. Gait Modulation for Neurological Disease

Gait and balance disturbance is common, difficult to treat despite rehabilitation, and a cause of significant morbidity and mortality. Parkinson's disease is a common cause of gait and postural instability and although it is defined pathologically by the loss of dopaminergic neurons in the substantia nigra, much of the long-term disability is related to symptoms that do not respond to levodopa [3]. We therefore sought to apply noninvasive brain stimulation techniques using a novel electrode montage in patients with Parkinson's disease to improve gait and balance.

In Parkinson's disease, an overactivity of inhibitory efferents from basal ganglia to the thalamus results in suppression on thalamocortical projections, with reduced activity in premotor and primary motor cortical regions [4, 5]. The motor cortex may thus be an important therapeutic neurostimulatory target in these patients.

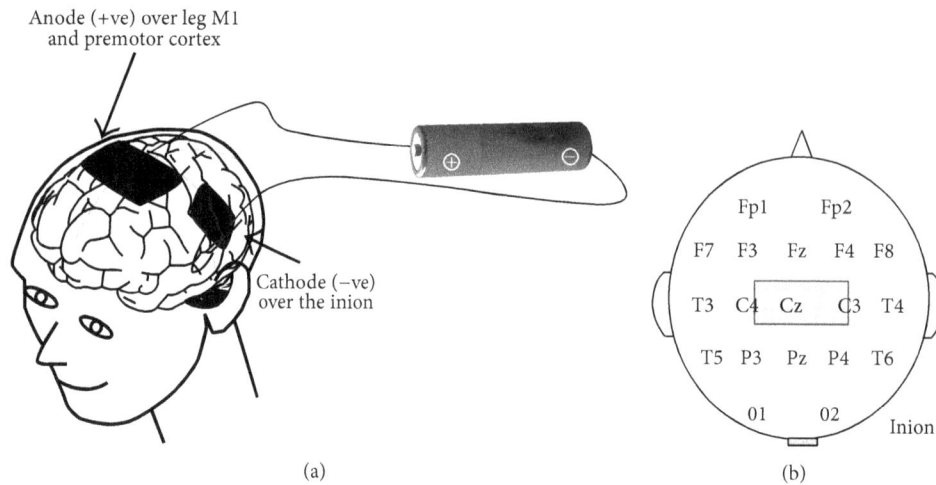

FIGURE 1: (a) A novel bihemispheric tDCS montage targeting right and left lower limb motor cortices simultaneously. (b) Illustrative tDCS montage using the international 10–20 EEG electrode placement. The anodal (stimulating) electrode was placed over Cz and covered a region 10–20% anterior to Cz as measured from the midpoint of the electrode. The cathode was placed over the inion.

From a cortical perspective, human locomotion relies upon a distributed neural network including primary motor, premotor areas, and, importantly, white matter connections thereof [6]. Not surprisingly, changes in the cerebral white matter, associated with vascular risk factors and frequently detected on imaging in the elderly [7], are associated with gait and balance dysfunction [8, 9]. Clinically, these patients have a low gait velocity due to reduced stride length, long double support time, and broad based gait [10]. Small vessel disease (SVD) is an increasing cause of falls in the ageing population for which, critically, there is currently no treatment. The relevance of the primary motor and premotor cortices in the control of gait in relation to SVD has been demonstrated using fMRI [11] and cerebral perfusion techniques [12, 13]. Given the lack of treatment options for this growing problem, we attempted to improve gait and balance function in these patients using noninvasive electrical stimulation that as we found can alter gait learning in healthy subjects [14].

3. Current Treatments for Gait Disturbance

Neurological gait and balance impairment has proved notoriously difficult to treat. For example, although some evidence suggests that freezing of gait in patients with Parkinson's disease may improve with levodopa [15], one study indicated that gait may worsen in medicated patients, perhaps as a result of drug-induced dyskinesia [16]. As a result, there has been a drive towards nonpharmacological therapies. Deep brain stimulation (DBS) has revolutionized the management of dopaminergic motor features in many patients with severe Parkinson's disease, and whilst there is some evidence in support of DBS in the treatment of gait disorders in these patients [17], its effect on the nondopaminergic motor features of Parkinson's disease, such as gait and balance, has been variable. Thus, one study showed that approximately 50% of freezers convert to nonfreezers after subthalamic nucleus DBS [18], although freezing of gait has also been shown to worsen after bilateral DBS [19]. In patients with resistant gait

disturbance stimulation of the substantia nigra pars reticulata appears to improve axial motor features [20], including freezing of gait [21]. More recently DBS of the pedunculopontine nucleus (PPN) has shown variable outcomes on gait and balance [22–25].

Noninvasive treatment options, in particular repetitive transcranial magnetic stimulation, showed early promise in the treatment of gait in this group of patients [26, 27], but subsequent studies using intermittent magnetic stimulation [28] and tDCS [29] have yielded negative results. Physical therapy remains the mainstay of treatment for patients with neurological gait and balance dysfunction [30, 31] and is known to induce long-lasting plastic changes in the cerebral cortex [32]. We addressed an important but as yet unanswered question of whether the beneficial effects of physical training can be enhanced using noninvasive brain stimulation techniques. To do this we applied tDCS during physical training.

4. Transcranial Direct Current Stimulation

tDCS is a noninvasive neurostimulation technique that consists of delivering a weak current via the use of saline-soaked electrodes applied over the scalp. This has been shown to induce bidirectional polarity-dependent changes in cortical excitability of the underlying cortex. In general terms, anodal tDCS increases cortical excitability, and cathodal tDCS decreases it [33]. The physiological and behavioural effects of tDCS have been shown to last for up to one hour, implying that tDCS also modulates the synaptic microenvironment, modulating the synaptic strength of NMDA receptors, altering GABA-ergic activity, and modulating intracortical and corticospinal neurons [33–35].

5. Bihemispheric tDCS for Gait

Most studies using tDCS in the field of locomotor control have focused on stimulation over the lower limb primary motor cortex (M1) of a single hemisphere. So-called bihemispheric tDCS, however, aims to deliver cathodal stimulation to one motor cortex and anodal tDCS to the opposite hemisphere in an attempt to restore the interhemispheric imbalance caused by discrete cortical lesions (e.g., stroke) and to thus improve walking through its effects on the function of the hemiparetic limb.

Although there is some evidence that DBS reprogramming techniques such as "better side reduction" can reduce lower limb akinesia asymmetry and thus improve gait freezing [36], the cortical influences over locomotion are not lateralized. It is perhaps then surprising that there have not been attempts at applying electrical stimulation to both motor cortices simultaneously, particularly for nonstroke neurological gait disorders. We therefore attempted to modulate gait by applying tDCS to the primary motor and premotor cortices of both hemispheres *simultaneously* using a large midline electrode (Figure 1). Whilst the relative lack of focus of tDCS is an apparent disadvantage for physiological experiments, this may be welcomed when attempting to modulate complex and distributed cortical networks such as those involved in gait.

6. Can tDCS Modulate Locomotor Activity in Healthy Individuals?

Before tDCS can be considered as a therapeutic tool to treat patients with gait disorder, its effect upon lower limb excitability in healthy individuals needs to be evaluated. We posed two associated questions: first, can anodal tDCS over M1 and premotor cortex alter locomotor adaptation? Second, are the putative behavioural changes associated with tDCS related to neurophysiological changes in M1 cortical excitability of the legs?

To address the first question, we explored the effect of anodal tDCS over primary motor and premotor leg cortices on a locomotor adaptation task: the "broken escalator" paradigm—a laboratory reconstruction of the unusual sensation and physical stumble many people experience when stepping onto an escalator that is out-of-order [37–41]. This paradigm induces a locomotor aftereffect (forward trunk displacement and increased gait velocity) that reflects motor learning. We predicted that increasing the excitability of the primary motor and premotor cortical leg areas using anodal tDCS would increase the amplitude of the locomotor aftereffect. We further hypothesized that anodal tDCS over M1 would prolong the aftereffect given the role of M1 in memory retention. To address the second question we used TMS in a separate group of subjects to probe changes in cortical leg excitability before and after tDCS to M1.

For the gait experiments, we recruited 30 healthy participants that were allocated to 2 separate groups for testing. The "real tDCS" group received tDCS at 2 mA over 15 minutes, and "sham tDCS" group received sham stimulation for 15 minutes. Both groups performed 5 "BEFORE" trials by stepping onto a stationary sled, 5 MOVING (learning) trials stepping onto a moving platform, and 5 AFTER trials. The aftereffect is typically seen only in the 1st AFTER trial.

We applied tDCS to these subjects using a novel electrode montage that was determined using evidence from MRI studies [42] and three-dimensional probabilistic anatomic correlation techniques [43] showing that the scalp topography of Cz (international 10–20 EEG system [44]) corresponds to lower limb primary motor cortex. Thus a DC stimulating rectangular saline-soaked sponge electrode (10×4 cm; surface area 40 cm^2) was placed centrally across the scalp to cover a region 10–20% anterior to Cz as measured from the midline of the stimulating electrode (Figure 1). The reference electrode (4×4 cm) was positioned at the inion. A 2-mA current was delivered by a battery-driven Magstim Eldith DC stimulator (neuroConn, Ilmenau, Germany) between the end of the BEFORE trials and the beginning of the MOVING trials (i.e., just before the adaptation period). The current was initially increased by a ramp input over 10 s until reaching 2 mA (current density 0.05 mA/cm^2). Stimulation duration of 15 min, as chosen, can result in an excitability change lasting up to 90 min [33]. The sham stimulation used for control purposes and is identical to the real stimulation condition except that the current drops off to zero after 30 s.

We recorded forward trunk displacement and gait approach velocity using a position tracking device (Fastrak) attached to the subjects' back at C7 and electromyograms of the anterior tibialis and gastrocnemius muscles.

How can one be sure that tDCS as used here was having an effect on lower limb excitability? In a separate series of experiments we used transcranial magnetic stimulation that delivers a magnetic pulse to depolarise the cortical membrane over leg M1 and evaluating the effect of tDCS on TMS-induced motor-evoked potentials (MEPs) and silent period durations in tibialis anterior bilaterally in 16 additional healthy subjects. Magnetic stimuli were delivered to the motor cortex using an angled double-cone coil positioned over the tibialis anterior hotspot. TMS-induced MEPs from the tibialis anterior were recorded before and after tDCS (real stimulation in 8 subjects, sham in 8).

Finally, in a separate series of experiments we assess what effect, if any, cathodal stimulation over the inion (Figure 1) could have had on cerebellar structures, given the recognized role of the cerebellum in motor learning and adaptation [45]. We predicted that our electrode montage would spare cerebellar structures, as this is a suboptimal placement to stimulate the cerebellar cortex [46]. Eyeblink classic conditioning (EBC) is a well-characterized experimental paradigm that is conserved across species and is dependent on the cerebellum [47] and consists of pairing a weak conditioning stimulus with a strong unconditioning stimulus repeatedly to produce conditioned responses consisting of an eyeblink starting before the US. EBC was evaluated in 8 subjects after receiving tDCS as applied in the main gait experiment.

The main finding was that the real tDCS group, compared with sham, displayed a 80% larger trunk sway ($P = 0.04$) and increased gait velocity (although not statistically significant; $P = 0.15$) in the first AFTER trial (aftereffect) and a persistence of the trunk sway aftereffect into the second AFTER trial ($P = 0.0013$). Neither gait velocity nor trunk sway was

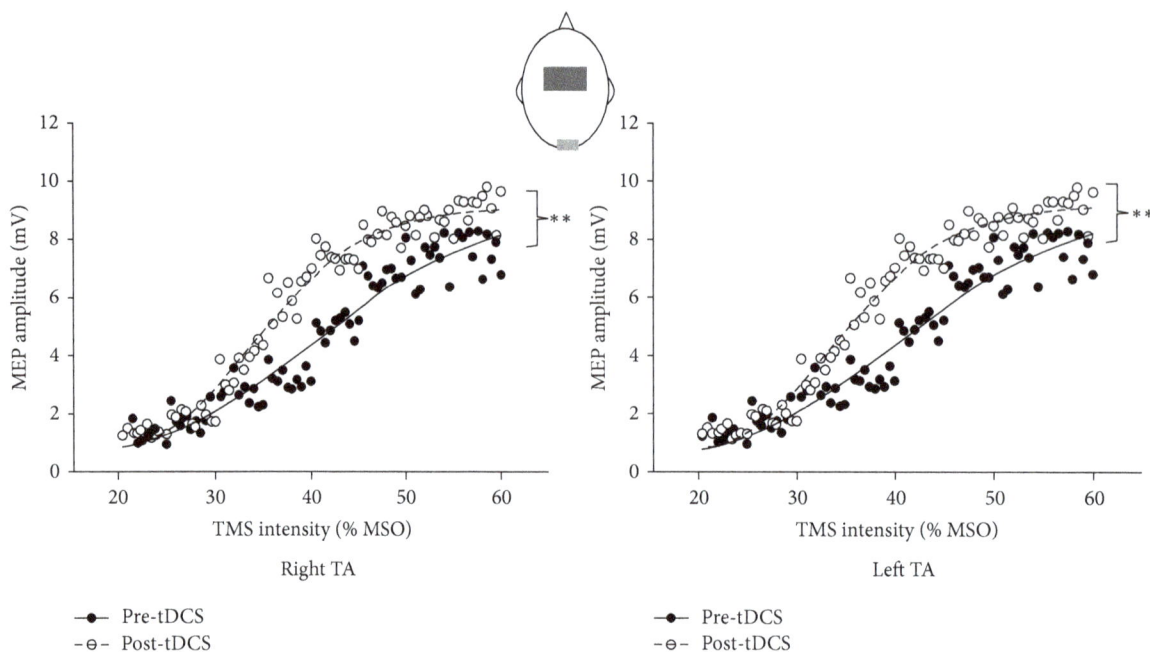

FIGURE 2: TMS-induced motor-evoked potential (MEP) amplitudes in right and left tibialis anterior (TA) muscles before and after tDCS or sham. *Top*: MEP amplitudes before (black spots) and after (white spots) real tDCS. *Bottom*: MEP amplitudes before and after sham stimulation. MSO, maximum stimulator output.

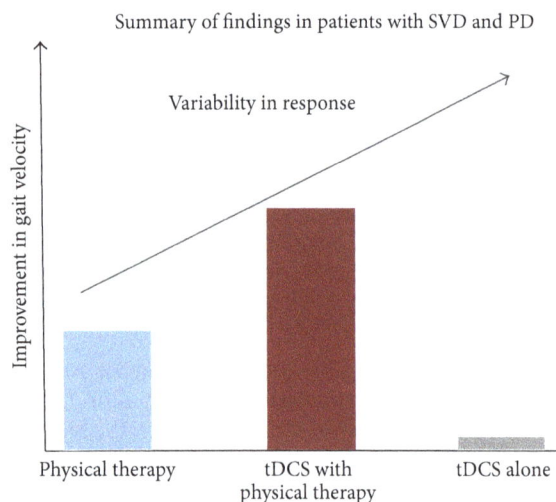

FIGURE 3: Summary of findings. The combination of tDCS with physical therapy resulted in the greatest improvements in gait velocity in patients with Parkinson's disease and small vessel disease; physical therapy improved gait, but tDCS alone had no significant effect. Notably, the variability in response was greatest in patients receiving tDCS, indicating that some patients improved more than others.

significantly different between stimulation groups during the learning trials ($P = 0.67$). The EMG signals were rectified and integrated over a 500 ms time window after foot-sled contact and normalized with respect to mean BEFORE (trials 3–5) values. In keeping with results from forward trunk sway, EMG activity was significantly raised in the left and right medial gastrocnemius (MG) muscles in the tDCS group in

the aftereffect trial ($P < 0.001$ for left MG and $P = 0.03$ for right MG). Note that the left MG is the muscle involved in breaking the forward momentum during the aftereffect as it is the left leg that makes the first contact on the sled.

Our TMS data revealed a significant increase in MEP amplitudes in right ($P < 0.001$) and left TA muscles ($P < 0.001$) following 15 min of 2 mA anodal tDCS using an inion reference electrode (as used in the broken escalator experiment) but not for sham stimulation (Figure 2). Concordantly, silent-period durations increased with real stimulation but not with sham.

Cathodal effects over the cerebellum would be expected to impair conditioned eyeblink responses. All subjects in the real tDCS group, however, and 7 subjects in the sham group ($n = 8$) acquired the conditioned response, indicating that placing the cathode electrode over the inion does not appear to have significant cerebellar effects.

In summary, we showed that stimulation of M1 and premotor cortex before skill acquisition increases the trunk overshoot component of the locomotor aftereffect, thus modulating locomotor adaptation. When the brain encounters environmental or sensory changes in the body, it must choose the most appropriate response for the current situation, using a Bayesian motor decision-making process [48]. Such a process of "risk assessment" may be subject to interactions from the physical properties of the sled and the individual's state of arousal. tDCS as used in this study may thus prevent the selection of a motor program that is contextually appropriate in favor of a cautious approach "the sled may move after all", thus generating a larger aftereffect. Alternatively, anodal tDCS may have increased neuronal excitability in a widespread cortical network with reinforcement of synaptic changes appropriate for stepping onto a moving sled as a result of the repetitive locomotor task. This in turn could lead to an enhanced expression of the adaptation aftereffect when stepping onto the stationary platform.

An interesting observation is that no significance was found for the gait velocity component of the locomotor aftereffect following tDCS. Data from previous work exploring the relationship between gait velocity and trunk overshoot components of the locomotor aftereffect have shown that they are dissociable [49]. Different neural mechanisms may underlie the trunk overshoot and gait velocity components of the aftereffect and may thus be subject to differential effects from tDCS although such a hypothesis warrants further exploration.

Our results could have clinical implications. The finding of an effect of cortical modulation on involuntary locomotor control is of potential interest for patients with gait disorders as tDCS offers the advantage of ease of access. Whilst there is evidence supporting the use of tDCS in upper limb rehabilitation following stroke [50] and Parkinson's disease [29], this is the first study to assess specifically the effect of bihemispheric anodal tDCS on gait. Results from the current finding suggest that direct noninvasive stimulation of primary motor cortex and premotor areas may be suitable sites to target locomotor adaptive learning [14]. Accordingly, our findings in healthy subjects support the use of tDCS for experimental treatment of neurological gait disorders.

7. The Use of tDCS in Patients with Parkinson's Disease

Based on our findings that tDCS was able to increase excitability in lower limb motor cortex and increase locomotor adaptation, we next applied anodal tDCS using the same bihemispheric tDCS montage in patients with Parkinson's disease (PD). PD is a common cause of gait and postural instability but it is generally accepted that these features are largely levodopa resistant [3, 51–54]. An early study assessing levodopa responsiveness for various gait parameters identified that temporal parameters such as stride and swing duration and stride duration variability were levodopa resistant, whereas stride length was levodopa sensitive [55]. More recent evidence suggests that levodopa may differentially improve proximal more than distal lower limb kinematics [56]. Interestingly, levodopa appears to have no effect on locomotor adaptation [57].

Given the reduced activity in premotor and primary motor cortical regions in Parkinson's disease [58], these areas may be important therapeutic noninvasive neurostimulatory targets for patients with Parkinson's disease and gait disturbance [59].

It is recognized that physical therapy induces physiological changes in the primary motor cortex of patients with Parkinson's disease [32]. tDCS has also been shown to improve motor learning and rehabilitation in PD [60], although outcomes have been mixed [61]. Previous studies using noninvasive brain stimulation in patients with PD did not find reproducible benefits on gait [28, 29], although stimulation paradigms were not combined with physical therapy.

We hypothesised that anodal tDCS time locked to physical training would improve gait and balance in Parkinson's disease above and beyond the effects of tDCS in isolation. Our primary gait outcome was gait velocity as this is a functional marker of disease severity, and our primary balance outcome was recovery of stance in the pull test [62], with postural instability being a common cause of falls in these patients.

Sixteen patients were recruited (average age 76.4, (SD = 5.7); disease duration 10.4 yrs (3.0); UPDRS III 25.8 (5.7)). Patients were assigned to one of two groups; Group I "physical-training" (n = 8) and Group II "no physical-training" (n = 8). Patients in Group I received tDCS during a fifteen-minute period of physical training and those in Group II received only tDCS, without physical training. For both groups, the application of tDCS was also randomised to either real tDCS stimulation or sham stimulation in the first session. All subjects returned 1 week later, to allow an appropriate wash-out period for the neurostimulation. In this second session subjects in the "physical training" group again received physical therapy, but those that had received real stimulation in the first session were given sham stimulation, and vice versa. Patients in the "No physical training" group again received only neurostimulation in this second session, with those that received real stimulation in the first session given sham stimulation, and vice versa. Outcomes were recorded prior to any intervention (baseline) and after intervention (final assessment). The physical therapy protocol lasted 15 minutes with a focus on improving gait initiation, stride length, gait velocity, arm swing, and balance.

Statistical analysis consisted of paired student t-tests, with appropriate Bonferroni correction. To assess the effect of combining tDCS with physical training we compared the average % change in performance in patients receiving real stimulation in Group I versus real stimulation in Group II. We compared the average % change in performance in patients receiving real versus sham stimulation in Group II to assess the isolated effect of tDCS stimulation (independent of physical training). Lastly, to assess the isolated effect of physical training (independent of tDCS) we compared the average % change in performance in patients receiving sham in Group I versus patients receiving sham stimulation in Group II. Where an isolated effect of physical training was observed, we compared the average % change in performance in patients receiving real stimulation in Group I versus sham stimulation in Group I, to assess the effect of combining tDCS with physical training—above and beyond the effect of physical training alone.

We used an identical tDCS montage and stimulation protocol as described in the initial healthy subject study above. The current was delivered for 15 minutes during training ("physical training" group) or during the execution of the gait and balance tasks ("No physical training" group). Electrodes were secured onto the scalp during the assessments using a modified diving head cap and tDCS battery fitted on a lightweight backpack.

The primary outcome for gait was gait velocity. Secondary outcomes included stride length, 3 m "Timed Up and Go," 6 m walk. The primary balance outcome was a quantitative pull test that is a clinical tool used to evaluate postural instability in patients with Parkinson's disease [63].

We found that the combination of anodal tDCS with concurrent physical therapy increased gait velocity ($P < 0.001$), stride length ($P = 0.01$), the time taken to complete the "Timed Up and Go" ($P = 0.04$), and the 6 m walk ($P = 0.04$). Whilst there were modest benefits in patients receiving only physical therapy, these were comparatively less than when therapy was combined with tDCS. We did not observe any benefits of isolated tDCS (i.e., without physical therapy) [64].

For balance, the combination of tDCS and physical therapy reduced the time taken to regain stability following the retropulsion stimulus compared to tDCS alone ($P = 0.01$). Again, there was no isolated effect of stimulation ($P = 0.94$) or physical therapy ($P = 0.87$).

In summary, we found a significant benefit of combining tDCS with physical training for gait velocity (primary gait outcome) and the performance on the pull test (primary balance outcome), but there was no isolated effect for tDCS or physical training [64].

Physical training in Parkinson's disease normalises cortical excitability in M1 [32], whilst tDCS may lower the threshold for these changes to occur (Figure 5). Thus, combining physical gait and balance therapy with tDCS over primary motor and premotor cortex has a physiological basis.

One interesting finding from this study was that patients with more severe motor symptoms (UPDRS III and Hoehn Yahr scale) tended to show a greater improvement in walking time with tDCS compared to patients with milder disease [64]. Although the number of patients tested is insufficient to draw firm conclusions from a correlation analysis, our data suggest that patients with more advanced disease are more likely to benefit from combined DC stimulation and physical therapy than patients with mild disease. In contrast, individual gait outcomes did not correlate with age, the degree of leukoaraiosis, or cognitive impairment, suggesting that individual patients at the extremes of the disease process may be less likely to respond to neurostimulation.

Whilst our patient sample size lacks the power to draw conclusive results, our preliminary data suggests that the tDCS may be a useful adjunct to physical therapy to improve gait in patients with Parkinson's disease. Unfortunately, the lack of follow-up assessments meant that we were unable to comment on possible longer-term benefit of the interventions, or indeed whether repeated tDCS sessions lead to greater and sustained improvements.

8. Combining tDCS and Dance Therapy in a Single Patient with Parkinson's Disease

A hallmark of progression of PD is postural instability and associated falls [65]. Dance and movement therapy has been shown to improve balance and gait in patients with gait disturbances [66], with the Argentine tango receiving particular interest in patients with PD [67]. There is evidence that tango dancing may alter cortical excitability, with increased activity over supplementary motor and premotor cortices in healthy subjects during imagined walking following a tango lesson [68]. Given our findings that tDCS improves gait in patients with PD, we decided to explore the effect of applying anodal tDCS over primary motor and premotor cortex on trunk kinematics in a patient with moderate PD during tango dancing.

We applied transcranial direct current stimulation (tDCS) in a 79-year-old male patient with moderate PD (UPDRS III = 34, HY scale = stage 3; disease duration 7 yrs) during tango dancing to assess its effect on trunk motion and balance [69]. The patient performed a total of four dances ("The butterfly," Osvaldo Pugliese orquestra, music by Pedro Maffia, and lyrics by Celedonio Flores) over two days; two "tango and tDCS" and two "tango and sham" in a randomised double-blind fashion.

We recorded the average sagittal (pitch) and coronal (roll) trunk peak-to-peak velocity was measured across the whole dance using digitally based angular-velocity transducers attached to the patients lower back [70]. We also recorded a Tinetti Gait index questionnaire [71] (which is performed on a three-point ordinal scale assessing task-oriented gait and balance parameters, such as the ability to rise from a chair, standing balance, step symmetry, etc.) and obtained a subjective measure of performance before and after each dance session from the patient's professional dance partner, who was blinded to the intervention.

As in the studies reported above, a DC stimulating rectangular saline-soaked sponge electrode ($10 \text{ cm} \times 4 \text{ cm}$) was placed centrally across the scalp to cover a region 10–20% anterior to Cz as measured from the midline of the stimulating electrode. The reference electrode ($4 \text{ cm} \times 4 \text{ cm}$) was positioned at the inion (Figure 1). A 2 mA current was delivered by a battery-driven Magstim Eldith DC stimulator (NeuroConn, Germany) during the Tango dance. The current was initially increased by a ramp input over 10 s until reaching 2 mA (current density 0.05 mA/cm^2).

We found that trunk peak velocity during tango was significantly greater during tDCS compared to sham stimulation [69] (Figure 4(a)). The questionnaire data revealed subjective improvements in dance performance, and the dance partner commented that the patient performed an unusually greater number of choreographed steps in one of the sessions, which was later found to correspond to a tDCS (rather than sham) session. Improvements were also seen in the semiquantitative gait function assessment (Tinetti Gait Index: t-test; $P = 0.04$).

Our findings suggest that tDCS may be a useful adjunct to gait rehabilitation for patients with PD, although studies in a larger group of patients are needed to evaluate the therapeutic use of noninvasive brain stimulation during dance therapy.

9. The Use of tDCS in Patients with Small Vessel Disease with Gait Disturbance

Whilst physical therapy has been used in conjunction with tDCS to augment the effects of gait training [72] and lower

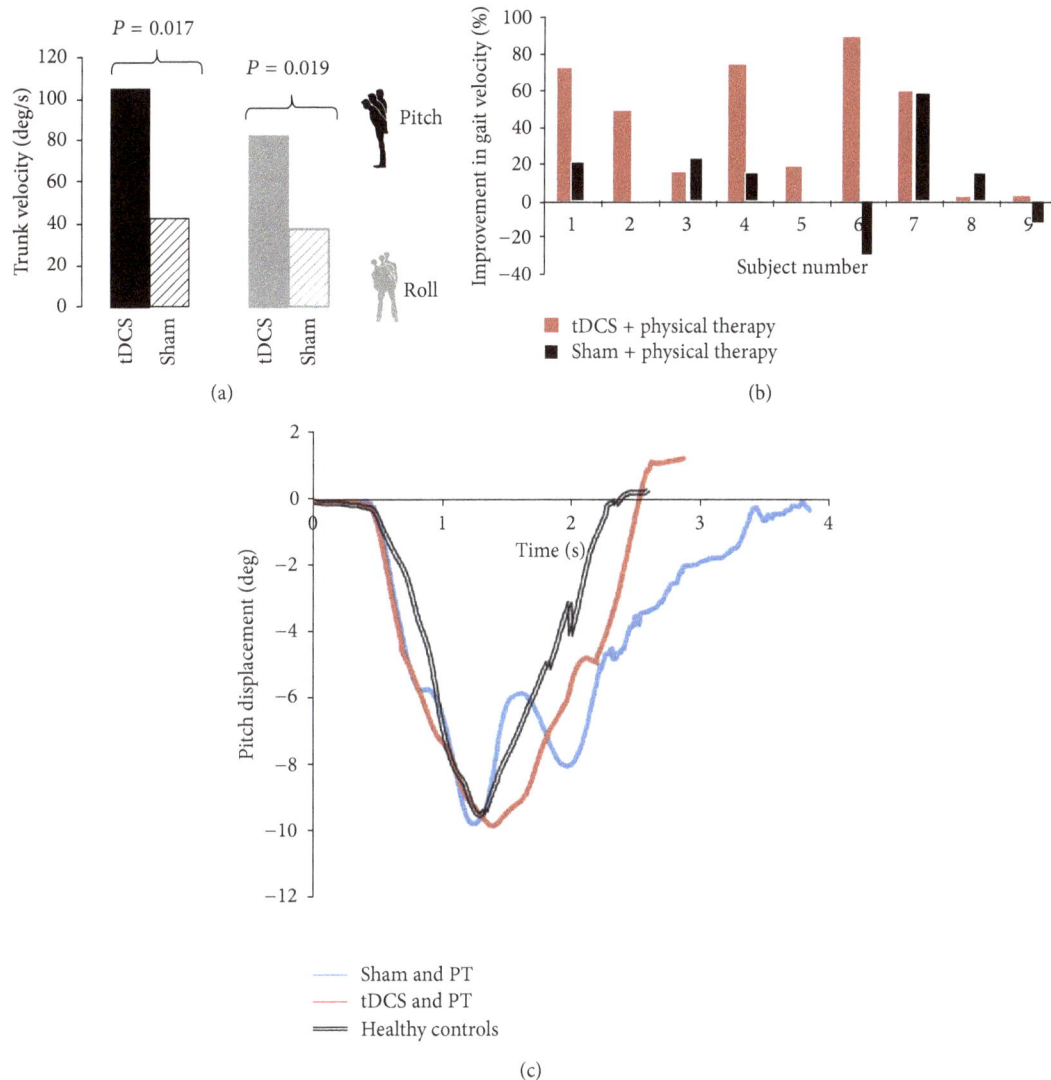

FIGURE 4: (a) Averaged data for the 4 tango dances showing increased trunk velocity in coronal (roll) and sagittal (pitch) planes in the real tDCS sessions, compared to sham. (b) Individual data from patients with small vessel disease showing percentage change in gait velocity following real tDCS (red) and sham stimulation (blue). (c) Time taken to regain a pitch angular displacement of +/− 2 cm of baseline following a backward pull on the shoulders for tDCS with physical therapy, sham with physical therapy in patients with Parkinson's disease, and healthy aged-matched controls.

limb rehabilitation [73] in patients with hemiparesis following established cortical strokes, the combination of noninvasive stimulation with simultaneous physical therapy has not been previously studied in patients with primary gait disorders such as small vessel disease.

Small vessel disease (white matter lesions or leukoaraiosis) describes hyperintensities in the cerebral subcortical white matter and is associated with gait and balance dysfunction and falls in the elderly [8] for which there are no evidence-based treatments.

Primary motor and premotor cortices are relevant to the control of gait in relation to small vessel disease [11, 12]. We attempted to facilitate neural activity in this network by combining physical training with tDCS of the primary motor leg area and premotor cortex bilaterally [14]. We recruited

9 patients with SVD (mean age 79.4 years, SD = 5.5; mean minimental state examination score 27.0; Fazekas score 2.4).

The primary gait outcomes were gait velocity and stride length, which correlate with disease severity in these patients [74]. The primary balance outcome was recovery of stance in the retropulsion test, with postural instability being a feature of small vessel disease and a common cause of falls in these patients [75]. Secondary outcomes were timed walk (a surrogate measure of gait velocity) and angular trunk velocity and amplitude.

Subjects performed a 6 m walk, Timed Up and Go (TUG), and retropulsion test twice in each session: "baseline" and "final" assessments. Following "baseline" assessments patients underwent a 15-minute balance and gait training session *concurrently* with anodal tDCS stimulation (real or

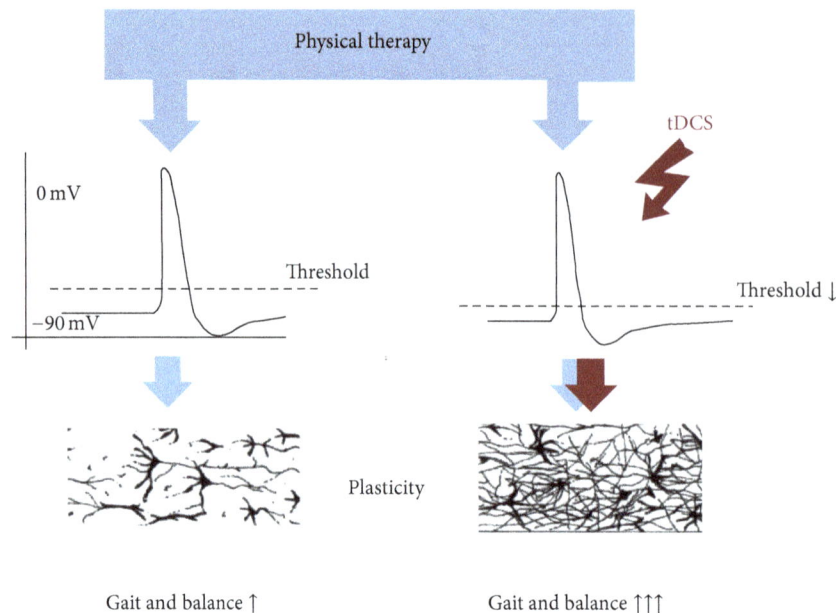

FIGURE 5: Proposed neural mechanism for combining tDCS with physical therapy. Physical therapy induces cortical changes that are thought to underlie the functional improvement in motor function. tDCS alters cortical excitability, perhaps reducing the threshold for these changes to occur when combined with physical therapy, resulting in greater cortical plasticity and better motor outcomes than physical therapy alone.

sham). Subjects then immediately repeated the gait and balance tests ("final" assessment). Assessments took on average approximately 15 minutes to complete.

A device encompassing two digitally based angular-velocity transducers arranged to measure angular trunk displacement and velocity in the roll (coronal) and pitch (sagittal) planes (SwayStar System, Balance Int. Innovations GmbH, Switzerland) was used in all subjects. The transducers were encased in a lightweight Bluetooth cordless device attached to an elasticised motorcycle belt, which was easily fitted on the subjects back at the L2-3 level. Angular deviations were calculated using online-trapezoid integration of the angular velocities [70].

Anodal tDCS was applied to the motor cortex of both hemispheres simultaneously using the same electrode montage and protocol previously described (Figure 1). The current was delivered during the exercise session for 15 minutes. Sham stimulation was identical to real stimulation except that the current was delivered for only 30 seconds and then switched off [76]. As part of a proof-of-principle study each patient received a single session of active (and sham) tDCS rather than repeated treatment sessions.

The principal result was that the combination of tDCS and locomotor training improves clinically relevant locomotor performance as measured by stride length ($P = 0.047$), stride length variability ($P = 0.001$), and gait velocity ($P = 0.008$; Figure 4(b)) in patients with leukoaraiosis [77]. We also observed improvements in the time taken to regain posture following a retropulsive stimulus in the tDCS and physical therapy group, but not with tDCS or physical therapy alone ($P = 0.045$; Figure 4(c)).

Our results support the finding that tDCS applied *during* the motor practice ("voluntary drive" [78]) improves performance [73, 79]. Although we cannot comment on whether this effect relates to motor practice or motor learning, our previous work described here has shown improvements in motor adaptive learning in healthy subjects using an identical tDCS montage [14].

This result suggests that targeting neocortical regions involved with gait using noninvasive stimulation may be one therapeutic strategy to overcome the corticosubcortical disconnection caused by white matter lesions in leukoaraiosis [77].

One explanation for our findings is that the voluntary motor activity (versus external involuntary robotic assistance, e.g.) occurring during physical training induces changes in excitability in relevant motor cortex [80]. Such neural activity strengthens corticospinal and intracortical networks, and tDCS may lower the threshold for these plastic changes to occur (Figure 5). Although the magnitude of the increase in gait velocity observed was somewhat unexpected, motor improvements of this magnitude have been previously observed within single sessions combining noninvasive brain stimulation techniques with peripheral nerve stimulation [81]. Further studies in a larger cohort of patients will help determine the everyday clinical applicability of this technique.

The effect of tDCS on balance in such patients has not been previously investigated. Whilst the response to the retropulsion test undoubtedly involves a coordinated neuronal network including cortical (M1) and subcortical (basal ganglia) structures and vestibular and spinal reflexes, one unanswered question was whether tDCS could impact on this network, either through direct actions on the motor cortex, or as a result of the more widespread effects of tDCS that are increasingly recognised [82]. Nevertheless, given that the retropulsion test is abnormal in patients with frontobasal ganglia disorders, the observed effects of tDCS most likely reflect changes to corticosubcortical networks. The combination of physical therapy and offline tDCS (applied during learning rather than execution of the task) improves balance in patients with leukoaraiosis that may be related to preferential effects on reflex activity, rather than voluntary motor performance [83]. Alternatively, neurostimulatory effects over phasic execution of movement such as a postural response may result from an increase in spontaneous neuronal firing rate [84]. Further studies dissecting the underlying mechanisms involved are warranted.

10. The Use of tDCS in Patients with Gait Disturbance following Subacute Stroke

A third of stroke survivors become unable to walk as a consequence of their stroke [85]. This functional deficit imposes a significant burden upon patients and carers and explains why gait recovery is a major focus of poststroke rehabilitation [86]. Despite the impact of gait impairment upon quality of life, most evidence that tDCS may boost the efficacy of conventional physical therapy has been obtained for poststroke upper limb motor recovery [87–89].

The application of tDCS to improve gait in patients with stroke necessarily differs from its application in patients with diffuse cortical or subcortical neurological disease. Thus, in bihemispheric tDCS the anode and cathode are placed over separate hemispheres [90] to simultaneously upregulate and downregulate activity in opposite hemispheres. Such tDCS-induced activity is theorised to temporarily restore the interhemispheric excitability balance that is disrupted following unilateral stroke [91]. A rebalancing of interhemispheric activity may be pivotal to promote functional recovery poststroke. Bihemispheric tDCS applied in this way enhances upper limb recovery in both chronic and subacute stroke patients [88]. Whether such effects extend to gait rehabilitation has not been explored. The subacute stroke phase represents a period of considerable neural plasticity [92] and thus a prime opportunity to influence such adaptive mechanisms using noninvasive brain stimulation.

Fourteen patients with subacute hemispheric stroke (2–8 weeks after stroke) were randomised to either active ($n = 7$; mean age 67.5 years (SD = 11.8); modified Rankin scale 2.1 (SD = 1.1)) or sham ($n = 7$; 56.4 years (SD = 12.4); modified Rankin scale 2.6 (SD = 1.1)) tDCS. The anode was placed over the ipsilesional lower limb primary motor cortex and the cathode over the contralesional leg motor cortex. A blinded assessor measured performance in the Timed Up and Go (TUG) test and the Performance Oriented Mobility Assessment (POMA; a 0–28 point ordinal scale where 28 is indicative of independent mobility and balance, with a low falls risk and 0 is most impaired). Assessments were performed before and after active tDCS or sham tDCS.

The average difference scores (i.e., posttest minus pretest) for the TUG test showed that, despite their older age, the active group was significantly faster following tDCS by 4.64 s whereas the sham group improved by only 0.01 s following sham stimulation ($P = 0.02$ for tDCS versus sham).

There was no significant difference between the two groups when comparing the difference in POMA scores after stimulation (POMA difference score for active group = 0.3; POMA difference score for sham group = 0.3; $P = 0.90$; Mann-Whitney U-test). In the sham group, no participant improved by a clinically meaningful amount; however, one subject in the active tDCS group did improve by a clinically meaningful level (4 points).

We found that active tDCS is safe and uniformly reduced walking time in patients with subacute stroke compared to sham. In contrast, the gait and balance subscale scores of the performance-orientated mobility assessment were not improved by tDCS. The differential benefits of tDCS on gait speed versus no effect on the POMA score may reflect the fact that the POMA is an ordinal scale, whereas gait speed is a continuous measure and may thus be more sensitive to detect change.

Notably, the two patients showing greatest improvements with tDCS also had comparatively worse baseline scores for the TUG, suggesting that the effects of tDCS may be more pronounced in more severely affected patients. One subject from the sham stimulation group showed a nearly 4-second improvement in the time to complete the TUG. This may represent a large placebo effect in a patient who may not have felt confident to walk to his maximum capability before the stimulation. Alternatively, the effect size may reflect the nature of the subcortical stroke-gait function in patients with subcortical white matter disease can be more variable [74], perhaps relating to fluctuating attentional drive directed towards walking.

Overall, we have shown that a single session of anodal bihemispheric tDCS can improve gait speed in patients with subacute stroke [93]. Additional larger studies will be required to see if these benefits can be replicated and sustained with repeated treatment sessions and if there is indeed a differential response to tDCS between subcortical versus cortical stroke.

11. Summary of Findings and Future Work

There are surprisingly few studies addressing the use of noninvasive cortical stimulation for the treatment of neurological gait disorders. Repetitive transcranial magnetic stimulation, for example, showed early promise in the treatment of gait in patients with Parkinson's disease [26, 27], but subsequent studies using intermittent magnetic stimulation [28] and tDCS [29] have yielded negative results. One study assessed the effect of tDCS when applied concomitantly with gait rehabilitation in patients with chronic stroke finding no additional benefit over and above rehabilitation alone [72].

Studies assessing the effect of tDCS in upper limb rehabilitation variously report benefit in both chronic and subacute strokes [87, 88]. In contrast, one large study [94] found no improvement in clinical outcome with acute (i.e., 48 hours) tDCS.

Firstly, this work has shown that it is possible to target lower limb muscles cortically, and that this can be done for both legs simultaneously by placing a central large anodal electrode over the motor strip and a smaller cathode electrode over the inion. Using a combination of TMS with tDCS it has been possible to show that such a montage increases cortical excitability of lower limb muscles of both legs.

Secondly, such cortical stimulation can be combined with physical therapy to enhance the effects of physical activity alone, for patients with Parkinson's disease and with small vessel disease and gait disturbance—an increasingly common cause of falls in the elderly.

Whilst the findings of these studies suggest that noninvasive electrical stimulation techniques may be a useful adjunct to physical therapy in patients with neurological gait disorders, there remains a need for further large mutlicentre randomized sham-controlled studies to evaluate the clinical relevance of such therapies. One striking feature across these and many other studies using noninvasive electrical stimulation is the intra- and interindividual variability in the behavioural responses following stimulation (Figure 3). One problem is that tDCS-related behavioural outcome measures are presumably dependent on factors outside the stimulation, such as motivation and attention that are difficult to control experimentally. As such, large numbers of patients and perhaps a range of electrode montages with computational modeling and direct imaging of current flow will be required to enable a translation of tDCS from experimental use into mainstream clinical practice for the treatment of gait disorders.

Conflict of Interests

The authors declare that there is no conflict of interests regarding the publication of this paper.

References

[1] J. G. Nutt, C. D. Marsden, and P. D. Thompson, "Human walking and higher-level gait disorders, particularly in the elderly," *Neurology*, vol. 43, no. 2, pp. 268–279, 1993.

[2] J. G. Nutt, "Classification of gait and balance disorders," *Advances in Neurology*, vol. 87, pp. 135–141, 2001.

[3] M. A. Hely, J. G. L. Morris, W. G. J. Reid, and R. Trafficante, "Sydney Multicenter Study of Parkinson's disease: non-L-dopa-responsive problems dominate at 15 years," *Movement Disorders*, vol. 20, no. 2, pp. 190–199, 2005.

[4] H. Fukuyama, Y. Ouchi, S. Matsuzaki et al., "Brain functional activity during gait in normal subjects: a SPECT study," *Neuroscience Letters*, vol. 228, no. 3, pp. 183–186, 1997.

[5] I. Miyai, H. C. Tanabe, I. Sase et al., "Cortical mapping of gait in humans: a near-infrared spectroscopic topography study," *NeuroImage*, vol. 14, no. 5, pp. 1186–1192, 2001.

[6] G. E. Alexander and M. D. Crutcher, "Preparation for movement: neural representations of intended direction in three motor areas of the monkey," *Journal of Neurophysiology*, vol. 64, no. 1, pp. 133–150, 1990.

[7] O. Franch, L. Calandre, J. Alvarez-Linera, E. D. Louis, F. Bermejo-Pareja, and J. Benito-Leon, "Gait disorders of unknown cause in the elderly: clinical and MRI findings," *Journal of the Neurological Sciences*, vol. 280, no. 1-2, pp. 84–86, 2009.

[8] C. Blahak, H. Baezner, L. Pantoni et al., "Deep frontal and periventricular age related white matter changes but not basal ganglia and infratentorial hyperintensities are associated with falls: cross sectional results from the LADIS study," *Journal of Neurology, Neurosurgery and Psychiatry*, vol. 80, no. 6, pp. 608–613, 2009.

[9] R. A. Bhadelia, L. L. Price, K. L. Tedesco et al., "Diffusion tensor imaging, white matter lesions, the corpus callosum, and gait in the elderly," *Stroke*, vol. 40, no. 12, pp. 3816–3820, 2009.

[10] K. Iseki, T. Hanakawa, K. Hashikawa et al., "Gait disturbance associated with white matter changes: a gait analysis and blood flow study," *NeuroImage*, vol. 49, no. 2, pp. 1659–1666, 2010.

[11] P. Linortner, F. Fazekas, R. Schmidt et al., "White matter hyperintensities alter functional organization of the motor system," *Neurobiology of Aging*, vol. 33, no. 1, pp. 197.e1–197.e9, 2012.

[12] P. Linortner, F. Fazekas, R. Schmidt et al., "White matter hyperintensities alter functional organization of the motor system," *Neurobiology of Aging*, vol. 33, no. 1, pp. 197–e9, 2012.

[13] H.-J. Freund and H. Hummelsheim, "Lesions of premotor cortex in man," *Brain*, vol. 108, no. 3, pp. 697–733, 1985.

[14] D. Kaski, S. Quadir, M. Patel, N. Yousif, and A. M. Bronstein, "Enhanced locomotor adaptation aftereffect in the "broken escalator" phenomenon using anodal tDCS," *Journal of Neurophysiology*, vol. 107, no. 9, pp. 2493–2505, 2012.

[15] S. Fahn, "Levodopa and the progression of Parkinson's disease," *The New England Journal of Medicine*, vol. 351, no. 24, pp. 2498–2566, 2004.

[16] Q. J. Almeida, J. S. Frank, E. A. Roy, A. E. Patla, and M. S. Jog, "Dopaminergic modulation of timing control and variability in the gait of Parkinson's disease," *Movement Disorders*, vol. 22, no. 12, pp. 1735–1742, 2007.

[17] A. Stefani, A. Peppe, M. Pierantozzi et al., "Multi-target strategy for Parkinsonian patients: the role of deep brain stimulation in the centromedian-parafascicularis complex," *Brain Research Bulletin*, vol. 78, no. 2-3, pp. 113–118, 2009.

[18] S. Vercruysse, W. Vandenberghe, L. Münks, B. Nuttin, H. Devos, and A. Nieuwboer, "Effects of deep brain stimulation of the subthalamic nucleus on freezing of gait in Parkinson's disease: a prospective controlled study," *Journal of Neurology, Neurosurgery and Psychiatry*, vol. 85, no. 8, pp. 871–877, 2014.

[19] A. M. S. Muniz, J. Nadal, K. E. Lyons, R. Pahwa, and W. Liu, "Long-term evaluation of gait initiation in six Parkinson's disease patients with bilateral subthalamic stimulation," *Gait and Posture*, vol. 35, no. 3, pp. 452–457, 2012.

[20] N. Chastan, G. W. M. Westby, J. Yelnik et al., "Effects of nigral stimulation on locomotion and postural stability in patients with Parkinson's disease," *Brain*, vol. 132, no. 1, pp. 172–184, 2009.

[21] D. Weiss, M. Walach, C. Meisner et al., "Nigral stimulation for resistant axial motor impairment in Parkinson's disease? A randomized controlled trial," *Brain*, vol. 136, no. 7, pp. 2098–2108, 2013.

[22] D. Nosko, M. U. Ferraye, V. Fraix et al., "Low-frequency versus high-frequency stimulation of the pedunculopontine nucleus area in Parkinson's disease: a randomised controlled trial," *Journal of Neurology, Neurosurgery, and Psychiatry*, 2014.

[23] M. U. Ferraye, B. Debû, V. Fraix et al., "Effects of pedunculopontine nucleus area stimulation on gait disorders in Parkinson's disease," *Brain*, vol. 133, part 1, pp. 205–214, 2010.

[24] P. Plaha and S. S. Gill, "Bilateral deep brain stimulation of the pedunculopontine nucleus for Parkinson's disease," *NeuroReport*, vol. 16, no. 17, pp. 1883–1887, 2005.

[25] E. Moro, C. Hamani, Y.-Y. Poon et al., "Unilateral pedunculopontine stimulation improves falls in Parkinson's disease," *Brain*, vol. 133, no. 1, pp. 215–224, 2010.

[26] E. M. Khedr, J. C. Rothwell, O. A. Shawky, M. A. Ahmed, and A. Hamdy, "Effect of daily repetitive transcranial magnetic stimulation on motor performance in Parkinson's disease," *Movement Disorders*, vol. 21, no. 12, pp. 2201–2205, 2006.

[27] M. P. Lomarev, S. Kanchana, W. Bara-Jimenez, M. Iyer, E. M. Wassermann, and M. Hallett, "Placebo-controlled study of rTMS for the treatment of Parkinson's disease," *Movement Disorders*, vol. 21, no. 3, pp. 325–331, 2006.

[28] D. H. Benninger, B. D. Berman, E. Houdayer et al., "Intermittent theta-burst transcranial magnetic stimulation for treatment of Parkinson disease," *Neurology*, vol. 76, no. 7, pp. 601–609, 2011.

[29] D. H. Benninger, M. Lomarev, G. Lopez et al., "Transcranial direct current stimulation for the treatment of Parkinson's disease," *Journal of Neurology, Neurosurgery and Psychiatry*, vol. 81, no. 10, pp. 1105–1111, 2010.

[30] I. Boers, W. Gerschlager, P. A. Stalenhoef, and B. R. Bloem, "Falls in the elderly II. Strategies for prevention," *Wiener Klinische Wochenschrift*, vol. 113, no. 11-12, pp. 398–407, 2001.

[31] K. H. Deane, D. Jones, E. D. Playford, Y. Ben-Shlomo, and C. E. Clarke, "Physiotherapy for patients with Parkinson's Disease: a comparison of techniques," *The Cochrane Database of Systematic Reviews*, no. 3, Article ID CD002817, 2001.

[32] B. E. Fisher, A. D. Wu, G. J. Salem et al., "The effect of exercise training in improving motor performance and corticomotor excitability in people with early Parkinson's disease," *Archives of Physical Medicine and Rehabilitation*, vol. 89, no. 7, pp. 1221–1229, 2008.

[33] M. A. Nitsche and W. Paulus, "Sustained excitability elevations induced by transcranial DC motor cortex stimulation in humans," *Neurology*, vol. 57, no. 10, pp. 1899–1901, 2001.

[34] D. Liebetanz, M. A. Nitsche, F. Tergau, and W. Paulus, "Pharmacological approach to the mechanisms of transcranial DC-stimulation-induced after-effects of human motor cortex excitability," *Brain*, vol. 125, no. 10, pp. 2238–2247, 2002.

[35] M. A. Nitsche, L. G. Cohen, E. M. Wassermann et al., "Transcranial direct current stimulation: state of the art 2008," *Brain Stimulation*, vol. 1, no. 3, pp. 206–223, 2008.

[36] A. Fasano, J. Herzog, E. Seifert et al., "Modulation of gait coordination by subthalamic stimulation improves freezing of gait," *Movement Disorders*, vol. 26, no. 5, pp. 844–851, 2011.

[37] R. F. Reynolds and A. M. Bronstein, "The broken escalator phenomenon: aftereffect of walking onto a moving platform," *Experimental Brain Research*, vol. 151, no. 3, pp. 301–308, 2003.

[38] K. L. Bunday, R. F. Reynolds, D. Kaski, M. Rao, S. Salman, and A. M. Bronstein, "The effect of trial number on the emergence of the "broken escalator" locomotor aftereffect," *Experimental Brain Research*, vol. 174, no. 2, pp. 270–278, 2006.

[39] A. M. Bronstein, K. L. Bunday, and R. Reynolds, "What the "broken escalator" phenomenon teaches us about balance," *Annals of the New York Academy of Sciences*, vol. 1164, pp. 82–88, 2009.

[40] K. L. Bunday and A. M. Bronstein, "Locomotor adaptation and aftereffects in patients with reduced somatosensory input due to peripheral neuropathy," *Journal of Neurophysiology*, vol. 102, no. 6, pp. 3119–3128, 2009.

[41] D. A. Green, K. L. Bunday, J. Bowen, T. Carter, and A. M. Bronstein, "What does autonomic arousal tell us about locomotor learning?" *Neuroscience*, vol. 170, no. 1, pp. 42–53, 2010.

[42] T. D. Lagerlund, F. W. Sharbrough, C. R. Jack Jr. et al., "Determination of 10-20 system electrode locations using magnetic resonance image scanning with markers," *Electroencephalography and Clinical Neurophysiology*, vol. 86, no. 1, pp. 7–14, 1993.

[43] M. Okamoto, H. Dan, K. Sakamoto et al., "Three-dimensional probabilistic anatomical cranio-cerebral correlation via the international 10-20 system oriented for transcranial functional brain mapping," *NeuroImage*, vol. 21, no. 1, pp. 99–111, 2004.

[44] G. H. Klem, H. O. Lüders, H. H. Jasper, and C. Elger, "The ten-twenty electrode system of the International Federation. The International Federation of Clinical Neurophysiology," *Electroencephalography and Clinical Neurophysiology*, vol. 52, pp. 3–6, 1999.

[45] J. M. Galea, A. Vazquez, N. Pasricha, J.-J. O. de Xivry, and P. Celnik, "Dissociating the roles of the cerebellum and motor cortex during adaptive learning: the motor cortex retains what the cerebellum learns," *Cerebral Cortex*, vol. 21, no. 8, pp. 1761–1770, 2011.

[46] K. Ohtsuka and T. Enoki, "Transcranial magnetic stimulation over the posterior cerebellum during smooth pursuit eye movements in man," *Brain*, vol. 121, no. 3, pp. 429–435, 1998.

[47] M. Gerwig, F. P. Kolb, and D. Timmann, "The involvement of the human cerebellum in eyeblink conditioning," *Cerebellum*, vol. 6, no. 1, pp. 38–57, 2007.

[48] D. M. Wolpert, "Probabilistic models in human sensorimotor control," *Human Movement Science*, vol. 26, no. 4, pp. 511–524, 2007.

[49] K.-S. Tang, D. Kaski, J. H. J. Allum, and A. M. Bronstein, "The effect of gait approach velocity on the broken escalator phenomenon," *Experimental Brain Research*, vol. 226, no. 3, pp. 335–346, 2013.

[50] Y.-H. Kim, S. H. You, M.-H. Ko et al., "Repetitive transcranial magnetic stimulation-induced corticomotor excitability and associated motor skill acquisition in chronic stroke," *Stroke*, vol. 37, no. 6, pp. 1471–1476, 2006.

[51] G. Ebersbach, C. Moreau, F. Gandor, L. Defebvre, and D. Devos, "Clinical syndromes: parkinsonian gait," *Movement Disorders*, vol. 28, no. 11, pp. 1552–1559, 2013.

[52] W. C. Koller, S. Glatt, B. Vetere-Overfield, and R. Hassanein, "Falls and Parkinson's disease," *Clinical Neuropharmacology*, vol. 12, no. 2, pp. 98–105, 1989.

[53] M. Weinrich, K. Koch, F. Garcia, and R. W. Angel, "Axial versus distal motor impairment in Parkinson's disease," *Neurology*, vol. 38, no. 4, pp. 540–545, 1988.

[54] H. L. Klawans, "Individual manifestations of Parkinson's disease after ten or more years of levodopa," *Movement Disorders*, vol. 1, no. 3, pp. 187–192, 1986.

[55] O. Blin, A. M. Ferrandez, J. Pailhous, and G. Serratrice, "Dopa-sensitive and dopa resistant gait parameters in Parkinson's disease," *Journal of the Neurological Sciences*, vol. 103, no. 1, pp. 51–54, 1991.

[56] K. B. Foreman, M. L. Singer, O. Addison, R. L. Marcus, P. C. LaStayo, and L. E. Dibble, "Effects of dopamine replacement therapy on lower extremity kinetics and kinematics during a rapid force production task in persons with Parkinson disease," *Gait and Posture*, vol. 39, no. 1, pp. 638–640, 2014.

[57] R. T. Roemmich, N. Hack, U. Akbar, and C. J. Hass, "Effects of dopaminergic therapy on locomotor adaptation and adaptive learning in persons with Parkinson's disease," *Behavioural Brain Research*, vol. 268, pp. 31–39, 2014.

[58] E. D. Playford, I. H. Jenkins, R. E. Passingham, J. Nutt, R. S. J. Frackowiak, and D. J. Brooks, "Impaired mesial frontal and putamen activation in Parkinson's disease: a positron emission tomography study," *Annals of Neurology*, vol. 32, no. 2, pp. 151–161, 1992.

[59] A. Pascual-Leone, J. Valls-Solé, J. P. Brasil-Neto, A. Cammarota, J. Grafman, and M. Hallett, "Akinesia in Parkinson's disease. II. Effects of subthreshold repetitive transcranial motor cortex stimulation," *Neurology*, vol. 44, no. 5, pp. 892–898, 1994.

[60] J. A. Williams, M. Imamura, and F. Fregni, "Updates of the use of non-invasive brain stimulation in physical and rehabilitation medicine," *Journal of Rehabilitation Medicine*, vol. 41, no. 5, pp. 305–311, 2009.

[61] G. Alon, D. A. Yungher, L. M. Shulman, and M. W. Rogers, "Safety and immediate effect of noninvasive transcranial pulsed current stimulation on gait and balance in parkinson disease," *Neurorehabilitation and Neural Repair*, vol. 26, no. 9, pp. 1089–1095, 2012.

[62] A. L. Hunt and K. D. Sethi, "The pull test: a history," *Movement Disorders*, vol. 21, no. 7, pp. 894–899, 2006.

[63] A. Lang, "Clinical rating scales and videotape analysis," in *Therapy of Parkinson's Disease*, W. C. Koller and G. Paulson, Eds., pp. 21–46, Marcel Dekker, New York, NY, USA, 1995.

[64] D. Kaski, R. Dominguez, J. Allum, A. Islam, and A. Bronstein, "Combining physical training with transcranial direct current stimulation to improve gait in Parkinson's disease: a pilot randomized controlled study," *Clinical Rehabilitation*, vol. 28, no. 11, pp. 1115–1124, 2014.

[65] B. R. Bloem, J. P. van Vugt, and D. J. Beckley, "Postural instability and falls in Parkinson's disease," *Advances in Neurology*, vol. 87, pp. 209–223, 2001.

[66] R. R. Pratt, "Art, dance, and music therapy," *Physical Medicine & Rehabilitation Clinics of North America*, vol. 15, no. 4, pp. 827–841, 2004.

[67] M. E. Hackney and G. M. Earhart, "Effects of dance on gait and balance in Parkinsons disease: a comparison of partnered and nonpartnered dance movement," *Neurorehabilitation and Neural Repair*, vol. 24, no. 4, pp. 384–392, 2010.

[68] K. Sacco, F. Cauda, L. Cerliani, D. Mate, S. Duca, and G. C. Geminiani, "Motor imagery of walking following training in locomotor attention. The effect of "the tango lesson"," *NeuroImage*, vol. 32, no. 3, pp. 1441–1449, 2006.

[69] D. Kaski, J. H. Allum, A. M. Bronstein, and R. O. Dominguez, "Applying anodal tDCS during tango dancing in a patient with Parkinson's disease," *Neuroscience Letters*, vol. 568, pp. 39–43, 2014.

[70] J. H. J. Allum and M. G. Carpenter, "A speedy solution for balance and gait analysis: angular velocity measured at the centre of body mass," *Current Opinion in Neurology*, vol. 18, no. 1, pp. 15–21, 2005.

[71] M. E. Tinetti, "Performance-orientated assessment of mobility problems in elderly patients," *Journal of the American Geriatrics Society*, vol. 34, no. 2, pp. 119–126, 1986.

[72] C. Geroin, A. Picelli, D. Munari, A. Waldner, C. Tomelleri, and N. Smania, "Combined transcranial direct current stimulation and robot-assisted gait training in patients with chronic stroke: a preliminary comparison," *Clinical Rehabilitation*, vol. 25, no. 6, pp. 537–548, 2011.

[73] S. Madhavan, K. A. Weber II, and J. W. Stinear, "Non-invasive brain stimulation enhances fine motor control of the hemiparetic ankle: implications for rehabilitation," *Experimental Brain Research*, vol. 209, no. 1, pp. 9–17, 2011.

[74] K. F. de Laat, A. G. W. van Norden, R. A. R. Gons et al., "Gait in elderly with cerebral small vessel disease," *Stroke*, vol. 41, no. 8, pp. 1652–1658, 2010.

[75] C. R. G. Guttmann, R. Benson, S. K. Warfield et al., "White matter abnormalities in mobility-impaired older persons," *Neurology*, vol. 54, no. 6, pp. 1277–1283, 2000.

[76] P. C. Gandiga, F. C. Hummel, and L. G. Cohen, "Transcranial DC stimulation (tDCS): a tool for double-blind sham-controlled clinical studies in brain stimulation," *Clinical Neurophysiology*, vol. 117, no. 4, pp. 845–850, 2006.

[77] D. Kaski, R. O. Dominguez, J. H. Allum, and A. M. Bronstein, "Improving gait and balance in patients with leukoaraiosis using transcranial direct current stimulation and physical training: an exploratory study," *Neurorehabilitation and Neural Repair*, vol. 27, no. 9, pp. 864–871, 2013.

[78] M. Lotze, C. Braun, N. Birbaumer, S. Anders, and L. G. Cohen, "Motor learning elicited by voluntary drive," *Brain*, vol. 126, no. 4, pp. 866–872, 2003.

[79] J. M. Galea and P. Celnik, "Brain polarization enhances the formation and retention of motor memories," *Journal of Neurophysiology*, vol. 102, no. 1, pp. 294–301, 2009.

[80] M. A. Perez, B. K. Lungholt, K. Nyborg, and J. B. Nielsen, "Motor skill training induces changes in the excitability of the leg cortical area in healthy humans," *Experimental Brain Research*, vol. 159, no. 2, pp. 197–205, 2004.

[81] P. Celnik, N.-J. Paik, Y. Vandermeeren, M. Dimyan, and L. G. Cohen, "Effects of combined peripheral nerve stimulation and brain polarization on performance of a motor sequence task after chronic stroke," *Stroke*, vol. 40, no. 5, pp. 1764–1771, 2009.

[82] N. Roche, A. Lackmy, V. Achache, B. Bussel, and R. Katz, "Effects of anodal transcranial direct current stimulation over the leg motor area on lumbar spinal network excitability in healthy subjects," *Journal of Physiology*, vol. 589, no. 11, pp. 2813–2826, 2011.

[83] F. Fregni, P. S. Boggio, M. C. Santos et al., "Noninvasive cortical stimulation with transcranial direct current stimulation in Parkinson's disease," *Movement Disorders*, vol. 21, no. 10, pp. 1693–1702, 2006.

[84] D. P. Purpura and J. G. McMurtry, "Intracellular activities and evoked potential changes during polarization of motor cortex," *Journal of Neurophysiology*, vol. 28, pp. 166–185, 1965.

[85] H. Muramatsu and K. Koike, "Stroke rehabilitation therapy in a patient with a cardiac pacemaker for chronic atrial fibrillation," *International Journal of Rehabilitation Research*, vol. 26, no. 4, pp. 317–321, 2003.

[86] R. Dickstein, "Rehabilitation of gait speed after stroke: a critical review of intervention approaches," *Neurorehabilitation and Neural Repair*, vol. 22, no. 6, pp. 649–660, 2008.

[87] D.-Y. Kim, J.-Y. Lim, E. K. Kang et al., "Effect of transcranial direct current stimulation on motor recovery in patients with subacute stroke," *The American Journal of Physical Medicine and Rehabilitation*, vol. 89, no. 11, pp. 879–886, 2010.

[88] R. Lindenberg, V. Renga, L. L. Zhu, D. Nair, and G. Schlaug, "Bihemispheric brain stimulation facilitates motor recovery in chronic stroke patients," *Neurology*, vol. 75, no. 24, pp. 2176–2184, 2010.

[89] G. Jayaram and J. W. Stinear, "The effects of transcranial stimulation on paretic lower limb motor excitability during walking," *Journal of Clinical Neurophysiology*, vol. 26, no. 4, pp. 272–279, 2009.

[90] A. R. Brunoni, M. A. Nitsche, N. Bolognini et al., "Clinical research with transcranial direct current stimulation (tDCS): challenges and future directions," *Brain Stimulation*, vol. 5, no. 3, pp. 175–195, 2012.

[91] N. Murase, J. Duque, R. Mazzocchio, and L. G. Cohen, "Influence of interhemispheric interactions on motor function in chronic stroke," *Annals of Neurology*, vol. 55, no. 3, pp. 400–409, 2004.

[92] R. J. Nudo, "Recovery after brain injury: mechanisms and principles," *Frontiers in Human Neuroscience*, vol. 7, article 887, 2013.

[93] V. Tahtis, D. Kaski, and B. M. Seemungal, "The effect of single session bi-cephalic transcranial direct current stimulation on gait performance in sub-acute stroke: a pilot study," *Restorative Neurology and Neuroscience*, vol. 32, no. 4, pp. 527–532, 2014.

[94] C. Rossi, F. Sallustio, S. Di Legge, P. Stanzione, and G. Koch, "Transcranial direct current stimulation of the affected hemisphere does not accelerate recovery of acute stroke patients," *European Journal of Neurology*, vol. 20, no. 1, pp. 202–204, 2013.

10

Reelin in the Years: Controlling Neuronal Migration and Maturation in the Mammalian Brain

Gabriella D'Arcangelo

Department of Cell Biology and Neuroscience, Rutgers, The State University of New Jersey, Piscataway, NJ 08854, USA

Correspondence should be addressed to Gabriella D'Arcangelo; darcangelo@dls.rutgers.edu

Academic Editor: Abdallah Hayar

The extracellular protein Reelin was initially identified as an essential factor in the control of neuronal migration and layer formation in the developing mammalian brain. In the years following its discovery, however, it became clear that Reelin is a multifunctional protein that controls not only the positioning of neurons in the developing brain, but also their growth, maturation, and synaptic activity in the adult brain. In this review, we will highlight the major discoveries of the biological activities of Reelin and the underlying molecular mechanisms that affect the development and function of the mammalian brain, from embryonic ages to adulthood.

1. The *reeler* Mouse and *Reelin* Gene Discovery

Reelin was identified in 1995 as the gene disrupted in two mouse strains carrying the autosomal recessive mutation *reeler*, a transgenic and a spontaneous strain that originated in Edinburgh [1]. While a newly generated transgenic strain was instrumental in the cloning of the gene, the classic, spontaneous Edinburgh *reeler* mutant strain had been well known for decades to developmental neurobiologists for the distinct neurological phenotype observed in homozygous mice, which includes tremors, ataxia, cerebellar hypoplasia, and widespread disruption of cellular layers throughout the brain [2–10]. Upon cloning and mapping of the gene, it turned out that a large deletion in the *Reelin* gene had occurred in the Edinburgh strain, resulting in the complete loss of transcript expression [1]. Around the same time, a portion of the *Reelin* coding sequence was also identified in another spontaneous *reeler* strain that originated in Orleans [11]. In this strain, however, a truncated transcript predicted to encode a C terminal deletion mutant protein was stably expressed. To date, several additional *reeler* mouse mutant strains carrying mutations in the *Reelin* gene have been identified, all resulting in the loss of transcript expression. Like the original Edinburgh mutation (now called B6C3Fe

ala-Reln^rl/J), these strains exhibit essentially the same *reeler* phenotype and are made commercially available from The Jackson Laboratory. As *Reelin* gene orthologs were identified in other vertebrate species, other *reeler*-like mutations were quickly characterized. In the rat, for example, two mutant strains, the Shaking Rat Kawasaki and the Komed Zucker Creeping rat, that exhibited a *reeler*-like phenotype were reported to carry *Reelin* gene mutation [12, 13]. The human *REELIN* gene was also quickly cloned [14], and human subjects carrying *REELIN* mutations in homozygousity were identified few years later [15]. These patients exhibit lissencephaly with cerebellar hypoplasia (LCH), a phenotype that is very reminiscent of that observed in *reeler* mice.

One of the most intriguing aspects of the *reeler* phenotype is that many neuronal populations are born in normal numbers, at the right time and in the right place, but fail to reach the appropriate position and to form cellular layers in laminated cortical structures of the brain, such as the cerebral cortex, the hippocampus, or the cerebellum [6]. Additionally, failure of specific neuronal populations to reach appropriate locations and to assemble into distinct nuclei was reported in the brain stem and in the spinal cord [5, 16]. These observations strongly suggested that the gene mutated in *reeler* mice had to be an essential regulator of neuronal migration and ultimately determines neuronal position within cortical structures and other anatomically distinct cellular aggregates of the central nervous system. Indeed, several studies have shown that *Reelin* plays important roles in the development of the spinal cord [16–18] and the retinal circuitry [19]. Here, we will discuss primarily its role in brain development and focus especially on recent advances related to the control of neuronal migration, which was the first recognized biological function of *Reelin* and, perhaps still to these days, its best-characterized activity. However, this is by no means its only function. In fact, it was noted early on that additional defects are present in the *reeler* mutant, including subtle connectivity abnormalities in the cerebellum [7] and fiber segregation abnormalities in the hippocampus [20, 21], suggesting that *Reelin* plays multiple roles in brain development.

How does *Reelin* control different aspects of brain development and function? Almost twenty years after its discovery, we still do not know everything to be known about this remarkable protein, but we have made tremendous progress in elucidating its structure, expression, and biochemical properties and ultimately in understanding how *Reelin* exerts its diverse functions, not only during embryonic and postnatal brain development, but also in the adult brain.

2. The *Reelin* Gene

Shortly after the identification of the *Reelin* coding sequence, the genomic organization of the mouse *Reelin* gene and its promoter region on chromosome 5 was unraveled [22]. This study revealed that the *Reelin* gene is very large and complex, containing 65 exons spanning approximately 450 kb of genomic DNA. The study also identified different *Reelin* transcripts generated by alternative splicing of a microexon although the significance of this splicing event remains obscure to these days. Furthermore, two different polyadenylation sites and a promoter region lacking canonical TATA and CAAT boxes, but containing putative recognition sites for transcription factors Sp1 and AP2, were defined. The promoter region of human *REELIN* gene was also cloned and characterized shortly thereafter, revealing the presence not only of Sp1 site, but also of binding sites for additional transcription factors, such as the cyclic AMP responsive element binding protein (CREB), T brain 1 (Tbr1), and paired homeobox 6 (Pax6) [23]. These and other follow-up studies led to the recognition that *REELIN* expression is heavily regulated by promoter methylation and that this epigenetic event may play an important role in controlling *Reelin* expression levels [23, 24]. Since reduced expression of *REELIN* has been reported in patients with schizophrenia [25], bipolar disorder [26], and autism [27], these findings have potentially important implications for the treatment of these disorders. The intriguing association between *REELIN* expression and cognitive disorders, as well as the possible use of pharmacological agents that decrease methylation and restore normal levels of *REELIN* in these patients, has been extensively discussed in several review articles [28–30]. Therefore, we will not address this topic here, except to underscore the importance of furthering our understanding

of *Reelin* activities in processes that take place during brain development and beyond.

3. The *Reelin* Protein

The cloning of mouse *Reelin* coding sequence predicted that the encoded protein was likely to be large and secreted. Indeed, a full-length *Reelin* protein of approximately 385 kDA was found to be secreted in the culture medium of wild type mouse neurons or clonal cells transfected with an expression vector containing the newly assembled coding sequence [31]. The secreted protein also was shown to be glycosylated. A remarkably similar protein was deduced from the sequence of the human *REELIN* cDNA, which resulted to be 388 kDA in size and 94.2% identical to the mouse protein at the amino acid level [14]. However, since the sequence of *Reelin* did not extensively match other known sequences in the database, the cloning of *Reelin* revealed little about its biochemical function. The predicted protein had a modular structure composed of a series of unique repeats, flanked by distinct N- and C-terminal regions. The N-terminal region contains a signal peptide, which is required for secretion, a small region of similarity to the extracellular protein F-spondin, and an epitope region that is recognized by the CR-50 monoclonal antibody. This antibody was developed concurrently with the cloning of *Reelin*, based on the presence of an antigen expressed by Cajal-Retzius cells which was absent in the embryonic forebrain of *reeler* mice [32]. Upon cloning of *Reelin*, the CR-50 antibody was shown to recognize the N-terminal of the native protein [31]. This antibody turned out to be an excellent reagent to study not only the distribution of the *Reelin* protein in brain tissue slices, but also its function, since it interfered with many *Reelin*-induced cellular and molecular events [20, 32–35]. Biochemical studies revealed that the interfering activity of the CR-50 antibody most likely lies in its ability to mask an N-terminal region of *Reelin* that is necessary for disulfide-linked homodimer formation [36]. The main body of the *Reelin* protein is composed of eight consecutive repeats, each composed of two subrepeats separated by a cysteine pattern commonly found in extracellular proteins, the EGF-like repeat [1]. The boundaries of these repeats have now been clearly defined, and the crystal structure of two central repeats 5 and 6 has been resolved in recent years [37]. The C terminal region of *Reelin* is highly conserved and contains a positively charged stretch of amino acids which appears to be important for optimal signaling [38]. Following the development of a battery of monoclonal antibodies [39], a biochemical analysis of the processing of *Reelin* became possible. It is now established that, after secretion in the extracellular environment, full-length *Reelin* is rapidly cleaved by proteases at two specific sites, generating three major proteolytic fragments [40]. Among these, the central fragment composed of repeats 3 to 6 is the only one that appears to be necessary and sufficient to induce layer formation in a cortical slice culture assay [40]. This fragment also contains amino acid residues that are required for receptor binding and is sufficient to induce signal transduction, albeit to a reduced extent compared to the entire *Reelin* moiety [37, 40, 41]. Together, the data suggest that proteolytic processing is important *in vivo* to produce *Reelin* fragments, which can either diffuse away from the site of origin or assemble locally into large protein aggregates or homodimers capable of activating signal transduction to the full extent [36, 41, 42].

4. *Reelin* Expression during Brain Development

In situ hybridization experiments gave an initial overview of *Reelin* expression in the mouse brain and spinal cord [43, 44]. These studies also revealed that *Reelin* is expressed in many organs outside the central nervous system, during development and also in adult ages , suggesting that *Reelin* may be important not only for the initial cellular organization, but also for the stabilization and remodeling of these different tissues [43]. However, since only the brain was obviously disrupted in *reeler* mice, most studies of *Reelin* naturally focused on the development of this organ. Immunolabeling studies with the CR-50 antibody and double-labeling studies demonstrated that an early and transient neuronal population, the Cajal-Retzius cells, expresses high levels of *Reelin* during the embryonic development of forebrain structures [1, 20, 32, 44, 45]. These cells occupy the marginal zone of the cerebral cortex and hippocampus throughout embryonic development and die 1-2 weeks after birth, as neuronal migration and layer formation in these structures are completed. It is interesting to note that Cajal-Retzius cells had been described since the late 1800s, and their unique and complex morphology was carefully reconstructed, but it was not until the discovery of *Reelin* that the essential role of these cells in the control of neuronal migration during forebrain development was finally appreciated. In the embryonic cerebellum, *Reelin* is expressed by granule cell precursors in the external granule layer [1, 45, 46]. These cells eventually migrate inwardly to form the internal granule cell layer as the cerebellum continues to grow in size and becomes foliated at early postnatal ages. Thus, a similar scenario is present in all laminated embryonic cortical structures of the murine brain, where transient neurons express and secrete *Reelin* in superficial regions to promote neuronal migration and cellular layer formation in the cortical plate that is developing underneath them. This general pattern of expression is highly conserved in other rodents such as the rat [47, 48]. In this species, *Reelin* is expressed not only by Cajal-Retzius cells but also by another cell population of the forebrain marginal zone, the subpial pyriform cells. With the development of new monoclonal antibodies that recognized human *Reelin* [39], more immunochemical studies became possible. These studies showed that, like in the rat, two major cell populations of *Reelin*-expressing cells are present in the marginal zone of the prenatal human neocortex: classic Cajal-Retzius and Cajal-Retzius-like cells [49]. The presence of additional *Reelin*-producing cells types in the embryonic marginal zone correlates with a more complex and protracted development of the neocortex in more cognitively competent species.

5. Functions of *Reelin* during Brain Development

What is the role of *Reelin* during early brain development? Clearly, the expression of *Reelin* by Cajal-Retzius and Cajal-Retzius-like cells in the embryonic forebrain is linked to the control of neuronal migration in the cortical plate. In the embryonic cerebral cortex, it specifically directs the radial migration and the formation of cellular layers by principal, excitatory cortical neurons born in the ventricular zone. The cellular and molecular mechanisms that underlie this critical biological function of *Reelin* in the embryonic forebrain will be discussed in detail below. Similar to the cerebral cortex, *Reelin* also directs the radial migration and layer formation of pyramidal neurons in the embryonic hippocampus proper. The essential function of *Reelin* in the establishment of cortical cellular layers is maintained postnatally in the dentate gyrus. In this structure, neurogenesis and granule neuron migration continues after birth and into adulthood. Thus, in this unique brain region, *Reelin*, produced by Cajal-Retzius cells in the outer molecular layer, continues to function as a major regulator of neuronal migration and cellular layer formation throughout life [50]. The importance of *Reelin* in the postnatal dentate gyrus as a positional clue is underscored by the finding that loss of *Reelin* is associated with granule cell dispersion in patients, as well as in animal models of temporal lobe epilepsy [51, 52]. This observation has potential clinical implications, since follow-up studies have shown that addition of recombinant *Reelin* can rescue granule cell dispersion, at least in animal models [53]. Recent studies further suggested that granule cell dispersion results from impaired *Reelin* processing and the consequent lack of secretion by Cajal-Retzius cells of the dentate gyrus and not from cell death or expression deficits, raising renewed interest in the identification of the proteases that carry out *Reelin* proteolytic cleavage [51]. In the cerebellum, *Reelin* produced by granule cells in the external granule layer is required for the radial migration of Purkinje cells, which are born in the cerebellar ventricular zone and form initially a plate and then a single-cell layer. This view stems from the extensive analysis of cerebellar development in *reeler* mice [7, 54–56], from *Reelin* gene and protein expression data [1, 46], and from functional studies in organotypic cultures [34]. Taken together, this body of work indicates that *Reelin*, expressed by transient cells in superficial layers, specifically regulates radial neuronal migration in all developing laminated brain structures.

In addition to cellular layer formation, *Reelin* produced by Cajal-Retzius cells has been shown to promote the initial growth of axonal and dendrite processes. The formation of hippocampal fiber layers was first recognized as a perinatal function of *Reelin* [57]. In the early postnatal hippocampus, Cajal-Retzius cells continue to secrete large amounts of *Reelin* in the stratum lacunosum moleculare (SLM) and the outer molecular layer (OML) of the dentate gyrus. These regions represent the main targets of the entorhinohippocampal pathway. Using an organotypic coculture system, investigators elegantly demonstrated that *Reelin* is not essential for targeting these axons to the SLM and OML, but it is required for their early growth and branching [20]. Furthermore, Cajal-Retzius-produced *Reelin* was shown to promote synaptogenesis by entorhinal afferents [58]. These studies implicated *Reelin* in axon maturation and indirectly implicated this protein in the formation of synaptic structures. However, the ability of *Reelin* to stimulate axon growth appears to be limited in time and place. Indeed, defects in the branching of entorhinohippocampal axons were only found in the developing, but not in the adult, *reeler* hippocampus [20]. Furthermore, no defects have been reported in other axonal pathways of *reeler* mice so far. Building on the early observation that dendrite growth and cellular orientation are abnormal in *reeler* [59–61], other studies implicated *Reelin* in the control of the growth of these cellular processes. Using a fluorescent transgene to facilitate visualization *in vivo*, the development of apical processes of dentate granule cells was found to be delayed in *reeler* mice [62]. Furthermore, using cultured immature hippocampal neurons of wild type and *reeler* mice, this study demonstrated that *Reelin* is directly required for normal dendritic elongation and branching. Altogether, these findings suggested that *Reelin* promotes the early growth of apical dendrites of hippocampal neurons, which grow toward the Cajal-Retzius-cell-containing layers at early postnatal ages. Similarly, in the developing cerebral cortex, *Reelin* signaling was shown to promote the outgrowth of apical dendrites originating from cortical neurons contacting Cajal-Retzius cells in the marginal zone [63, 64]. *In vitro* studies largely supported *in vivo* observations and helped defining the molecular mechanisms underlying dendrite outgrowth by forebrain neurons [62, 65]. Recent studies further demonstrated that *Reelin* induces the extension of the Golgi apparatus in apical dendrites, thus stimulating dendrite growth and cell polarization [66]. However, as for axonal processes, the role of *Reelin* may be limited to promoting the initial dendrite outgrowth that occurs during development. This idea is supported by the observation that Reelin signaling is not required for the full maturation of pyramidal hippocampal neurons in long-term *in vitro* cultures [67].

Besides growth of cellular processes, synapse formation represents an important step in postnatal brain development, which occurs during the late phase of dendrite and axon maturation. During these later times, approximately corresponding to 2-3 weeks after birth in rodents, the expression of Reelin in the forebrain is no longer exclusively localized to superficial layers but is widespread throughout all cellular layers due to the gradual appearance of Reelin-expressing interneurons [1, 32, 44, 45, 68, 69]. However, some Cajal-Retzius cells persist in the postnatal hippocampus and thus may play a role in later aspects of the development of this structure. Indeed, using fluorescence imaging techniques *in vivo* and *in vitro*, further studies demonstrated that Reelin promotes the development of dendritic spines [70]. This study specifically identified a defect in spine density in young adult heterozygous and homozygous *reeler* mice *in vivo* and in organotypic slice cultures *in vitro*, which was rescued by the addition of exogenous *Reelin*. However, as for the growth effect on hippocampal axonal and dendrites, spine density was only transiently impaired in young adult Reelin-deficient mice (less than 1 month old), was very slightly reduced at 2 months [71], and was no longer affected in adult animals older than 6 months of age.

Taken together, the evidence so far indicates that Reelin plays multiple roles in brain development: it plays a unique and major role in controlling radial neuronal migration in cortical structures during embryonic ages and also contributes to promoting the growth of some axonal projections in the hippocampus, apical dendrite development and synapse formation in forebrain cortical structures at postnatal ages. In the adult brain, it also modulates synaptic function and plasticity, as discussed later in this review (Figure 1).

6. Cellular Targets of *Reelin* Signaling during Early Brain Development

Decades of neuroanatomical analysis of the homozygous *reeler* mouse, which preceded the discovery of the *Reelin* gene, had set the stage for understanding the role of this protein in brain development. The reported widespread defects in cellular layer formation in all cortical structures implied that Reelin is essential for the migration of many neuronal populations, including most cortical and hippocampal neurons [2, 8, 59, 60, 72–75]. A careful examination of the progression of the anatomical defects during cerebellar development also indicated that the layer organization of Purkinje cells in the cerebellar cortex represented the step that was directly affected by the absence of Reelin [7, 54–56, 76]. Thus, the failure of granule cells to proliferate, which ultimately leads to the lack of foliation and cerebellar hypoplasia in *reeler* mice, was recognized as a secondary defect due to the malposition of Purkinje cells, which failed to enter the cerebellar cortex after leaving the ventricular zone and remained localized in a deep cerebellar mass. This insightful observation also suggested that Purkinje cells are the direct targets of Reelin and that Reelin primarily promotes the final steps in the radial migration of principal neurons in cortical structures. However, examination of the anatomical phenotype of *reeler* mice in other structures led to different interpretations. For example, in the *reeler* hippocampus, pyramidal neurons and dentate granule cells appeared to migrate past their normal position, leading to the hypothesis that Reelin represents a stop signal necessary to arrest radial migration rather than promoting it [57]. The cellular complexity of cerebral cortex made it even more difficult to predict, based on anatomical phenotype and expression data alone, the identity of the cellular targets of Reelin and its mechanism of action with regard to the control of radial migration. This determination required a deeper understanding of molecular mechanisms of Reelin activity on migration, which originated from advances in the wider field of brain development and the development of new genetic approaches that occurred over the course of two decades.

At the end of the 1900s, the prevailing view of neocortical development was that principal neurons, born in the ventricular zone, migrate radially into the cortical plate following the guidance of radial glial cells, which provide a scaffold for migration. Thus, a reasonable expectation around this time was that Reelin would affect the development or

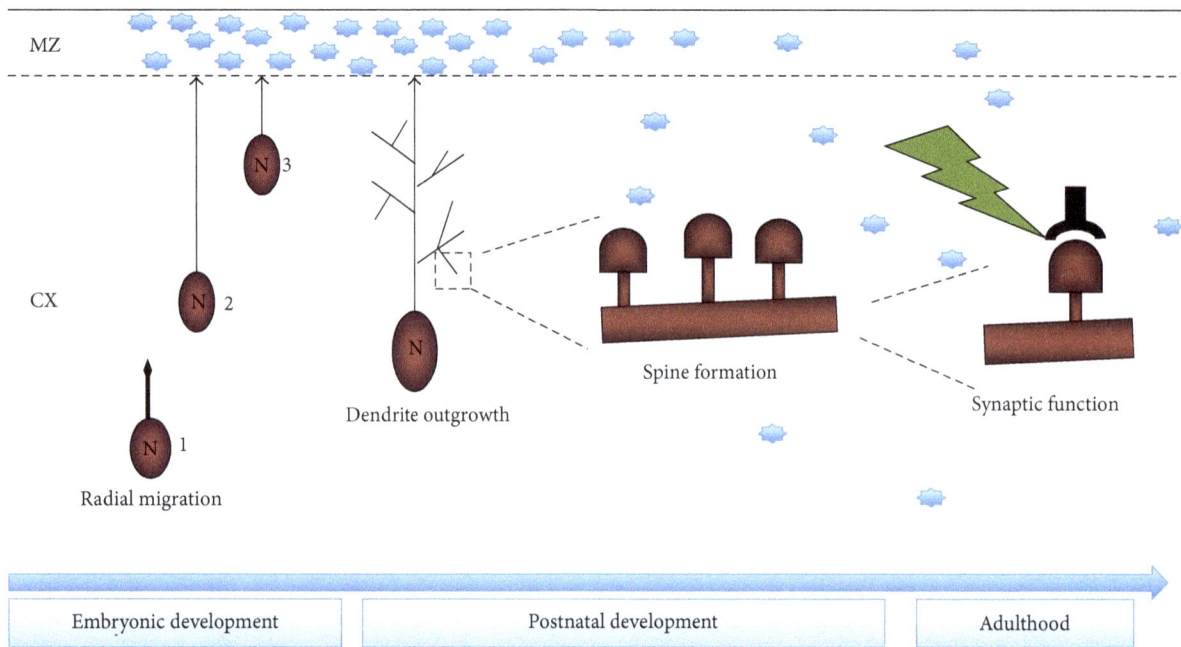

FIGURE 1: Schematic representation of the multiple activities of Reelin in the developing and adult forebrain. Blue octagons represent secreted Reelin molecules, and red ovals represent the cell bodies of principal forebrain neurons (N). During embryonic development, Reelin is mostly localized to the marginal zone (MZ) and directs radial migration by affecting multiple steps, such as radial orientation (1), attachment of the leading edge to the MZ (2), and somal translocation (3). During postnatal development, Reelin becomes expressed throughout cortical forebrain structures (CX), where it promotes mainly the growth of apical dendrites and spine formation. In the adult brain, Reelin modulates synaptic function and plasticity.

the integrity of radial glia scaffold and thus indirectly affect neuronal migration. Indeed, this scenario appears to be the predominant mechanism of action in at least one structure, the dentate gyrus of the hippocampus, where the radial glial scaffold is severely disrupted in *reeler* mutants [77]. In the *reeler* forebrain, some evidence of impaired radial glial cell development was also found [78]. However, based on the early observation that the CR-50 interfering antibody blocked neuronal aggregation in cortical explants lacking a true radial glia scaffold [32], the alternative hypothesis that Reelin may primarily affect principal cortical neurons directly, especially during the last phase of their migration inside the cortical plate, began to take hold [10]. Furthermore, new crucial discoveries in the field of cortical development provided a framework for this latter hypothesis. First, it became clear that radial glia cells are actually neural progenitor cells that give rise to many principal neurons of the neocortex [79, 80]. Second, new imaging studies demonstrated that, in addition to glial-guided locomotion, neurons could also migrate independently of radial support, by somal translocation or a multipolar mechanism [81, 82]. However, the clear identification of the cellular targets of Reelin during radial migration required a better knowledge of the molecules necessary to transduce the signal.

In addition to its major function in the control of radial neuronal migration in cortical structures, Reelin was also shown to affect the migration of neuronal precursors in the rostromigratory stream [83]. These precursors engage in tangential chain migration from the subventricular zone of the cerebral cortex on route to the olfactory bulb. Reelin causes the detachment of these precursors from their substrate, thus disrupting their migration. Thus, neuronal precursors in the rostromigratory stream appear to be direct cellular targets of Reelin, even though Reelin exerts a negative effect on their migration.

7. Molecular Mechanisms: The Discovery of the Dab1 Adaptor Protein

The first essential transducer of the Reelin signal to be identified was the mammalian homolog of Drosophila *Disabled-1* (Dab1), an intracellular adaptor protein that, when phosphorylated on tyrosine residues, was capable of interacting with Src-homology (SH2) domains of Src-family kinases (SFKs) [84]. Dab1 contains a phosphotyrosine binding (PTB) domain, which also enables this adaptor protein to bind not only tyrosine-phosphorylated proteins, but also phosphoinosites and receptor internalization domains [85–87]. Spontaneous mutations in the Dab1 gene were identified in *scrambler* and *yotari*, two independent lines of mutant mice that exhibited a phenotype remarkably similar to *reeler* [88–91]. Furthermore, an engineered Dab1 knockout mouse also exhibited the *reeler*-like phenotype [92]. The similarity between Dab1 and Reelin mutant mouse phenotypes strongly suggested that Dab1 functioned downstream of Reelin in the same linear signaling pathway. In addition, biochemical studies revealed that recombinant Reelin rapidly induces the phosphorylation of Dab1 on multiple tyrosine residues in cultured cortical neurons [93–95]. This event is mediated mainly by Fyn and Src, two SFKs that are activated by Reelin [96, 97]. Dab1 phosphorylation on tyrosine residues is essential for signal transduction, since point mutations in these sites result in the appearance of a *reeler*-like phenotype *in vivo* [98]. Dab1 tyrosine phosphorylation is also coupled to its ubiquitination by the Cbl ligase and to its degradation by the proteasome system [99, 100]. This degradation represents a mechanism for signal termination and explains why Dab1 protein levels are elevated in the brain of *reeler* as well as Fyn/Src double knockout mice [89, 101, 102]. Taken together, these findings indicate that Reelin promotes the activation of Dab1 in target cells, but protein degradation mechanisms ensure that the signal is transient. This sequence of activation and shutoff may be crucial for the execution of multiple steps in neuronal migration. Indeed, different models have been proposed to explain how the Reelin function may change dynamically from a permissive, attractive clue during the initial phases of migration to a detachment from radial glia and thus a stop signal during later phases [103–106].

Expression studies indicated that Dab1 is expressed at high levels by principal neurons of the embryonic cerebral cortex and hippocampus and by Purkinje cells in the cerebellum, in a pattern that is largely complementary to that of Reelin [107, 108]. This pattern suggested that forebrain principal neurons and Purkinje cells are the direct targets of Reelin during migration and cellular layer formation. In the forebrain, however, Dab1 expression was also reported in radial glia cells [109], and the morphology of these cells was shown to be affected by Reelin [110], raising the possibility that Reelin may target both principal neurons and radial glia cells, to regulate migration and cellular layer formation.

8. Cellular Mechanisms of *Reelin*-Dependent Neuronal Migration

With the development of novel techniques that enabled investigators to manipulate gene expression *in vivo* and to observe neuronal migration in cultured organotypic slices, new functional studies became possible. Using the GFP-labeling retroviral and confocal imaging approach pioneered by the Kriegstein Lab to study cortical migration in rat cultures [80], investigators reported that Dab1 mutant (*scrambler*) neurons maintain an increased adhesion to radial glia fibers which prevents them from reaching the upper cortical layers [111]. This view seemed to lend support to earlier hypotheses postulating that the *reeler* defect was essentially due to excessive cellular adhesion, leading to an inability of newborn neurons to bypass previously generated cohorts and causing a traffic jam along radial fibers [9, 112]. This interpretation was challenged by later studies employing more sophisticated genetic tools [113]. Nevertheless, the first analysis of the migratory behavior of *scrambler* cortical neurons provided some important mechanistic insights into Reelin activity. Indeed, this study was the first to demonstrate that Dab1 is required to extend the leading processes of migrating neurons into the developing cortical plate. However, it did not identify

the target cells directly affected by Reelin, since the *scrambler* cortical slices lacked Dab1 in migrating cortical neurons as well as in radial glia. This issue was addressed in a following study, which utilized the newly developed technique of *in utero* electroporation [114] and RNA interference (RNAi) to suppress Dab1 expression specifically in a subset of migrating neurons [64]. Dab1 knockdown neurons were found to be deficient in their ability to extend the leading process and to translocate their cell bodies into the upper cortical layers. In addition to pointing out a mode of migration that may be exquisitely affected by Dab1 deficiency, this study also suggested that the apical processes of migrating neuron are essentially immature dendrites, and, in this context, Reelin stimulates the dendrite outgrowth, of neocortical pyramidal neurons, as it had been previously shown for hippocampal neurons [62]. Indeed, further studies demonstrated that Reelin controls neuronal orientation and polarized dendritic growth in the cortical plate as well as the developing cerebellum [63, 115, 116]. Together, these studies underscored the close functional link between cellular polarization, early dendrite outgrowth and neuronal migration. Despite these advances, many questions remained unanswered regarding the specific mode of migration affected by Reelin and Dab1 and the identity of the direct targets of Reelin during radial migration in the neocortex. These questions were finally answered through the development of a novel set of genetic tools, which enabled investigators to conditionally delete the *Dab1* gene in either early or late cortical neurons and examine their ability to undergo somal or glial-guide locomotion in cultured slices [113]. This study conclusively demonstrated that Reelin affects primarily somal translocation and that Dab1 is required in migrating neurons to extend their apical process into the superficial areas of the neocortex, thus enabling both somal translocation of early-born neurons from the ventricular zone and also the terminal translocation of late-born neurons that initially move by glial-guided locomotion past cohorts of previously generated neurons. A following study demonstrated that Reelin in the marginal zone promotes the adhesion, stabilization, and branching of Dab1-expressing apical processes by a cell-matrix adhesion mechanism mediated by Integrin $\alpha5\beta1$ [117]. However, this integrin may function in radial glia cells rather than in migrating neurons. Recently, another study documented heterotypic cell-cell interactions between migrating neurons and Cajal-Retzius cells, which are mediated by adhesion molecules nectin1 and nectin3 and by Cadherin 2 [118]. Cajal-Retzius cells express nectin1, which binds nectin3 on the cell surface of migrating neurons. Nectin3 and its associated effector afadin then mediate homophilic cell-cell adhesion via Cadherin 2 molecules, which are expressed by both cell types. These adhesion mechanisms allow for somal translocation to occur, bringing the cell bodies of migrating neurons just underneath the marginal zone, and explain why Reelin must be so strikingly localized to this zone during corticogenesis. They also reveal how Reelin (presumably in the form of a full-length protein, dimer, or insoluble multimer aggregate) conveys its short-range promigratory cue to neurons that come in contact with superficial layers via their apical process. But what about neurons that do not contact the marginal zone and are located in the deep regions of the intermediate zone during the development of the cortical plate? Most of these neurons exhibit an initial multipolar morphology and normally acquire a bipolar morphology just prior to engaging in radial migration. Are they responsive to Reelin, and how do they receive the signal? Earlier work using cortical slices demonstrated that soluble Reelin added to the culture medium was able to promote migration and layer formation, albeit not as neatly as *in vivo* [40]. This activity seemed unlikely to be spatially restricted to the marginal zone, but how would Reelin come in contact with these distant neurons *in vivo*? With the development of novel epitope-specific antibodies, it became possible to visualize Reelin fragments in brain sections [41]. These immunolabeling studies revealed that the central fragment of Reelin could reach the depth of the cortical plate, suggesting that the cleavage of the Reelin protein generates signaling molecules that may function at long range, away from the marginal zone. Consistently, a recent study revealed that Reelin affects the migratory behavior of neurons that are located deep into the developing cortical plate, by promoting the conversion from a multipolar to a bipolar morphology [119].

In summary, the data so far indicate that Reelin in the marginal zone promotes somal translocation of Dab1-expressing principal cortical neurons directly from the ventricular zone, or terminal translocation from the developing cortical plate, and thus acts directly on migrating neurons as long as they make contact with the marginal zone through an apical process. This function may be induced by full-length Reelin or fragments that assemble into oligomers to maximize signaling activity through the phosphorylation of Dab1. Reelin fragments may also diffuse into the depth of the cortical plate to promote the bipolar transformation and the oriented migration of Dab1-expressing neurons that do not contact the marginal zone. While it seems likely that these direct effects of Reelin on migrating cortical neurons do not require a radial glia scaffold, the possibility that Reelin also functions by affecting the stability and branching of the radial glia end feet cannot be excluded, particularly in structures such as the dentate gyrus where the radial scaffold could significantly contribute to the efficiency of migration.

9. Dab1 Signaling in the Control of *Reelin*-Dependent Neuronal Migration

In the section above, we discussed the crucial role of the adaptor protein Dab1 in Reelin-dependent neuronal migration. Here, we will discuss the molecular mechanisms linking Reelin to Dab1 activation and the downstream events that link Dab1 to the execution of the migration function.

Early studies demonstrated that full-length Reelin or its central fragment alone induces the phosphorylation of Dab1 on specific tyrosine residues [40, 94, 95]. These phosphorylation events are mediated by the SFKs *Fyn* and *Src*, since they are blocked by the pharmacological inhibitor PP2 and by the genetic deletion of *Fyn* and *Src* genes [96, 101]. The appearance of a *reeler*-like phenotype in phospho-mutant Dab1 mice [98], as well as double Fyn/Src knockout

mice [101], further demonstrated that these tyrosine phosphorylation events are crucial for Reelin-induced neuronal migration and layer formation. Given the importance of this signaling event, considerable efforts have been devoted over the years to understand how Dab1 phosphorylation is stimulated and what are the molecular consequences of this protein modification. However, signal transduction is often the result of a nonlinear series of intersecting events, and it soon became clear that Reelin signaling was not going to be an exception. Indeed, Reelin was found to stimulate Src phosphorylation (presumably reflecting an activation of multiple SFKs) in a manner that is dependent on the presence of Dab1 [97, 120]. Thus, it appears that a positive feedback mechanism potentiates SFK and Dab1 activation in response to Reelin. SFK activation likely plays a major role in Reelin signal transduction. For example, it was shown to be required for the activation of other downstream events such as the activation of the PI3K by Reelin. The activation of PI3K was deduced from the induction of downstream events, such as the phosphorylation of Akt and the phosphorylation of GSK3β on an Akt-dependent site (Ser9) and from the ability of the PI3K pharmacological inhibitor LY294002 to block both of these events [121]. It was later demonstrated that Reelin also increases the levels of Akt phosphorylation on the Thr308 residue, a site which is directly phosphorylated by the PI3K-dependent kinase Pdk1 [71]. In addition, Dab1 was found to interact directly with the PI3K regulatory subunit p85α in response to Reelin stimulation [122]. Further downstream of Akt, other phosphorylation events were identified linking Reelin signaling to the mTOR pathway. The mTOR kinase participates in two complexes: mTORC1, which is primarily implicated in the control of protein translation and cell growth, and mTORC2, which is principally involved in the regulation of cytoskeletal dynamics [123]. Reelin was found to stimulate mTOR phosphorylation and to promote the mTORC1-dependent phosphorylation of p70S6K and the ribosomal protein S6 [65, 71]. Thus, Reelin stimulates mTORC1 activity likely through SFK, PI3K, and Akt since p70S6K and S6 phosphorylation is blocked by the SFK inhibitor PP2 and by the PI3K inhibitor LY294002, in addition to the mTORC1 inhibitor rapamycin [71]. However, it should be noted that, since biochemical studies identified mTORC2 as the complex that directly phosphorylates Akt on Ser473 [124] and Reelin stimulates this phosphorylation event, mTORC2 may also participate in Reelin signaling. The mechanism of activation of mTORC2 by many extracellular signals is not completely clear; however, SFK, PI3K, and Akt are also likely to mediate Reelin-induced mTORC2 activation, since Ser473 Akt phosphorylation is blocked by SFK and PI3K inhibitors. Despite the abundance of biochemical evidence, the biological significance of PI3K and Akt activation in Reelin signaling is not entirely clear. *In vitro* pharmacological studies using cultures cortical slices initially suggested that the activation of PI3K and Akt may be important for the control of neural migration during early brain development, while the activation of the mTOR pathway may be more relevant to postnatal functions of Reelin, such as the modulation of dendrite elongation [65].

However, a genetic requirement for PI3K and Akt in neuronal migration has not been demonstrated. Furthermore, the analysis of recent knockout models lacking PI3K modulators, such as the Pten phosphatase (a suppressor of PI3K) [125] or PIKE (an enhancer of PI3K) suggests that this kinase is likely to be primarily involved in the control of neuronal growth, dendritogenesis, and survival rather than migration or layer formation [126]. Finally, it should be noted that Akt phosphorylation defects have not been reported in the embryonic brain of *reeler* or Dab1 mutant mice. Recent studies provided evidence that mTORC1 is involved in the NMDA-dependent rescue of synaptic plasticity and behavioral defects in juvenile *reeler* heterozygous mice [127]. Finally, basal levels of Akt phosphorylation were shown to be reduced in adult forebrain-specific conditional Dab1 knockout mice, which also exhibit plasticity and behavioral defects [128]. Together, these findings suggest that activation of the PI3K/Akt/mTOR pathway by Reelin may not play a crucial role in the early events leading to layer formation and corticogenesis but is likely to be involved in the postnatal control of neuronal maturation and synaptic plasticity.

Early efforts to identify potential downstream effectors of Dab1 in the control of migration pointed to components of the platelet activating factor (PAF) acetyl hydrolase 1b (Pafah1b) complex. This complex functions as a phospholipase and catalyzes the PAF lipid through the activity of two catalytic α subunits. The complex also contains a regulatory subunit, Lis1, which is involved in neuronal migration [129] and human lissencephaly [130, 131]. Genetic interactions and biochemical experiments indicated that Reelin promotes the interaction between Dab1 and Lis1 and that the absence of these two proteins cooperated to increase the frequency of hydrocephalus [132]. Further studies also demonstrated that the catalytic subunit of Pafah1b α2 binds to Dab1 and suppresses the hydrocephalus phenotype of Reelin/Lis double mutant mice [133, 134]. However, Lis1 turned out to control many aspects of neurogenesis and neuronal migration through a mechanism that involves the coupling of the centrosome to the nucleus [135]. This mechanism appears to be independent of both the catalytic activity of the Pafah1b complex and Reelin. Furthermore, genetic ablation of the catalytic subunits of Pafah1b did not result in neuronal migration defects [133]. Thus, this complex does not appear to be involved in the control of migration or corticogenesis; however, it may play a role in as yet unidentified mechanisms that contribute to normal brain development by preventing the onset of hydrocephalus.

Other biochemical studies identified several molecules that bind Dab1 and thus may potentially function in Reelin signaling. These include proteins that affect the actin cytoskeleton, such as Nckβ [136] and N-WASP [100], proteins that modulate the activity of the Ras/Rap family of GTP-binding proteins, such as the GTPase activating protein (GAP) Dab2IP [137], and Crk family proteins [93, 138]. Recent RNA interference studies and knockout studies suggest that Dab2IP is required for neuronal migration in the neocortex [139] and for dendrite and synapse development

in the cerebellum [140]. However, its direct involvement in Reelin signaling has not yet been established. Crk family proteins, on the other hand, have been shown to play a significant role in Reelin-dependent migration, likely by binding the GTP exchange factor (GEF) C3G, which then activates Rap1 [93]. Three members of this family, CrkI, Crk II, and CrkL, were shown to bind phospho-Dab1, and Reelin was shown to induce the phosphorylation of C3G and the activation of Rap1. This study suggested that the CrkL/C3G/Rap1 pathway operates downstream of Dab1 in Reelin-stimulated neurons. However, CrkI and II, but not CrkL, were also shown to promote Dab1 phosphorylation in an SFK-dependent manner, suggesting a more complex signaling mechanism [138]. The biological relevance of Crk family proteins in neuronal migration was demonstrated *in vivo* by the conditional double knockout of Crk and CrkL in neural progenitor cells. In a situation analogous to that of Fyn and Src, single Crk or CrkL mutant mice displayed mild neuroanatomical phenotypes, but double Crk/CrkL mutant mice displayed a *reeler*-like phenotype [141]. The absence of Crk and CrkL did not affect Dab1 phosphorylation but, surprisingly, hindered the ability of Reelin to phosphorylate not only C3G, but also Akt on Ser473. Because this site is a target of mTORC2, these findings raise the possibility that Crks transduce Reelin signaling downstream to Rap1 as well as mTORC2.

The role of Rap1 in Reelin signaling and radial migration was further explored in multiple *in vivo* studies. In one study, Rap1 was shown to regulate the expression of cell adhesion molecules of the Cadherin family in migrating neurons, an event that is required for glia-independent migration [113]. Specifically, in this study, it was proposed that Rap1 promotes Cadherin expression, which in turn favors the extension and attachment of leading processes of migrating neurons and enables terminal translocation near the upper cortical plate. In a second study, Rap1 was shown to regulate the membrane localization of N-Cadherin [119]. This event was linked specifically to the acquisition of proper cellular orientation, which is also required for glia-independent neuronal migration, but occurs in the deeper regions of the developing cortical plate. Building on these observations, recent studies further investigated the role of the Crk/C3G/Rap1 pathway in Reelin-dependent migration and provided a comprehensive view of its molecular mechanisms [117, 118]. This work suggested that Rap1 has a dual function in migration. In deep regions of the cortical plate, Rap1 functions through N-Cadherins to orient cell bodies and enable entry into the cortical plate, but this activity may not be stimulated by C3G. Near the upper cortical plate, Reelin strongly activates C3G and Rap1, and this in turn leads to the activation of $\alpha5\beta1$ integrins, which mediate the attachment of apical processes to fibronectin in the marginal zone, and the recruitment of cell adhesion molecules such as nectins and Cadherin 2, which mediate cell-cell interactions in the marginal zone. Together, these secreted and contact-dependent mechanisms enable terminal translocation and the completion of radial migration near the Reelin-rich marginal zone.

10. *Reelin* Receptors and the Control of Neuronal Migration

The body of work discussed above described in considerable detail the cellular and molecular mechanisms of neuronal migration which operate immediately upstream and downstream of Dab1 during Reelin signal transduction. This section will address the receptor activation mechanisms leading to Dab1 recruitment at the plasma membrane. What are the Reelin receptors, and how do they cause SFK activation and Dab1 phosphorylation?

Based on extensive genetic and biochemical studies, two high-affinity Reelin receptors have been identified and shown to play a major role in Reelin signaling. They are the apolipoprotein E receptor 2 (ApoER2) and the very-low-density lipoprotein receptor (VLDLR) [33, 142]. These two receptors are members of the lipoprotein receptor superfamily [143], and their involvement in Reelin signaling was first suggested by the observation that double Apoer2/Vldlr knockout mice exhibit a *reeler*-like neuroanatomic phenotype [102]. Single knockout mice displayed a milder layer phenotype, suggesting that they have partially overlapping functions in mediating the activity of Reelin on neuronal migration. Biochemical experiments *in vivo* and *in vitro* demonstrated that ApoER2 and VLDLR are each capable of binding Reelin with similar affinity [33, 142, 144]. Like all members of the lipoprotein receptor superfamily, ApoER2 and VLDLR can also bind lipoproteins and other extracellular ligands with lower affinity. Upon binding, these receptors internalize their ligand, including Reelin, a process that requires the NPxY motif, an internalization domain present on the cytoplasmic tail of the receptors. The receptors also bind Dab1 on their cytoplasmic tail near their NPxY motif [86, 145]. On the Dab1 side, binding to the receptors is mediated by the pleckstrin homology/phosphotyrosine binding domain (PH/PTB) [87, 145, 146]. ApoER2 and VLDLR actively traffic between the plasma membrane and the endosomes, and their translocation to the plasma membrane is facilitated by Dab1 binding [146]. Upon Reelin binding, the receptors cluster and internalize [147], thereby causing the activation of Fyn and Src, which then phosphorylate Dab1 and initiate downstream signaling events crucial for migration. Despite their partially redundant function, there are differences between ApoER2 and VLDLR signaling. Some of the differences can be attributed to relative receptor expression. For example, VLDLR is more highly expressed in the Purkinje cells of the cerebellum, and single VLDLR knockout mice exhibit defects in this structure, whereas ApoER2 is preferentially expressed in cortical and hippocampal neurons, correlating with defects in forebrain structures of single *ApoER2* knock out mice [102]. However, the two receptors can bind distinct signaling proteins, in addition to Dab1. Indeed, VLDLR, but not ApoER2, has been found to bind subunits of the Pafah1b complex [148], whereas ApoER2, but not VLDLR, can bind JNK and activate the p38MAP kinase pathway [149]. However, it is not clear whether these unique interactions participate in the control of neuronal migration. Both ApoER2 and VLDLR bind Reelin through a similar extracellular domain that contains a conserved lysine residue [37]. It is thought that the strongest signal activation is achieved when the receptors bind multimeric aggregates of full-length Reelin, presumably leading to massive receptor clustering and SFK activation [42]. However, it has been shown that ApoER2 and VLDLR can also bind a central fragment of Reelin that is generated by proteolytic cleavage [40]. Functional studies demonstrated that binding of this fragment is sufficient to induce Dab1 phosphorylation and lead to layer formation in cultured cortical slices. These findings raised the question of whether Reelin cleavage is an event that dampens activity by reducing the levels of the more active full-length protein or enables activity by releasing the active central fragment from a precursor full-length protein. This question has not yet been resolved and awaits the identification of the specific sites of cleavage, as well as the identification of the proteases responsible for Reelin cleavage. In the meantime, the fact that N- and C-terminal Reelin fragments are generated by cleavage and that they do not bind ApoER2 and VLDLR raised the possibility that other receptors or coreceptors may participate in Reelin signaling and contribute to migration control.

Some of the earliest candidates as alternative Reelin receptors were integrins. Integrins $\alpha 3/\beta 1$ and $\alpha 5/\beta 1$ in particular were implicated in Reelin signaling by binding experiments [150]. However, this finding has not been replicated by others, and the analysis of knockout mice lacking several integrin subunits suggested that, while these proteins contribute to migration and layer formation, they may not be directly required for Reelin-dependent migration. Rather, knockout studies suggested that $\beta 1$ integrins are primarily required for the integrity of the glia limitans [151]. Thus, their loss disrupts cellular layer formation through disruption of the radial scaffold; however, it does not directly affect neuronal migration, and it does not result in a *reeler*-like phenotype, suggesting that $\beta 1$ integrins are not essential for Reelin signaling in neurons [152]. Given the recent studies discussed above [117], the role of integrins in Reelin signaling cannot be completely dismissed. However, it seems likely that $\beta 1$-containing integrins in the cerebral cortex function in radial glial cells rather than in migrating neurons. This view is consistent with previous data demonstrating that Reelin and $\beta 1$ integrins are required for the formation of the radial glial scaffold in the hippocampus [153].

Another family of proteins that have been proposed to function as Reelin receptors is the Cadherin-related neuronal receptor (CNR) family, particularly CNR1 [154]. CNR proteins were found to be expressed in migrating neurons, bind the N terminal region of Reelin, and also associate with the SFK Fyn on the intracellular side. Their expression pattern and binding properties made them excellent candidates as Reelin receptors or coreceptors. However, the binding of CNR1 to Reelin was not replicated by other investigators [40].

In the past couple of years, new potential Reelin receptor systems have surfaced. Ephrin B proteins were reported to bind the N terminal region of Reelin and claimed to be essential components of the Reelin pathway in the control of neuronal migration [155]. However, as evident from the published corrigendum and the multitude of online comments related to this paper, many questions about the validity of the findings have been raised. Nevertheless, further investigations of these receptors have been conducted. Since ephrin B proteins bind to the EphB family of transmembrane receptor tyrosine kinases, which transduce bidirectional tyrosine kinase-mediated signals to both the Eph receptor-expressing (forward signaling) and the ephrin-expressing cell (reverse signaling), the potential role of these kinases in brain development and Reelin signaling was also investigated. One study found that ephrin-B1 interacting with EphB2 controls the migration of dentate progenitor cells into the dorsal half of the developing dentate gyrus, perhaps in part by affecting Reelin expression [156]. Recently, a new study showed that the N terminal region of Reelin binds to the extracellular domains of EphB transmembrane proteins, inducing receptor clustering and activation of EphB forward signaling in neurons, independently of ApoER2 and VLDLR [157]. However, mice lacking EphBs displayed a very mild migration phenotype that was limited to a modest positioning defect of CA3 hippocampal-pyramidal neurons. Thus, even though there appears to be some signal integration between Reelin and ephrin/EphB receptors, the physiological significance of this interaction for neuronal migration is rather limited. Based on a recent study, it appears that ephrin/Eph signaling may be more important for mediating contact repulsion among Cajal-Retzius cells to ensure the even distribution of these neurons in the brain [158].

Overall, the data available so far indicate that the activity of Reelin in the control of neuronal migration is predominantly mediated by ApoER2 and VLDLR receptors, whose functions are overlapping but not identical. Both receptors are involved in the activation of SFKs, Dab1 phosphorylation on tyrosine residues, and the recruitment of Crk/CrkL, which lead to the activation of downstream events discussed above, which are essential for radial migration (Figure 2).

11. *Reelin*-Regulated Growth of Cellular Processes

In addition to controlling neuronal migration and layer formation in embryonic cortical structures, Reelin also plays an important role in promoting the growth and maturation of specific neuronal populations in the postnatal brain. As we mentioned above, the cellular source of Reelin in forebrain structures changes after birth. While Cajal-Retzius cells are the predominant population of Reelin-expressing cells in the marginal zone of the embryonic cerebral cortex and hippocampus, a subset of inhibitory, GABA-synthesizing neurons express Reelin and gradually become the predominant source of Reelin in the postnatal and adult forebrain [45, 68]. However, Cajal-Retzius cells are still present and remain the major source of Reelin during the first 1-2 weeks after birth in the early postnatal hippocampus. Transplantation studies demonstrated that this early postnatal source of Reelin is needed to promote the branching of axonal projections from the entorhinal-hippocampal pathway, which terminates in the marginal zone of the hippocampus and dentate gyrus (the outer molecular layer) [20, 58]. However, since Reelin is a secreted protein, its functional range needs not to be

limited to the growth of cellular processes that develop in the same layers that contain Reelin-expressing cells, that is, the marginal layers. Indeed, early studies had revealed extensive dendrite abnormalities throughout the hippocampus of homozygous *reeler* mice [60]. However, it was unclear from these anatomical observations whether dendrite defects were due primarily to cellular ectopia or were the direct result of Reelin deficiency. This issue was revised in recent years with a combination of novel *in vivo* and *in vitro* approaches. Taking advantage of a fluorescent transgene that was expressed in the postnatal forebrain, developing apical dendrites of dentate granule neurons were visualized in *reeler* mutant and control littermates. From this comparison, it was apparent that dendrite growth was delayed in *reeler* mice [62]. Furthermore, *in vitro* studies demonstrated that dendrite elongation and branching proceed at a reduced rate in immature hippocampal neurons obtained from *reeler* or Dab1 knockout mice and kept for 3–6 days *in vitro* (DIV), irrespective of neuronal positioning [62]. In this experimental assay, the addition of recombinant Reelin to the culture medium rescued the *reeler* defect in a manner that was dependent on the activity of lipoprotein receptors and Dab1. Thus, the same signaling pathway that controls neuronal migration before birth also mediated an early postnatal function of Reelin in the control of dendrite outgrowth, at least in immature hippocampal neurons. Following *in vitro* studies further revealed that the trophic effect of Reelin on dendrite outgrowth is dependent not only on Dab1 and lipoprotein receptors, but also on other previously identified components of Reelin signaling, including Src kinases, Crks, PI3K, and Akt [65, 159]. These studies also demonstrated that Reelin, acting through the well-known PI3K/Akt pathway, positively modulates the activity of the mTOR kinase, which is required for the stimulation of dendrite outgrowth, and activates downstream proteins, such as the p70S6K, that are known to participate in the control of protein translation. Few years later, other studies confirmed the activation of mTOR by Reelin and further demonstrated the increased phosphorylation of p70S6K and the downstream ribosomal protein S6, events that are completely dependent on SFK and PI3K activity [71]. To these days, however, the effects of Reelin on protein translation and its significance in terms of cell growth and dendrite morphogenesis have not been fully investigated.

In addition to the previously identified signaling cascade, the analysis of the molecular mechanisms of cellular and fiber layer formation led to the identification of potentially new players in Reelin signal transduction. A study revealed that serum response factor (SRF), a transcription factor that regulates synaptic-activity-induced immediate-early gene (IEG) induction and cytoskeleton-based neuronal motility, is important for hippocampal lamination and that this factor mediates the effect of Reelin on dendrite development [160]. This finding raised the intriguing possibility that Reelin might enhance F-actin stability by elevating IEG mRNA levels via SRF-dependent gene transcription. All the studies mentioned above utilized immature hippocampal cultures (3–6 DIV) and demonstrated a trophic effect of Reelin on the initial growth of dendrites. However, it should

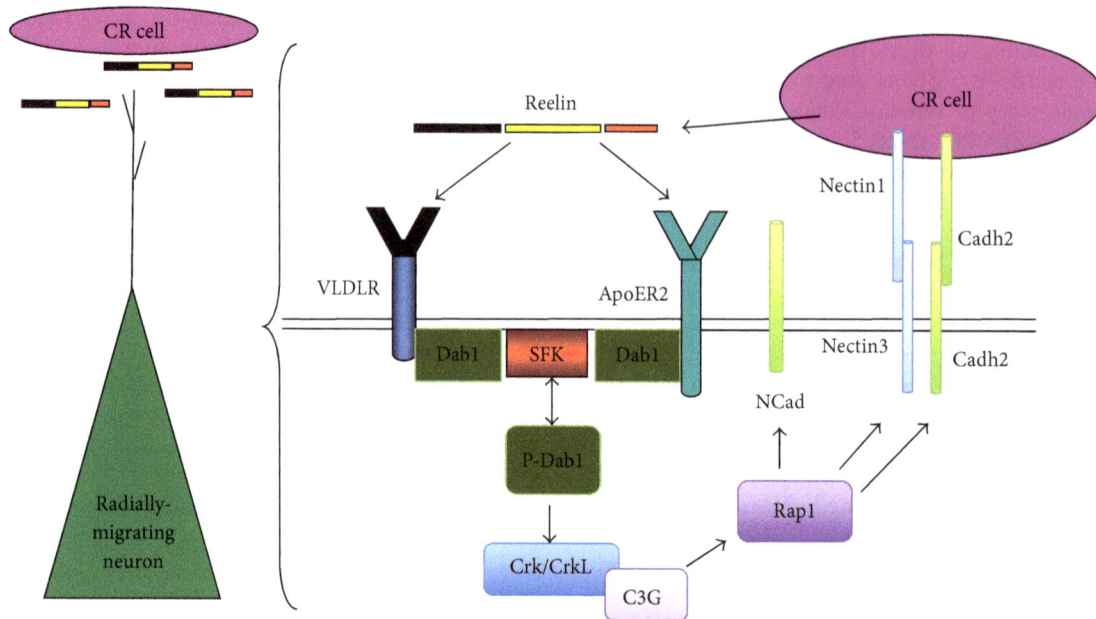

FIGURE 2: Diagram depicting the relationship between Reelin-secreting surface neurons and radially migrating neurons expressing the core signaling machinery (right). Surface neurons such as Cajal-Retzius cells (CR) secrete Reelin, which through its central region (yellow region) binds VLDLR and ApoER2 receptors on the surface of radially-migrating neurons. Ligand binding causes the activation of SFKs Src and Fyn, and the phosphorylation of the Dab1 adaptor protein. This event results in the recruitment of Crk/CrkL adaptor proteins mediate further downstream signaling through C3G and Rap1, resulting in the surface expression of N-Cadherin (Ncad), which is required for radial orientation, and activation of Nectin1-Nectin3, and homophilic Cadherin 2 (Cadh2) cell-cell interactions that are required to complete radial migration by somal translocation.

be noted that *in vitro* studies utilizing mature hippocampal cultures (18–20 DIV) obtained from Dab1 knockout mice demonstrated that, although Reelin-Dab1 signaling promotes initial hippocampal dendrite development, it is not required for neurons to reach full maturity [67]. Thus, as for entorhi-nohippocampal axons, hippocampal dendrite outgrowth is stimulated by Reelin during early neuronal development, but neurons do not require Reelin signaling to reach their full morphological maturity, as other growth factors likely compensate and promote the growth of these processes even in the absence of Reelin signaling.

What cellular mechanisms underlie the control of neurite development by Reelin? Recent studies showed that the Golgi apparatus is abnormal in *reeler* and Dab1 knockout mice and that Reelin treatment rapidly induced the deployment of the Golgi apparatus into dendrites of cultured neurons [66]. Mechanistically, it was demonstrated that Reelin-Dab1 signaling antagonizes the effects of Stk25, a scaffolding protein that links the LKB1-STRAD-GM130 complex to neuronal polarization. Other studies have shown that Reelin increases growth cone motility and filopodia formation, through activation of the Rho GTPase Cdc42, in an ApoER2-, Dab1-, and PI3K-dependent manner [161]. Building on these findings, a recent study further demonstrated that the Cdc42/Rac1 guanine nucleotide exchange factor αPIX/Arhgef6 promoted translocation of Golgi cisternae into developing dendrites of hippocampal neurons [162]. Reelin increased the αPIX-dependent effect and promoted the translocation of the Golgi apparatus into the dendrite that was most proximal to the Reelin source. These observations led to the interesting

conclusion that the spatial distribution of Reelin may contribute to the selection of the neuritic process that becomes the apical dendrite.

In addition to *in vitro* studies, *in vivo* studies demonstrated that the effect of Reelin on dendrite development is closely coupled to neuronal migration and is an important aspect of cellular layer formation. An examination of the morphology of Dab1 knockdown neurons in the late embryonic and early postnatal neocortex revealed simplified leading processes that were less likely to contact the Reelin-rich marginal zone [64]. These data confirmed a cell-autonomous role of Dab1 in dendritogenesis in the neocortex and suggested that remodeling of the leading process of a migrating neuron into a nascent dendrite by Reelin/Dab1 signaling plays an important role in final cell positioning. Furthermore, it was shown that Reelin injection *in vivo* caused deep cortical neurons to reorient their nuclei and polarize their Golgi toward the pia while initiating exuberant dendritic outgrowth within few hours [63]. Thus, Reelin exerts a direct role in promoting the rapid morphological differentiation and orientation of deep cortical neurons during early corticogenesis.

Finally, other *in vivo* studies indicated that Reelin not only promotes growth but also promotes the selective pruning of dendritic process in cortical neurons [163]. This study implicated serotonin 5-HT(3) receptor and Reelin signaling in the control of the complexity of apical dendrites of cortical layer II/III pyramidal neurons. Relevant to Reelin activity, these authors found that injection of Reelin antibodies resulted in increased dendritic complexity, whereas the application of recombinant full-length Reelin rescued this defect. Surprisingly, however, they found that pruning was also achieved when the N-terminal fragment, but not the central fragment of Reelin, was injected. This study also suggested that the N terminal region of Reelin mediates dendrite refinement through receptors other than ApoER2 and VLDLR, consistent with previous observations that only the central fragment of Reelin can bind and engage these receptors [40]. The mechanisms of the Reelin-mediated regulation of dendrite growth may thus be more complex than initially envisioned, and it may vary depending on the cell type examined. For example, other investigators found that the amyloid precursor protein (APP) promotes the growth of cortical dendrites *in vivo* and is required for Reelin-induced dendrite growth in cultured hippocampal neurons [164]. This finding builds on previous reports that APP family members interact with Dab1 due to their NPxY motif [85, 86] and that Reelin signaling affects APP processing [165]. Mechanistically, the new study found that APP interacts with the central fragment of Reelin and with $\alpha 3\beta 1$ integrin. Since an $\alpha 3\beta 1$ antibody prevented APP and Reelin-induced neurite outgrowth, this study implicated integrins in Reelin signaling controlling neurite development.

12. Reelin Functions in Synaptogenesis and Spine Formation

As postnatal development continues and Cajal-Retzius cells progressively disappear from the forebrain, the expression of Reelin becomes predominantly localized to interneurons. A subset of GABAergic interneurons express Reelin throughout all cellular layers of the rodent neocortex and hippocampus at postnatal and adult ages [45, 68]. Since its early discovery, the physiological role of this new pattern of expression has been the subject of intense inquiry, given that the function of Reelin in the late postnatal and adult forebrain could no longer be related to neuronal migration or dendrite development in these brain regions. Attention turned to synapse development and function, since these biological processes predominate at later postnatal ages. The first documented evidence that Reelin plays a role in synapse formation in the forebrain related to the development of entorhinohippocampal connections [58]. Since Reelin had previously been implicated in the branching of this axonal projection, the finding appeared to be a logical extension of previous observations: the more axonal terminals are formed, the more they can synapse on hippocampal target cells. Therefore, the effect on synapse development initially appeared indirect and secondary to that on axonal branching. Nevertheless, adding support to a role for Reelin signaling in synaptogenesis, few years later came the observation that Reelin and Dab1 modulate the structure and function of retinal synaptic circuitry [19]. This paper showed that, even though there is no cellular ectopia in the highly laminated structure of the retina in *reeler* or Dab1 mutant mice, connectivity defects are present which ultimately lead to altered physiological responses. Thus, this paper was significant because it highlighted a role for the Reelin pathway in the formation and functional output of a specific synaptic circuitry, independent of cell position. In

the retina, Reelin is expressed not only by retinal ganglion cells, but also by some amacrine and cone bipolar cells, whereas Dab1 is expressed almost exclusively by AII amacrine cells [19]. These Dab1-positive cells play an essential role in mediating Reelin signaling and establishing retinal synaptic circuitry. A recent study revealed that, as in other parts of the central nervous system, ApoER2 and VLDLR function as Reelin receptors and are both required for the establishment and maintenance of normal retinal synaptic connectivity [166]. However, they appear to contribute differently to the development and maintenance of retinal synaptic connectivity. ApoER2 is predominantly expressed by both AII amacrine cells and other amacrine or bipolar cells in the developing retina and plays a role in the development of the rod bipolar pathway, whereas VLDLR is required for the establishment of oscillatory potentials [166].

In the forebrain, studies of heterozygous *reeler* mice emphasized a direct role for Reelin in the control of synaptogenesis, particularly in the formation of the excitatory postsynaptic structures. Heterozygous *reeler* mice express half the *Reln* mRNA levels of wild type mice and appear phenotypically normal in that they do not exhibit ataxia or layer defects in any brain region [1]. However, these mice exhibit behavioral and cognitive defects reminiscent of those found in human psychoses [167, 168] and are thus considered animal models for the disease [169]. The behavioral phenotype of heterozygous *reeler* mice has been challenged by other investigators [170] however, these mice do appear to have subtle anatomical abnormalities that would account for functional connectivity problems. For example, they exhibit delayed growth of dendritic processes in hippocampal neurons [62] and a reduction in the density of synaptic contacts in the frontal [171] and prefrontal cortex [127]. Defects in dendritic spine density were also found in the hippocampus of heterozygous *reeler* and Dab1 knockout mice, accompanied by altered molecular composition of the synaptosomes [70]. This study also showed that Reelin treatment rescued spine density defects of *reeler* organotypic hippocampal slices in a manner that was dependent on all core components of the signaling pathway, namely, the lipoprotein receptors ApoER2 and VLDLR, SFKs and Dab1 [70]. Follow-up studies revealed that defects in spine density are transient in heterozygous *reeler* mice and essentially disappear in adult mice by 2 months of age; however, the expression of postsynaptic proteins, including NMDA receptor subunits, remains altered [71]. In a complementary study, other investigators examined spine density and size in transgenic mice that overexpressed Reelin and found that Reelin overexpression caused an increase in spine size but did not change spine density in hippocampal regions [75]. Consistent with this view, a recent study in which a single dose of Reelin was injected in the hippocampus of live adult mice indicated that acute administration of Reelin alters dendritic spine morphology but not spine density [172]. In contrast, long-term administration (5 days) of Reelin *in vivo* also increases spine density [173]. Taken together, these studies suggest that subthreshold levels of Reelin are deleterious because they delay the normal development of excitatory synapses, but a chronic excess of Reelin may also be disruptive because it alters spine morphology and number. Finally, it should be noted that reduced spontaneous inhibitory postsynaptic potentials have been reported in adult *reeler* heterozygous mice [167], suggesting that Reelin may play a significant role in the development of inhibitory synapses. However, this topic has not been yet investigated at a cellular and molecular level.

13. Adult Function of *Reelin* in the Modulation of Synaptic Activity

Reelin-expressing interneurons in the adult forebrain were identified as a heterogeneous population of bitufted, horizontal, and multipolar cells coexpressing either calretinin, calbindin, somatostatin, or NPY but not parvalbumin [45, 68]. A similar pattern of Reelin expression in selected interneurons was also observed in primates at postnatal ages [174]. In humans, the selective expression of Reelin in interneurons, together with the observed decrease in the expression of Reelin [25] and other interneuron markers in the postmortem brains of schizophrenic patients, led to the hypothesis that Reelin deficiency contributes to interneuron dysfunction in this disorder [30]. Reelin deficiency is recapitulated in the heterozygous *reeler* mouse, which exhibited subtle neuroanatomical abnormalities, such as decreased neuropil and dendritic spine density [70, 171], reminiscent of the changes reported in the brain of schizophrenia patients [175]. Heterozygous *reeler* mice also exhibit altered hippocampal synaptic function [167] and multiple behavioral abnormalities that parallel those noted in schizophrenia, such as defects in executive function [170, 176], contextual fear conditioning learning, and crossmodal prepulse inhibition [167, 177]. Thus, these mutant mice are useful models for understanding the cellular basis of behavioral and cognitive defects characterizing schizophrenia [169].

What is the significance of normal adult Reelin expression? Histochemical and ultrastructural studies revealed that extracellular Reelin accumulates around synapses [174, 178–180], leading to the suggestion that it may play a role in synaptic function. Indeed, a large body of evidence now suggests that this is the main function of Reelin in the adult brain. The first direct evidence that Reelin regulates synaptic function came from physiological studies using hippocampal slice cultures. In this acute *in vitro* system, Reelin treatment was shown to promote robust long-term potentiation (LTP) [181]. This study also showed that Reelin promotes hippocampal LTP in a manner that is dependent on both VLDLR and ApoER2. However, a following study further revealed that a particular splicing variant of ApoER2 capable of interacting with the NMDA receptor through PSD95 was required for Reelin-induced LTP [149, 181]. A number of electrophysiological studies using dissociated neuronal cultures demonstrated that Reelin increases synaptic activity by affecting postsynaptic NMDA and AMPA receptor activity [182–186] and also promotes neurotransmitter release [187]. Long-term Reelin treatment was found to alter the subunit composition of the NMDA receptor, favoring maturation of this receptor, and to increase AMPA receptor insertion

in the plasma membrane, thus reducing the number of silent synapses. Other studies further demonstrated that the LTP enhancement by brief Reelin stimulation is associated with increased Ca^{++} influx through the NMDA receptor [149, 183, 186]. Using an *in vivo* approach, the effect of chronic exposure was examined in transgenic mice that overexpressed Reelin under the control of the adult-forebrain specific CamKIIα promoter [75]. Reelin overexpressing mice displayed a dramatic dendritic spine hypertrophy but no changes in synaptic density, suggesting a specific function in the control of the size of excitatory synapses, which is highly related to their level of activity. Physiological recordings from hippocampal slices further documented an increase in LTP responses as well as neuronal activity during classical conditioning [75]. Using a different *in vivo* approach, other investigators injected Reelin directly into the hippocampus of adult mice and documented increases in synaptic plasticity, which correlated with enhanced cognitive performance in hippocampal-dependent tasks [173]. The role of Dab1 signaling in adult synaptic plasticity and learning was very recently addressed in a study that also utilized the adult-forebrain specific CamKIIα promoter, this time to drive conditional *Dab1* gene deletion [128]. This study demonstrated the critical role of Dab1, not only in mediating hippocampal LTP and especially the enhancing effect of Reelin on LTP, but also in modulating basal and plasticity-induced Erk signaling, and promoting hippocampal-dependent associative learning and the consolidation of long-term spatial memory.

Taken together, these findings indicate that Reelin-Dab1 signaling plays an important role in modulating synaptic function in the adult forebrain and significantly affects memory formation and cognitive function. The observed effects of Reelin signaling on synaptic development and function suggest that this pathway is potentially an excellent target for intervention in the treatment of cognitive diseases associated with Reelin deficiency, such as schizophrenia, autism, epilepsy, or Alzheimer's disease. The involvement of Reelin in neurodevelopmental or neurodegenerative disease and the potential implications for treatment have been recently reviewed and discussed in detail [28, 188]. However, further studies are needed to fully understand the impact of the Reelin signaling pathway on brain development and function in order to develop effective and safe therapeutic agents.

Conflict of Interests

The author declares that there is no conflict of interests regarding the publication of this paper.

References

[1] G. D'Arcangelo, G. G. Miao, S.-C. Chen, H. D. Soares, J. I. Morgan, and T. Curran, "A protein related to extracellular matrix proteins deleted in the mouse mutant reeler," *Nature*, vol. 374, no. 6524, pp. 719–723, 1995.

[2] J. B. Angevine Jr. and R. L. Sidman, "Autoradiographic study of cell migration during histogenesis of cerebral cortex in the mouse," *Nature*, vol. 192, no. 4804, pp. 766–768, 1961.

[3] V. S. Caviness Jr. and P. Rakic, "Mechanisms of cortical development: a view from mutations in mice," *Annual Review of Neuroscience*, vol. 1, pp. 297–326, 1978.

[4] D. S. Falconer, "Two new mutants, "trembler" and "reeler", with neurological actions in the house mouse (Mus musculus L.)," *Journal of Genetics*, vol. 50, no. 2, pp. 192–205, 1951.

[5] A. M. Goffinet, "Events governing organization of postmigratory neurons: studies on brain development in normal and reeler mice," *Brain Research*, vol. 319, no. 3, pp. 261–296, 1984.

[6] C. Lambert de Rouvroit and A. M. Goffinet, "The reeler mouse as a model of brain development," *Advances in Anatomy, Embryology, and Cell Biology*, vol. 150, pp. 1–106, 1998.

[7] J. Mariani, F. Crepel, K. Mikoshiba, J. P. Changeux, and C. Sotelo, "Anatomical, physiological and biochemical studies of the cerebellum from Reeler mutant mouse," *Philosophical Transactions of the Royal Society of London. Series B*, vol. 281, no. 978, pp. 1–28, 1977.

[8] K. Mikoshiba, S. Kohsaka, and K. Takamatsu, "Morphological and biochemical studies on the cerebral cortex from reeler mutant mice: development of cortical layers and metabolic mapping by the deoxyglucose method," *Journal of Neurochemistry*, vol. 34, no. 4, pp. 835–844, 1980.

[9] M. C. Pinto Lord, P. Evrard, and V. S. Caviness Jr., "Obstructed neuronal migration along radial glial fibers in the neocortex of the Reeler mouse: a Golgi-EM analysis," *Developmental Brain Research*, vol. 4, no. 4, pp. 379–393, 1982.

[10] P. Rakic and V. S. Caviness Jr., "Cortical development: view from neurological mutants two decades later," *Neuron*, vol. 14, no. 6, pp. 1101–1104, 1995.

[11] S. Hirotsune, T. Takahara, N. Sasaki et al., "The reeler gene encodes a protein with an EGF-like motif expressed by pioneer neurons," *Nature Genetics*, vol. 10, no. 1, pp. 77–83, 1995.

[12] S. Kikkawa, T. Yamamoto, K. Misaki et al., "Missplicing resulting from a short deletion in the reelin gene causes reeler-like neuronal disorders in the mutant shaking rat Kawasaki," *Journal of Comparative Neurology*, vol. 463, no. 3, pp. 303–315, 2003.

[13] N. Yokoi, M. Namae, H.-Y. Wang et al., "Rat neurological disease creeping is caused by a mutation in the reelin gene," *Molecular Brain Research*, vol. 112, no. 1-2, pp. 1–7, 2003.

[14] U. DeSilva, G. D'Arcangelo, V. V. Braden et al., "The human reelin gene: isolation, sequencing, and mapping on chromosome 7," *Genome Research*, vol. 7, no. 2, pp. 157–164, 1997.

[15] S. E. Hong, Y. Y. Shugart, D. T. Huang et al., "Autosomal recessive lissencephaly with cerebellar hypoplasia is associated with human RELN mutations," *Nature Genetics*, vol. 26, no. 1, pp. 93–96, 2000.

[16] P. E. Phelps, R. Rich, S. Dupuy-Davies, Y. Ríos, and T. Wong, "Evidence for a cell-specific action of Reelin in the spinal cord," *Developmental Biology*, vol. 244, no. 1, pp. 180–198, 2002.

[17] M. D. Kubasak, R. Brooks, S. Chen, S. A. Villeda, and P. E. Phelps, "Developmental distribution of reelin-positive cells and their secreted product in the rodent spinal cord," *Journal of Comparative Neurology*, vol. 468, no. 2, pp. 165–178, 2004.

[18] J. W. Yip, Y. P. L. Yip, K. Nakajima, and C. Capriotti, "Reelin controls position of autonomic neurons in the spinal cord," *Proceedings of the National Academy of Sciences of the United States of America*, vol. 97, no. 15, pp. 8612–8616, 2000.

[19] D. S. Rice, S. Nusinowitz, A. M. Azimi, A. Martínez, E. Soriano, and T. Curran, "The Reelin pathway modulates the structure and fof retinal synaptic circuitry," *Neuron*, vol. 31, no. 6, pp. 929–941, 2001.

[20] J. A. Del Río, B. Heimrich, V. Borrell et al., "A role for Cajal-retzius cells and reelin in the development of hippocampal connections," *Nature*, vol. 385, no. 6611, pp. 70–74, 1997.

[21] T. Deller, A. Drakew, B. Heimrich, E. Förster, A. Tielsch, and M. Frotscher, "The hippocampus of the reeler mutant mouse: fiber segregation in area CA1 depends on the position of the postsynaptic target cells," *Experimental Neurology*, vol. 156, no. 2, pp. 254–267, 1999.

[22] I. Royaux, C. L. De Rouvroit, G. D'Arcangelo, D. Demirov, and A. M. Goffinet, "Genomic organization of the mouse reelin gene," *Genomics*, vol. 46, no. 2, pp. 240–250, 1997.

[23] Y. Chen, R. P. Sharma, R. H. Costa, E. Costa, and D. R. Grayson, "On the epigenetic regulation of the human reelin promoter," *Nucleic Acids Research*, vol. 30, no. 13, pp. 2930–2939, 2002.

[24] C. P. Mitchell, Y. Chen, M. Kundakovic, E. Costa, and D. R. Grayson, "Histone deacetylase inhibitors decrease reelin promoter methylation in vitro," *Journal of Neurochemistry*, vol. 93, no. 2, pp. 483–492, 2005.

[25] F. Impagnatiello, A. R. Guidotti, C. Pesold et al., "A decrease of reelin expression as a putative vulnerability factor in schizophrenia," *Proceedings of the National Academy of Sciences of the United States of America*, vol. 95, no. 26, pp. 15718–15723, 1998.

[26] A. Guidotti, J. Auta, J. M. Davis et al., "Decrease in reelin and glutamic acid decarboxylase67 (GAD67) expression in schizophrenia and bipolar disorder: a postmortem brain study," *Archives of General Psychiatry*, vol. 57, no. 11, pp. 1061–1069, 2000.

[27] S. H. Fatemi, "The role of Reelin in pathology of autism," *Molecular Psychiatry*, vol. 7, no. 9, pp. 919–920, 2002.

[28] T. D. Folsom and S. H. Fatemi, "The involvement of Reelin in neurodevelopmental disorders," *Neuropharmacology*, vol. 68, pp. 122–135, 2012.

[29] D. R. Grayson, Y. Chen, E. Costa et al., "The human reelin gene: transcription factors (+), repressors (−) and the methylation switch (+/−) in schizophrenia," *Pharmacology and Therapeutics*, vol. 111, no. 1, pp. 272–286, 2006.

[30] A. Guidotti, J. Auta, J. M. Davis et al., "GABAergic dysfunction in schizophrenia: new treatment strategies on the horizon," *Psychopharmacology*, vol. 180, no. 2, pp. 191–205, 2005.

[31] G. D'Arcangelo, K. Nakajima, T. Miyata, M. Ogawa, K. Mikoshiba, and T. Curran, "Reelin is a secreted glycoprotein recognized by the CR-50 monoclonal antibody," *Journal of Neuroscience*, vol. 17, no. 1, pp. 23–31, 1997.

[32] M. Ogawa, T. Miyata, K. Nakajima et al., "The realer gene-associated antigen on cajal-retzius neurons is a crucial molecule for laminar organization of cortical neurons," *Neuron*, vol. 14, no. 5, pp. 899–912, 1995.

[33] G. D'Arcangelo, R. Homayouni, L. Keshvara, D. S. Rice, M. Sheldon, and T. Curran, "Reelin is a ligand for lipoprotein receptors," *Neuron*, vol. 24, no. 2, pp. 471–479, 1999.

[34] T. Miyata, K. Nakajima, K. Mikoshiba, and M. Ogawa, "Regulation of Purkinje cell alignment by Reelin as revealed with CR-50 antibody," *Journal of Neuroscience*, vol. 17, no. 10, pp. 3599–3609, 1997.

[35] M. Sinagra, D. Verrier, D. Frankova et al., "Reelin, very-low-density lipoprotein receptor, and apolipoprotein E receptor 2 control somatic NMDA receptor composition during hippocampal maturation in vitro," *Journal of Neuroscience*, vol. 25, no. 26, pp. 6127–6136, 2005.

[36] K.-I. Kubo, K. Mikoshiba, and K. Nakajima, "Secreted Reelin molecules form homodimers," *Neuroscience Research*, vol. 43, no. 4, pp. 381–388, 2002.

[37] N. Yasui, T. Nogi, T. Kitao, Y. Nakano, M. Hattori, and J. Takagi, "Structure of a receptor-binding fragment of reelin and mutational analysis reveal a recognition mechanism similar to endocytic receptors," *Proceedings of the National Academy of Sciences of the United States of America*, vol. 104, no. 24, pp. 9988–9993, 2007.

[38] Y. Nakano, T. Kohno, T. Hibi et al., "The extremely conserved C-terminal region of Reelin is not necessary for secretion but is required for efficient activation of downstream signaling," *Journal of Biological Chemistry*, vol. 282, no. 28, pp. 20544–20552, 2007.

[39] V. de Bergeyck, B. Naerhuyzen, A. M. Goffinet, and C. Lambert de Rouvroit, "A panel of monoclonal antibodies against reelin, the extracellular matrix protein defective in reeler mutant mice," *Journal of Neuroscience Methods*, vol. 82, no. 1, pp. 17–24, 1998.

[40] Y. Jossin, N. Ignatova, T. Hiesberger, J. Herz, C. Lambert De Rouvroit, and A. M. Goffinet, "The central fragment of Reelin, generated by proteolytic processing in vivo, is critical to its function during cortical plate development," *Journal of Neuroscience*, vol. 24, no. 2, pp. 514–521, 2004.

[41] Y. Jossin, L. Gui, and A. M. Goffinet, "Processing of Reelin by embryonic neurons is important for function in tissue but not in dissociated cultured neurons," *Journal of Neuroscience*, vol. 27, no. 16, pp. 4243–4252, 2007.

[42] N. Utsunomiya-Tate, K.-I. Kubo, S.-I. Tate et al., "Reelin molecules assemble together to form a large protein complex, which is inhibited by the function-blocking CR-50 antibody," *Proceedings of the National Academy of Sciences of the United States of America*, vol. 97, no. 17, pp. 9729–9734, 2000.

[43] Y. Ikeda and T. Terashima, "Expression of reelin, the gene responsible for the Reeler mutation, in embryonic development and adulthood in the mouse," *Developmental Dynamics*, vol. 210, pp. 157–172, 1997.

[44] S. N. Schiffmann, "Reelin mRNA expression during mouse brain development," *European Journal of Neuroscience*, vol. 9, no. 5, pp. 1055–1071, 1997.

[45] S. Alcántara, M. Ruiz, G. D'Arcangelo et al., "Regional and cellular patterns of reelin mRNA expression in the forebrain of the developing and adult mouse," *Journal of Neuroscience*, vol. 18, no. 19, pp. 7779–7799, 1998.

[46] T. Miyata, K. Nakajima, J. Aruga et al., "Distribution of the reeler gene-related antigen in the developing cerebellum: an immunohistochemical study with an allogenic antibody CR-50 on normal and reeler mice," *Journal of Comparative Neurology*, vol. 372, pp. 215–228, 1996.

[47] A. Drakew, M. Frotscher, T. Deller, M. Ogawa, and B. Heimrich, "Developmental distribution of a reeler gene-related antigen in the rat hippocampal formation visualized by CR-50 immunocytochemistry," *Neuroscience*, vol. 82, no. 4, pp. 1079–1086, 1997.

[48] G. Meyer, J. M. Soria, J. R. Martinez-Galan, B. Martin-Clemente, and A. Fairen, "Different origins and developmental histories of transient neurons in the marginal zone of the fetal and neonatal rat cortex," *Journal of Comparative Neurology*, vol. 397, pp. 493–518, 1998.

[49] G. Meyer and A. M. Goffinet, "Prenatal development of Reelin-immunoreactive neurons in the human neocortex," *Journal of Comparative Neurology*, vol. 397, pp. 29–40, 1998.

[50] E. Förster, S. Zhao, and M. Frotscher, "Laminating the hippocampus," *Nature Reviews Neuroscience*, vol. 7, no. 4, pp. 259–267, 2006.

[51] V. Duveau, A. Madhusudan, M. Caleo, I. Knuesel, and J.-M. Fritschy, "Impaired reelin processing and secretion by Cajal-Retzius cells contributes to granule cell dispersion in a mouse model of temporal lobe epilepsy," *Hippocampus*, vol. 21, no. 9, pp. 935–944, 2011.

[52] C. A. Haas, O. Dudeck, M. Kirsch et al., "Role for reelin in the development of granule cell dispersion in temporal lobe epilepsy," *Journal of Neuroscience*, vol. 22, no. 14, pp. 5797–5802, 2002.

[53] C. Heinrich, N. Nitta, A. Flubacher et al., "Reelin deficiency and displacement of mature neurons, but not neurogenesis, underlie the formation of granule cell dispersion in the epileptic hippocampus," *Journal of Neuroscience*, vol. 26, no. 17, pp. 4701–4713, 2006.

[54] A. M. Goffinet, "The embryonic development of the cerebellum in normal and reeler mutant mice," *Anatomy and Embryology*, vol. 168, no. 1, pp. 73–86, 1983.

[55] Y. Inoue, N. Maeda, T. Kokubun et al., "Architecture of Purkinje cells of the reeler mutant mouse observed by immunohistochemistry for the inositol 1,4,5-trisphosphate receptor protein P400," *Neuroscience Research*, vol. 8, no. 3, pp. 189–201, 1990.

[56] K. Mikoshiba, K. Nagaike, and S. Kohsaka, "Developmental studies on the cerebellum from reeler mutant mouse in vivo and in vitro," *Developmental Biology*, vol. 79, no. 1, pp. 64–80, 1980.

[57] M. Frotscher, "Dual role of Cajal-Retzius cells and reelin in cortisal development," *Cell and Tissue Research*, vol. 290, no. 2, pp. 315–322, 1997.

[58] V. Borrell, J. A. Del Río, S. Alcántara et al., "Reelin regulates the development and synaptogenesis of the layer-specific entorhino-hippocampal connections," *Journal of Neuroscience*, vol. 19, no. 4, pp. 1345–1358, 1999.

[59] M. C. Pinto Lord and V. S. Caviness Jr., "Determinants of cell shape and orientation: a comparative Golgi analysis of cell-axon interrelationships in the developing neocortex of normal and reeler mice," *Journal of Comparative Neurology*, vol. 187, no. 1, pp. 49–70, 1979.

[60] B. B. Stanfield and W. M. Cowan, "The development of the hippocampus and dentate gyrus in normal and reeler mice," *Journal of Comparative Neurology*, vol. 185, no. 3, pp. 423–459, 1979.

[61] B. B. Stanfield and W. M. Cowan, "The morphology of the hippocampus and dentate gyrus in normal and reeler mice," *Journal of Comparative Neurology*, vol. 185, no. 3, pp. 393–422, 1979.

[62] S. Niu, A. Renfro, C. C. Quattrocchi, M. Sheldon, and G. D'Arcangelo, "Reelin promotes hippocampal dendrite development through the VLDLR/ApoER2-Dab1 pathway," *Neuron*, vol. 41, no. 1, pp. 71–84, 2004.

[63] A. J. Nichols and E. C. Olson, "Reelin promotes neuronal orientation and dendritogenesis during preplate splitting," *Cerebral Cortex*, vol. 20, no. 9, pp. 2213–2223, 2010.

[64] E. C. Olson, S. Kim, and C. A. Walsh, "Impaired neuronal positioning and dendritogenesis in the neocortex after cell-autonomous Dab1 suppression," *Journal of Neuroscience*, vol. 26, no. 6, pp. 1767–1775, 2006.

[65] Y. Jossin and A. M. Goffinet, "Reelin signals through phosphatidylinositol 3-kinase and Akt to control cortical development and through mTor to regulate dendritic growth," *Molecular and Cellular Biology*, vol. 27, no. 20, pp. 7113–7124, 2007.

[66] T. Matsuki, R. T. Matthews, J. A. Cooper et al., "Reelin and Stk25 have opposing roles in neuronal polarization and dendritic Golgi deployment," *Cell*, vol. 143, no. 5, pp. 826–836, 2010.

[67] S. A. MacLaurin, T. Krucker, and K. N. Fish, "Hippocampal dendritic arbor growth in vitro: regulation by Reelin-disabled-1 signaling," *Brain Research*, vol. 1172, no. 1, pp. 1–9, 2007.

[68] C. Pesold, F. Impagnatiello, M. G. Pisu et al., "Reelin is preferentially expressed in neurons synthesizing γ-aminobutyric acid in cortex and hippocampus of adult rats," *Proceedings of the National Academy of Sciences of the United States of America*, vol. 95, no. 6, pp. 3221–3226, 1998.

[69] O. Yabut, A. Renfro, S. Niu, J. W. Swann, O. Marín, and G. D'Arcangelo, "Abnormal laminar position and dendrite development of interneurons in the reeler forebrain," *Brain Research*, vol. 1140, no. 1, pp. 75–83, 2007.

[70] S. Niu, O. Yabut, and G. D'Arcangelo, "The reelin signaling pathway promotes dendritic spine development in hippocampal neurons," *Journal of Neuroscience*, vol. 28, no. 41, pp. 10339–10348, 2008.

[71] A. Ventruti, T. M. Kazdoba, S. Niu, and G. D'Arcangelo, "Reelin deficiency causes specific defects in the molecular composition of the synapses in the adult brain," *Neuroscience*, vol. 189, pp. 32–42, 2011.

[72] V. S. Caviness Jr. and R. L. Sidman, "Time of origin or corresponding cell classes in the cerebral cortex of normal and reeler mutant mice: an autoradiographic analysis," *Journal of Comparative Neurology*, vol. 148, no. 2, pp. 141–151, 1973.

[73] V. S. Caviness Jr., "Time of neuron origin in the hippocampus and dentate gyrus of normal and reeler mutant mice: an autoradiographic analysis," *Journal of Comparative Neurology*, vol. 151, no. 2, pp. 113–120, 1973.

[74] A. M. Goffinet, "An early developmental defect in the cerebral cortex of the reeler mouse. A morphological study leading to a hypothesis concerning the action of the mutant gene," *Anatomy and Embryology*, vol. 157, no. 2, pp. 205–216, 1979.

[75] L. Pujadas, A. Gruart, C. Bosch et al., "Reelin regulates postnatal neurogenesis and enhances spine hypertrophy and long-term potentiation," *Journal of Neuroscience*, vol. 30, no. 13, pp. 4636–4649, 2010.

[76] T. Terashima, K. Inoue, and Y. Inoue, "Observations on the cerebellum of normal-reeler mutant mouse chimera," *Journal of Comparative Neurology*, vol. 252, no. 2, pp. 264–278, 1986.

[77] K. H. Weiss, C. Johanssen, A. Tielsch et al., "Malformation of the radial glial scaffold in the dentate gyrus of reeler mice, scrambler mice, and ApoER2/VLDLR-deficient mice," *Journal of Comparative Neurology*, vol. 460, no. 1, pp. 56–65, 2003.

[78] K. E. Hunter-Schaedle, "Radial glial cell development and transformation are disturbed in reeler forebrain," *Journal of Neurobiology*, vol. 33, pp. 459–472, 1997.

[79] P. Malatesta, E. Hartfuss, and M. Götz, "Isolation of radial glial cells by fluorescent-activated cell sorting reveals a neural lineage," *Development*, vol. 127, no. 24, pp. 5253–5263, 2000.

[80] S. C. Noctor, A. C. Flint, T. A. Weissman, R. S. Dammerman, and A. R. Kriegstein, "Neurons derived from radial glial cells establish radial units in neocortex," *Nature*, vol. 409, no. 6821, pp. 714–720, 2001.

[81] B. Nadarajah, J. E. Brunstrom, J. Grutzendler, R. O. L. Wong, and A. L. Pearlman, "Two modes of radial migration in early development of the cerebral cortex," *Nature Neuroscience*, vol. 4, no. 2, pp. 143–150, 2001.

[82] H. Tabata and K. Nakajima, "Multipolar migration: the third mode of radial neuronal migration in the developing cerebral cortex," *Journal of Neuroscience*, vol. 23, no. 31, pp. 9996–10001, 2003.

[83] I. Hack, M. Bancila, K. Loulier, P. Carroll, and H. Cremer, "Reelin is a detachment signal in tangential chain-migration during postnatal neurogenesis," *Nature Neuroscience*, vol. 5, no. 10, pp. 939–945, 2002.

[84] B. W. Howell, F. B. Gertler, and J. A. Cooper, "Mouse disabled (mDab1): a Src binding protein implicated in neuronal development," *The MBO Journal*, vol. 16, no. 1, pp. 121–132, 1997.

[85] R. Homayouni, D. S. Rice, M. Sheldon, and T. Curran, "Disabled-1 binds to the cytoplasmic domain of amyloid precursor-like protein 1," *Journal of Neuroscience*, vol. 19, no. 17, pp. 7507–7515, 1999.

[86] B. W. Howell, L. M. Lanier, R. Frank, F. B. Gertler, and J. A. Cooper, "The disabled 1 phosphotyrosine-binding domain binds to the internalization signals of transmembrane glycoproteins and to phospholipids," *Molecular and Cellular Biology*, vol. 19, no. 7, pp. 5179–5188, 1999.

[87] P. C. Stolt, H. Jeon, H. K. Song, J. Herz, M. J. Eck, and S. C. Blacklow, "Origins of peptide selectivity and phosphoinositide binding revealed by structures of disabled-1 PTB domain complexes," *Structure*, vol. 11, no. 5, pp. 569–579, 2003.

[88] D. Goldowitz, R. C. Gushing, E. Laywell et al., "Cerebellar disorganization characteristic of reeler in scrambler mutant mice despite presence of reelin," *Journal of Neuroscience*, vol. 17, no. 22, pp. 8767–8777, 1997.

[89] M. Sheldon, D. S. Rice, G. D'Arcangelo et al., "Scrambler and yotari disrupt the disabled gene and produce a reeler-like phenotype in mice," *Nature*, vol. 389, no. 6652, pp. 730–733, 1997.

[90] M. L. Ware, J. W. Fox, J. L. González et al., "Aberrant splicing of a mouse disabled homolog, mdab1, in the scrambler mouse," *Neuron*, vol. 19, no. 2, pp. 239–249, 1997.

[91] H. Yoneshima, E. Nagata, M. Matsumoto et al., "A novel neurological mutant mouse, yotari, which exhibits reeler-like phenotype but expresses CR-50 antigen/Reelin," *Neuroscience Research*, vol. 29, no. 3, pp. 217–223, 1997.

[92] B. W. Howell, R. Hawkes, P. Soriano, and J. A. Cooper, "Neuronal position in the developing brain is regulated by mouse disabled-1," *Nature*, vol. 389, no. 6652, pp. 733–737, 1997.

[93] B. A. Ballif, L. Arnaud, W. T. Arthur, D. Guris, A. Imamoto, and J. A. Cooper, "Activation of a Dab1/CrkL/C3G/Rap1 pathway in Reelin-stimulated neurons," *Current Biology*, vol. 14, no. 7, pp. 606–610, 2004.

[94] B. W. Howell, T. M. Herrick, and J. A. Cooper, "Reelin-induced tyrosine phosphorylation of disabled 1 during neuronal positioning," *Genes and Development*, vol. 13, no. 12, pp. 643–648, 1999.

[95] L. Keshvara, D. Benhayon, S. Magdaleno, and T. Curran, "Identification of Reelin-induced sites of tyrosyl phosphorylation on disabled 1," *Journal of Biological Chemistry*, vol. 276, no. 19, pp. 16008–16014, 2001.

[96] L. Arnaud, B. A. Ballif, E. Förster, and J. A. Cooper, "Fyn tyrosine kinase is a critical regulator of disabled-1 during brain development," *Current Biology*, vol. 13, no. 1, pp. 9–17, 2003.

[97] H. H. Bock and J. Herz, "Reelin activates Src family tyrosine kinases in neurons," *Current Biology*, vol. 13, no. 1, pp. 18–26, 2003.

[98] B. W. Howell, T. M. Herrick, J. D. Hildebrand, Y. Zhang, and J. A. Cooper, "Dab1 tyrosine phosphorylation sites relay positional

signals during mouse brain development," *Current Biology*, vol. 10, no. 15, pp. 877–885, 2000.

[99] L. Arnaud, B. A. Ballif, and J. A. Cooper, "Regulation of protein tyrosine kinase signaling by substrate degradation during brain development," *Molecular and Cellular Biology*, vol. 23, no. 24, pp. 9293–9302, 2003.

[100] S. Suetsugu, T. Tezuka, T. Morimura et al., "Regulation of actin cytoskeleton by mDab1 through N-WASP and ubiquitination of mDab1," *Biochemical Journal*, vol. 384, no. 1, pp. 1–8, 2004.

[101] G. Kuo, L. Arnaud, P. Kronstad-O'Brien, and J. A. Cooper, "Absence of Fyn and Src causes a Reeler-like phenotype," *Journal of Neuroscience*, vol. 25, no. 37, pp. 8578–8586, 2005.

[102] M. Trommsdorff, M. Gotthardt, T. Hiesberger et al., "Reeler/disabled-like disruption of neuronal migration in knockout mice lacking the VLDL receptor and ApoE receptor 2," *Cell*, vol. 97, no. 6, pp. 689–701, 1999.

[103] G. D'Arcangelo, "Reelin mouse mutants as models of cortical development disorders," *Epilepsy and Behavior*, vol. 8, no. 1, pp. 81–90, 2006.

[104] L. Feng and J. A. Cooper, "Dual functions of Dab1 during brain development," *Molecular and Cellular Biology*, vol. 29, no. 2, pp. 324–332, 2009.

[105] G. Kerjan and J. G. Gleeson, "A missed exit: Reelin sets in motion Dab1 polyubiquitination to put the break on neuronal migration," *Genes and Development*, vol. 21, no. 22, pp. 2850–2854, 2007.

[106] S. Zhao and M. Frotscher, "Go or stop? Divergent roles of reelin in radial neuronal migration," *Neuroscientist*, vol. 16, no. 4, pp. 421–434, 2010.

[107] D. S. Rice, M. Sheldon, G. D'Arcangelo, K. Nakajima, D. Goldowitz, and T. Curran, "Disabled-1 acts downstream of Reelin in a signaling pathway that controls laminar organization in the mammalian brain," *Development*, vol. 125, no. 18, pp. 3719–3729, 1998.

[108] G. Meyer, C. L. De Rouvroit, A. M. Goffinet, and P. Wahle, "Disabled-1 mRNA and protein expression in developing human cortex," *European Journal of Neuroscience*, vol. 17, no. 3, pp. 517–525, 2003.

[109] J. M. Luque, J. Morante-Oria, and A. Fairén, "Localization of ApoER2, VLDLR and Dab1 in radial glia: groundwork for a new model of reelin action during cortical development," *Developmental Brain Research*, vol. 140, no. 2, pp. 195–203, 2003.

[110] E. Hartfuss, E. Förster, H. H. Bock et al., "Reelin signaling directly affects radial glia morphology and biochemical maturation," *Development*, vol. 130, pp. 4597–4609, 2003.

[111] K. Sanada, A. Gupta, and L.-H. Tsai, "Disabled-1-regulated adhesion of migrating neurons to radial glial fiber contributes to neuronal positioning during early corticogenesis," *Neuron*, vol. 42, no. 2, pp. 197–211, 2004.

[112] R. M. Hoffarth, J. G. Johnston, L. A. Krushel, and D. Van der Kooy, "The mouse mutation reeler causes increased adhesion within a subpopulation of early postmitotic cortical neurons," *Journal of Neuroscience*, vol. 15, no. 7, pp. 4838–4850, 1995.

[113] S. J. Franco, I. Martinez-Garay, C. Gil-Sanz, S. R. Harkins-Perry, and U. Müller, "Reelin regulates cadherin function via Dab1/Rap1 to control neuronal migration and lamination in the neocortex," *Neuron*, vol. 69, no. 3, pp. 482–497, 2011.

[114] H. Tabata and K. Nakajima, "Efficient in utero gene transfer system to the developing mouse brain using electroporation: visualization of neuronal migration in the developing cortex," *Neuroscience*, vol. 103, no. 4, pp. 865–872, 2001.

[115] T. Miyata, Y. Ono, M. Okamoto et al., "Migration, early axonogenesis, and Reelin-dependent layer-forming behavior of early/posterior-born Purkinje cells in the developing mouse lateral cerebellum," *Neural Development*, vol. 5, no. 1, article 23, 2010.

[116] R. S. O'Dell, C. J. Ustine, D. A. Cameron et al., "Layer 6 cortical neurons require Reelin-Dab1 signaling for cellular orientation, Golgi deployment, and directed neurite growth into the marginal zone," *Neural Development*, vol. 7, p. 25, 2012.

[117] K. Sekine, T. Kawauchi, K. Kubo et al., "Reelin controls neuronal positioning by promoting cell-matrix adhesion via inside-out activation of integrin $\alpha5\beta1$," *Neuron*, vol. 76, pp. 353–369, 2012.

[118] C. Gil-Sanz, S. J. Franco, I. Martinez-Garay, A. Espinosa, S. Harkins-Perry, and U. Muller, "Cajal-Retzius cells instruct neuronal migration by coincidence signaling between secreted and contact-dependent guidance cues," *Neuron*, vol. 79, pp. 461–477, 2013.

[119] Y. Jossin and J. A. Cooper, "Reelin, Rap1 and N-cadherin orient the migration of multipolar neurons in the developing neocortex," *Nature Neuroscience*, vol. 14, no. 6, pp. 697–703, 2011.

[120] B. A. Ballif, L. Arnaud, and J. A. Cooper, "Tyrosine phosphorylation of disabled-1 is essential for Reelin-stimulated activation of Akt and Src family kinases," *Molecular Brain Research*, vol. 117, no. 2, pp. 152–159, 2003.

[121] U. Beffert, G. Morfini, H. H. Bock, H. Reyna, S. T. Brady, and J. Herz, "Reelin-mediated signaling locally regulates protein kinase B/Akt and glycogen synthase kinase 3β," *Journal of Biological Chemistry*, vol. 277, no. 51, pp. 49958–49964, 2002.

[122] H. H. Bock, Y. Jossin, P. Liu et al., "Phosphatidylinositol 3-kinase interacts with the adaptor protein Dab1 in response to reelin signaling and is required for normal cortical lamination," *Journal of Biological Chemistry*, vol. 278, no. 40, pp. 38772–38779, 2003.

[123] M. Laplante and D. M. Sabatini, "mTOR signaling at a glance," *Journal of Cell Science*, vol. 122, no. 20, pp. 3589–3594, 2009.

[124] D. D. Sarbassov, D. A. Guertin, S. M. Ali, and D. M. Sabatini, "Phosphorylation and regulation of Akt/PKB by the rictor-mTOR complex," *Science*, vol. 307, no. 5712, pp. 1098–1101, 2005.

[125] T. M. Kazdoba, C. N. Sunnen, B. Crowell, G. H. Lee, A. E. Anderson, and G. D'Arcangelo, "Development and characterization of NEX-Pten, a novel forebrain excitatory neuron-specific knockout mouse," *Developmental Neuroscience*, vol. 34, no. 2-3, pp. 198–209, 2012.

[126] C. B. Chan, X. Liu, S. Pradoldej et al., "Phosphoinositide 3-kinase enhancer regulates neuronal dendritogenesis and survival in neocortex," *Journal of Neuroscience*, vol. 31, no. 22, pp. 8083–8092, 2011.

[127] J. Iafrati, M. J. Orejarena, O. Lassalle, L. Bouamrane, and P. Chavis, "Reelin, an extracellular matrix protein linked to early onset psychiatric diseases, drives postnatal development of the prefrontal cortex via GluN2B-NMDARs and the mTOR pathway," *Molecular Psychiatry*, 2013.

[128] J. Trotter, G. H. Lee, T. M. Kazdoba et al., "Dab1 is required for synaptic plasticity and associative learning," *The Journal of Neuroscience*, vol. 33, pp. 15652–15668, 2013.

[129] S. Hirotsune, M. W. Fleck, M. J. Gambello et al., "Graded reduction of Pafah1b1 (Lis1) activity results in neuronal migration defects and early embryonic lethality," *Nature Genetics*, vol. 19, no. 4, pp. 333–339, 1998.

[130] M. Hattori, H. Adachi, M. Tsujimoto, H. Arai, and K. Inoue, "Miller-Dieker lissencephaly gene encodes a subunit of brain

platelet-activating factor," *Nature*, vol. 370, no. 6486, pp. 216–218, 1994.

[131] O. Reiner, R. Carrozzo, Y. Shen et al., "Isolation of a Miller-Dieker lissencephaly gene containing G protein β-subunit-like repeats," *Nature*, vol. 364, no. 6439, pp. 717–721, 1993.

[132] A. H. Assadi, G. Zhang, U. Beffert et al., "Interaction of reelin signaling and Lis1 in brain development," *Nature Genetics*, vol. 35, no. 3, pp. 270–276, 2003.

[133] A. H. Assadi, G. Zhang, R. McNeil, G. D. Clark, and G. D'Arcangelo, "Pafah1b2 mutations suppress the development of hydrocephalus in compound Pafah1b1; Reln and Pafah1b1; Dab1 mutant mice," *Neuroscience Letters*, vol. 439, no. 1, pp. 100–105, 2008.

[134] G. Zhang, A. H. Assadi, M. Roceri, G. D. Clark, and G. D'Arcangelo, "Differential interaction of the Pafah1b alpha subunits with the Reelin transducer Dab1," *Brain Research*, vol. 1267, pp. 1–8, 2009.

[135] L.-H. Tsai and J. G. Gleeson, "Nucleokinesis in neuronal migration," *Neuron*, vol. 46, no. 3, pp. 383–388, 2005.

[136] A. Pramatarova, P. G. Ochalski, K. Chen et al., "Nckβ interacts with tyrosine-phosphorylated disabled 1 and redistributes in Reelin-stimulated neurons," *Molecular and Cellular Biology*, vol. 23, no. 20, pp. 7210–7221, 2003.

[137] R. Homayouni, S. Magdaleno, L. Keshvara, D. S. Rice, and T. Curran, "Interaction of disabled-1 and the GTPase activating protein Dab2IP in mouse brain," *Molecular Brain Research*, vol. 115, no. 2, pp. 121–129, 2003.

[138] Y. Huang, S. Magdaleno, R. Hopkins, C. Slaughter, T. Curran, and L. Keshvara, "Tyrosine phosphorylated disabled 1 recruits Crk family adapter proteins," *Biochemical and Biophysical Research Communications*, vol. 318, no. 1, pp. 204–212, 2004.

[139] G. H. Lee, S. H. Kim, R. Homayouni, and G. D'Arcangelo, "Dab2ip regulates neuronal migration and neurite outgrowth in the developing neocortex," *PLoS ONE*, vol. 7, Article ID e46592, 2012.

[140] S. Qiao, S. H. Kim, D. Heck, D. Goldowitz, M. S. LeDoux, and R. Homayouni, "Dab2IP GTPase activating protein regulates dendrite development and synapse number in cerebellum," *PLoS ONE*, vol. 8, Article ID e53635, 2013.

[141] T.-J. Park and T. Curran, "Crk and Crk-like play essential overlapping roles downstream of disabled-1 in the reelin pathway," *Journal of Neuroscience*, vol. 28, no. 50, pp. 13551–13562, 2008.

[142] T. Hiesberger, M. Trommsdorff, B. W. Howell et al., "Direct binding of Reelin to VLDL receptor and ApoE receptor 2 induces tyrosine phosphorylation of disabled-1 and modulates tau phosphorylation," *Neuron*, vol. 24, no. 2, pp. 481–489, 1999.

[143] J. Herz, "The LDL receptor gene family: (Un)expected signal transducers in the brain," *Neuron*, vol. 29, no. 3, pp. 571–581, 2001.

[144] D. Benhayon, S. Magdaleno, and T. Curran, "Binding of purified Reelin to ApoER2 and VLDLR mediates tyrosine phosphorylation of disabled-1," *Molecular Brain Research*, vol. 112, no. 1-2, pp. 33–45, 2003.

[145] M. Trommsdorff, J.-P. Borg, B. Margolis, and J. Herz, "Interaction of cytosolic adaptor proteins with neuronal apolipoprotein E receptors and the amyloid precursor protein," *Journal of Biological Chemistry*, vol. 273, no. 50, pp. 33556–33560, 1998.

[146] T. Morimura, M. Hattori, M. Ogawa, and K. Mikoshiba, "Disabled1 regulates the intracellular trafficking of reelin receptors," *Journal of Biological Chemistry*, vol. 280, no. 17, pp. 16901–16908, 2005.

[147] V. Strasser, D. Fasching, C. Hauser et al., "Receptor clustering is involved in Reelin signaling," *Molecular and Cellular Biology*, vol. 24, no. 3, pp. 1378–1386, 2004.

[148] G. Zhang, A. H. Assadi, R. S. McNeil et al., "The Pafah1b complex interacts with the reelin receptor VLDLR," *PLoS ONE*, vol. 2, no. 2, article e252, 2007.

[149] U. Beffert, E. J. Weeber, A. Durudas et al., "Modulation of synaptic plasticity and memory by Reelin involves differential splicing of the lipoprotein receptor Apoer2," *Neuron*, vol. 47, no. 4, pp. 567–579, 2005.

[150] L. Dulabon, E. C. Olson, M. G. Taglienti et al., "Reelin binds $\alpha 3\beta 1$ integrin and inhibits neuronal migration," *Neuron*, vol. 27, no. 1, pp. 33–44, 2000.

[151] D. Graus-Porta, S. Blaess, M. Senften et al., "$\beta 1$-Class integrins regulate the development of laminae and folia in the cerebral and cerebellar cortex," *Neuron*, vol. 31, no. 3, pp. 367–379, 2001.

[152] R. Belvindrah, D. Graus-Porta, S. Goebbels, K.-A. Nave, and U. Müller, "$\beta 1$ integrins in radial glia but not in migrating neurons are essential for the formation of cell layers in the cerebral cortex," *Journal of Neuroscience*, vol. 27, no. 50, pp. 13854–13865, 2007.

[153] E. Förster, A. Tielsch, B. Saum et al., "Reelin, disabled 1, and $\beta 1$ integrins are required for the formation of the radial glial scaffold in the hippocampus," *Proceedings of the National Academy of Sciences of the United States of America*, vol. 99, no. 20, pp. 13178–13183, 2002.

[154] K. Senzaki, M. Ogawa, and T. Yagi, "Proteins of the CNR family are multiple receptors for reelin," *Cell*, vol. 99, no. 6, pp. 635–647, 1999.

[155] A. Sentürk, S. Pfennig, A. Weiss, K. Burk, and A. Acker-Palmer, "Ephrin Bs are essential components of the Reelin pathway to regulate neuronal migration," *Nature*, vol. 472, no. 7343, pp. 356–360, 2011.

[156] T. Catchpole and M. Henkemeyer, "EphB2 tyrosine kinase-dependent forward signaling in migration of neuronal progenitors that populate and form a distinct region of the dentate niche," *Journal of Neuroscience*, vol. 31, no. 32, pp. 11472–11483, 2011.

[157] E. Bouche, M. I. Romero-Ortega, M. Henkemeyer et al., "Reelin induces EphB activation," *Cell Research*, vol. 23, pp. 473–490, 2013.

[158] V. Villar-Cervino, M. Molano-Mazon, T. Catchpole et al., "Contact repulsion controls the dispersion and final distribution of Cajal-Retzius cells," *Neuron*, vol. 77, pp. 457–471, 2013.

[159] T. Matsuki, A. Pramatarova, and B. W. Howell, "Reduction of Crk and CrkL expression blocks reelin-induced dendritogenesis," *Journal of Cell Science*, vol. 121, no. 11, pp. 1869–1875, 2008.

[160] C. Stritt and B. Knöll, "Serum response factor regulates hippocampal lamination and dendrite development and is connected with reelin signaling," *Molecular and Cellular Biology*, vol. 30, no. 7, pp. 1828–1837, 2010.

[161] J. Leemhuis and H. H. Bock, "Reelin modulates cytoskeletal organization by regulating Rho GTPases," *Communicative and Integrative Biology*, vol. 4, no. 3, pp. 254–257, 2011.

[162] M. Meseke, G. Rosenberger, and E. Forster, "Reelin and the Cdc42/Rac1 guanine nucleotide exchange factor alphaPIX/Arhgef6 promote dendritic Golgi translocation in hippocampal neurons," *European Journal of Neuroscience*, vol. 37, pp. 1404–1412, 2013.

[163] P. Chameau, D. Inta, T. Vitalis, H. Monyer, W. J. Wadman, and J. A. van Hooft, "The N-terminal region of reelin regulates

postnatal dendritic maturation of cortical pyramidal neurons," *Proceedings of the National Academy of Sciences of the United States of America*, vol. 106, no. 17, pp. 7227–7232, 2009.

[164] H.-S. Hoe, J. L. Kea, R. S. E. Carney et al., "Interaction of Reelin with amyloid precursor protein promotes neurite outgrowth," *Journal of Neuroscience*, vol. 29, no. 23, pp. 7459–7473, 2009.

[165] H.-S. Hoe, T. S. Tran, Y. Matsuoka, B. W. Howell, and G. W. Rebeck, "DAB1 and reelin effects on amyloid precursor protein and ApoE receptor 2 trafficking and processing," *Journal of Biological Chemistry*, vol. 281, no. 46, pp. 35176–35185, 2006.

[166] J. H. Trotter, M. Klein, U. K. Jinwal et al., "ApoER2 function in the establishment and maintenance of retinal synaptic connectivity," *Journal of Neuroscience*, vol. 31, no. 40, pp. 14413–14423, 2011.

[167] S. Qiu, K. M. Korwek, A. R. Pratt-Davis, M. Peters, M. Y. Bergman, and E. J. Weeber, "Cognitive disruption and altered hippocampus synaptic function in Reelin haploinsufficient mice," *Neurobiology of Learning and Memory*, vol. 85, no. 3, pp. 228–242, 2006.

[168] P. Tueting, E. Costa, Y. Dwivedi et al., "The phenotypic characteristics of heterozygous reeler mouse," *NeuroReport*, vol. 10, no. 6, pp. 1329–1334, 1999.

[169] E. Costa, Y. Chen, J. Davis et al., "REELIN and schizophrenia: a disease at the interface of the genome and the epigenome," *Molecular Interventions*, vol. 2, no. 1, pp. 47–57, 2002.

[170] D. D. Krueger, J. L. Howell, B. F. Hebert, P. Olausson, J. R. Taylor, and A. C. Nairn, "Assessment of cognitive function in the heterozygous reeler mouse," *Psychopharmacology*, vol. 189, no. 1, pp. 95–104, 2006.

[171] W. S. Liu, C. Pesold, M. A. Rodriguez et al., "Down-regulation of dendritic spine and glutamic acid decarboxylase 67 expressions in the reelin haploinsufficient heterozygous reeler mouse," *Proceedings of the National Academy of Sciences of the United States of America*, vol. 98, no. 6, pp. 3477–3482, 2001.

[172] J. T. Rogers, L. Zhao, J. H. Trotter et al., "Reelin supplementation recovers sensorimotor gating, synaptic plasticity and associative learning deficits in the heterozygous reeler mouse," *Journal of Psychopharmacology*, vol. 27, pp. 386–395, 2013.

[173] J. T. Rogers, I. Rusiana, J. Trotter et al., "Reelin supplementation enhances cognitive ability, synaptic plasticity, and dendritic spine density," *Learning and Memory*, vol. 18, no. 9, pp. 558–564, 2011.

[174] M. A. Rodriguez, C. Pesold, W. S. Liu et al., "Colocalization of integrin receptors and reelin in dendritic spine postsynaptic densities of adult nonhuman primate cortex," *Proceedings of the National Academy of Sciences of the United States of America*, vol. 97, no. 7, pp. 3550–3555, 2000.

[175] L. A. Glantz and D. A. Lewis, "Decreased dendritic spine density on prefrontal cortical pyramidal neurons in schizophrenia," *Archives of General Psychiatry*, vol. 57, no. 1, pp. 65–73, 2000.

[176] J. L. Brigman, K. E. Padukiewicz, M. L. Sutherland, and L. A. Rothblat, "Executive functions in the heterozygous reeler mouse model of schizophrenia," *Behavioral Neuroscience*, vol. 120, no. 4, pp. 984–988, 2006.

[177] A. M. Barr, K. N. Fish, A. Markou, and W. G. Honer, "Heterozygous reeler mice exhibit alterations in sensorimotor gating but not presynaptic proteins," *European Journal of Neuroscience*, vol. 27, no. 10, pp. 2568–2574, 2008.

[178] V. Martínez-Cerdeño, M. J. Galazo, C. Cavada, and F. Clascá, "Reelin immunoreactivity in the adult primate brain: intracellular localization in projecting and local circuit neurons of the cerebral cortex, hippocampus and subcortical regions," *Cerebral Cortex*, vol. 12, no. 12, pp. 1298–1311, 2002.

[179] C. Pesold, W. S. Liu, A. Guidotti, E. Costa, and H. J. Caruncho, "Cortical bitufted, horizontal, and Martinotti cells preferentially express and secrete reelin into perineuronal nets, nonsynaptically modulating gene expression," *Proceedings of the National Academy of Sciences of the United States of America*, vol. 96, no. 6, pp. 3217–3222, 1999.

[180] R. C. Roberts, L. Xu, J. K. Roche, and B. Kirkpatrick, "Ultrastructural localization of reelin in the cortex in post-mortem human brain," *Journal of Comparative Neurology*, vol. 482, no. 3, pp. 294–308, 2005.

[181] E. J. Weeber, U. Beffert, C. Jones et al., "Reelin and apoE receptors cooperate to enhance hippocampal synaptic plasticity and learning," *Journal of Biological Chemistry*, vol. 277, no. 42, pp. 39944–39952, 2002.

[182] C. G. Campo, M. Sinagra, D. Verrier, O. J. Manzoni, and P. Chavis, "Reelin secreted by GABAergic neurons regulates glutamate receptor homeostasis," *PloS ONE*, vol. 4, no. 5, Article ID e5505, 2009.

[183] Y. Chen, U. Beffert, M. Ertunc et al., "Reelin modulates NMDA receptor activity in cortical neurons," *Journal of Neuroscience*, vol. 25, no. 36, pp. 8209–8216, 2005.

[184] L. Groc, D. Choquet, F. A. Stephenson, D. Verrier, O. J. Manzoni, and P. Chavis, "NMDA receptor surface trafficking and synaptic subunit composition are developmentally regulated by the extracellular matrix protein reelin," *Journal of Neuroscience*, vol. 27, no. 38, pp. 10165–10175, 2007.

[185] S. Qiu and E. J. Weeber, "Reelin signaling facilitates maturation of CA1 glutamatergic synapses," *Journal of Neurophysiology*, vol. 97, no. 3, pp. 2312–2321, 2007.

[186] S. Qiu, L. F. Zhao, K. M. Korwek, and E. J. Weeber, "Differential reelin-induced enhancement of NMDA and AMPA receptor activity in the adult hippocampus," *Journal of Neuroscience*, vol. 26, no. 50, pp. 12943–12955, 2006.

[187] S. Hellwig, I. Hack, J. Kowalski et al., "Role for reelin in neurotransmitter release," *Journal of Neuroscience*, vol. 31, no. 7, pp. 2352–2360, 2011.

[188] I. Knuesel, "Reelin-mediated signaling in neuropsychiatric and neurodegenerative diseases," *Progress in Neurobiology*, vol. 91, no. 4, pp. 257–274, 2010.

11

How Basal Ganglia Outputs Generate Behavior

Henry H. Yin

Department of Psychology and Neuroscience and Department of Neurobiology, Center for Cognitive Neuroscience, Duke University, P.O. Box 91050, Durham, NC 27708, USA

Correspondence should be addressed to Henry H. Yin; hy43@duke.edu

Academic Editor: Xiang-Ping Chu

The basal ganglia (BG) are a collection of subcortical nuclei critical for voluntary behavior. According to the standard model, the output projections from the BG tonically inhibit downstream motor centers and prevent behavior. A pause in the BG output opens the gate for behavior, allowing the initiation of actions. Hypokinetic neurological symptoms, such as inability to initiate actions in Parkinson's disease, are explained by excessively high firing rates of the BG output neurons. This model, widely taught in textbooks, is contradicted by recent electrophysiological results, which are reviewed here. In addition, I also introduce a new model, based on the insight that behavior is a product of closed loop negative feedback control using internal reference signals rather than sensorimotor transformations. The nervous system is shown to be a functional hierarchy comprising independent controllers occupying different levels, each level controlling specific variables derived from its perceptual inputs. The BG represent the level of transition control in this hierarchy, sending reference signals specifying the succession of body orientations and configurations. This new model not only explains the major symptoms in movement disorders but also generates a number of testable predictions.

1. Introduction

The basal ganglia (BG) have been implicated in functions as diverse as movement, learning, and motivation [1–5]. Damage to these nuclei impair or even abolish voluntary behavior. But after decades of research it remains unclear how the BG generate behavior.

I shall argue that the BG occupy a specific level in a functional hierarchy. Unlike traditional models, which are based on the linear causation paradigm [6], the proposed hierarchy is based on the principle of cascade control [7]. Unfortunately control theory is currently misunderstood in neuroscience, mainly due to conceptual confusions introduced by cybernetics and engineering control theory. To understand the role of the BG in behavior, it would be necessary to explain the principles of control and the organization of the functional hierarchy.

I shall first discuss current models of the BG and recent results that begin to challenge these models. I shall then explain how control theory, correctly applied, can help us understand behavior, and how different control systems can be arranged in a hierarchy using the principle of cascade control. Finally, I shall discuss the neural implementation of cascade control and the distinct contributions of the BG in this functional hierarchy.

2. What Are the Basal Ganglia?

The rapid accumulation of facts on the BG has added new pieces of the puzzle without revealing how the pieces are to fit together. The facts are often isolated and, in the absence of a coherent theory, incomprehensible. Rather than giving a detailed review of the physiology and anatomy, I shall only outline the most salient features that are relevant to our understanding of behavior.

First, the terminology is confusing and daunting to beginning students. Conventional names for parts of the BG are usually Latin descriptions of their visual appearance, independent of the functional significance of the signals being transmitted by these parts. From a functional perspective, it would be more useful to classify brain regions on the basis of the neurotransmitter released by the projection neurons [8]. In any brain region there is typically one type of projection neuron with axons leaving the structure of origin and targeting other brain regions (and multiple

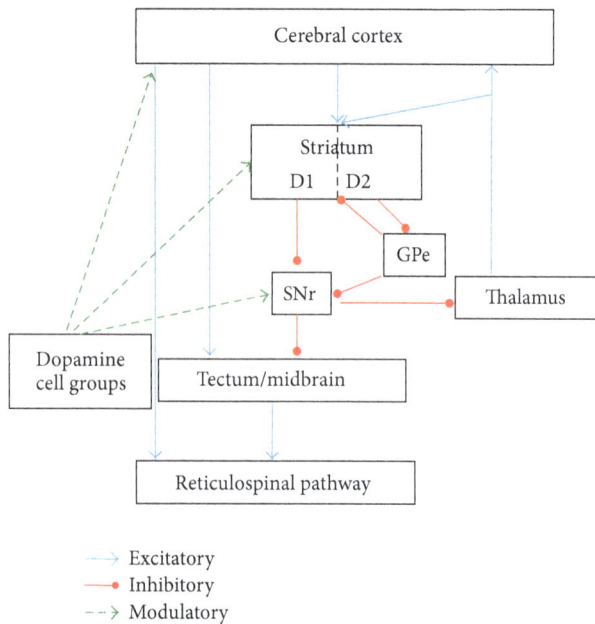

FIGURE 1: Highly simplified illustration of the inputs and outputs of the basal ganglia.

types of interneurons whose axons stay within the region). For example, cortical pyramidal neurons, which release glutamate as a neurotransmitter, excite target structures. In contrast, the projection neurons in the striatum, the input nucleus of the BG, are the medium spiny projection neurons, which release GABA and inhibit their targets. The projection neurons in the pallidum, the output nucleus of the BG, are also GABAergic. The BG appear to be one of the few areas in the nervous system with inhibitory projection neurons (Figure 1). Although recent work has shown some exceptions [9], this rule appears to apply in most cases. It should also be noted that an area like the subthalamic nucleus, although traditionally considered to belong to the BG, is not classified as such here, because it contains glutamatergic projection neurons like the cerebral cortex.

Here the term BG refers to three general classes of nuclei: input, intrinsic, and output.

(1) The input nucleus is the striatum. The striatum receives projections from the entire cortical mantle and from multiple diencephalic regions, especially the intralaminar thalamus. Various terms, such as caudate, putamen, and nucleus accumbens core, have been used to describe various regions of the input nucleus. Most of these can be grouped on the basis of the region of origin of the massive corticostriatal projections. Just as diverse cortical regions are characterized by pyramidal projection neurons, which are glutamatergic and excitatory, the striatal regions share the spiny projection neurons, which are GABAergic and inhibitory. They possess large dendritic arbors with thousands of spines, which are the sites of glutamatergic synapses made by the cortical and thalamic inputs [10].

(2) The intrinsic nucleus is the globus pallidus, often called the globus pallidus external segment (GPe), to be distinguished from the internal segment (GPi), which is found in primates. The entopeduncular nucleus is often considered the rodent version of GPi [11]. It is an output nucleus along with substantia nigra pars reticulata (SNr). Only the GPe is considered the "intrinsic nucleus" here, as its inputs and outputs are largely restricted to other BG nuclei [12]. It is the major target of the striatopallidal projections, from striatal neurons that coexpress D2 class dopamine receptors and A2A adenosine receptors. Traditionally called the "indirect pathway," this projection is the subject of a vast literature [13]. The output of the GPe can inhibit the SNr neurons [14]. The GPe also sends projections back to the striatum, but the functional significance of these pallidostratal projections remains unknown [15].

(3) The output nuclei include entopeduncular nucleus (rodents), GPi, and SNr. These nuclei generally inhibit downstream targets. The entopeduncular nucleus and GPi are both believed to be critical for limb movements, whereas the SNr may be more critical for movements of the head and trunk [16]. Throughout this review, the focus will be on the SNr, which project to the tectum, thalamus, and brainstem.

The excitatory inputs to the BG reach the striatum from the cerebral cortex (corticostriatal projections) and the intralaminar thalamus (thalamostriatal projections). Ascending projections from the midbrain and brainstem also reach the striatum, releasing neuromodulators such as dopamine [17]. Other inputs can also reach the striatum indirectly, via the thalamus, for example, projections from the dentate nucleus in the cerebellum [18] and from the vestibular nucleus [19].

Most striatal outputs target the output nuclei of the BG, which are inhibitory and often fire at high rates (e.g., 20–80 Hz in SNr neurons). Thus the input nucleus (striatum) and the output nucleus (e.g., SNr) have distinct sets of connections with other brain regions, but the main connection between them is the GABAergic projection from the input nucleus to output nucleus [20]. When the striatum is activated, the output of the medium spiny projection neurons inhibits the SNr neurons. Consequently, the downstream targets of nigral outputs, for example, superior colliculus, can be disinhibited [14, 21, 22].

Interestingly, such a circuit organization is similar to the model proposed by Von Holst and Lorenz long ago, purely based on behavioral observations: "the basic central nervous organisation consists of a cell permanently producing endogenous stimulation, but prevented from activating its effector by another cell which, also producing endogenous stimulation, exerts an inhibiting effect. It is this inhibiting cell which is influenced by the receptor and ceases its inhibitory activity at the biologically "right" moment [23]." The inhibiting cell, in this case, is the nigral projection neuron that ceases at the right moment, allowing the target structures of the nigral output to be disinhibited [24, 25].

This model of disinhibition, widely taught in introductory courses, is the foundation of current models of BG function [26, 27]. For example, Hikosaka wrote: "...GABAergic output acts as a gate for motor signals such that there should be no motor output as long as the gate is closed. For this gating function to work properly, the level of the GABAergic output must, by default, be maintained at a steady level" [16]. Normally the gate is locked, and the pause in nigral activity unlocks the behavior. The activation of the striatum, however, can inhibit the BG output neurons, thus disinhibiting behavior. As we shall see below, this model of the BG is inadequate for several reasons.

Much work has also been devoted to the understanding of the functional roles of the so-called direct and indirect pathways in the BG. The medium spiny projection neurons comprise over 90% of the neurons in the striatum. Two major populations have been identified based on their anatomical targets and on differential expression of various receptors [10, 13]. Dopamine can have different effects on striatonigral and striatopallidal neurons, depending on the class of dopamine receptors expressed. The striatonigral pathway originates from spiny neurons expressing D1-like receptors, whereas the striatopallidal pathway originates from those expressing D2-like receptors. The modulation is not only restricted to the glutamatergic transmission but also critical for the GABAergic lateral inhibition by the axon collaterals of striatal projection neurons [17, 28]. Such differences between the direct and indirect pathways are the focus of extensive research [17, 29–33]. Although much is now known regarding the properties of these pathways, so far their functional role remains controversial. There are a number of speculations on the functional distinction between the direct and indirect pathways [34, 35], but most of these are too qualitative and vaguely formulated to qualify as genuine models.

3. Opponent Output from the BG

We recently recorded from the SNr output neurons in mice performing an operant task [36]. We trained mice to hold down a lever for a minimum duration in order to receive a food reward. Once the lever is released, a food pellet is delivered if the press duration exceeds a minimum criterion determined by the experimenter (Figure 2). In this "temporal differentiation" procedure, antecedent stimuli (e.g., discriminative stimuli) are not manipulated. The mice must learn to generate behaviors that satisfy some arbitrary criterion in order to receive the reward [37, 38]. The action duration is used to tag neural activity related to the holding.

We found nigral neurons that increased their firing rate during the holding period. This increase lasted as long as the press duration and immediately returned to prepress baseline levels following the release of the lever (Figure 2). Such a sustained increase in firing rate appears to support the idea that an increase in the inhibitory output from the SNr should prevent movement. But, at the same time, other neurons exhibited the opposite pattern—pausing during the holding period. This result is more surprising. According to the gate model, a pause in nigral output disinhibits target structures in the tectum and thalamus and permits the initiation of movement. Yet when the mouse is holding down the lever, in the absence of any overt "movement," there is a clear pause in nigral activity.

It could be argued that our results agree with the "focused selection" theory [3], according to which the BG output selects a motor program while inhibiting competing programs. The competing actions are presumably inhibited by an increase in nigral output, whereas the selected action of lever pressing is enabled by a decrease in nigral output. According to this model, an action is a change in position (e.g., reaching with one's arm), which is achieved by inhibiting postural control that allows the arm to stay still. But, in our task, movement is only observed before the holding period, as the mouse presses down the lever or afterwards as the mouse releases it. During the holding period itself, there is no overt movement. Moreover, the increase and decrease in firing rate during the holding period appear to be similar in magnitude but opposite in polarity.

Why should there be such opponent activity in the BG output neurons? One interpretation is that these represent bidirectional signals from a tonic baseline. In electronics this is common in amplifier design. In neurobiology, one example of bidirectional outputs is found at the lowest level of the motor system, in the reciprocal inhibition circuit [39]. The primary or Ia afferents that excite the alpha motor neurons also project to inhibitory interneurons that inhibit alpha motor neurons innervating the antagonist muscle. A pair of push-pull signals is generated and sent to the final common path. As one muscle tightens, the opposing one relaxes. Of course, there is no pushing, only a reduction in pulling, because muscles can only pull by contracting. Different muscles pull the joint in different directions, so push-pull can be achieved with muscles that are in some antagonistic relationship, for example, biceps and triceps. The torque generated depends on the difference between the pair of signals. When the two signals are equal, there is no movement. The joint angle stops changing, but the opposing muscles still have "tone," both being activated without producing any net torque. The balance between the antagonistic muscles, analogous to the "common mode" signal in electronics, can be reached at different values. With movement, the output signal turns either positive or negative relative to the common mode value.

To send a pair of push-pull signals, one cannot use a single neural signal varying from negative to positive, because spike rates can never be negative. Subtraction is possible in neural signaling mainly through inhibition—the reduction of a positive signal (spike rate).

The use of a common mode signal, akin to muscle tone, allows the increase and decrease from the baseline to represent a pair of push-pull signals. Just as the muscle tone allows a smooth transition from a force in one direction to a force in the opposite direction, the common mode signal from the BG outputs will permit bidirectional control of their target systems. Increases and decreases from the average rate of firing will provide a pair of opposite signals to activate antagonistic pairs of control systems.

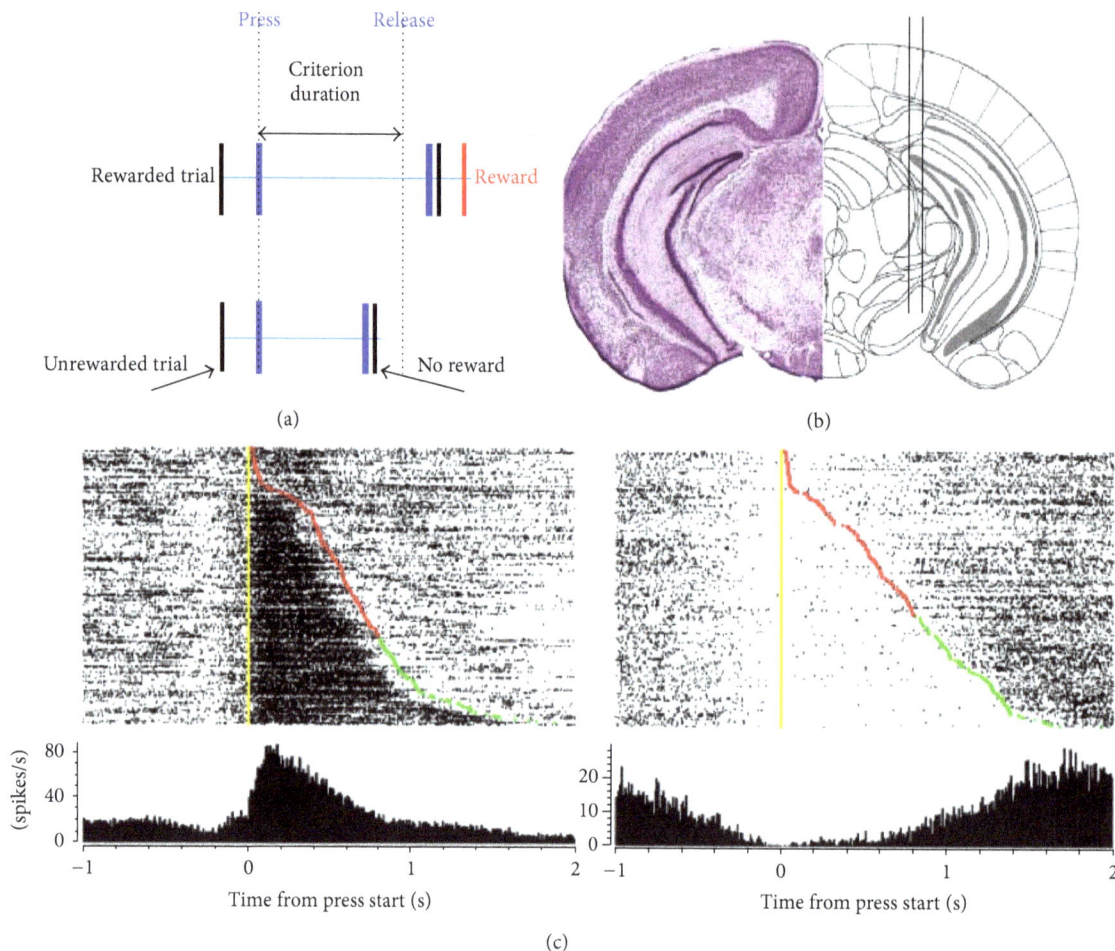

FIGURE 2: Opponent outputs during temporal differentiation [36]. (a) Illustration of the behavioral task. A food reward is delivered after the release of the lever, if the press duration exceeds the criterion duration set by the experimenter. (b) Location of the electrode array in the substantia nigra. (c) Perievent raster plots illustrating opponent output from the nigral GABAergic projection neurons. Yellow markers indicate start of lever press. Red markers indicate end of lever press on unrewarded trials. Green markers indicate end of lever press on rewarded trials. The press durations are sorted from shortest to longest.

With reciprocal inhibition, bidirectional signals to the alpha motor neurons clearly alter the contraction of the relevant muscles, but what can the BG outputs do? Since the BG do not innervate motor neurons directly, signals from the SNr cannot command individual muscles. What do the target systems represent, if not antagonistic muscles pulling a joint in different directions? That is the key question.

One clue is suggested by our results from the temporal differentiation task. That both "increasing" and "decreasing" neurons did not change their rate of firing during the lever press suggests that their outputs, in fact, are correlated with the fixed position of the animal [40]. From the initiation of the press, the mouse reaches a new posture or body configuration and is required to hold it for brief time period. Because the animal is not moving during this period, the position is largely fixed. The BG output is also fixed at the same time.

But, to test this idea, it would be necessary to introduce disturbances to the posture in opposite directions. If indeed the opponent outputs represent signals sent to bidirectional

control systems, they should reverse when the direction of disturbance is also reversed. Indeed, this is what we observed in a different set of studies. To test the hypothesis that BG output sends antiphasic signals for antagonistic lower systems, we recorded from SNr during continuous and cyclical postural disturbances (Figure 3). The mouse stood on an elevated and covered platform and experienced tilting disturbance in the roll plane (7 degrees of tilt to either side of the animal). To control posture, the mouse simply has to remain standing. In order to resist tilting to one side of the body, the mouse must produce the appropriate outputs. To avoid cables, which can introduce unexpected torques to the animal, we used wireless multielectrode recording to record single unit activity from many neurons simultaneously [41].

The output of most SNr neurons is quantitatively related to the tilt disturbance. Again we observed opponent outputs from the putative GABAergic projection neurons [42]. Some neurons were inhibited with tilt to the left and excited with tilt to the right, yet other neurons exhibited the opposite pattern (Figure 4). Neurons that reduced firing to tilt in one direction

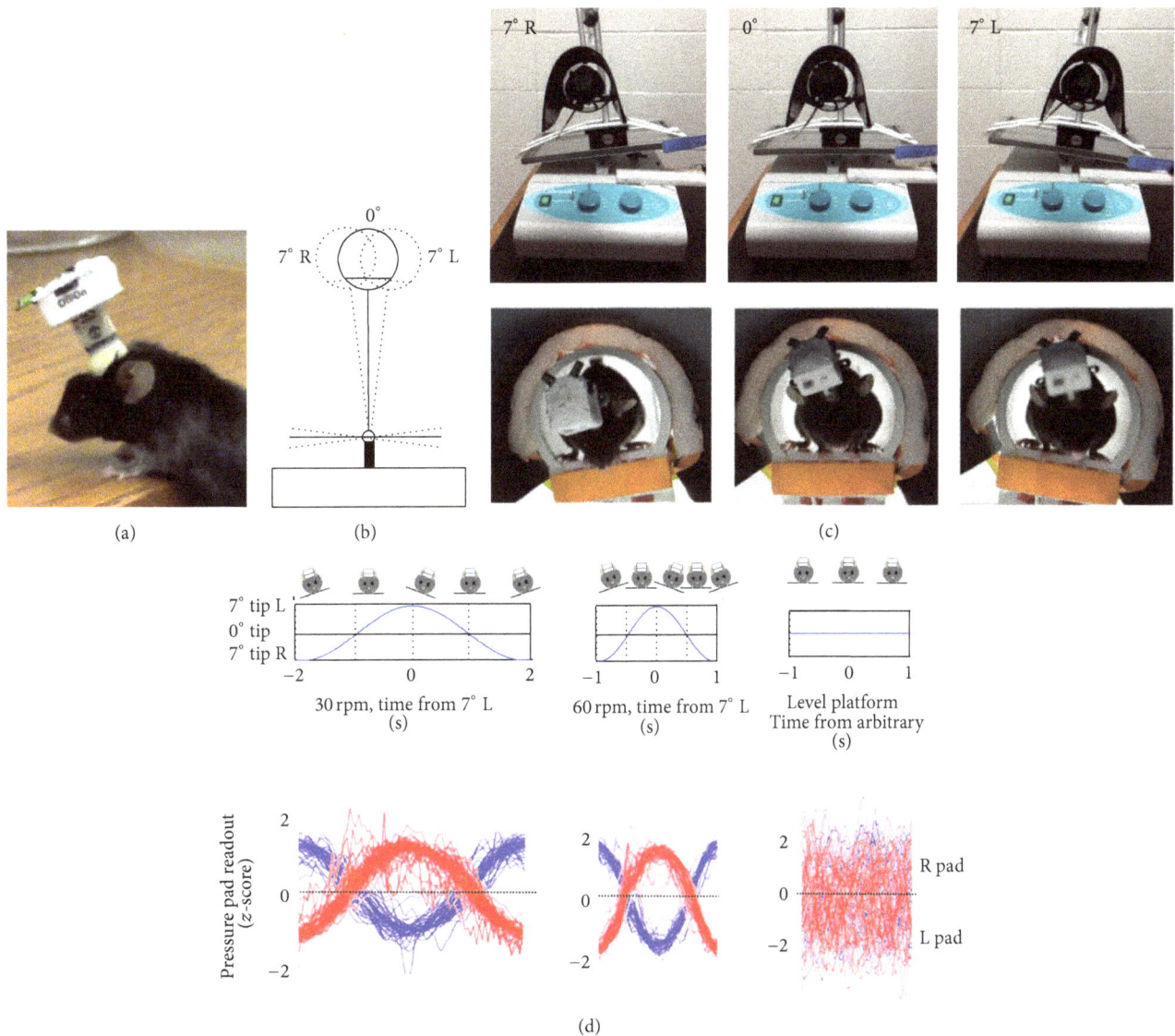

FIGURE 3: Design and behavioral results from the posture task [42]. (a) Photo of the mouse with wireless recording headstage. (b) The elevated platform with tilt disturbances (7 degrees to each side of the animal in the roll plane). (c) Pictures of the mouse during postural disturbances. (d) Left, pressure pad readings (left and right pressure pads placed underneath the mouse) on the platform, detecting the force exerted by the animal during slow postural disturbances (30 rpm). Center, pressure pad readings during fast disturbances (60 rpm). Right, pressure pad readings during rest period, in the absence of tilt in either direction.

always increased firing to tilt in the opposite direction. These two groups of neurons appear to be roughly 180 degrees out of phase.

Moreover, the relationship between neural activity and postural disturbance is highly linear, at least for the range of disturbances used in our study. In the absence of the tilt disturbance, the signals from these two populations of neurons are balanced. This reflects the common mode signal. With z-score normalization, the mean firing rate is zero—the effective zero signal for the BG output. From this baseline an increase in one output signal is paired with a corresponding decrease in another signal. These two signals are presumably sent to antagonistic downstream systems.

It is possible that these opponent signals are related to Newton's third law of motion. Since for every action there is an equal reaction, the generation of force in any direction will also produce a disturbance to the body in the opposite direction, requiring posture control. When pushing on a wall, for example, one is also experiencing the force from the wall in the opposite direction. Without resisting the reactive force, the posture will either collapse or, like astronauts in space, the body will be pushed away.

Our demonstration of the continuous relationship between neural activity and postural disturbances questions the assumptions of the "focused selection" model. BG output is not used to generate movements while inhibiting postural

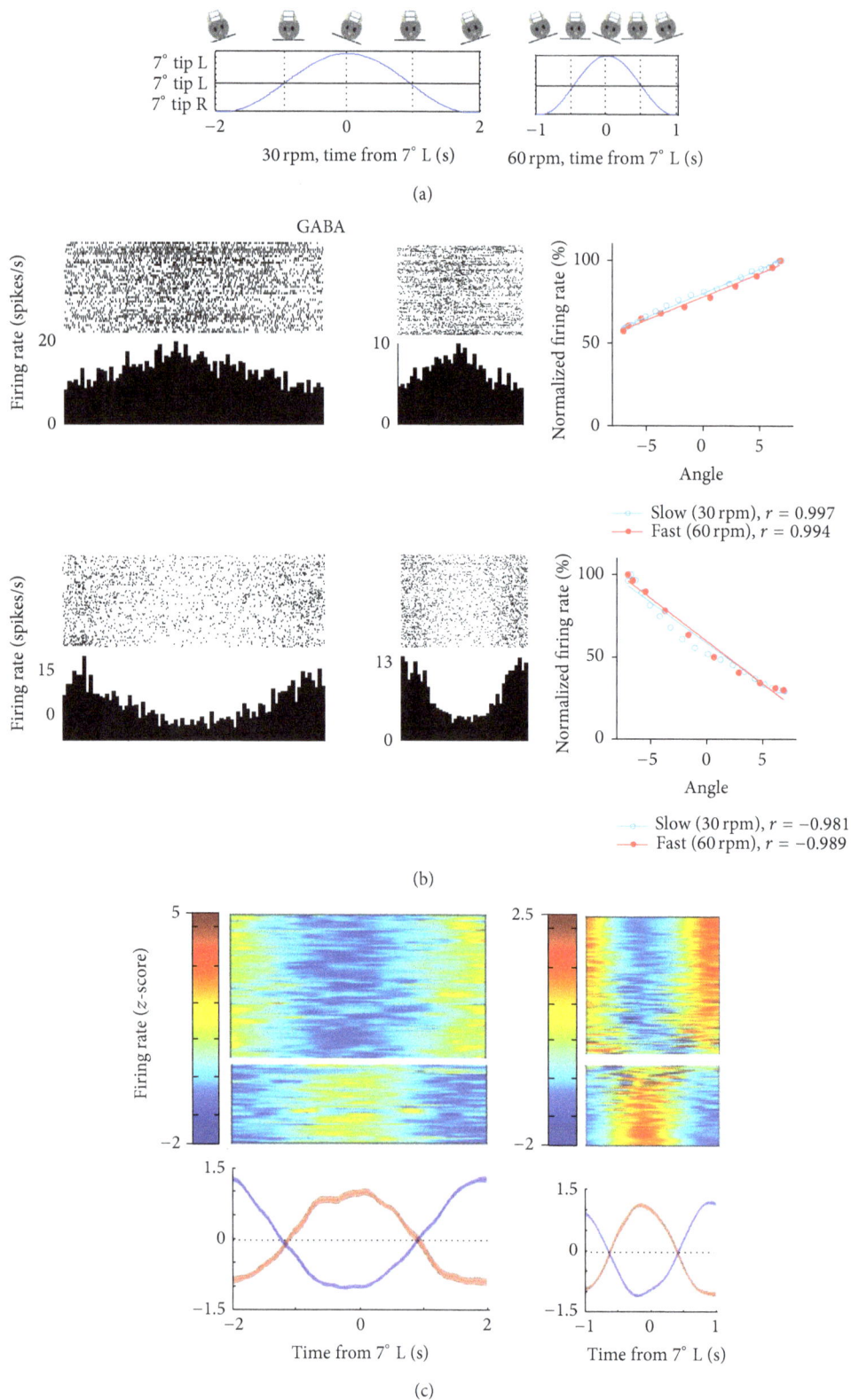

FIGURE 4: Neural activity from the SNr during postural disturbances [42]. (a) Pattern of postural disturbances. (b) Left, raster plots of two representative nigral GABAergic projection neurons. Right, correlation between the tilt disturbance and firing rate. (c) Spike density functions illustrating the two major populations of nigral neurons. Their firing rate in relation to the postural disturbance is 180 degrees out of phase.

control. Opponent signals are needed for any movement or posture. Movement and posture are not antagonistic but share the same mechanisms. Rather the antagonistic relationship exists between downstream systems that act in different directions.

But it could be argued that our results support the earlier idea that opponent BG pathways can scale the intended movements in a "push-pull" manner by grading the movement parameters such as speed and amplitude [43, 44]. Increased BG output results in hypokinesia (e.g., Parkinson's disease). Reduced BG output, by contrast, results in hyperkinesia (e.g., hemiballismus). In Parkinson's patients, the abnormally low velocity and amplitude of movements is thought to be a result of excessive BG output, which inhibits thalamocortical activation. This model actually assumes that there is a monolithic BG output and that the magnitude of this output is modulated by the direct (striatonigral) and indirect (striatopallidal) pathways, as water temperature (a single magnitude) is adjusted by the cold and hot water handles for a faucet. High BG output results in small and slow movements, whereas low BG output results in fast and large movements. But this model does not predict the pattern of bidirectional outputs we observed, and it neglects the role of the common mode signal or tonic activity in SNr neurons, which according to the present account represents the neutral position or body configuration. Push-pull signals are not used to adjust the amplitude and speed of movement but to command antagonistic downstream systems. Greater BG output does not result in larger or faster movements.

4. Behavior and Feedback

In both the temporal differentiation task and the posture control task, the critical data come from a period when there is no apparent movement of the animal. Yet lack of overt movement does not indicate a lack of neural activity. Whether holding the lever, fixating on a target, or standing, the nervous system must produce outputs to counter continuous disturbances to achieve position control. In studies that examined neural activity during rest, when the subject is not performing any task, it is common to call the neural activity the "default mode" to mask ignorance of the underlying processes [45].

Although it is easy for the naïve observer to ignore the continuous neural output in the absence of any overt movement, the role of posture control becomes abundantly clear when it fails. For example, as one dozes off, the head drops as the neck muscles become incapable of maintaining the upright posture. In neurological disorders simply maintaining a posture such as standing or keeping one's arm raised seems an impossible task.

Anyone attempting to build a system that can maintain a standing posture in a skeleton on a tilting platform will appreciate the tremendous computational challenges in posture control. Unlike a tank or robots with a stable base designed to obviate the computational challenges of postural control, there is no inherent postural stability in the skeleton, which is balancing on ball-and-socket joints. No engineer has

succeeded in building anything that can balance a skeleton in an environment with unpredictable disturbances. Yet any deviation from the vertical, in a living man, is corrected exactly by the pattern of muscle contractions needed to restore balance, with these corrections happening so quickly that they are almost imperceptible to the casual observer.

Based on his studies of patients with BG damage, Martin argued that the postural deficits found in BG-related disorders are also responsible for the movement deficits [46]. To understand BG function, it would be critical to understand, at a computational level, exactly what posture control entails and how it can be related to movement.

4.1. Negative Feedback as the Solution to the Calculation Problem. When someone is standing, to the casual observer there appears to be no behavior. But this appearance is misleading. Any perturbation, such as a push, is met with resistance from the organism. Not only a push, but invisible and unpredictable disturbances everywhere—gravity, wind, changes in effector properties such as the spring properties of the muscles. These disturbances must be overcome, by varying output. This is an example of position control.

The term "control" means that posture stays the same, despite environmental disturbances. The naïve assumption that whatever neural signals are sent to our muscles determine the effects we exert on the environment, that is, observable behavior, was demolished by Bernstein nearly a century ago [47]. Bernstein wrote: "There are no situations in which muscle shortening is the cause of a movement" [48]. The actual effect of the muscular contraction is not the product of our neural output. Behavior can never be equated with the output of the nervous system, because it is the joint product of unknown environmental influences and neural signals. To the motor neurons producing muscle contraction, even fatigue or slight changes in the properties of the muscles can become a major source of disturbance. Consequently, a measure of muscle contraction (e.g., electromyography) can never define the actual behavior or the posture. That the output does not equal behavior raises the question of how the neural output can be adjusted as unknown and unpredictable disturbances vary. This is the "calculation problem," the key problem that the nervous system must solve [49].

It is often believed that the calculation problem can be solved by computing inverse kinematics and dynamics or by feedforward computation to predict the future effects of actions using sophisticated mathematics. If only we can calculate the needed force output, it would be possible to produce movements [50, 51]. This feedforward approach requires enormous computational power and completely accurate knowledge of the physical interactions in the environment, if not omniscience. This is never found in any biological organism. Yet the calculation problem, after all, is solved by virtually all organisms. The solution is closed loop negative feedback, the only known organization to reduce error between the desired and the actual. Unfortunately feedback is widely misunderstood, even though the term is used frequently. Due to such misunderstanding, it is often considered a crude mechanism that has been replaced by modern developments. Because feedback is often incorrectly applied to the analysis of biological systems [52–54], it is useful to correct some common misconceptions at the outset.

4.2. Control of Input.

A control system always controls its input, not output [7]. Only perceivable consequences of behavior can be controlled. The control system contains internal reference signals, which indicate the desired state of some input variable. It varies its outputs until the consequence matches the reference signal. The output is proportional to the difference between input and reference. It is not determined by either perceptual inputs or reference signal, but by both simultaneously.

According to mainstream engineering control theory, a control system controls its outputs, not its input. This is perhaps the most common fallacy today, both in engineering and in the life sciences [49, 55, 56]. This fallacy, an unfortunate legacy of cybernetics, is the result of imposing the perspective of the observer rather than using the perspective of the organism or controller. The mistake is to assume that what the engineer perceives and records, the "objective" effect of the system, is the output of the system.

The goal of the engineer, when designing a controller, is to compute the output required—the "control signal" sent to the "motor plant" to move it in a certain way. For example, to move something to a preselected position, the engineer can compute the outputs that must be generated in order to produce the change in position, including inverse kinematics and dynamics, and send the signals to the transducers. To the organism, however, feedback through sensory channels is the only way it can know about the consequences of its behavior. There is no alternative way to discover the "objective" effects.

The common assumption that output is controlled ignores the perspective of the organism that is doing the controlling. By imposing his own desire and perspective, the engineer ignores the autonomy of the negative feedback controller, for he is always trying to make the machine do what he wants. He can only accomplish this by adjusting the reference signal, as the user operates a thermostat by adjusting the temperature setting. Since this is the signal generated by the user, it is usually labeled as the input to the system. In a biological organism, however, the reference signal is always internal to the organism.

The real input is the perceptual variable that can be affected by feedback [49]. In a temperature controller using negative feedback, the perceptual input is from the temperature sensors. Of course, in a man-made thermostat, the user can adjust the "set point," but that is a unique feature of these systems, because that is the only way to use a negative feedback control system. The man-made controller, at least so far, is not designed to adjust its own references. Rather it is designed as a "servo," to serve the needs of the user. A biological organism, in contrast, has reference signals of its own, not accessible to any user. It is autonomous, because it does not serve the needs of another, but those of itself only and always.

From the perspective of the engineer, negative feedback control is about injecting an error signal to get the desired output. In traditional cybernetic applications of control theory to the study of behavior, the comparison between error and reference is placed outside of the organism, where the engineer designing the system also performs the comparison function. Thus for decades such control systems have been treated as stimulus-response or input-output devices: error in, behavior out. The tendency to resort to linear causation is so strong that even closed loop controllers have been treated as devices that receive error signals and generate behaviors. This is only true of a component of the loop, namely, the output function when it is isolated [49]. It could never be true of the closed loop negative feedback controller.

In the end, the appropriate output signals must be computed somehow. The question is how. The negative feedback organization simply eliminates the effects of disturbance by subtracting them from the internal reference. The effect of its own output is monitored with its own sensors and actively controlled. This elegant solution to the calculation problem avoids calculations on the disturbances in advance. Whatever their effects, they are simply rejected by the negative feedback. The inverse kinematics and dynamics are realized by the physical interaction between organism and environment, in the forward equations describing how muscle contractions interact with the external environment. None of these calculations are performed inside the nervous system.

The misidentification of the inputs and outputs of a control system resulted in persistent mistakes in the application of control theory even when the correct mathematical equations were used. What is worse is that it has made it impossible to perform the appropriate experiments to measure the actual properties of the living control systems. Consequently, many myths have been propagated, for example, the idea that negative feedback controllers are slow [59], when speed is a chief advantage of such a system. Given a small error, the high loop gain can produce a rapid response, instantly removing any small deviation from the desired reference condition. High gain does not mean that a large response will be generated, as the response is always determined by the magnitude of the error. As error is self-reducing in a closed loop, the negative feedback necessarily limits the response, preventing it from becoming too large. But the time it takes for the output to reduce the error is greatly reduced by the high gain. When the input and output of the output function are incorrectly identified, as in all traditional diagrams illustrating the control loop, loop gain cannot be measured accurately [60–63].

As a result of these conceptual confusions, in traditional models negative feedback is always misunderstood. Placing the comparator outside the organism has the unintended effect of inverting the inside and outside of the system (Figure 5). What should be part of the organism is considered to be a part of the environment, and what should be part of the environment, namely, the feedback function, is considered a part of the organism. Consequently, the equations that describe how forces act on loads and accelerations and decelerations of the loads are assumed to be computed by the nervous system [50]. These conceptual confusions have largely prevented any progress in the study of behavior for many decades.

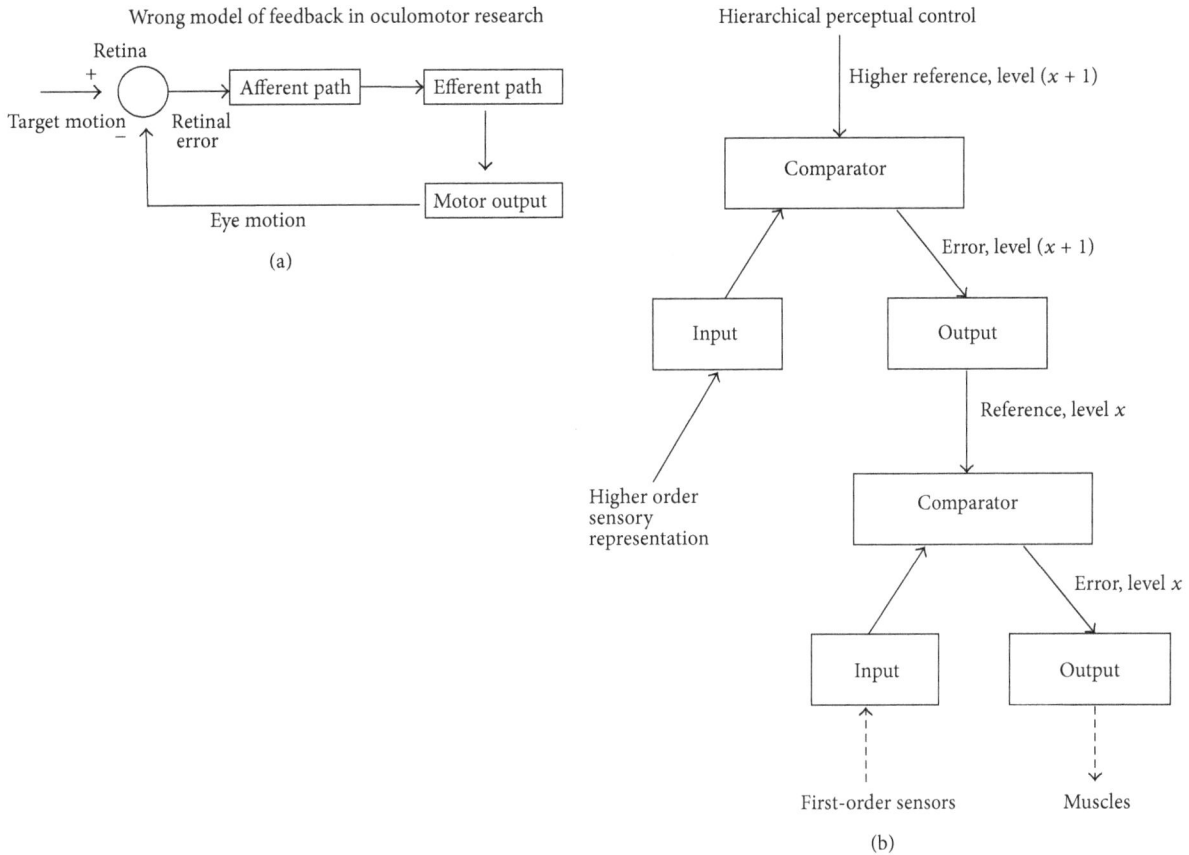

FIGURE 5: Negative feedback and control. (a) An example of the wrong application of control theory to the study of behavior in oculomotor studies [57]. In this diagram, there is no reference signal internal to the organism. The comparison function is performed in the external environment. Consequently, what is computed inside the organism is attributed to the external environment. And instead of receiving perceptual inputs, the input function receives error signals. This incorrect application of control theory has misled researchers for decades, leading to repeated rejections of negative feedback as an explanatory principle. (b) Illustration of cascade control proposed here. Two closed loop negative feedback control systems arranged hierarchically. Note that what is controlled is the perceptual variable, and the reference signal always comes from within the organism. In a hierarchy the higher level can adjust the reference of a lower level by sending a projection to the comparator function of the latter [58].

5. Posture/Movement Problem and Cascade Control

Posture control is an example of negative feedback control. The controlled variable is the perception of the current body configuration. The relevant perceptual signals are a set of perceptual signals sensed by the organism, using sensors distributed all over the body.

A body configuration may be defined as a collection of joint angles, but joint angles alone are not always sufficient to define a posture. The body configuration may be similar whether standing erect or lying supine, but the relation to environmental disturbances such as gravity is quite different. Perceptions like the sense of effort, related to proprioceptive perception of muscle tension, may also be involved.

The same effectors, the same final common path from motor neuron to muscle, must be used to defend a given posture and to change that posture. That postural control is

a prerequisite for normal movements is commonly acknowledged [64, 65]. A fundamental question, first raised by Von Holst and Mittelstaedt, is how movement is possible when posture is in fact defended against environmental disturbances [66]. Clearly animals can maintain a particular posture. But movements require a change in posture. With a self-initiated movement, why is not the current posture also defended? Why are self-initiated movements not treated as disturbances to the controller?

Posture control is traditionally viewed as a result of "postural reflexes," fast adjustments in muscle output in response to any disturbance. With voluntary movements such lower postural reflexes are assumed to be inhibited [66]. In a postural reflex, the output is highly correlated with the input. The high correlation between stimulus and response gave rise to the concept of the reflex. Yet students of behavior have often noticed the variability in such reflexes; the same stimulus sometimes produces one output and sometimes another, and sometimes opposite outputs can be produced (reflex reversal). Baffled by such variability, some attempted to eliminate it using techniques like decerebration, by removing the descending influence of the brain. Using decerebration, Sherrington was unwittingly forcing control systems to behave like input/output devices, though necessarily in vain [39, 67].

In an input/output device, the output is a function of input. If the output varies given the same input or if different inputs can produce the same output, the standard explanation is that the function relating sensory information to behavior is not fixed but somehow modifiable depending on "contexts" that higher levels can turn off reflexes that get in the way of behavior, or that the processing of perceptual inputs can be "noisy." The currently popular focused selection model of BG function, for example, assumes that BG output is needed to turn off the postural reflexes while selecting some action [3, 20].

Control theory, however, offers a very different explanation of the lack of correspondence between inputs and outputs. It shows that the output cannot possibly be a function of the input, even when it appears to be correlated, as in Sherrington's decerebrate dogs [39]. Because the output is generated from the error signal, which is the difference between reference and input, there is simply no function relating the input to the output in this system. Anyone trying to find the function relating the temperature sensor reading to the output of the thermostat is simply wasting his time, because there is none [49]. To find the output, it is necessary to know both the input and the reference.

Consequently, there is no such thing as sensorimotor transformation. Concepts like sensory or neural noise are also irrelevant [51], since the circuit only processes signals and does not make any distinction between noise and nonnoise. In neuroscience, noise is just a term usually used to describe signals that the observer does not understand or want. This confusion arises largely because neither behavior nor neural signal makes sense when viewed from the perspective of input/output systems. They almost always appear to be more variable than what is acceptable to the experimenter. This is mainly because a critical determinant of behavior, namely the internal reference, is left out of the traditional paradigm. Behavior and neural activity vary, but this variation is not due to noise or inconsistencies in the sensorimotor transformations. It varies because of the attempt to control desired perceptual variables by canceling the effects of environmental disturbances.

5.1. Behavioral Illusion and the Myth of the Reflex.
Gain in the output function in a negative feedback system is not used to convert input into output. The typical mistake is to measure gain by calculating the ratio between input and output, but input in this case is incorrectly identified: it is actually defined from the observer's perspective, which is usually a disturbance to a controlled variable [61].

When the input/output correlation appears to be high, it produces a powerful illusion: the illusion that what is observed is the behavior of an input/output device, in which output is generated by the input [68]. In a control system, the effects of disturbance are rejected with output through a feedback function. But what counts as disturbance depends on the reference signal. As soon as the reference is altered, the definition of disturbance also changes, and the input that used to generate output suddenly ceases to do so.

Decerebration alters descending reference signals permanently, so that these signals can no longer influence lower systems. Even then, the lower systems can still have reference signals, whether by default or from some other still intact sources, and error signals can still be generated. With the feedback path still intact, the output can still alter the perceptual signal. The correlation between input and output may seem to be high, but one can easily change the output by altering the feedback path in the environment.

Although reflexes can create the illusion of high input/output correlation, of antecedent automatically "causing" responses from the organism, a closer examination shows this is an illusion [68]. A change in the environment can produce what appears to be a change in the sensorimotor transformation inside the organism. This is because the disturbance is reflected in the error (and output), which reduces the effect of the disturbance, but any manipulation of the feedback function will necessarily change how effective the output will be in rejecting the effects of disturbance on the controlled variable. Systematic manipulations of the feedback function will change how the system "responds" to the input, even when neither the stimulus nor the organism has changed. This behavioral illusion is the first trap that students of behavior must understand and avoid, though unfortunately so far it has victimized even the best investigators.

5.2. The Control Hierarchy.
If postural mechanisms are not turned off during voluntary movements, then how can the brain generate movement? In the present model, a change in body position is produced by changing the reference signal of the position controller. Instead of a user injecting this reference signal, as in adjusting the temperature setting of a thermostat, it must come from within the organism.

Where then does the reference signal come from? The answer is suggested by cascade control or hierarchical perceptual control [58], in which the reference signal comes from the output of another controller. Thus there is a hierarchical relationship between the higher controller that sends the reference and the lower controller that receives it, much as an order is given in a chain of command.

At every level of the hierarchy, only inputs can be controlled. When the output of a control system serves as the reference signal of another control system, it does not specify the output of the lower system, but its input. Altering the output directly without altering the reference would affect the controlled variable via the feedback path, creating error that would cancel the effect of the output. Outputs from higher levels determine the type of perceptions the lower levels should achieve [58]. The lower controller will vary its output to produce the input determined by the descending reference signal, serving as an extension of the output function of higher levels (Figure 5).

If the reference signal of the posture control system is altered, the current posture will not be defended. Rather the system will defend the new value of the reference signal at any moment. There will then be a transition from the old posture to new posture, a movement.

The nervous system comprises a hierarchy of negative feedback control systems, each controlling its own perceptual input [58]. The higher systems do not have direct access to the actual actions or most of the perceptual inputs and error signals from lower levels. It only senses the variable to be controlled and generates error signals which become the reference signals for lower levels. To see where the BG fit on this control hierarchy, we must first outline, if only briefly, the functions of the lower levels. This may appear to be a circuitous route to understanding, but as we shall see a major problem with existing theories of BG function is their false assumptions about what behavior is and about the functions of the hierarchically lower systems.

6. Control of Muscle Tension and Length

The lowest level of the neural hierarchy controls muscle tension. The output function of this controller is the muscle. Projections from alpha motor neuron to muscle fibers send error signals in the tension controller [7]. The alpha motor neuron, as a comparator, receives signals from multiple sources. The major source of negative feedback is the Golgi tendon organ, which detects muscle tension produced by contraction of extrafusal fibers. The tension signal is fed back to the alpha motor neuron through the inhibitory Ib interneuron that inverts the sign of the signal, so that it is the opposite of the excitatory Ia afferent to the alpha motor neurons. This inversion creates negative feedback, as the inhibitory effect is subtracted from the excitatory effect. When the muscle contracts, the negative feedback keeps the tension in check. This is traditionally called an inverse myotatic reflex or the Golgi tendon reflex. The contraction creates the feedback, which restricts the contraction. Additional rate feedback can come from Renshaw cells, inhibitory interneurons that are excited by the alpha motor neurons, but in turn inhibit alpha motor neurons [69, 70].

On the other hand, muscle length itself can be controlled independently while tension varies. The relationship between length and tension is hierarchical. The higher length level specifies the tension to be reached. Tension can be varied to maintain a desired length. The difference between desired length and actual length, the error in length control, is turned into a reference signal to the tension controller.

The so-called myotatic or kneejerk reflex is a type of stretch reflex, in which the lengthening of the muscle is resisted by muscle contraction and shortening. This phenomenon reflects the action of a muscle length controller. A major signal driving the alpha motor neuron (and hence contraction of extrafusal muscle fibers) comes from the Ia afferent. This signal is often interpreted as representing muscle length. But the Ia afferent signal can be independent

of muscle length. When the extrafusal muscle fibers are stretched, the parallel muscle spindle, a stretch sensor, is also stretched and activates the alpha motor neuron (i.e., stretch reflex). But the Ia afferent can also generate a signal as a result of gamma motor neuron output, which activates the contractile part of the spindle, thus "simulating" a stretch. To the alpha motor neuron, it does not matter how the Ia afferent signal is produced, by actual stretch or by gamma activation. The function of the gamma mechanism is not to keep the spindle taut and maintain sensitivity to changes in muscle length, as described in textbooks [26]. Rather the arrangement produces a comparison between current muscle length (via Ia and II fibers) and the length "demanded" by the reference signals from the gamma motor neuron. The muscle spindle does not directly contribute to the generation of muscle tension but functions as a mechanical comparator of desired and actual muscle length signals. The Ia afferent thus carries an error signal for the length controller, which in turn activates the alpha motor neurons and generates shortening of the extrafusal muscle fibers and muscle tension.

This arrangement is traditionally called a "follow-up servo" model, first proposed by Merton [71]. Yet, although Merton correctly identified the comparator, he failed to take into account the hierarchical relationship between length control and tension control, the key feature also neglected by subsequent models [53, 62, 71, 72]. This failure led to subsequent rejection of servo models of the motor system. Instead, it is common to claim, incorrectly, that the gamma motor neuron output functions simply to keep the muscle spindle sensitive to stretch [26].

According to the model presented here, the length controller achieves control of desired length specified by the gamma motor neurons by varying the reference signal to the tension controller, which varies muscle tension as needed. Tension control at the lowest level is always used for posture control and all other behaviors, but tension is not the controlled variable of the higher levels, which achieve their respective purposes by varying reference signals for tension. The higher levels all adjust muscle tension ultimately but not directly. Directly they all attempt to control their own respective perceptual variables, whether muscle length or joint angle. One possible exception is the direct projection to alpha motor neurons from the motor cortex or more commonly projections to the spinal interneurons. The importance of corticospinal (pyramidal tract) projections, especially for movements of the digits, cannot be denied. These descending projections can directly affect tension or force control, but their functions are poorly understood. In the present review, the focus is on movements of the whole body, rather than distal joints like digits.

6.1. Joint Angle and Body Configuration. In any movement, the length of the relevant muscles must be changed. This changes the angular position of the segments at the joint at which all the forces are balanced. The segments accelerate toward the new position with various damping factors, such as viscosity within muscles as well as negative rate feedback from proprioceptors to prevent overshoot. The new position changes during the movement, and the sensed joint angle smoothly approaches the angle set by the descending reference signal; the segments automatically decelerate as the desired position is approached. This behavior is the necessary result of how the hierarchy is organized. During movement, all the required variations in neural signals to the muscles are created by continuous feedback at various levels, not by forward planning or computation of inverse dynamics and kinematics.

Actions of the length controller ("stretch reflexes") can facilitate posture control by bracing the knees, keeping the hip joints extended and the trunk upright, to minimize forces required for balance. But muscle length control is not sufficient for posture control. Patients with BG pathology often show intact stretch reflexes, yet they are still impaired in response to tilt [46].

Muscle length control in any controller is not sufficient to define posture. Multiple length controllers are needed just to define a joint angle, for example, biceps and triceps at the elbow joint. Moreover, any signal representing muscle length does not correspond exactly to the angle at the joint spanned by the muscle. The mechanical advantage changes with the angle, and loads can make the actual angle deviate from the angle represented by muscle length or tension. Without sensing the joint angle directly, controlling joint angle by relying only on muscle length would not be very effective. In addition to information from muscle length and tension sensors, joint angles can be perceived with specialized sensors located in the joints and stretch receptors that can detect rate of change.

It is also not sufficient to control posture simply by cocontraction of muscles, that is, "stiffness" or "impedance" control [73]. In muscles with spring constants that are an exponential function of tension, output gain in position control depends on the resting tension in opposing muscles. The common mode signal to both agonist and antagonist muscles can increase spring constants, thereby increasing the force applied to the tendons by a given amount of muscle shortening without generating net force. With continuous disturbances, the muscles across a joint can indeed appear to be stiff, but this apparent stiffness is mostly a result of rate feedback. It varies according to the disturbance applied to the sensed position. Without negative feedback, adjustment of stiffness alone is a poor method for achieving position control.

6.2. From Posture to Movement. At levels above joint angle control, the controlled variable is not the length of a single muscle or a single joint angle but a collection of joint angles coupled with the effort required to resist disturbances. With a complex body geometry, posture control requires a higher level that simultaneously adjusts joint angle in several joints at once, that is, body configuration. Movement can simply be defined as a change in body configuration, produced by a change in the reference signal to the comparator in the configuration controller. However, higher levels can produce movements by sending reference signals to any of the lower level controllers, for tension, length, or joint angle. The

purpose of each movement will differ depending on which level is initiating the change in reference signal. For example, one can either activate the tension controller directly, via direct projections to the alpha motor neurons, or by activating the gamma motor neurons specifying muscle length, so that the error signal from the length controller activates the alpha motor neurons. Often both alpha and gamma motor neurons can be activated simultaneously [74].

The above description of the lower levels of the neural hierarchy shows three important features not found in any other model of the nervous system. Familiarity with these properties is necessary for understanding the contributions of the BG.

(1) Control of perceptual inputs is the key principle in the hierarchical organization. Typically the higher levels receive higher order transformations of perceptual inputs compared to the lower levels and control these more abstract and global variables by varying reference signals sent to lower levels.

(2) The higher levels can use the lower levels without turning them off. For example, in length control, tension is still controlled, except that the tension is specified by the reference signal sent from the length controller. The same is true of higher levels that control other variables.

(3) Hierarchical organization allows one control system to command another. But it does so not by adjusting the output of the lower control system directly, but by sending a reference signal. The effect of this descending reference signal is to tell the lower system to achieve a particular level of perception. The actual output generated by the lower level will vary according to the comparison between the new reference signal and lower level perceptions. Thus the command signal in a control hierarchy never contains information about the actual outputs to be generated.

7. Reticulospinal System and Posture Control

In disorders implicating the BG, abnormal postures are common (e.g., somersault postures, bending of the spine). These could simply reflect abnormal reference signals to body configuration systems [46]. Position control is intact, but the reference signals for positions have extreme and fixed values. A fixed reference signal to body configuration would produce a fixed body configuration. In the most extreme condition, it would produce complete freezing of the body [75]. Consequently, the patient is continuously controlling a fixed position, still varying neural outputs in downstream controllers appropriately, until the effectors are exhausted.

Patients with BG pathology are also impaired in response to tilting of the body [46]. In particular, Martin found that, during tilt disturbances, the reaction of the trunk was much reduced. This observation suggests the involvement of the reticulospinal pathway, the most primitive motor system in vertebrates, and a major pathway influenced by the BG outputs [76, 77]. Although the BG output to the thalamus also eventually activates cortical regions giving rise to the corticospinal pathway [43], the latter pathway in most organisms is not critical for posture control.

As shown by lesion studies, the reticulospinal pathway is especially important for axial movements, rather than hand and finger movements that require the corticospinal pathway [46, 78]. The reticulospinal pathway is a major source of descending reference signals for joint angles and simple body configurations. It is therefore critical to consider the functional organization of this pathway before discussing the contributions of the higher levels.

The reticulospinal pathway has been extensively studied in lampreys [79–83]. In the lamprey, movement of the axial musculature involves alternation of muscles on two sides of the body, for example, left-right alternation or dorsal-ventral alternation. Muscles on one side lengthen while muscles on the opposite side are shortened. Activation on one side will produce contraction and bending of the muscles and inhibition of the contralateral circuit, that is, relaxation or lengthening of the contralateral segment. The reticulospinal neurons innervating one side can be excited by sensory inputs, but the reticulospinal neurons on the other side are inhibited by the same input. The disturbances sensed by the comparator produce error signals in body configuration, which become reference signals for joint angle control.

The reticulospinal neurons can receive inputs from the vestibular and proprioceptive sensors, which report the current values of the relevant sensory variables, and send projections to motor neurons, which in turn produce movements that resist the effect of disturbances to postural reference signals. They are activated by disturbances in pitch, roll, and yaw planes [84, 85]. If a reticulospinal neuron was activated by a turn in a given plane, it is also involved in generating a torque opposing the turn. For example, the neuron excited by the nose-up pitch tilts activates both left and right ventral muscles, which produce the nose-down body bending, the output that compensates for the initial postural disturbance of nose-up tilt [84, 86, 87]. The reticulospinal pathway can generate movements that counteract the effects of postural disturbances in any direction [85]. Two complimentary types of reticulospinal neurons were found to control posture in a particular axis of rotation: they were activated by rotation in opposite directions and produced movements generating torques counteracting the postural disturbances.

The reticulospinal system can control body orientation, in relation to gravity, by sending reference signals to joint angle controllers. There are obvious parallels between the reticulospinal activity and the nigral activity during postural disturbances [42]. As described below, the BG represent a higher level of the hierarchy.

It is sometimes claimed that the reticulospinal projections have general excitatory or inhibitory effects [88, 89], yet the evidence suggests otherwise. For example, with reticulospinal stimulation, the effects on posture show simultaneous action on pairs of muscles, for example, leg flexed or extended with reciprocal inhibition of the antagonists [90]. Ipsilateral flexion and contralateral extension could be produced with medial reticular stimulation, whereas the opposite pattern of ipsilateral extension and contralateral flexion could be

produced by more lateral stimulation. It appears that multiple reciprocal inhibition circuits can be engaged, probably by the activation of spinal interneurons. These behavioral observations are in accordance with the known anatomy. Reticulospinal neurons send branching projections to multiple regions in the spinal cord; for example, axons traveling to the cervical enlargement also project to lumbar levels. A single reticulospinal axon can project to several different spinal levels corresponding to different body parts and to neurons on both sides of the spinal cord [91, 92]. These projections are capable of producing coordinated contraction or relaxation of muscles in several body parts [90, 93, 94].

The reticulospinal pathway, then, implements the body configuration control systems that can adjust references to multiple joint angle controllers. Inputs to this level come from multiple joint angle sensors and muscle length sensors; they are compared with references for body configuration, and error signals are in turn sent to joint angle controllers in different body parts. If the reference signals are fixed, then a stable posture or body configuration will be assumed. By changing reference signals to this level, movements can be created.

8. Orientation Control in the Midbrain

Given the role of the reticulospinal pathway in posture control, the obvious question is how can higher order systems vary descending reference signals in order to generate movements. BG outputs are certainly in a position to do so via direct projections, yet much of the BG output does not reach the reticulospinal pathway directly. Instead there are extensive projections to the midbrain and parts of the diencephalon, which in turn projects to the reticulospinal pathway. Some of these areas, such as the tectum and pedunculopontine/mesencephalic locomotor region, project to reticulospinal neurons. I will focus on the tectum because more is known about its organization [95–97]. The nigrothalamic projections are not discussed, because the functions of the thalamocortical system remain obscure.

8.1. Organization of the Tectum. The tectum (superior and inferior colliculi) is chiefly concerned with orientation of the head and body and thereby with steering during locomotion. It is most commonly associated with the orienting reaction, in which any salient stimulus can result in orienting towards that stimulus. This reaction allows one to detect changes in the environment, in preparation for possible behavioral engagement, whether to approach or to avoid [98]. The superficial tectal layers receive perceptual inputs from multiple sensory modalities [95, 99], and stimulation of the tectum can produce a variety of movements (of eyes, ears, head, and muscles) [100–104].

Although only a subset of the output neurons from the intermediate and deep layers are related to eye movements [105], these neurons have been studied extensively. Studies of the monkey superior colliculus have shown a retinotopically organized map that receives inputs from the superficial layers above. Some deep layer collicular neurons fire just before the onset of a saccade that would bring the image to the center of the fovea [106].

It is believed that the tectum contains a map of angular deviations [107–109].The tectal output somehow allows the organism to orient towards the distal target that is the source of the stimulus. For oculomotor behavior, the question is how to produce a sudden gaze shift to a target off center. The target is selected by moving attention away from the foveated part of the visual field.

The remarkable accuracy in final position of eye movements, despite variability in actual movements, is exactly what we would expect in a position control system. Yet, after decades of study, eye movements are still described in terms of sensorimotor transformation. The fact that negative feedback control and error terms are often mentioned in the oculomotor literature, as mechanisms for sensorimotor transformations, only betrays ignorance of how control works, since control and sensorimotor transformation are mutually exclusive.

Traditional analysis of eye movements has been misguided by the fallacy, discussed above, of misassigning components of a negative feedback system to the organism-environment interaction while missing the one critical ingredient, namely, internal reference signals. Robinson, a pioneer in the study of eye movements, was perhaps chiefly responsible for propagating this fallacy. As he wrote: "The retina senses the error between the eye (fovea) and the target, and the system turns the eye until the error is zero—a simple negative feedback scheme" [110]. The mistake here is to place the comparator function outside the organism. The actual movement is compared with disturbance, and the difference is considered to be the error that is fed into the controller. The controller then becomes an input-output device that transforms the retinal error into neural output. Unfortunately this mistake has dominated oculomotor research [57].

Although the controller reduces the error between fovea and target, it is important to determine where this error signal is generated, by the nervous system or elsewhere. The only relevant visual input is detected by the retina. That self-motion reduces the actual "slip" on the retina simply describes the feedback function, the effect of the behavioral output on the perceived variable. This is the negative feedback. But there is no such thing as "retinal error." The retina cannot report the error between eye and target. That error is generated inside the brain, using internal comparison functions. Motion is only a disturbance to a control system with a reference signal representing zero motion or simply a particular position. Consequently, any detected motion can generate an error signal that results in movement of the eyes and body.

What is overlooked in the traditional analysis, then, is the internal reference that specifies how much perceived deviation of the target is tolerated. Object motion constitutes a disturbance to the organism precisely because it forces some perceptual inputs to deviate from the values specified by this internal reference signal. The key comparison is done inside the system, not at the retina. This behavioral illusion resulted in a complete reversal of the inside and outside of the control system, forcing theorists to use equations that describe physical processes in the environment to describe

the computational processes inside the brain [57]. Robinson, for example, thought it was necessary to use internal computations to generate a signal that represents the target motion, that is, the disturbance [63]. But one of the chief features of the negative feedback controller is that the actual perceptual variable is protected from the effects of the disturbance by producing the appropriate behavior. In other words, its function is to reject the effects of disturbance, in order not to sense it directly.

8.2. The Tectal Orientation Controller. The optic tectum is critical for maintaining foveation. The angular deviation is the difference between the current eye position and the eye position needed to foveate on the visual target. The controlled variable is roughly the distance between target and fovea. The intermediate and deep tectal layers contain neurons that serve as comparators and send error signals in position control. The units at a particular location on the tectal map can activate the appropriate downstream controllers to reduce the position error. The reference level for this variable is close to zero. Any deviation is promptly corrected. This can be called orientation control. There are a few differences from posture control.

(1) As control systems are characterized by the input variables they control directly, orientation control involves different types of sensory inputs. Tectal controllers rely on perceptual inputs unavailable to the lower levels such as the reticulospinal pathway. These are primarily the sensory modalities (e.g., vision and audition) for the detection of distal stimuli away from the organism, whereas posture control relies more strongly on proximal kinesthetic senses. Exteroceptive inputs are therefore needed for orientation control. The sensors involved are usually visual and auditory but also include vibrissae in rodents. The main goal is to produce movements to receive the relevant signals, much like adjusting an antenna to optimize signal reception.

(2) The use of the distal senses creates a representation of the external environment and of the relationship between one's own body and this environment (egocentric reference frame). This allows orientation and steering towards things in the environment at a distance from the organism [103, 106, 109, 111]. This level is where the sense of direction becomes relevant, as one is no longer simply changing the body configuration, but changing it in order to achieve some relationship with some other object locations in space. Without the distal senses, this would be nearly impossible. Imagine the difficulty of orienting or goal-directed behavior in complete darkness and in silence.

(3) This level is also where the head becomes extremely important. Because the head contains the distal sensory systems, orienting with the head is the equivalent of sensory target acquisition with the relevant receptors, hence the importance of the tectum in foveation control. But target acquisition is not limited to the

visual modality. According to the present model, the tectum is also critical for acquiring targets in other sensory modalities. With the head orientation defined with respect to objects perceived by the distal senses, certain concepts used to describe behavior only become meaningful at this level of the hierarchy: straight ahead, towards, and away from. These descriptions cannot be applied to the lower body configuration controllers in the reticulospinal pathway precisely because perceptual signals representing the distal environment do not reach the lower levels, which only receive information about the body.

The tectum, then, controls the orientation of the head and body in relation to some target in the environment. In the orienting reaction, the target is just any salient stimulus. For such control to be possible, both the current location of the fovea and the location of the visual target are needed. In the retinotopically organized tectal map, the fovea represents the origin, that is, $(0, 0)$ in polar or Cartesian coordinates. It also represents the default reference condition for visual tracking. Directions of movement are determined from this starting point. Without knowing the current position, it would be impossible to move towards any location in space.

In foveation control, the outputs vary to minimize deviation from fovea. By visually acquiring the target, the new target location becomes the origin. From the perspective of control theory, fixation, pursuit, and saccades are different modes of operation of the same controller. Fixation, for example, is pursuit tracking on a stationary target. Most differences can probably be attributed to descending reference signals from higher level controllers that have access to additional perceptual variables, such as representation of motion from cortical regions [112]. In smooth pursuit, when the target moves with a certain velocity, position control requires eye movement at a similar velocity as the rate of change in target position on the retina. The smoothness could be the result of additional velocity control, which requires velocity feedback not readily available at the level of the tectum. But current data cannot dissociate velocity control from position control. Both can produce the type of outputs observed in oculomotor studies.

In the rostral end of the tectal map, corresponding to the foveal representation, there are neurons that fire during fixation. Their activity appears to be proportional to position error, the mismatch between a parafoveal stimulus and the currently foveated location [113]. Krauzlis et al. concluded that the activity of these neurons represents a position error signal rather than a motor command [114]. What they failed to realize is that, in control systems, a position error signal is exactly what is needed to produce a motor output, being transformed into a descending reference signal for a lower level controller. These rostral neurons mediate microsaccades, small eye movements that maintain foveation [115]. In caudal tectal regions, neurons fire before and during saccades—large changes in eye position. The difference between rostral and caudal neurons seems to be one of degree, not of kind [116]. The function is to acquire

visual targets by placing the light pattern on the fovea in the center of the visual field.

The deep layers of the superior colliculus contain tectoreticulospinal neurons that project to contralateral brainstem regions that generate eye and head movements [117–119]. In cats that are free to move their heads, these projections appear to be critical for gaze shifts, using coordinated movements of the eyes and head. During a gaze shift, there is evidence for a zone of activity moving across the tectal map [120]. The gaze is controlled throughout the trajectory of activity on the motor map. Tectal output seems to reflect instantaneous gaze error. Just before the shift, caudal neurons reflect the initial error. Selection of caudal neurons as the goal target initiates the movement, until the rostral fovea region "captures" the target. The location of the activity at any moment during the gaze shift reflects the remaining error to the target. As the gaze shifts, this zone moves towards the rostral pole. The location of the activity reflects the remaining error to the target. As the gaze shift terminates, the active zone enters the rostral pole. These findings suggest that the activation of any point off center in the deep tectal map produces the output needed for position control. The output reflects position error at any moment; this error signal can be computed by subtracting the current target position from the center of the visual field.

At the level of the tectum, the controlled variable is not body configuration per se, but body configuration in relation to some perceived distal stimulus. In other words, any number of body parts (eyes, neck, trunk, etc.) will vary their position in order to reduce this discrepancy. This amounts to varying multiple joint angles, the lengths of many more muscles, and ultimately the sensed tension of many muscles.

The known anatomy suggests that the superficial layer contains the input function and the deep layers contain the comparator function. The projections from the deep layers to the reticulospinal neurons send an error signal, which is turned into a reference signal for the lower level.

A key question is how the position of the neuron on the tectal map can determine the actual movement vector. In polar coordinates, the position of any point on the map can be defined as (r, θ), where r is the radial deviation and θ is the angle. Experiments using electrical stimulation have shown that, in the brainstem targets of tectal projections, there are independent controllers for horizontal and vertical movements [103, 121]. Movement in any direction can be determined by a combination of outputs from these distinct controllers. Since deep layer tectal neurons at any location can project to both horizontal and vertical movement controllers, the ratio between the synaptic weights of these projections can determine θ [106]. The tectal map, then, reflects a map of varying synaptic weights from the deep layer neurons to the independent controllers below. On the other hand, the degree of activation, that is, pulses injected into the system, can determine the amplitude of the movement. Since the radial deviation from the origin in the map is the position error signal, the number of pulses reflects the magnitude of the error.

Stimulation of the tectum can generate coordinated movements of the eyes, neck, and body [101, 120, 122]. The eyes are in the best position to correct this error, but all the relevant controllers probably generate outputs proportional to the error. Consequently, in unrestrained animals, manipulations of the tectum can create sequential activation of orienting movements in a rostral-to-caudal direction (eyes, neck, and body).

The reference signal in this system represents the goal position. Changing the reference signal for a foveation control system moves the eyes to the new kinesthetically sensed configuration, after which the tracking system is again locked onto the visual field. Injection of the GABA-A receptor agonist muscimol can mimic the effect of a change in reference signal. But as GABA receptors are blocked by muscimol, the change is not transient but sustained. That is, we should expect a long-lasting offset in the reference signal and eye position. When injected into the rostral tectum, muscimol indeed creates offset towards the location of injection [123]: instead of foveating on the target, the eye is locked on a nearby region close to the site of injection. Thus the position reference for the foveation system can be altered by injecting an inhibitory signal into the comparator. The injected reference becomes the new center.

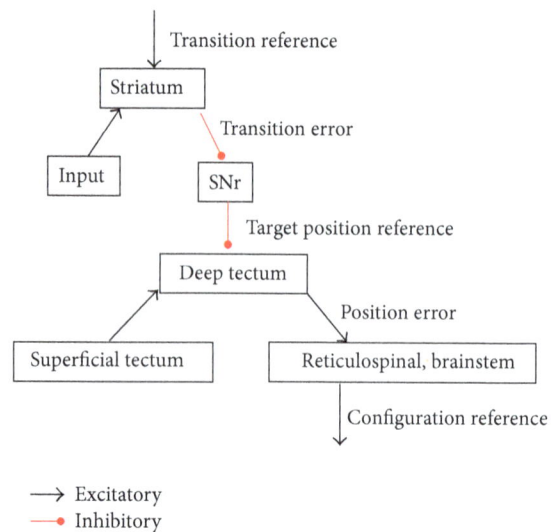

FIGURE 6: Illustration of the role of the nigrotectal projections in orientation control. The nigral output sends reference signals representing target position for the orientation control system in the tectum.

9. Nigral Outputs

If enhancing inhibition of the tectum can artificially create an offset in the fixation position, then normally an inhibitory reference signal may be sent to the tectal comparator. Interestingly, the deep tectum is one of the major targets of the BG outputs [96, 97, 99, 124]. The SNr sends strong GABAergic projections to the deep layers of the tectum. The dorsolateral and ventromedial outflows from the SNr terminate in the rostrolateral and caudomedial intermediate layers of the optic tectum, respectively. Nigrotectal channels map onto tectal map output cells with distinct brainstem projection zones [125].

That the nigrotectal projection sends an inhibitory reference signal to the tectal controller provides a clue about tectal function, for control systems with inhibitory reference signals have unique properties. First, the controller does not produce any output unless the perceptual signal exceeds the reference, creating a threshold-like effect. Unlike input/output devices, however, once the "threshold" is reached, negative feedback is used. An inhibitory reference signal does not allow the input to exceed the reference, so that the output of such a system will act to reduce its input to be less than or equal to its reference. Thirdly, the perceptual input should have a positive sign, because the perceptual signal and the reference signal must be opposite in sign (Figure 6), in order to produce the error signal. In the tectal controller, for example, the perceptual signals coming from the superficial layers to the tectal comparator are excitatory [126], and nigrotectal projections provide the inhibitory reference signals. This arrangement enables the comparison function. The reference signal is then subtracted from the perceptual signal.

Any retinal input can activate the corresponding input function in the superficial tectum, which in turn activates the relevant comparator unit, but the error is determined by a comparison between reference and input. During fixation, perceptual input to the comparator for peripheral units is lower than the inhibitory nigral reference signal, generating little error. A salient stimulus from the periphery can generate a perceptual signal that exceeds the inhibitory reference, generating an error signal that results in orienting towards the new target. Whenever the input exceeds the reference, that input is acquired as the target of foveation.

With a constant reference signal, any salient stimulus off center in the visual field can generate a sufficiently strong input to elicit orienting behavior. This creates the illusion of an input/output device. But when the reference signal is altered, the orienting reaction will also change. Habituation, for example, is common when the salient input is repeatedly presented with no significant consequences. An increase in the inhibitory reference signal can explain habituation.

According to the present model, the "baseline" rate of the nigral output would reflect the position control reference. A constant rate of firing corresponds to a fixed body configuration and orientation. For the oculomotor system, the currently foveated target can be viewed as the origin of the map. A change in the nigral reference signal reestablishes the origin. The BG output is hypothesized to send a reference signal for the desired position in Cartesian coordinates (x, y). The reference signal indicates goal location, whereas the center of the tectal map, the current reference point, indicates the current position. More generally, the "baseline" BG output corresponds to the neutral position when the animal is not moving (or simply maintaining foveation). From this position, increase or decrease in firing rate of different types of nigral output neurons can generate movements in different directions. The rate of change in the reference signals determines movement velocity.

If the inhibitory reference signal is set to zero, any perceptual input can generate errors. This would be the case if the SNr is lesioned or inactivated, or when GABAergic transmission in the nigrotectal pathway is blocked completely [127, 128]. A reduction in nigrotectal inhibition increases the error signal from the tectal comparator even if the perceptual input does not change. Of course, to control antagonistic systems, both a decrease and an increase will be necessary, but pharmacological manipulations like muscimol are not specific enough to reveal the function of opponent outputs.

According to the present model, the tectoreticulospinal system makes it possible to define body configuration and posture in relation to distal target in the environment. At a lower level, the reticulospinal pathway is responsible for generating reference signals for multiple joint angles. The requisite changes in joint angles allow position control in three-dimensional space (x, y, z), using independent controllers for yaw, pitch, and roll. The reticulospinal system itself cannot achieve orientation control or steering, because it lacks inputs from the distal senses.

Nigral outputs are not the only projections that reach the tectum. Nor is the tectum the only target of the nigral output. The pedunculopontine/mesencephalic locomotor region and ventral thalamus also receive extensive nigral projections [129]. The lower levels below the BG output rely on perceptual inputs from multiple modalities to orient towards the critical aspect of the environment and to coordinate the movements of the relevant body parts. The ventral thalamus, a major target of the BG output, also appears to contain certain body configuration controllers [7, 130], but its functional role remains poorly understood. The mesencephalic locomotor region and pedunculopontine nucleus are critical for the alternation and modulation of locomotor patterns and relevant posture control [76, 77]. References reaching these regions can modulate pattern generators for locomotion. Thus, when the locomotor circuit is engaged, orientation control serves a steering function, so that locomotion becomes directed at specific targets in the environment.

10. BG Circuits and Transition Control

I hypothesize that the BG implement the level of transitions in the control hierarchy [7]. This possibility was first suggested nearly three decades ago by Cools [122], but it was unknown at the time how outputs from the BG can use lower levels, because the opponent outputs from the BG were not known and the functions of the lower levels were poorly defined [4, 49].

In transition control, the relevant variable is not configuration, but the rate of change in any configuration. An example of a visual configuration is the perception of a photograph or a drawing. An example of a kinesthetic configuration is a posture. Each is a unitary representation at the configuration level. Transition is simply a change in that particular configuration, as animation is a succession of images.

The inputs to the transition level represent changes in perceptual variables from multiple modalities. This is the level at which the perceptual variables are "objects" and "things"; for example, a rose is perceived as a rose no matter what the viewing angle may be. The cerebral cortices, especially the secondary cortices, contain "gnostic units," invariant representations of lower level inputs, and the requisite higher order reference signals [98, 131]. These are sent to the transition controller in the BG via the corticostriatal projections.

The final outputs from the transition level are reference signals for orientation and body configuration controllers. The rate of change of this output signal, for example, a change in the firing rate of SNr neurons, represents movement velocity [40].

10.1. Distinct BG Networks Classified by Perceptual Input Signals. I hypothesize that the striatum serves as a comparator in the transition controller. Striatal output represents the error signal, while the pallidum (including the SNr) contains the output function of the transition controller.

The major projections to the striatum come from the cerebral cortex and intralaminar thalamus [132–135]. The corticostriatal and thalamostriatal projections are roughly organized in a topographical fashion. The sensorimotor cortex projects to the sensorimotor striatum. The associative cortex projects to the associative striatum and the limbic cortex, including basolateral amygdala and hippocampus, to the limbic striatum. This projection pattern is the basis for functional heterogeneity within the striatum [40, 136].

The complexity of the cerebral cortico-BG networks is due to the variety of perceptual variables, constructed from lower-order inputs. These higher order perceptual representations are achieved by the cerebral cortex. The organization of the cortex and the corticostriatal projections allows many perceptual variables to be controlled. At least in principle, any variable that can be perceived can also be controlled.

Different striatal regions are therefore associated with transition control of specific classes of perceptual variables [4]. The three major classes are exteroceptive (associative), interoceptive (limbic), and proprioceptive/somatosensory (sensorimotor). Exteroceptive inputs are primarily concerned with perceptions of objects and space. Interoceptive inputs are concerned with internal bodily sensors, which report the state of essential variables (e.g., thirst and hunger). On the other hand, proprioceptive/somatosensory perceptions come from the muscle and tendon sensors as well as sensors from the body surface.

Cortical areas are highly similar in their basic microcircuitry, with relatively minor variations [137]. Whether some cortical region is classified as visual or auditory, for example, is largely attributed to the ultimate source of its inputs. Striatal and pallidal regions, though often bearing many names, are also similar to their circuit organization [10, 138, 139]. To control transitions, different cortico-BG networks therefore perform similar computations on different types of perceptual variables [4, 40]. The computations performed by neural circuits are mathematical functions often used in analog computing. For example, the function $2x + b$ is the same, regardless of the value of x. The content of the signal is independent of the computations performed.

10.2. Control of Movement Velocity. The simplest type of transition control is the control of succession of proprioceptive signals or movement velocity control [40]. In velocity control, the controlled variable is the rate of transition in body configurations, whether in locomotion or in postural transitions or orienting movements. The error signal in velocity control changes the reference signal of the body configuration controller. In velocity control, all changes of position, velocity, and acceleration are necessary consequences of how the control hierarchy is organized. The load accelerates toward the final position and then starts decelerating before it gets there, as if it knows it is about to reach the desired position. But it has no such knowledge. Even though nobody is telling the system when to accelerate or decelerate, it does so at the right moments with just the right amounts. This is an important yet surprising property of negative feedback control systems.

By integrating the error signal from the velocity comparator, the descending reference signal for body configuration and orientation can be obtained. According to this model, the magnitude (firing rate) of the velocity error signal is proportional to the rate of change of the BG output from the SNr. A larger signal produces a faster rate of change in the orientation/configuration reference. The neural implementation of the leaky integrator is the projection from the striatum to the BG output nuclei such as the SNr.

Velocity control is hypothesized to be a major function of the sensorimotor cortico-BG network. In neurological disorders implicating the BG, velocity control is often impaired. For example, in bradykinesia, a common symptom after dopamine depletion in Parkinson's disease, movement is abnormally slow [140, 141], though position control is still effective. This deficit is a result of reduced rate of change in the body configuration reference signal. If the reference signal reaching the comparator is reduced, the movement will eventually correct the position error, but it will be slower [40]. If the reference signal is zero, there is akinesia. The effect is similar to playing a video in slow motion: the frame rate is reduced when the velocity reference signal is too low.

Bradykinesia could be a result of reduced velocity reference signal, though abnormalities in the input function or comparator are also possible [40]. The magnitude of the velocity reference signal could be determined by excitatory inputs to the striatum, from the cortex and perhaps thalamus, and by a modulatory signal from the midbrain dopamine neurons. With dopamine depletion in Parkinson's disease, the velocity controller is impaired, reducing the peak output of the velocity controller. Consequently, the rate of change in the BG output will be reduced, leading to slower transitions in body configurations.

The effect of dopamine is "modulatory" in the engineering sense (not in the conventional neurophysiological sense, which just means change). Playing the role of "volume control," dopamine is proposed to have a multiplicative effect on the glutamatergic signal arriving at the spines of the striatal projection neurons. The magnitude of the error signal entering the leaky integrator in the output function depends on both the glutamatergic input and the simultaneous dopamine signal. When dopamine is depleted, the glutamatergic signal has a reduced effect on the output. A reduced signal enters the leaky integrator that transforms the velocity reference signal into a rate of change in position reference. Position reference (from the SNr output), in turn, will change more slowly.

Recent work suggests that the sensorimotor striatum is a key component of the velocity controller. The firing rate of sensorimotor striatal projection neurons is highly correlated with movement velocity, though it is still difficult to ascertain whether the signals they carry reflect velocity reference, input, or error [142].

It remains unclear what the role of the striatonigral (direct) and striatopallidal (indirect) pathways is in the transition control network. It has been argued that the direct pathway serves to select desired actions, while the indirect pathway suppresses competing actions. But this model makes a number of questionable assumptions about behavior, in particular the relationship between posture and movement. It cannot be defended in light of recent data on opponent BG outputs. An important question is how these opponent outputs, which are needed for downstream controllers that move in opposite directions, are generated by the intrinsic circuitry. One obvious possibility is that they are generated by the direct and indirect pathways [36, 42]. There are common inputs to the striatonigral and striatopallidal neurons, for at least a large proportion of corticostriatal projections. This circuit can function as a phase splitter, in which a uniform input signal to the BG (e.g., carried by the corticostriatal projection) is transformed into a pair of output signals, one increasing and the other decreasing at the same time (Figure 2). Accordingly the rate of change in these outputs will correspond to movement velocity in different directions. This possibility remains to be tested.

11. Above Transition Control

The transition level is where voluntary or goal-directed behavior emerges. In traditional terms, this is where the will in the brain is translated into actions. According to the current model, the will can be viewed as a particular type of reference signal entering the comparator function of the transition controller. A common symptom after damage to the BG is abulia or lack of will [143]. This is a consequence of reduced reference signals to the transition control system.

A simple movement such as raising one's hand can serve multiple purposes: to scratch the neck, to fix the hair, to ask a question, and so forth. The kinematics of the arm movement per se is ambiguous, for it does not tell us which level of the hierarchy is responsible for initiating the action. Nevertheless, despite the fundamental ambiguity in interpreting the purpose of actions, the purpose of any control system can be determined experimentally.

What is needed is an explicit test for the controlled variable in question [144], by manipulating feedback functions and assessing the consequent changes in behavioral output. Control systems share an important property: whenever a variable is controlled, disturbance to this variable will be resisted by its output. Thus the hypothetical controlled variable will change less than one would expect had there been no feedback at all.

The entire motor hierarchy can be viewed as the final common path for actions, just as the neuromuscular junction is the final common path for specific muscle contractions. When we analyze actions, we ignore all the details at lower levels (e.g., joint angle or muscle length control in the spinal cord and brainstem). By analyzing the output of the transition controller we can see how a particular action is performed, but an equally important question is why it is performed. That is a question about the higher levels that can alter the reference signal of the transition controllers. When we ascend the control hierarchy, we ask "why" certain outputs are generated by trying to identify the reference signal, which is proportional to the error signal of a higher level.

The transition level is the highest level of the motor hierarchy, but we can still ask why a particular action is performed. For example, the reference signal for the velocity controller comes from still higher levels. The rate at which the configurations are altered appears to be related to the motivational urgency, that is, magnitude of error at still higher systems that becomes the reference signal for the velocity control system. The presence of reward can significantly increase the velocity reference signal, which reduces the latency and increases the firing rate of striatal neurons [145]. How do goals of actions affect the actions themselves? This is a question to be addressed below.

11.1. Relationship Control.

The feedback path between muscles and the loads they accelerate is short and relatively direct. Proprioceptive signals are automatically affected by the effectors. But this is not true of other types of transitions. For example, we perceive a cat running across the visual field. This perception is not automatically controlled by our behavior. The lowest levels of the oculomotor system can exert some effect on the perception, as the eyes track the running cat, but in a second the cat is gone. To have full control of the "cat perception," some feedback path can be discovered, so that our own movements can alter this perception, for example, by chasing the cat.

"Chasing" is the output of a controller that controls one perceptual variable, namely, transition of a set of proprioceptive configurations. Yet in this case the transition level is in the service of a still higher level, with its own controlled variable, which can be described as closing the distance to the cat. The same behavior can be described in different ways. It can be described as a series of changes in muscle tension, in muscle length, in joint angle, or in posture or as running or chasing. Which of these descriptions is the appropriate one? Strictly speaking, all of them are true, but they describe the actions of the control hierarchy at different levels. The most appropriate one here is chasing, because that describes the appropriate control variable. If one is simply running with no target, then the controlled variable is not "closing the distance between self and target." These two possibilities can be tested experimentally by manipulating the feedback function or introducing a disturbance to the controlled variable. If chasing is the appropriate description, then stopping the target would also stop the behavior, which would not be the case if running were the appropriate description. The key question is not only which perceptual variable is being controlled (as all levels of the hierarchy are controlling their local perceptual variables), but also which level of the control hierarchy is the "lead" level. This level controls its own perception by commanding the lower levels.

The level just above the transition is the relationship level, where the controlled variable is a relationship between at least two perceptual variables. In most cases, this relationship is between two transitions, that is, two changing configurations. In chasing a cat, the distance between the self and the cat is a relationship. Likewise, in a tracking task, one has to move the mouse cursor to follow a moving target [7], so the distance between the cursor and target is a relationship. In driving, the relationship between the car and various other perceptions, for example, the road, lane markers, or red lights, must also be controlled. Humans can readily choose any arbitrary distance, which means that the reference signal for the relationship control can be set at some arbitrary value. To control this value, the relationship level must have access to both perceptual variables and send some error signal that activates lower level controllers, that is, to initiate the appropriates types of transition control.

11.2. Sequence.

Another type of controlled variable may be called "sequence" or "serial order." An action such as "drinking a glass of water" can be broken down into multiple components: gaze shift, reaching, holding, moving the cup to the mouth, drinking, and so forth. It is necessary for these components to be ordered appropriately for the sequence to be effective. Serial order itself is a controlled variable. The sequence AB is different from BA, even though the same elements are involved.

Sequence, in this sense, is different from stereotyped alternation as in locomotor pattern generation, mediated by brainstem and diencephalic structures below the level of the BG [77]. The latter does not require learning of arbitrary serial order, relying instead on innately organized circuits for stereotyped sequences, for example, flexor extensor alternation. Serial order, the arbitrary ordering of individual action primitives, requires learning. This is evident in the lack of proper serial order in the actions of infants, for whom an action as simple as "drinking a glass of water" can be impossible.

Unsurprisingly, the learning of serial order also depends on the sensorimotor cortico-BG network [136, 146]. Lesions of the sensorimotor striatum or of secondary motor cortical regions that project to this region can impair the learning of serial order. Mice were trained to perform two actions sequentially (e.g., press the left lever first and right lever second) in order to earn some food reward. Lesions of the sensorimotor striatum can impair learning of the serial order without impairing the learning of individual actions. In other earlier studies, it was found that dopamine antagonists can also impair sequence control [147, 148]. Exactly how serial order control is implemented by neural circuits remains unclear.

11.3. Learning and Recruitment. So far we have considered how the proposed hierarchy of neural circuits can implement cascade control. One important question that remains is how these systems can be modified through learning.

At the level of transition control, an important phenomenon is observed, traditionally called reinforcement. As Thorndike first stated in his "law of effect," if a behavior is followed by a good consequence or effect, it is more likely to be repeated in the future; if it is followed by some bad effect, it is more likely to be eliminated or reduced in frequency [149]. This phenomenon is studied most commonly in the field of operant or instrumental conditioning, in which animals are trained to perform specific actions like pressing a lever in order to obtain food. The critical role of the cortico-BG networks in instrumental learning is supported by many studies [36, 150–153].

In relationship control, rate of change in one variable is related to that of another. This is similar to the "related rates problem" in calculus, where it is solved with implicit differentiation using the chain rule. Operant conditioning provides a good example. If one learns to press a lever for food, both the action of lever pressing and the outcome of food delivery are transitions in perceptual variables. There is a feedback function relating the rate of pressing to the rate of reward [154]. The organism can only become aware of this action-outcome contingency at the relationship level, where both perceptual variables (action transition and outcome transition) are available.

The key feature of such relationships or contingencies is that they do not reflect stable physical dependencies, in the same way that, for example, joint angle depends on muscle length. Rather they reflect ever-changing and arbitrary relationships in the environment. Exploiting this type of relationship, the organism can generate output to control one variable in order to control another. Precisely because such relationships are fleeting properties of the environment, learning and experience will be needed to acquire them. Learning to control one transition variable in order to control another is therefore the most important type of learning. There is a hierarchical relationship between these two variables. Only one is directly under the control of the organism before learning, whereas the other is not. Control over the new variable is acquired. Using this indirect method, any variable can be controlled provided that it can be perceived and that a feedback path exists between it and a currently controllable variable.

In the absence of experience, for example, in a newborn infant, many types of control systems are still functional, and a rudimentary control hierarchy is already in place. The essential variables necessary for life are, by definition, already controlled using existing homeostatic controllers in the body and the autonomic nervous system. But the extent of control is limited. For example, despite extremely sophisticated body temperature control in the infant, he is quite unable to perform specific actions to put out a fire. His ability to defend the essential variable against environmental disturbances is limited. To do that learning is required, and such learning is initially driven by the error signals in primary controllers, when essential variables are disturbed.

11.4. Trouble with Reinforcement. In recent years, models of reinforcement learning have had a major impact on neuroscience, especially on researchers studying the function of the BG [35, 155, 156]. It is widely believed that the BG circuits implement specific models of reinforcement learning, which are largely based on Thorndike's law of effect [157]. Reinforcement is what makes behavior repeat. Food reward, for example, is called a reinforcer when the preceding behavior can be reliably repeated.

What is lacking in reinforcement models is the internal reference [158–160]. Consequently, it is impossible to determine when to start or stop any behavior. When will a rat start pressing a lever for food? When will it stop pressing? Why is food reinforcing when the rat is hungry but not when it is sated?

The implicit assumption of the reinforcement model is that the organism maximizes rewards or good effects and that more reinforcement causes more behavior [155]. This belief persists partly because almost all studies in this field use food or water deprivation to generate behavior. The goal of the experimenter is to create conditions when the behavior in question can be observed. From the perspective of control theory, this means that error is high, and the animal strives to reduce error by performing the action. Drastic deprivation guarantees responding and creates the illusion of reward maximization during the period when the error is large. Yet the rate of reward in instrumental conditioning is a controlled variable. Changing the feedback function (i.e., reinforcement schedule) dramatically changes the rate of lever pressing, but in a predictable fashion because the rate of food delivery is relatively constant [49]. More reinforcement does not produce more behavior. In fact, when the schedule is leaner, as has been known for decades, the rate of pressing increases. The fluctuation in behavior may appear to be random, but it is understandable in light of what is happening to the variable being controlled, namely, the rate of reward delivery.

The reinforcement model also confounds learning and performance. The implicit model of the organism is a stimulus-response device. Behavior is a function of what happens to the organism. The only possible change in organization is in the strength of the bond connecting stimuli (or states) with responses, as originally proposed by Thorndike, regardless of how many intervening variables are inserted between these two. But clearly motivational state can also affect performance, as a sated rat stops pressing the lever. Consequently, whether a change in associative strength or motivational drive is responsible for the change in performance is impossible to ascertain. Early investigators like Hull at least attempted to solve this problem, but in recent years it has been ignored entirely [158, 159].

The absurdity of explaining behavior by their antecedent conditions has already been discussed above. Knowing how control systems function, it is impossible to define learning simply as a change in behavior. For an important property of control systems is that they can produce new behaviors without ever changing their parameters.

According to the model proposed here, deprivation creates large error signals in the essential variables [55]. The primary deficit in energy homeostasis is the ultimate source for the error signal that initiates the food seeking behavior. What is traditionally called reinforcement is a reduction in error signals in systems that control the essential variables. Behaviors are repeated because they reduce error signals created by deprivation and other disturbances.

In a rat that has already learned to press a lever for food, the action of lever pressing is the means by which the error is reduced as the rat becomes less hungry. But the question is how did the rat ever learn to press the lever in the first place. Such learning requires a change in the properties of the control systems, such as construction of new references signals or establishing or modifying links between levels in a labile hierarchy [4, 7].

Instrumental learning consists of multiple phases [153]. Initially, as a result of large error signals in controllers for the essential variables, the organism generates random variation in system parameters. This is manifested in behavioral variability, which leads, by chance, to the action that reduces the error [161]. The error reduction is what is traditionally called reinforcement. It reduces the rate of variation, preserving the effective set of parameters in the control system. Next time, when the error signal increases again, the system that has been reorganized to reduce it most quickly will be selected.

This process of reorganization is the opposite of the reinforcement mechanism. The reinforcer does not strengthen some existing connection between sensory input and motor output. Rather the error signal in controllers for essential variables starts an active process of reorganization, during which the system parameters simply vary at a high rate. This process, however, is stopped by the error reduction. That saves the set of system parameters.

Performance always depends on the amount of error present, but learning explains which lower level systems are actually recruited to reduce the error and why. In an operant conditioning experiment, to satisfy its hunger the rat must press the lever in the operant chamber. The error signal from the food pellet controller is used as a reference signal for the action. Thus during reorganization the controller for food recruits the controller for lever pressing. This process of "recruitment" is critical in instrumental learning. It involves establishing or strengthening the connection between two independent controllers, so that one will serve the other. The relationship between them is hierarchical, so that the higher controller can use the lower one by sending a reference signal to the comparator function of the latter. This learning process explains what happens, in traditional terms, when an action is associated with an outcome [162]. The action-outcome link is established so that the error of the outcome control system can reliably set a reference for a lower system that specifies some action to be performed. The higher level, therefore, recruits a lower one to reduce its error.

There are important differences between the type of feedback function in operant conditioning and feedback function between, say, the output of motor neurons and muscle tension. There are no first-order sensors for "reward" or "reward rate" as there are for muscle tension. Rather these are highly abstract variables constructed from multiple perceptual signals from lower levels. By definition, to control a particular relationship it is necessary to perceive it. The detection of the instrumental contingency between action and outcome cannot be achieved by the lower levels below transition control. The lower levels are also incapable of instrumental control. Only at the highest levels can different transitions be related to each other and only there can such feedback functions be learned, so that the appropriate actions can be acquired to reach desired goals. The control of the outcome through instrumental actions, therefore, requires relationship control.

The action of pressing the lever, which is generated by a proprioceptive transition controller, can be used to serve many different purposes. There is no fixed relationship between the action and the variables the organism would like to control. One learns to control x in order to control y. But y could also be a variable that was acquired through experience. Its "value" was established very early on, through experience of error reduction in more primary control systems [163, 164].

The organism must form new goals or reference signals to reduce errors in essential variables corresponding to motivational states like hunger and thirst. It must also acquire specific actions to reach these goals. These secondary reference values explain the traditional notion of secondary reinforcement and signals that predict primary reinforcement also obtain incentive value. Value, in this sense, is an attempt to explain how often a behavior is performed. Thus in the traditional literature, stimuli and actions are often assigned value, which merely attempts to explain performance. If, given a particular stimulus, the rate of some behavior is high, this stimulus is endowed with value. Likewise, if the animal chooses to perform one action rather than another, the preferred action is said to have value [165, 166]. Such values can be understood as acquired reference conditions in a control hierarchy.

11.5. Cortico-BG Networks and the Motivational Hierarchy. Above the transition control level, there is no fixed hierarchy. Rather there is a labile motivational hierarchy, in which the levels are defined by acquired controlled variables and relationships between these variables. I hypothesize that the cortico-BG networks can implement this labile hierarchy.

As discussed earlier, inputs to the BG can be roughly divided into interoceptive, exteroceptive, and proprioceptive. Each class of perceptual signals is carried by cortical and possibly thalamic projections to the striatum. These glutamatergic and excitatory projections send the main feedback signals to the level of transitions. With proprioceptive transitions in the body sensors during movement, both interoceptive transitions and exteroceptive transitions can also change.

Imagine a hungry rat exploring its environment, proprioceptive feedback is sent to different levels of the hierarchy. At the same time, distal senses (e.g., visual and auditory) also detect transitions in space, and the interceptive senses detect transitions in autonomic variables, including those related to hunger. Given its motivational state, there will be large error signals in essential variables such as blood glucose controllers. When the rat learns to perform some action to obtain food, the parameters of the exteroceptive and proprioceptive transition controllers are saved (e.g., where food is found and how it can be obtained).

The relationship between interoceptive and exteroceptive transition controllers can therefore be hierarchical. The detection of distal changes usually occurs before the detection of proximal changes; for example, the sight and smell of food usually precedes its digestion. Likewise, for the animal to exert instrumental control on food, it must first produce movements or proprioceptive transitions. Thus the order of dependency is as follows.

(1) Exteroceptive, associative network depends on proprioceptive, sensorimotor network. Distal perceptions of the environment change as one moves.

(2) Interoceptive, limbic network depends on exteroceptive network. Internal states can also change as distal perceptions change; for example, food is seen, smelled, heard, and then consumed.

(3) Interoceptive network depends on proprioceptive network. The feedback in terms of transitions from proprioceptive transitions is mainly exteroceptive but could also be interoceptive. Normally, however, the dependence is more indirect.

The labile motivational hierarchy allows the proprioceptive transition controller to be in the service of higher levels that control any perceptual variable, provided a feedback function is present. The cortico-BG networks are the neural implementations of this hierarchy, as the anatomical connections allow the limbic and associative networks to affect the sensorimotor network, possibly through the striato-midbrain-striatal loops [167–169].

The striatonigral projections, at least for the sensorimotor network, transform proprioceptive transition control error into reference signals for configuration and position control systems. The projections from the substantia nigra back to the striatum are less direct. They are not from the GABAergic output neurons but from the dopaminergic neurons, which receive projections from the output neurons and send projections to striatal comparators in a lower level on the motivational hierarchy [134, 167, 170]. The errors from interoceptive transition control can thus be used to alter the reference signals of the exteroceptive transition controller, which in turn uses the proprioceptive transition controller.

Interoceptive inputs such as taste are mediated by limbic cortico-BG network, which is also important for orofacial movements [171, 172]. The inputs to the limbic striatum (nucleus accumbens and surrounding ventral striatum) come from limbic cortical regions such as medial and orbital frontal cortices and the basolateral amygdala [134, 173]. Its output through the ventral pallidum can affect the autonomic nervous system via the hypothalamus [8, 174, 175]. These connections may be sufficient to generate consummatory behaviors [176, 177]. Yet these outputs are not always sufficient for the control of interceptive inputs; for example, chewing is not sufficient to make food appear. If, however, some arbitrary instrumental action is required to obtain the reward, then the taste control system must recruit the associative network and sensorimotor network to generate the appropriate actions.

The limbic circuit by itself cannot acquire instrumental behaviors that lead to specific rewards [178]. But indirect projections to the associative and sensorimotor networks allow serial adaptation to recruit the requisite controllers to perform the task.

12. Summary and Conclusions

To understand the contributions of the BG to behavior, it is above all necessary to understand what behavior is. Here the traditional linear causation paradigm is the greatest obstacle to progress. Whenever behavior is conceived as the output of some input/output system with linear causation, as the result of sensorimotor transformation in multiple steps inside the organism, the attempt to understand its neural substrates is doomed at the outset.

I have argued instead that behavior is the outward manifestation of a more fundamental process of control, generated by a hierarchy of negative feedback control systems, each controlling its own perceptual inputs by varying outputs. It is not the result of sensorimotor transformations but is jointly determined by the perceptual input and the internal reference signal, in a mathematically precise way. Using cascade control, the output of a particular level specifies the input signal to be obtained by level immediately below. The loop is closed in the environment, as the output function of the lowest level in the hierarchy—muscles—acts on the environment to generate behavior. Although the basic unit of neural function—the closed loop negative feedback circuit—is simple, a hierarchy of these systems can generate exceedingly complex behavior. We are only now beginning to understand the properties of the control hierarchy.

The properties of negative feedback control systems are counterintuitive from the perspective of the linear causation paradigm. The striking failure to understand control theory in the life sciences so far only illustrates the fundamental difference between closed loop systems and input/output systems. Regardless of how many intervening variables are inserted between the stimulus and the response, an input/output system always lacks internal references, which are only found in negative feedback control systems. This is the crucial difference. The behavior of control systems is not caused by what happens to them. It can never be a function of inputs received or of internal representations of any kind.

For any control systems to function, reference signals are necessary, and negative feedback makes it possible to obtain inputs matching the reference by reducing the discrepancy between the two. The reference signal is the representation of some unrealized future state, but the system makes it possible for this state to be realized by varying its behavior. In this sense, the reference is simply the purpose of the controller, though purposes and goals in ordinary language usually refer to higher level reference signals at the transition level because few lower reference signals are available to conscious awareness. We are not aware of the reference signal for muscle tension in hundreds of muscles in the body at any moment, though these are the signals that ultimately close the loop by causing muscle contraction to act on the environment. We are usually aware of the higher goals of our actions, the reference signals sent to the transition level, for example, to get a cup of coffee. The higher purpose is achieved by elaborations as one descends the hierarchy; for example, the desire to get coffee affects the reference signal for sequence control of the action, which changes the reference for rate of change in body configurations, which then alters references for joint angles, which then alters references for muscle length, which finally alters references for muscle tension.

I have identified the neural implementations of the basic levels of the hierarchy: muscle tension, muscle length, joint angle, body configuration and orientation, and transition. In the proposed neural hierarchy, the BG occupy the highest level, receiving inputs representing rate of change in different perceptual variables, comparing these signals with reference signals, and generating error signals that alter the reference signals for downstream position controllers. Such a model suggests a new view of the relationship between the inputs and outputs. The BG are neither sensory nor motor. Rather their function is to control certain types of higher order perceptual variables, above all relationship, sequence, and transition.

Because traditional studies in systems and behavioral neuroscience rely on input/output methods to understand behavior, without identifying the controlled variable, their results are of limited utility. Given the lack of useful data, the hierarchical model proposed here is still incomplete. No attempt has been made to elucidate the function of many brain regions, such as the cerebellum and the diencephalon, that work closely with the BG in generating behavior. Although the proposed model is still incomplete, even in its present form it generates a number of testable predictions which can be useful in guiding future experiments:

(1) The BG produce signals related to movement kinematics: velocity, acceleration, and position. The striatal output, for example, reflects velocity, whereas the nigral output reflects position. This suggests that operations like addition, subtraction, integration, and differentiation are the primary computations performed in these circuits. We would also expect both reference signals and perceptual signals representing these signals. These will be similar, so long as there is successful control. Perturbation experiments will be needed to distinguish between these signals.

(2) From the striatum to the SNr or any other BG output nucleus, the neural circuit performs the equivalent of mathematical integration. In the neural integrator, the rate of change in the output will be proportional to the magnitude of the input. The outputs of the SNr (and GPi/entopeduncular nucleus) will be proportional to the time integral of striatal outputs. The presence of the integrator will also produce a roughly 90-degree phase shift in the BG output signal when compared to the striatal output. Although the existence of neural integrators has been known for a long time, often integration is misleadingly called a mechanism for memory [179, 180]. The crucial function performed by integration in the nervous system is not memory

but control, as integrators are often needed in building output functions of negative feedback controllers.

(3) Dopamine is a gain signal in the transition control system. It is neither a hedonic reward signal nor a reward prediction error signal [181, 182]. By modulating the glutamate signal, it can determine the velocity reference signal or velocity error. The primary function of dopamine is to alter the gain of different types of perceptual transitions. The sensorimotor striatum, which receives the strongest DA projections from the nigrostriatal pathway, is hypothesized to be critical for velocity control. But DA clearly can also be involved in the control of other types of transitions, transitions of any perceptual configuration.

(4) The output of the BG quantitatively determines posture and movement. The rate of firing in the output can determine position at any time. A change in firing rate represents a change in body configuration and orientation, that is, movement. From any stable position, opponent and antiphase signals are generated to create movement.

Conflict of Interests

The author declares that there is no conflict of interests regarding the publication of this paper.

Acknowledgments

The author is supported by NIH AA021074. The author would like to thank Joseph Barter, Peter Redgrave, and Mark Rossi for helpful discussions.

References

[1] J. A. Saint-Cyr, A. E. Taylor, and A. E. Lang, "Procedural learning and neostriatal dysfunction in man," *Brain*, vol. 111, no. 4, pp. 941–959, 1988.

[2] R. L. Albin, A. B. Young, and J. B. Penney, "The functional anatomy of basal ganglia disorders," *Trends in Neurosciences*, vol. 12, no. 10, pp. 366–375, 1989.

[3] J. W. Mink, "The basal ganglia: focused selection and inhibition of competing motor programs," *Progress in Neurobiology*, vol. 50, no. 4, pp. 381–425, 1996.

[4] H. H. Yin, "Cortico-basal ganglia network and the neural substrate of actions," in *Neurobiology of Alcohol Dependence*, A. Noronha, Ed., pp. 29–48, Academic Press, New York, NY, USA, 2014.

[5] M. A. Rossi, D. Fan, J. W. Barter, and H. H. Yin, "Bidirectional modulation of substantia nigra activity by motivational state," *PLoS ONE*, vol. 8, no. 8, Article ID e71598, 2013.

[6] J. M. Fuster, *Memory in the Cerebral Cortex*, The MIT Press, Cambridge, Mass, USA, 1995.

[7] W. T. Powers, *Behavior: Control of Perception*, Benchmark, New Canaan, Conn, USA, 1973.

[8] L. W. Swanson, "Cerebral hemisphere regulation of motivated behavior," *Brain Research*, vol. 886, no. 1-2, pp. 113–164, 2000.

[9] M. Antal, B. M. Beneduce, and W. G. Regehr, "The substantia nigra conveys target-dependent excitatory and inhibitory

outputs from the basal ganglia to the thalamus," *Journal of Neuroscience*, vol. 34, no. 23, pp. 8032–8042, 2014.

[10] C. J. Wilson, "Basal ganglia," in *The Synaptic Organization of the Brain*, G. M. Shephard, Ed., pp. 361–413, Oxford University Press, New York, NY, USA, 2004.

[11] D. A. Carter and H. C. Fibiger, "The projections of the entopeduncular nucleus and globus pallidus in rat as demonstrated by autoradiography and horseradish peroxidase histochemistry," *Journal of Comparative Neurology*, vol. 177, no. 1, pp. 113–123, 1978.

[12] K. J. Mastro, R. S. Bouchard, H. A. K. Holt, and A. H. Gittis, "Transgenic mouse lines subdivide external segment of the globus pallidus (GPe) neurons and reveal distinct GPe output pathways," *The Journal of Neuroscience*, vol. 34, no. 6, pp. 2087–2099, 2014.

[13] C. R. Gerfen, "The neostriatal mosaic: multiple levels of compartmental organization in the basal ganglia," *Annual Review of Neuroscience*, vol. 15, pp. 285–320, 1992.

[14] J. P. Bolam, Y. Smith, C. A. Ingham, M. Von Krosigk, and A. D. Smith, "Convergence of synaptic terminals from the striatum and the globus pallidus onto single neurones in the substantia nigra and the entopeduncular nucleus," *Progress in Brain Research*, vol. 99, pp. 73–88, 1993.

[15] N. Mallet, B. R. Micklem, P. Henny et al., "Dichotomous organization of the external globus pallidus," *Neuron*, vol. 74, no. 6, pp. 1075–1086, 2012.

[16] O. Hikosaka, "GABAergic output of the basal ganglia," *Progress in Brain Research*, vol. 160, pp. 209–226, 2007.

[17] C. R. Gerfen and D. J. Surmeier, "Modulation of striatal projection systems by dopamine," *Annual Review of Neuroscience*, vol. 34, pp. 441–466, 2011.

[18] E. Hoshi, L. Tremblay, J. Féger, P. L. Carras, and P. L. Strick, "The cerebellum communicates with the basal ganglia," *Nature Neuroscience*, vol. 8, no. 11, pp. 1491–1493, 2005.

[19] H. Lai, T. Tsumori, T. Shiroyama, S. Yokota, K. Nakano, and Y. Yasui, "Morphological evidence for a vestibulo-thalamo-striatal pathway via the parafascicular nucleus in the rat," *Brain Research*, vol. 872, no. 1-2, pp. 208–214, 2000.

[20] O. Hikosaka, Y. Takikawa, and R. Kawagoe, "Role of the basal ganglia in the control of purposive saccadic eye movements," *Physiological Reviews*, vol. 80, no. 3, pp. 953–978, 2000.

[21] G. Chevalier, S. Vacher, J. M. Deniau, and M. Desban, "Disinhibition as a basic process in the expression of striatal functions. I. The striato-nigral influence on tecto-spinal/tecto-diencephalic neurons," *Brain Research*, vol. 334, no. 2, pp. 215–226, 1985.

[22] J. M. Deniau and G. Chevalier, "Disinhibition as a basic process in the expression of striatal functions. II. The striato-nigral influence on thalamocortical cells of the ventromedial thalamic nucleus," *Brain Research*, vol. 334, no. 2, pp. 227–233, 1985.

[23] K. Lorenz, *Les Prix Nobel*, Stockholm, Sweden, 1973.

[24] G. Chevalier, J. M. Deniau, A. M. Thierry, and J. Feger, "The nigro-tectal pathway. An electrophysiological reinvestigation in the rat," *Brain Research*, vol. 213, no. 2, pp. 253–263, 1981.

[25] G. Chevalier, S. Vacher, and J. M. Deniau, "Inhibitory nigral influence on tectospinal neurons, a possible implication of basal ganglia in orienting behavior," *Experimental Brain Research*, vol. 53, no. 2, pp. 320–326, 1984.

[26] E. R. Kandel, J. H. Schwartz, and T. M. Jessell, *Principles of Neural Science*, vol. 4, McGraw-Hill, New York, NY, USA, 2000.

[27] D. Purves, G. J. Augustine, D. Fitzpatrick, W. C. Hall, A.-S. LaMantia, and L. E. White, *Neuroscience*, Sinauer Associates, Sunderland, Mass, USA, 2012.

[28] S. Taverna, E. Ilijic, and D. J. Surmeier, "Recurrent collateral connections of striatal medium spiny neurons are disrupted in models of Parkinson's disease," *Journal of Neuroscience*, vol. 28, no. 21, pp. 5504–5512, 2008.

[29] H. H. Yin and D. M. Lovinger, "Frequency-specific and D_2 receptor-mediated inhibition of glutamate release by retrograde endocannabinoid signaling," *Proceedings of the National Academy of Sciences of the United States of America*, vol. 103, pp. 8251–8256, 2006.

[30] H. H. Yin and R. M. Costa, "The generation and modification of adaptive behavior," in *Dopamine-Glutamate Interactions in the Basal Ganglia*, S. Jones, Ed., pp. 203–226, CRC Press, New York, NY, USA, 2011.

[31] M. S. Levine and C. Cepeda, "Dopamine modulation of responses mediated by excitatory amino acids in the neostriatum," *Advances in Pharmacology*, vol. 42, pp. 724–729, 1998.

[32] A. C. Kreitzer, "Physiology and pharmacology of striatal neurons," *Annual Review of Neuroscience*, vol. 32, pp. 127–147, 2009.

[33] G. O. Hjelmstad, "Dopamine excites nucleus accumbens neurons through the differential modulation of glutamate and GABA release," *The Journal of Neuroscience*, vol. 24, no. 39, pp. 8621–8628, 2004.

[34] M. J. Frank, L. C. Seeberger, and R. C. O'Reilly, "By carrot or by stick: cognitive reinforcement learning in Parkinsonism," *Science*, vol. 306, no. 5703, pp. 1940–1943, 2004.

[35] A. V. Kravitz, L. D. Tye, and A. C. Kreitzer, "Distinct roles for direct and indirect pathway striatal neurons in reinforcement," *Nature Neuroscience*, vol. 15, no. 6, pp. 816–818, 2012.

[36] D. Fan, M. A. Rossi, and H. H. Yin, "Mechanisms of action selection and timing in substantia nigra neurons," *Journal of Neuroscience*, vol. 32, no. 16, pp. 5534–5548, 2012.

[37] B. F. Skinner, *The Behavior of Organisms*, Appleton-Century-Crofts, New York, NY, USA, 1938.

[38] M. D. Zeiler, "Pure timing in temporal differentiation," *Journal of the Experimental Analysis of Behavior*, vol. 43, no. 2, pp. 183–193, 1985.

[39] C. S. Sherrington, *The Integrative Action of the Nervous System*, Yale University Press, New Haven, Conn, USA, 1906.

[40] H. H. Yin, "Action, time and the basal ganglia," *Philosophical Transactions of the Royal Society B: Biological Sciences*, vol. 369, no. 1637, Article ID 20120473, 2014.

[41] D. Fan, D. Rich, T. Holtzman et al., "A wireless multi-channel recording system for freely behaving mice and rats," *PLoS ONE*, vol. 6, no. 7, Article ID e22033, 2011.

[42] J. W. Barter, S. Castro, T. Sukharnikova, M. A. Rossi, and H. H. Yin, "The role of the substantia nigra in posture control," *European Journal of Neuroscience*, vol. 39, no. 9, pp. 1465–1473, 2014.

[43] G. E. Alexander and M. D. Crutcher, "Functional architecture of basal ganglia circuits: neural substrates of parallel processing," *Trends in Neurosciences*, vol. 13, no. 7, pp. 266–271, 1990.

[44] M. R. DeLong, "Primate models of movement disorders of basal ganglia origin," *Trends in Neurosciences*, vol. 13, no. 7, pp. 281–285, 1990.

[45] R. L. Buckner, J. R. Andrews-Hanna, and D. L. Schacter, "The brain's default network: anatomy, function, and relevance to disease," *Annals of the New York Academy of Sciences*, vol. 1124, pp. 1–38, 2008.

[46] J. P. Martin, *The Basal Ganglia and Posture*, Lippincott, Philadelphia, Pa, USA, 1967.

[47] N. Bernstein, *The Coordination and Regulation of Movements*, Pergamon Press, Oxford, UK, 1967.

[48] O. G. Meijer and S. M. Bruijn, "The loyal dissident: N.A. Bernstein and the double-edged sword of stalinism," *Journal of the History of the Neurosciences*, vol. 16, no. 1-2, pp. 206–224, 2007.

[49] H. H. Yin, "Restoring purpose in behavior," in *Computational and Robotic Models of the Hierarchical Organization of Behavior*, pp. 319–347, Springer, Berlin, Germany, 2013.

[50] D. M. Wolpert and M. Kawato, "Multiple paired forward and inverse models for motor control," *Neural Networks*, vol. 11, no. 7-8, pp. 1317–1329, 1998.

[51] A. Pouget and L. H. Snyder, "Computational approaches to sensorimotor transformations," *Nature Neuroscience*, vol. 3, pp. 1192–1198, 2000.

[52] T. Mergner, G. Schweigart, and L. Fennell, "Vestibular humanoid postural control," *Journal of Physiology Paris*, vol. 103, no. 3–5, pp. 178–194, 2009.

[53] J. McIntyre and E. Bizzi, "Servo hypotheses for the biological control of movement," *Journal of Motor Behavior*, vol. 25, no. 3, pp. 193–202, 1993.

[54] T. G. Deliagina, G. N. Orlovsky, P. V. Zelenin, and I. N. Beloozerova, "Neural bases of postural control," *Physiology*, vol. 21, no. 3, pp. 216–225, 2006.

[55] W. R. Ashby, *An Introduction to Cybernetics*, John Wiley and Sons, 1956.

[56] N. Wiener, *Cybernetics*, Hermann & Cie Editeurs, Paris, France, 1948.

[57] S. G. Lisberger, E. J. Morris, and L. Tychsen, "Visual motion processing and sensory-motor integration for smooth pursuit eye movements," *Annual Review of Neuroscience*, vol. 10, pp. 97–129, 1987.

[58] W. T. Powers, R. K. Clark, and R. L. McFarland, "A feedback model of human behavior: part I," *Perceptual and Motor Skills*, vol. 11, pp. 71–78, 1960.

[59] K. S. Lashley, "The problem of serial order in behavior," in *Cerebral Mechanisms in Behavior: The Hixon Symposium*, L. A. Jeffress, Ed., pp. 112–146, John Wiley & Sons, New York, NY, USA, 1951.

[60] P. M. Rack, Comprehensive Physiology, 2011.

[61] J. M. Camhi, *Neuroethology*, Sinauer, New York, NY, USA, 1984.

[62] J. C. Houk and W. Z. Rymer, Comprehensive Physiology, 2011.

[63] D. Robinson, *The Vision, Brain, and Cooperative Computation*, MIT, Cambridge, Mass, USA, 1990.

[64] N. Bernstein, *Dexterity and Its Development*, Lawrence Erlbaum Associates, Mahwah, NJ, USA, 1996.

[65] J. Massion, A. Alexandrov, and A. Frolov, "Why and how are posture and movement coordinated?" *Progress in Brain Research*, vol. 143, pp. 13–27, 2004.

[66] E. Von Holst and H. Mittelstaedt, *The Collected Papers of Erich von Holst*, University of Miami Press, Coral Gables, Fla, USA, 1950.

[67] L. Adrian, "The analysis of the nervous system," *Proceedings of the Royal Society of Medicine*, vol. 50, no. 12, pp. 991–998, 1957.

[68] W. T. Powers, "Feedback: beyond behaviorism: stimulus-response laws are wholly predictable within a control-system model of behavioral organization," *Science*, vol. 179, no. 4071, pp. 351–356, 1973.

[69] T. A. McMahon, *Muscles, Reflexes, and Locomotion*, Princeton University Press, Princeton, NJ, USA, 1984.

[70] F. J. Alvarez and R. E. W. Fyffe, "The continuing case for the Renshaw cell," *The Journal of Physiology*, vol. 584, no. 1, pp. 31–45, 2007.

[71] P. Merton, "Paper presented at the Ciba Foundation Symposium-The Spinal Cord, 1953," 1953.

[72] P. B. Matthews, *Mammalian Muscle Receptors and Their Central Actions*, Edward Arnold, 1972.

[73] N. Hogan, "Adaptive control of mechanical impedance by coactivation of antagonist muscles," *IEEE Transactions on Automatic Control*, vol. 29, no. 8, pp. 681–690, 1984.

[74] R. Granit, *The Basis of Motor Control: Integrating the Activity of Muscles, Alpha and Gamma Motoneurons and Their Leading Control Systems*, Academic Press, London, UK, 1970.

[75] O. Sacks, *Awakenings*, Pan Macmillan Adult, London, UK, 1991.

[76] K. Takakusaki, K. Saitoh, H. Harada, and M. Kashiwayanagi, "Role of basal ganglia-brainstem pathways in the control of motor behaviors," *Neuroscience Research*, vol. 50, no. 2, pp. 137–151, 2004.

[77] S. Grillner, P. Wallén, K. Saitoh, A. Kozlov, and B. Robertson, "Neural bases of goal-directed locomotion in vertebrates—an overview," *Brain Research Reviews*, vol. 57, no. 1, pp. 2–12, 2008.

[78] D. G. Lawrence and H. G. Kuypers, "The functional organization of the motor system in the monkey: II. The effects of lesions of the descending brain-stem pathways," *Brain*, vol. 91, no. 1, pp. 15–36, 1968.

[79] A. K. Kozlov, E. Aurell, G. N. Orlovsky et al., "Modeling postural control in the lamprey," *Biological Cybernetics*, vol. 84, no. 5, pp. 323–330, 2001.

[80] S. Grillner, A. Kozlov, P. Dario et al., "Modeling a vertebrate motor system: pattern generation, steering and control of body orientation," *Progress in Brain Research*, vol. 165, pp. 221–234, 2007.

[81] A. Kozlov, M. Huss, A. Lansner, J. H. Kotaleski, and S. Grillner, "Simple cellular and network control principles govern complex patterns of motor behavior," *Proceedings of the National Academy of Sciences of the United States of America*, vol. 106, no. 47, 2009.

[82] T. Wannier, T. G. Deliagina, G. N. Orlovsky, and S. Grillner, "Differential effects of the reticulospinal system on locomotion in lamprey," *Journal of Neurophysiology*, vol. 80, no. 1, pp. 103–112, 1998.

[83] T. G. Deliagina, P. V. Zelenin, P. Fagerstedt, S. Grillner, and G. N. Orlovsky, "Activity of reticulospinal neurons during locomotion in the freely behaving lamprey," *Journal of Neurophysiology*, vol. 83, no. 2, pp. 853–863, 2000.

[84] P. V. Zelenin, E. L. Pavlova, S. Grillner, G. N. Orlovsky, and T. G. Deliagina, "Comparison of the motor effects of individual vestibulo- and reticulospinal neurons on dorsal and ventral myotomes in lamprey," *Journal of Neurophysiology*, vol. 90, no. 5, pp. 3161–3167, 2003.

[85] P. V. Zelenin, G. N. Orlovsky, and T. G. Deliagina, "Sensory-motor transformation by individual command neurons," *Journal of Neuroscience*, vol. 27, no. 5, pp. 1024–1032, 2007.

[86] P. V. Zelenin, S. Grillner, G. N. Orlovsky, and T. G. Deliagina, "Heterogeneity of the population of command neurons in the lamprey," *Journal of Neuroscience*, vol. 21, no. 19, pp. 7793–7803, 2001.

[87] P. V. Zelenin, S. Grillner, G. N. Orlovsky, and T. G. Deliagina, "The pattern of motor coordination underlying the roll in the lamprey," *Journal of Experimental Biology*, vol. 206, no. 15, pp. 2557–2566, 2003.

[88] H. W. Magoun and R. Rhines, "An inhibitory mechanism in the bulbar reticular formation," *Journal of Neurophysiology*, vol. 9, pp. 165–171, 1946.

[89] K. Takakusaki, T. Habaguchi, J. Ohtinata-Sugimoto, K. Saitoh, and T. Sakamoto, "Basal ganglia efferents to the brainstem centers controlling postural muscle tone and locomotion: a new concept for understanding motor disorders in basal ganglia dysfunction," *Neuroscience*, vol. 119, no. 1, pp. 293–308, 2003.

[90] J. M. Sprague and W. W. Chambers, "Control of posture by reticular formation and cerebellum in the intract, anesthetized and unanesthetized and in the decerebrated cat," *The American Journal of Physiology*, vol. 176, no. 1, pp. 52–64, 1954.

[91] B. W. Peterson, "Reticulospinal projections to spinal motor nuclei," *Annual Review of Physiology*, vol. 41, pp. 127–140, 1979.

[92] S. Grillner and S. Lund, "The origin of a descending pathway with monosynaptic action on flexor motoneurones," *Acta Physiologica Scandinavica*, vol. 74, no. 3, pp. 274–284, 1968.

[93] M. B. Foreman and R. C. Eaton, "The direction change concept for reticulospinal control of goldfish escape," *Journal of Neuroscience*, vol. 13, no. 10, pp. 4101–4113, 1993.

[94] M. Shimamura and I. Kogure, "Discharge patterns of reticulospinal neurons corresponding with quadrupedal leg movements in thalamic cats," *Brain Research*, vol. 260, no. 1, pp. 27–34, 1983.

[95] M. F. Huerta and J. K. Harting, "Connectional organization of the superior colliculus," *Trends in Neurosciences*, vol. 7, no. 8, pp. 286–289, 1984.

[96] A. M. Graybiel, "Organization of the nigrotectal connection: an experimental tracer study in the cat," *Brain Research*, vol. 143, no. 2, pp. 339–348, 1978.

[97] R. L. M. Faull and W. R. Mehler, "The cells of origin of nigrotectal, nigrothalamic and nigrostriatal projections in the rat," *Neuroscience*, vol. 3, no. 11, pp. 989–1002, 1978.

[98] J. Konorski, *Integrative Activity of the Brain*, University of Chicago Press, Chicago, Ill, USA, 1967.

[99] I. Kilpatrick, G. Collingridge, and M. Starr, "Evidence for the participation of nigrotectal γ-aminobutyrate-containing neurons in striatal and nigral-derived circling in the rat," *Neuroscience*, vol. 7, no. 1, pp. 207–222, 1982.

[100] N. Sahibzada, P. Dean, and P. Redgrave, "Movements resembling orientation or avoidance elicited by electrical stimulation of the superior colliculus in rats," *the Journal of Neuroscience*, vol. 6, no. 3, pp. 723–733, 1986.

[101] S. M. King, P. Dean, and P. Redgrave, "Bypassing the saccadic pulse generator: possible control of head movement trajectory by rat superior colliculus," *European Journal of Neuroscience*, vol. 3, no. 8, pp. 790–801, 1991.

[102] J. McHaffie and B. E. Stein, "Eye movements evoked by electrical stimulation in the superior colliculus of rats and hamsters," *Brain Research*, vol. 247, no. 2, pp. 243–253, 1982.

[103] T. Masino, "Brainstem control of orienting movements: intrinsic coordinate systems and underlying circuitry," *Brain, Behavior and Evolution*, vol. 40, no. 2-3, pp. 98–111, 1992.

[104] K. Saitoh, A. Ménard, and S. Grillner, "Tectal control of locomotion, steering, and eye movements in lamprey," *Journal of Neurophysiology*, vol. 97, no. 4, pp. 3093–3108, 2007.

[105] D. L. Sparks and R. Hartwich-Young, "The deep layers of the superior colliculus," *Reviews of Oculomotor Research*, vol. 3, pp. 213–255, 1989.

[106] D. A. Robinson, "Eye movements evoked by collicular stimulation in the alert monkey," *Vision Research*, vol. 12, no. 11, pp. 1795–1808, 1972.

[107] C. R. Gallistel, *The Organization of Learning*, MIT Press, Cambridge, UK, 1990.

[108] D. L. Sparks, "The brainstem control of saccadic eye movements," *Nature Reviews Neuroscience*, vol. 3, no. 12, pp. 952–964, 2002.

[109] E. I. Knudsen, "Auditory and visual maps of space in the optic tectum of the owl," *The Journal of Neuroscience*, vol. 2, no. 9, pp. 1177–1194, 1982.

[110] D. A. Robinson, "Integrating with neurons," *Annual Review of Neuroscience*, vol. 12, pp. 33–45, 1989.

[111] U. C. Drager and D. H. Hubel, "Topography of visual and somatosensory projections to mouse superior colliculus," *Journal of Neurophysiology*, vol. 39, no. 1, pp. 91–101, 1976.

[112] W. T. Newsome and E. B. Pare, "A selective impairment of motion perception following lesions of the middle temporal visual area (MT)," *Journal of Neuroscience*, vol. 8, no. 6, pp. 2201–2211, 1988.

[113] R. J. Krauzlis, M. A. Basso, and R. H. Wurtz, "Shared motor error for multiple eye movements," *Science*, vol. 276, no. 5319, pp. 1693–1695, 1997.

[114] R. J. Krauzlis, M. A. Basso, and R. H. Wurtz, "Discharge properties of neurons in the rostral superior colliculus of the monkey during smooth-pursuit eye movements," *Journal of Neurophysiology*, vol. 84, no. 2, pp. 876–891, 2000.

[115] Z. M. Hafed, L. Goffart, and R. J. Krauzlis, "A neural mechanism for microsaccade generation in the primate superior colliculus," *Science*, vol. 323, no. 5916, pp. 940–943, 2009.

[116] N. J. Gandhi and H. A. Katnani, "Motor functions of the superior colliculus," *Annual Review of Neuroscience*, vol. 34, pp. 205–231, 2011.

[117] M. Paré and D. Guitton, "The fixation area of the cat superior colliculus: effects of electrical stimulation and direct connection with brainstem omnipause neurons," *Experimental Brain Research*, vol. 101, no. 1, pp. 109–122, 1994.

[118] S. Everling, M. Paré, M. C. Dorris, and D. P. Munoz, "Comparison of the discharge characteristics of brain stem omnipause neurons and superior colliculus fixation neurons in monkey: Implications for control of fixation and saccade behavior," *Journal of Neurophysiology*, vol. 79, no. 2, pp. 511–528, 1998.

[119] D. Guitton, "Control of eye-head coordination during orienting gaze shifts," *Trends in Neurosciences*, vol. 15, no. 5, pp. 174–179, 1992.

[120] D. P. Munoz, D. Pélisson, and D. Guitton, "Movement of neural activity on the superior colliculus motor map during gaze shifts," *Science*, vol. 251, no. 4999, pp. 1358–1360, 1991.

[121] K. Fukushima, C. R. S. Kaneko, and A. F. Fuchs, "The neuronal substrate of integration in the oculomotor system," *Progress in Neurobiology*, vol. 39, no. 6, pp. 609–639, 1992.

[122] A. R. Cools, *Perspectives in Ethology*, Springer, 1985.

[123] L. Goffart, Z. M. Hafed, and R. J. Krauzlis, "Visual fixation as equilibrium: evidence from superior colliculus inactivation," *The Journal of Neuroscience*, vol. 32, no. 31, pp. 10627–10636, 2012.

[124] P. Redgrave, L. Marrow, and P. Dean, "Topographical organization of the nigrotectal projection in rat: evidence for segregated channels," *Neuroscience*, vol. 50, no. 3, pp. 571–595, 1992.

[125] U. J. Niemi-Junkola and G. W. Max Westby, "Spatial variation in the effects of inactivation of substantia nigra on neuronal activity in rat superior colliculus," *Neuroscience Letters*, vol. 241, no. 2-3, pp. 175–179, 1998.

[126] T. Isa and W. C. Hall, "Exploring the superior colliculus in vitro," *Journal of Neurophysiology*, vol. 102, no. 5, pp. 2581–2593, 2009.

[127] O. Hikosaka and R. H. Wurtz, "Modification of saccadic eye movements by GABA-related substances. II. Effects of muscimol in monkey substantia nigra pars reticulata," *Journal of Neurophysiology*, vol. 53, no. 1, pp. 292–308, 1985.

[128] O. Hikosaka and R. H. Wurtz, "Modification of saccadic eye movements by GABA-related substances. I. Effect of muscimol and bicuculline in monkey superior colliculus," *Journal of Neurophysiology*, vol. 53, no. 1, pp. 266–291, 1985.

[129] K. Takakusaki, "Forebrain control of locomotor behaviors," *Brain Research Reviews*, vol. 57, no. 1, pp. 192–198, 2008.

[130] W. R. Hess, *The Functional Organization of the Diencephalon*, Grune & Stratton, New York, NY, USA, 1957.

[131] A. Luria, *Higher Cortical Functions in Man*, Basic Books, New York, NY, USA, 1966.

[132] G. J. Kress, N. Yamawaki, D. L. Wokosin, I. R. Wickersham, G. M. G. Shepherd, and D. J. Surmeier, "Convergent cortical innervation of striatal projection neurons," *Nature Neuroscience*, vol. 16, no. 6, pp. 665–667, 2013.

[133] A. J. McGeorge and R. L. M. Faull, "The organization of the projection from the cerebral cortex to the striatum in the rat," *Neuroscience*, vol. 29, no. 3, pp. 503–537, 1989.

[134] D. Joel and I. Weiner, "The organization of the basal ganglia-thalamocortical circuits: open interconnected rather than closed segregated," *Neuroscience*, vol. 63, no. 2, pp. 363–379, 1994.

[135] G. M. G. Shepherd, "Corticostriatal connectivity and its role in disease," *Nature Reviews Neuroscience*, vol. 14, no. 4, pp. 278–291, 2013.

[136] H. H. Yin, "The role of the murine motor cortex in action duration and order," *Frontiers in Integrative Neuroscience*, vol. 3, article 23, 2009.

[137] V. Mountcastle, "An organizing principle for cerebral function: the unit model and the distributed system," in *The Mindful Brain*, G. Edelman and V. Mountcastle, Eds., pp. 7–50, The MIT Press, Cambridge, Mass, USA, 1978.

[138] P. Voorn, L. J. M. J. Vanderschuren, H. J. Groenewegen, T. W. Robbins, and C. M. A. Pennartz, "Putting a spin on the dorsal-ventral divide of the striatum," *Trends in Neurosciences*, vol. 27, no. 8, pp. 468–474, 2004.

[139] J. P. Bolam, J. J. Hanley, P. A. C. Booth, and M. D. Bevan, "Synaptic organisation of the basal ganglia," *Journal of Anatomy*, vol. 196, no. 4, pp. 527–542, 2000.

[140] O. B. White, J. A. Saint Cyr, R. D. Tomlinson, and J. A. Sharpe, "Ocular motor deficits in Parkinson's disease. II. Control of the saccadic and smooth pursuit systems," *Brain*, vol. 106, no. 3, pp. 571–587, 1983.

[141] M. R. DeLong and A. P. Georgopoulos, *Comprehensive Physiology*, 2011.

[142] J. W. Barter, S. Castro, T. Sukharnikova, M. A. Rossi, and H. H. Yin, "The role of the substantia nigra in posture control," *European Journal of Neuroscience*, vol. 39, no. 9, pp. 1465–1473, 2014.

[143] K. P. Bhatia and C. D. Marsden, "The behavioural and motor consequences of focal lesions of the basal ganglia in man," *Brain*, vol. 117, no. 4, pp. 859–876, 1994.

[144] R. S. Marken, "Controlled variables: psychology as the center fielder views it," *The American Journal of Psychology*, vol. 114, pp. 259–281, 2001.

[145] R. Kawagoe, Y. Takikawa, and O. Hikosaka, "Expectation of reward modulates cognitive signals in the basal ganglia," *Nature Neuroscience*, vol. 1, no. 5, pp. 411–416, 1998.

[146] H. H. Yin, "The sensorimotor striatum is necessary for serial order learning," *Journal of Neuroscience*, vol. 30, no. 44, pp. 14719–14723, 2010.

[147] A. R. Cools, J. H. van den Bercken, M. W. Horstink, K. P. van Spaendonck, and H. J. Berger, "Cognitive and motor shifting aptitude disorder in Parkinson's disease," *Journal of Neurology, Neurosurgery & Psychiatry*, vol. 47, pp. 443–453, 1984.

[148] M. C. Vrijmoed-De Vries and A. R. Cools, "Differential effects of striatal injections of dopaminergic, cholinergic and GABAergic drugs upon swimming behavior of rats," *Brain Research*, vol. 364, no. 1, pp. 77–90, 1986.

[149] E. L. Thorndike, *Animal Intelligence: Experimental Studies*, Macmillan, New York, NY, USA, 1911.

[150] M. A. Rossi, T. Sukharnikova, V. Y. Hayrapetyan, L. Yang, and H. H. Yin, "Operant self-stimulation of dopamine neurons in the substantia Nigra," *PLoS ONE*, vol. 8, no. 6, Article ID e65799, 2013.

[151] H. H. Yin, S. B. Ostlund, B. J. Knowlton, and B. W. Balleine, "The role of the dorsomedial striatum in instrumental conditioning," *European Journal of Neuroscience*, vol. 22, no. 2, pp. 513–523, 2005.

[152] C. Yu, J. Gupta, J.-F. Chen, and H. H. Yin, "Genetic deletion of A2A adenosine receptors in the striatum selectively impairs habit formation," *Journal of Neuroscience*, vol. 29, no. 48, pp. 15100–15103, 2009.

[153] M. A. Rossi and H. H. Yin, "The roles of the dorsal striatum in instrumental conditioning," in *Animal Models of Movement Disorders*, pp. 55–69, Springer, New York, NY, USA, 2011.

[154] W. M. Baum, "The correlation based law of effect," *Journal of the Experimental Analysis of Behavior*, vol. 20, no. 1, pp. 137–153, 1973.

[155] P. W. Glimcher, "Understanding dopamine and reinforcement learning: the dopamine reward prediction error hypothesis," *Proceedings of the National Academy of Sciences of the United States of America*, vol. 108, pp. 1564–1565, 2011.

[156] N. D. Daw, Y. Niv, and P. Dayan, "Uncertainty-based competition between prefrontal and dorsolateral striatal systems for behavioral control," *Nature Neuroscience*, vol. 8, no. 12, pp. 1704–1711, 2005.

[157] R. S. Sutton and A. G. Barto, *Reinforcement Learning*, MIT Press, Cambridge, Mass, USA, 1998.

[158] C. Hull, *Principles of Behavior*, Appleton-Century-Crofts, New York, NY, USA, 1943.

[159] C. Hull, *A Behavior System*, Yale University Press, New Haven, Conn, USA, 1952.

[160] K. Spence, *Behavior Theory and Learning*, Prentice Hall, Englewood Cliffs, NJ, USA, 1960.

[161] A. L. Derusso, D. Fan, J. Gupta, O. Shelest, R. M. Costa, and H. H. Yin, "Instrumental uncertainty as a determinant of behavior under interval schedules of reinforcement," *Frontiers in Integrative Neuroscience*, vol. 4, article 17, 2010.

[162] A. Dickinson and N. J. Mackintosh, "Instrumental conditioning," in *Animal Learning and Cognition*, pp. 45–79, Academic Press, Orlando, Fla, USA, 1994.

[163] B. W. Balleine, "Incentive processes in instrumental conditioning," in *Handbook of Contemporary Learning Theories*, R. R. Mowrer and S. B. Klein, Eds., pp. 307–366, Lawrence Erlbaum Associates, Mahwah, NJ, USA, 2001.

[164] S. Freud, "Instincts and their vicissitudes," in *Collected Papers*, vol. 4, Basic Books, New York, NY, USA, 1915.

[165] J. W. Kable and P. W. Glimcher, "The neurobiology of decision: consensus and controversy," *Neuron*, vol. 63, no. 6, pp. 733–745, 2009.

[166] M. R. Roesch, T. Singh, P. Leon Brown, S. E. Mullins, and G. Schoenbaum, "Ventral striatal neurons encode the value of the chosen action in rats deciding between differently delayed or sized rewards," *Journal of Neuroscience*, vol. 29, no. 42, pp. 13365–13376, 2009.

[167] S. N. Haber, J. L. Fudge, and N. R. McFarland, "Striatonigrostriatal pathways in primates form an ascending spiral from the shell to the dorsolateral striatum," *Journal of Neuroscience*, vol. 20, no. 6, pp. 2369–2382, 2000.

[168] H. H. Yin and B. J. Knowlton, "The role of the basal ganglia in habit formation," *Nature Reviews Neuroscience*, vol. 7, pp. 464–476, 2006.

[169] S. N. Haber, "The primate basal ganglia: parallel and integrative networks," *Journal of Chemical Neuroanatomy*, vol. 26, no. 4, pp. 317–330, 2003.

[170] D. Joel and I. Weiner, "The connections of the dopaminergic system with the striatum in rats and primates: an analysis with respect to the functional and compartmental organization of the striatum," *Neuroscience*, vol. 96, no. 3, pp. 451–474, 2000.

[171] S. Peciña, K. S. Smith, and K. C. Berridge, "Hedonic hot spots in the brain," *Neuroscientist*, vol. 12, no. 6, pp. 500–511, 2006.

[172] E. P. Prinssen, W. Balestra, F. F. Bemelmans, and A. R. Cools, "Evidence for a role of the shell of the nucleus accumbens in oral behavior of freely moving rats," *Journal of Neuroscience*, vol. 14, no. 3, pp. 1555–1562, 1994.

[173] G. J. Mogenson, D. L. Jones, and C. Y. Yim, "From motivation to action: functional interface between the limbic system and the motor system," *Progress in Neurobiology*, vol. 14, no. 2-3, pp. 69–97, 1980.

[174] L. W. Swanson, G. J. Mogenson, C. R. Gerfen, and P. Robinson, "Evidence for a projection from the lateral preoptic area and substantia innominata to the "mesencephalic locomotor region" in the rat," *Brain Research*, vol. 295, no. 1, pp. 161–178, 1984.

[175] C. J. Swanson and P. W. Kalivas, "Regulation of locomotor activity by metabotropic glutamate receptors in the nucleus accumbens and ventral tegmental area," *Journal of Pharmacology and Experimental Therapeutics*, vol. 292, no. 1, pp. 406–414, 2000.

[176] S. A. Taha and H. L. Fields, "Encoding of palatability and appetitive behaviors by distinct neuronal populations in the nucleus accumbens," *Journal of Neuroscience*, vol. 25, no. 5, pp. 1193–1202, 2005.

[177] L. H. Corbit and B. W. Balleine, "The general and outcome-specific forms of pavlovian-instrumental transfer are differentially mediated by the nucleus accumbens core and shell," *Journal of Neuroscience*, vol. 31, no. 33, pp. 11786–11794, 2011.

[178] H. H. Yin, S. B. Ostlund, and B. W. Balleine, "Reward-guided learning beyond dopamine in the nucleus accumbens: the integrative functions of cortico-basal ganglia networks," *European Journal of Neuroscience*, vol. 28, no. 8, pp. 1437–1448, 2008.

[179] A. Compte, N. Brunel, P. S. Goldman-Rakic, and X. J. Wang, "Synaptic mechanisms and network dynamics underlying spatial working memory in a cortical network model," *Cerebral Cortex*, vol. 10, no. 9, pp. 910–923, 2000.

[180] H. S. Seung, "How the brain keeps the eyes still," *Proceedings of the National Academy of Sciences of the United States of America*, vol. 93, no. 23, pp. 13339–13344, 1996.

[181] W. Schultz, Current Opinion in Neurobiology, 2012.

[182] R. A. Wise, "Dopamine, learning and motivation," *Nature Reviews Neuroscience*, vol. 5, no. 6, pp. 483–494, 2004.

12

The Role of Habenula in Motivation and Reward

Marc Fakhoury and Sergio Domínguez López

Department of Neuroscience, Faculty of Medicine, University of Montreal, Montreal, QC, Canada H2V 2S9

Correspondence should be addressed to Marc Fakhoury; marc_fakhoury@hotmail.com

Academic Editor: Daniela Schulz

Located centrally along the dorsal diencephalic system, the habenula is divided into two structures: the medial and the lateral portions. It serves as an important relay between the forebrain and several hindbrain sites. In the last few years, a huge attention has been devoted to this structure, especially the lateral habenula (LHb), which seems to play an important role in emotion, motivation, and reward. Recent studies using techniques such as electrophysiology and neuroimaging have shown that the LHb is involved in motivational control of behavior. Its dysfunction is often associated with depression, schizophrenia, and mood disorder. This review focuses on providing a neuroanatomical and behavioral overview of some of the research previously done on the LHb. First, we describe the anatomical structure of the habenula and we explain how it is involved in reward and motivation. Then, we will discuss how this structure is linked to the limbic system, to finally provide a comparison between several studies that have used electrolytic lesions.

1. Introduction

The study of the habenula started in the early 1980s [1], and it was known that this structure has the potential to control several regions of the midbrain. However, it was just recently that scientists discovered the influence of the habenula in motivational states, mood disorders, and several other mental problems [2, 3]. The habenula, which is part of the epithalamus, is composed of the lateral habenula (LHb) and the medial habenula (MHb), each having distinct functions and a unique anatomical structure. Here, we will focus on the LHb, which is more involved with pain processing, reward, motivation, and learning [4, 5]. In rodents, studies have shown that lesions at the level of the habenula cause cognitive impairment, attention deficits, hyperreactivity to stress, and schizophrenic-like symptoms [6]. Moreover, additional studies have linked the activity of the LHb to the regulation of serotonin (5-HT) and norepinephrine, suggesting that this structure modulates multiple regions in the brain [7–9]. It was also shown that neurons in the habenula are responsive to peripheral nociceptive stimulation, and when exposed to stress, the level of c-fos in this structure significantly increases [10, 11].

The habenula receives its main afferents from the septum and stria medullaris (sm) [8]. Furthermore, the habenula projects towards many areas in the midbrain that are involved in the release of neuromodulators and also towards dopaminergic midbrain nuclei such as the ventral tegmental area (VTA) [2, 12]. Studies utilizing lesions of the afferent projections of the LHb have demonstrated an increase in the level of anxiety in rats, with neonatal rats exhibiting a higher state of anxiety compared to adult rats [13]. Lesions of the LHb also induce impairment of memory and attention in rats, suggesting a connection between the LHb and cognition [5, 6, 13]. Here, we will discuss how studies using lesions and electrical self-stimulation have been able to show that the LHb is an important component of the brain reward system. We will begin by describing how the activity of LHb neurons can be influenced by regulatory synapses and neuromodulators and how they interact with the limbic system in the brain, to finally discuss the ability of the LHb in encoding rewarding stimuli.

2. Anatomical Organization of the Habenula

The primary input regions to the LHb are the lateral preoptic area, the ventral pallidum, the lateral hypothalamus, and the internal segment of the globus pallidus (GPi) [14]. The habenula is connected to the anterior diencephalon in the epiphysis peduncle. While the MHb receives its main afferents from the septum, the LHb is connected to the striatum and projects onto the midbrain [9, 15]. The habenula is present across all species and is greater in size relative to the whole brain of most mammals [5]. It is a bilateral structure located above the thalamus at its posterior end and directly adjacent to the midline. Figure 1 illustrates coronal sections of the rat brain that clearly show that the habenula is a bilateral structure divided into a medial portion and a lateral portion.

Neurons in the habenula are heterogeneous in nature. In fact, studies using a Golgi staining showed that these neurons can adopt various morphologies. Neurons in the MHb are divided into two groups: the first group of neurons has piriform cell bodies with a mean diameter of 12 μm and two to five primary dendrites, while the second group is comprised of neurons that are fusiform in shape and have around three primary dendrites that arose from cell bodies [16]. Furthermore, the phenotype of neurons of the LHb differs from the neurons in the MHb. The MHb includes a dense aggregate of cholinergic neurons and neurons producing substance P [16, 17], whereas in the LHb, the majority of the neurons are glutamatergic [18]. In LHb neurons, GABAergic transmission arises from the medial globus pallidus (MGP). GABA receptors can be coupled to G protein-coupled inwardly-rectifying potassium channels (GIRK) for potassium ions intake [1]. Glutamate transmission also arises from MGP and to a lesser extent from the lateral hypothalamus. It largely relies on acid receptors that can be calcium-permeable (CP-AMPAR) or calcium-impermeable (CI-AMPAR). Moreover, the dopamine (DA) released from the VTA can bind to D2R and D4R receptors of dopaminergic cells. LHb neurons also express G-protein coupled receptors (GPCR) specific to glutamate in addition to 5-HT2C receptors that can detect 5-HT released from the dorsal raphe [1].

3. Role of the Habenula in Reward and Its Relationship with the Limbic System

The LHb is considered to be the highway to the midbrain for processing aversion and reward [1, 2]. Studies have shown that neurons in the LHb are "reward-negative," meaning that they can get activated by stimulus associated with no reward or unpleasing events [20]. Indeed, it has been demonstrated in monkeys that the omission of an expected reward leads to a strong increase in the activity of LHb neurons, while unexpected delivery of rewards decreases LHb neuron firing [21]. It was also shown that optogenetic activation of excitatory projections towards the LHb drives aversive behaviors [1]. The habenula receives its main afferents from the septum through the sm and is part of the epithalamus [8, 22]. The epithalamus, which is also composed of the pineal body, is connected to the basal ganglia and the limbic system. All afferents go to the LHb through the sm. However, the projections leaving the LHb go to the fasciculus retroflexus, which is composed of major axons that form a link between the projections of the habenula and midbrain structures.

Several other areas transmit information to the habenula from the sm, such as the lateral hypothalamus, the lateral preoptic area, the nucleus of diagonal band of Broca, and the septum. Also, the caudate transmits information to the GPi, which in turn sends projections to the LHb. Furthermore, the neurons of the LHb project towards many areas of the midbrain that send signals to the forebrain enabling the release of DA in the striatum [2, 12].

DA is a neurotransmitter that belongs to the class of catecholamines. It is synthesized from the amino acid tyrosine and is mainly produced in the substantia nigra and in the VTA [23]. A dysfunction of DA dopamine neuronal activity is associated with a variety of important diseases of the nervous system. Thus, a better understanding of the dopaminergic system will help scientists elucidate the biological and neurological mechanisms implicated in many neurodegenerative diseases. DA has received the most attention for its role in building rewarding behaviors, including behaviors that contribute to addiction and drug abuse [24, 25]. Located upstream of the mesolimbic dopaminergic pathway, the habenula is closely linked to reward because of its ability to activate dopaminergic neurons. Indeed, several studies show that the habenula has glutamatergic projections that establish their synaptic contacts with dopaminergic cells [26–28]. Moreover, the habenula is capable of communicating with dopaminergic neurons in the VTA (Figure 2) by activating the rostral medial tegmental nucleus (RMTg) [2, 29].

Input from the basal ganglia to the habenula, specifically the LHb, derives from the border region of the GPi, which receives inputs from the striosome subterritory of the striatum (Striatum-S) [2]. The habenula then influences DA neurons via inhibitory neurons in the RMTg. Activation of neurons in the LHb causes a decrease of the activity of dopaminergic neurons, whereas inhibition of the LHb accompanies activation of dopaminergic neurons [30]. As shown in Figure 2, motor activity is directly mediated by the substantia nigra pars reticulata (SNr) and the GPi, which are influenced by the innervation of the matrix subterritory of the striatum (Striatum-M), the DA neurons in the VTA, and in the substantia nigra pars compacta (SNc).

4. Role of the Habenula in Pain and Mood Disorders

The habenula is a structure involved in behavioral response to pain and is also implicated with psychiatric disorders such as depression and schizophrenia [2, 31]. Several animal studies support its role in pain and analgesia [32]. It has been shown that the habenula receives information from forebrain structures and the dorsal diencephalic conduction system, which is a major site that interconnects the limbic forebrain with the midbrain [33]. The habenula also modulates the intensity of pain, aversion, and motor responses. It receives projections from the spinal cord, the limbic system, and cortical structures, while its efferent pathways are in areas of the brainstem involved in pain modulation [5, 32]. The MHb projects predominantly to the interpeduncular nucleus (IPN) in the midbrain, while the LHb has projections to the VTA,

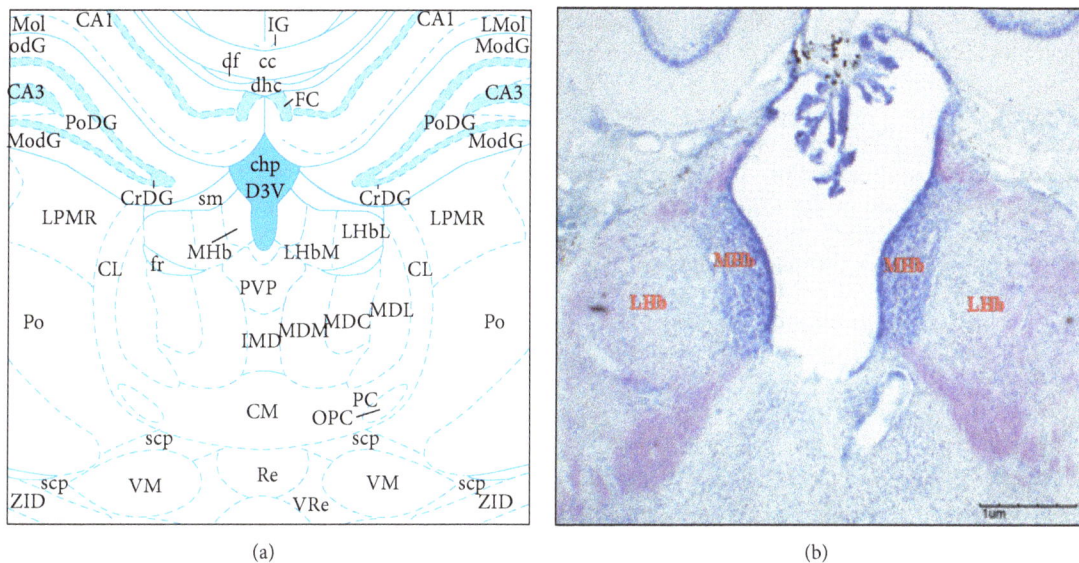

FIGURE 1: (a) Coronal section of the rat brain showing the habenula and its subdivision (taken from an atlas of the rat brain [19]). (b) A Thionin staining of a coronal section of the rat brain showing that the habenula is divided into a medial (MHb) portion and lateral (LHb) portion.

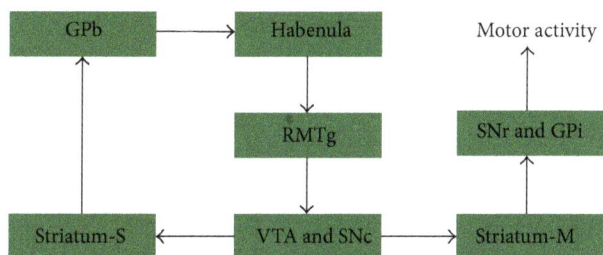

FIGURE 2: Dopamine-mediated circuit.

the dorsal raphe, and the SNc [34, 35]. The IPN modulates cells in the periaqueductal gray and the dorsal raphe, which both play a major role in descending modulation of pain. The dorsal raphe also sends afferents directly to the spinal cord via the raphe magnus in the medulla, through serotonergic mediated pain modulatory processing [5]. Studies using electrophysiology or electrostimulation have clear indication that the habenula may be involved in pain modulation. It was shown that the LHb responds to noxious stimuli that may be excitatory or inhibitory [11] and that this structure is a central target for the nociceptive input at the upper brainstem level [36, 37]. Moreover, studies using c-fos immunohisto-chemistry as a marker of neuronal activity show increases in neuronal stains in the LHb in experimental pain [38, 39]. Another study utilizing diabetes-induced pain in rats showed that the pain in diabetic neuropathy significantly decreased the activation of the habenula, suggesting that the latter structure represents part of a modulatory pain system [40].

It is also well documented that the LHb is hyperactive in individuals with mood disorder such as depression and in animal models of this psychiatric disorder [41, 42]. Indeed, the habenula plays a crucial role in regulating behavioral responses to stress and shows increased cerebral blood flow because of its hyperactivity [43, 44]. Consistent with these data, recent studies reported a decrease in the habenula volume of unmedicated patients with bipolar disorder and major depressive disorder (MDD) [45]. Also, deep brain stimulation of the LHb was found to induce remission of symptoms in patients with MDD [46, 47].

5. Comparison of Studies Done with Electrolytic Lesions

Several studies have done lesions in regions of the brain in order to determine the neural circuitry involved in motivation and reward. Lesioning is a technique in which a specific region of interest in the brain is destroyed to observe any resulting changes such as altered performance on some behavioral measure. Using a 3-dimensional atlas of the brain, one can stereotaxically implant electrodes with very high accuracy to produce a lesion. Another technique commonly employed is the infusion of excitotoxic drugs into the brain, which causes death of neurons with high accuracy and efficacy [48, 49]. However, most of the studies done to examine the function of the habenula relied on lesions to this site by passing an electric current through electrodes implanted in the brain of animals [3, 50]. Following the passage of the current, the cell bodies and axons that are located at the tip of the electrode are destroyed. Destruction of neuronal cells within a confined zone should be reflected in a deterioration of the effectiveness of brain stimulation reward: when the animal receives stimulation, the reward signal gets attenuated. This technique is very useful in research and is useful to determine how eliminating the activity of specific areas in the brain can change the behavior.

A study conducted in the University of Maryland in Baltimore has shown that the habenula can govern the attribution of incentive salience to reward predictive cues [51]. Incentive salience attribution endows a reward-predicting stimulus with the capacity to initiate goal-directed behaviour [52]. It is a type of motivation in the brain associated with an external stimuli or reward that drives the addictive behaviors. In this study, researchers used electrolytic lesions of the fasciculus retroflexus (fr), a pathway through which descending habenula efferents are conveyed. The results showed that lesioning the fr significantly increased incentive salience, suggesting that the habenula is involved in regulating the relative degree of incentive salience assigned to a given cue, which is critical for motivation and reward. Moreover, they showed that changing the activity of neurons in the LHb could result in avolition and depression-like symptoms [51]. Another study from Morissette and Boye [3] has used electrolytic lesions aimed at the LHb in order to demonstrate the role that this structure plays in motivation and reward. Following the implantation of stimulation and lesioning electrodes, the rats were trained at several currents and were put in a cage with a lever that could self-administer the stimulation. Each time the rat pressed the lever, the rewarding stimulation was transmitted to its brain. Behavioral curves correlating the number of presses with the frequency of the stimulation were then generated. From these curves, the number of presses required to obtain half-maximal responding, known as the reward threshold, was calculated. It was shown that lesioning the LHb significantly increases the reward threshold and alters the behavior of the rats. The increase in reward threshold was the result of destruction of habenular neurons that seem to be necessary in transmitting the reward signal.

By regulating the 5-HT and DA system, the habenula may also has an implication in Parkinson's disease [2, 12, 50]. Patients with Parkinson's disease suffer from motor disturbances, which result from the death of DA-generating cells in the substantia nigra. To test whether the habenula is implicated in this disease, scientists have monitored the behavior of rats after functionally suppressing the LHb activity [50]. The results of their study showed that hyperactivity in the LHb downregulates the serotonergic system, thus resulting in depressive symptoms in patients with Parkinson's disease. However, this process can be partially reversed by DA replacement therapy and habenula lesion. These findings provide a link between Parkinson's disease and depression and open up avenues for new therapeutic interventions.

6. Conclusion

Evidence collected in the last 20 years illustrated the potential of the LHb in controlling the midbrain, but not much was known of the anatomy of this structure and its synaptic organization. Only recently it is starting to become clear that this structure participates in the encoding of aversive and rewarding stimuli, influences motivational states, and contributes to pathologies such as mood disorders and addiction [1]. Such discoveries have the potential to rapidly advance our knowledge and can open up avenues for therapeutic interventions. Indeed, by understanding the function of the habenula and its implication in brain reward circuits, scientists could find new molecular and genetic targets that could potentially aid in the treatment of several neurological diseases. As presented in this review, the habenula is strongly connected to the limbic system and plays an important role in regulating directed behavior. It receives its main afferents from the septum through the sm and projects towards several areas of the midbrain involved in the release of neuromodulators. The presence of dopaminergic projections that innervate the LHb has also been described, suggesting that the habenula could be implicated in psychological disorders such as depression, addiction, and drug abuse. Finally, most of the understanding of the function of the LHb so far, has been done by observing how the behavior of subjects was altered after lesioning this structure. Several studies found that the LHb plays a critical part of the reward system and that a dysfunction of the LHb is often associated with psychiatric disorders [36, 37, 50]. The studies presented here discuss several pathways in which the habenula is involved and describe several neurotransmitters that act in the LHb, including amino acids such as glutamate and GABA. However, evidence suggests that other potentially relevant molecules may also act in the LHb, including orexins, acetylcholine, and vasopressin [1, 42]. Several studies have shown that the habenula is implicated in the release of neuromodulators such as DA and 5-HT, but the big challenge now is to determine the downstream implications of such changes on reward and motivation. There are several studies that still need to be done on the habenula, and what will be learned in the next few years will allow us to better understand how regulatory systems control motivated behavior and may offer a window to further develop therapeutic strategies.

Conflict of Interests

The authors declare no conflict of financial interests.

References

[1] F. J. Meye, S. Lecca, K. Valentinova, and M. Mameli, "Synaptic and cellular profile of neurons in the lateral habenula," *Frontiers in Human Neuroscience*, vol. 7, p. 860, 2013.

[2] O. Hikosaka, "The habenula: from stress evasion to value-based decision-making," *Nature Reviews Neuroscience*, vol. 11, no. 7, pp. 503–513, 2010.

[3] M. Morissette and S. M. Boye, "Electrolytic lesions of the habenula attenuate brain stimulation reward," *Behavioural Brain Research*, vol. 187, no. 1, pp. 17–26, 2008.

[4] K. H. Andres, M. V. During, and R. W. Veh, "Subnuclear organization of the rat habenular complexes," *The Journal of Comparative Neurology*, vol. 407, no. 1, pp. 130–150, 1999.

[5] L. Shelton, L. Becerra, and D. Borsook, "Unmasking the mysteries of the habenula in pain and analgesia," *Progress in Neurobiology*, vol. 96, no. 2, pp. 208–219, 2012.

[6] L. Lecourtier, H. C. Neijt, and P. H. Kelly, "Habenula lesions cause impaired cognitive performance in rats: implications for schizophrenia," *European Journal of Neuroscience*, vol. 19, no. 9, pp. 2551–2560, 2004.

[7] J. Amat, P. D. Sparks, P. Matus-Amat, J. Griggs, L. R. Watkins, and S. F. Maier, "The role of the habenular complex in the elevation of dorsal raphe nucleus serotonin and the changes in the behavioral responses produced by uncontrollable stress," *Brain Research*, vol. 917, no. 1, pp. 118–126, 2001.

[8] M. Herkenham and W. J. H. Nauta, "Efferent connections of the habenular nuclei in the rat," *Journal of Comparative Neurology*, vol. 187, no. 1, pp. 19–47, 1979.

[9] K. M. Velasquez, D. L. Molfese, and R. Salas, "The role of the habenula in drug addiction," *Frontiers in Human Neuroscience*, vol. 8, article 174, 2014.

[10] D. Wirtschafter, K. E. Asin, and M. R. Pitzer, "Dopamine agonists and stress produce different patterns of Fos-like immunoreactivity in the lateral habenula," *Brain Research*, vol. 633, no. 1-2, pp. 21–26, 1994.

[11] D. M. Gao, D. Huffman, and A. L. Benabid, "Simultaneous recording of spontaneous activities and nociceptive responses from neurons in the Pars compacta of Substantia nigra and in the lateral habenula," *European Journal of Neuroscience*, vol. 8, no. 7, pp. 1474–1478, 1996.

[12] P. Baldwin, R. Alanis, and R. Salas, "The role of the Habenula in nicotine addiction," *Journal of Addiction Research & Therapy*, vol. S1, article 002, 2001.

[13] C. A. Murphy, A. M. DiCamillo, F. Haun, and M. Murray, "Lesion of the habenular efferent pathway produces anxiety and locomotor hyperactivity in rats: a comparison of the effects of neonatal and adult lesions," *Behavioural Brain Research*, vol. 81, no. 1-2, pp. 43–52, 1996.

[14] S. Geisler and M. Trimble, "The lateral habenula: no longer neglected," *CNS Spectrums*, vol. 13, no. 6, pp. 484–489, 2008.

[15] O. Hikosaka, S. R. Sesack, L. Lecourtier, and P. D. Shepard, "Habenula: crossroad between the basal ganglia and the limbic system," *Journal of Neuroscience*, vol. 28, no. 46, pp. 11825–11829, 2008.

[16] N. Iwahori, "A Golgi study on the habenular nucleus of the cat," *Journal of Comparative Neurology*, vol. 171, no. 3, pp. 319–344, 1977.

[17] A. Claudio Cuello, P. C. Emson, G. Paxinos, and T. Jessell, "Substance P containing and cholinergic projections from the habenula," *Brain Research*, vol. 149, no. 2, pp. 413–429, 1978.

[18] K. Brinschwitz, A. Dittgen, V. I. Madai, R. Lommel, S. Geisler, and R. W. Veh, "Glutamatergic axons from the lateral habenula mainly terminate on GABAergic neurons of the ventral midbrain," *Neuroscience*, vol. 168, no. 2, pp. 463–476, 2010.

[19] G. Paxinos and C. Watson, *The Rat Brain in Stereotaxic Coordinates—The New Coronal Set*, Academic Press, 6th edition, 2007.

[20] S. Hong, T. C. Jhou, M. Smith, K. S. Saleem, and O. Hikosaka, "Negative reward signals from the lateral habenula to dopamine neurons are mediated by rostromedial tegmental nucleus in primates," *The Journal of Neuroscience*, vol. 31, no. 32, pp. 11457–11471, 2011.

[21] M. Matsumoto and O. Hikosaka, "Representation of negative motivational value in the primate lateral habenula," *Nature Neuroscience*, vol. 12, no. 1, pp. 77–84, 2009.

[22] L. W. Swanson and W. M. Cowan, "The connections of the septal region in the rat," *Journal of Comparative Neurology*, vol. 186, no. 4, pp. 621–655, 1979.

[23] J. H. Fallon and R. Y. Moore, "Catecholamine innervation of the basal forebrain. IV. Topography of the dopamine projection to the basal forebrain and neostriatum," *Journal of Comparative Neurology*, vol. 180, no. 3, pp. 545–572, 1978.

[24] R. A. Wise, "Roles for nigrostriatal—not just mesocorticolimbic—dopamine in reward and addiction," *Trends in Neurosciences*, vol. 32, no. 10, pp. 517–524, 2009.

[25] S. Ikemoto, "Brain reward circuitry beyond the mesolimbic dopamine system: a neurobiological theory," *Neuroscience & Biobehavioral Reviews*, vol. 35, pp. 129–150, 2010.

[26] N. Omelchenko, R. Bell, and S. R. Sesack, "Lateral habenula projections to dopamine and GABA neurons in the rat ventral tegmental area," *European Journal of Neuroscience*, vol. 30, no. 7, pp. 1239–1250, 2009.

[27] J. J. Balcita-Pedicino, N. Omelchenko, R. Bell, and S. R. Sesack, "Sesack inhibitory influence of the lateral habenula on midbrain dopamine cells: ultrastructural evidence for indirect mediation via the rostromedial mesopontine tegmental nucleus," *Journal of Comparative Neurology*, vol. 519, pp. 1143–1164, 2011.

[28] C. H. Good, H. Wang, Y. H. Chen, C. A. Mejias-Aponte, A. F. Hoffman, and C. R. Lupica, "Dopamine D4 receptor excitation of lateral habenula neurons via multiple cellular mechanisms," *The Journal of Neuroscience*, vol. 33, no. 43, pp. 16853–16864, 2013.

[29] T. C. Jhou, S. Geisler, M. Marinelli, B. A. Degarmo, and D. S. Zahm, "The mesopontine rostromedial tegmental nucleus: a structure targeted by the lateral habenula that projects to the ventral tegmental area of Tsai and substantia nigra compacta," *Journal of Comparative Neurology*, vol. 513, no. 6, pp. 566–596, 2009.

[30] M. Matsumoto and O. Hikosaka, "Lateral habenula as a source of negative reward signals in dopamine neurons," *Nature*, vol. 447, no. 7148, pp. 1111–1115, 2007.

[31] G. Ellison, "Stimulant-induced psychosis, the dopamine theory of schizophrenia, and the habenula," *Brain Research Reviews*, vol. 19, no. 2, pp. 223–239, 1994.

[32] L. Shelton, G. Pendse, N. Maleki et al., "Mapping pain activation and connectivity of the human habenula," *Journal of Neurophysiology*, vol. 107, no. 10, pp. 2633–2648, 2012.

[33] I. H. Bianco and S. W. Wilson, "The habenular nuclei: A conserved asymmetric relay station in the vertebrate brain," *Philosophical Transactions of the Royal Society B: Biological Sciences*, vol. 364, no. 1519, pp. 1005–1020, 2009.

[34] G. R. Christoph, R. J. Leonzio, and K. S. Wilcox, "Stimulation of the lateral habenula inhibits dopamine-containing neurons in the substantia nigra and ventral tegmental area of the rabbit," *Journal of Neuroscience*, vol. 6, no. 3, pp. 613–619, 1986.

[35] C. Sego, L. Gonɾalves, L. Lima, IC. Furigo, J. Donato Jr., and M. Metzger, "Lateral habenula and the rostromedial tegmental nucleus innervate neurochemically distinct subdivisions of the dorsal raphe nucleus in the rat," *Journal of Comparative Neurology*, vol. 522, no. 7, pp. 1454–1484, 2014.

[36] A. L. Benabid and L. Jeaugey, "Cells of the rat lateral habenula respond to high-threshold somatosensory inputs," *Neuroscience Letters*, vol. 96, no. 3, pp. 289–294, 1989.

[37] M. J. Millan, "The induction of pain: an integrative review," *Progress in Neurobiology*, vol. 57, no. 1, pp. 1–164, 1999.

[38] W. J. Smith, J. Stewart, and J. G. Pfaus, "Tail pinch induces fos immunoreactivity within several regions of the male rat brain: effects of age," *Physiology and Behavior*, vol. 61, no. 5, pp. 717–723, 1997.

[39] M. Lehner, E. Taracha, A. Skórzewska et al., "Sensitivity to pain and c-Fos expression in brain structures in rats," *Neuroscience Letters*, vol. 370, no. 1, pp. 74–79, 2004.

[40] P. E. Paulson, J. W. Wiley, and T. J. Morrow, "Concurrent activation of the somatosensory forebrain and deactivation of periaqueductal gray associated with diabetes-induced neuropathic pain," *Experimental Neurology*, vol. 208, no. 2, pp. 305–313, 2007.

[41] L. Welberg, "Psychiatric disorders: reining in the habenula?" *Nature Reviews Neuroscience*, vol. 14, no. 10, pp. 668–669, 2013.

[42] J. Shumake, E. Edwards, and F. Gonzalez-Lima, "Opposite metabolic changes in the habenula and ventral tegmental area of a genetic model of helpless behavior," *Brain Research*, vol. 963, no. 1-2, pp. 274–281, 2003.

[43] J. B. Savitz, O. Bonne, A. C. Nugent et al., "Habenula volume in post-traumatic stress disorder measured with high-resolution MRI," *Biology of Mood & Anxiety Disorders*, vol. 1, no. 1, article 7, 2011.

[44] J. P. Roiser, J. Levy, S. J. Fromm et al., "The effects of tryptophan depletion on neural responses to emotional words in remitted depression," *Biological Psychiatry*, vol. 66, no. 5, pp. 441–450, 2009.

[45] J. B. Savitz, A. C. Nugent, W. Bogers et al., "Habenula volume in bipolar disorder and major depressive disorder: a high-resolution magnetic resonance imaging study," *Biological Psychiatry*, vol. 69, no. 4, pp. 336–343, 2011.

[46] A. Sartorius, K. L. Kiening, P. Kirsch et al., "Remission of major depression under deep brain stimulation of the lateral habenula in a therapy-refractory patient," *Biological Psychiatry*, vol. 67, no. 2, pp. e9–e11, 2010.

[47] H. Meng, Y. Wang, M. Huang, W. Lin, S. Wang, and B. Zhang, "Chronic deep brain stimulation of the lateral habenula nucleus in a rat model of depression," *Brain Research*, vol. 1422, pp. 32–38, 2011.

[48] R. B. Whitelaw, A. Markou, T. W. Robbins, and B. J. Everitt, "Excitotoxic lesions of the basolateral amygdala impair the acquisition of cocaine-seeking behaviour under a second-order schedule of reinforcememt," *Psychopharmacology*, vol. 127, no. 3, pp. 213–224, 1996.

[49] E. D. Kirby, K. Jensen, K. A. Goosens, and D. Kaufer, "Stereotaxic surgery for excitotoxic lesion of specific brain areas in the adult rat," *Journal of Visualized Experiment*, no. 65, Article ID e4079, 2012.

[50] D. Sourani, R. Eitan, N. Gordon, and G. Goelman, "The habenula couples the dopaminergic and the serotonergic systems: application to depression in Parkinson's disease," *European Journal of Neuroscience*, vol. 36, no. 6, pp. 2822–2829, 2012.

[51] L. Carey, D. Danna Paul, and I. Greg, "The habenula governs the attribution of incentive salience to reward predictive cues," *Frontiers in Human Neuroscience*, vol. 7, article 781, 2013.

[52] R. A. Rescorla and R. L. Solomon, "Two-process learning theory: relationships between Pavlovian conditioning and instrumental learning," *Psychological Review*, vol. 74, no. 3, pp. 151–182, 1967.

13

Understanding Neural Population Coding: Information Theoretic Insights from the Auditory System

Arno Onken,[1] **P. P. Chamanthi R. Karunasekara,**[1,2]
Christoph Kayser,[3,4,5] **and Stefano Panzeri**[1]

[1] *Center for Neuroscience and Cognitive Systems @UniTn, Istituto Italiano di Tecnologia, Via Bettini 31, 38068 Rovereto, Italy*
[2] *Doctoral School in Cognitive and Brain Sciences, University of Trento, Via Bettini 31, 38068 Rovereto, Italy*
[3] *Institute of Neuroscience and Psychology, University of Glasgow, Glasgow G12 8QB, UK*
[4] *Max Planck Institute for Biological Cybernetics, Spemannstraße 38, 72076 Tübingen, Germany*
[5] *Bernstein Centre for Computational Neuroscience, 72076 Tübingen, Germany*

Correspondence should be addressed to Stefano Panzeri; stefano.panzeri@iit.it

Academic Editor: Xiang-Ping Chu

In recent years, our research in computational neuroscience has focused on understanding how populations of neurons encode naturalistic stimuli. In particular, we focused on how populations of neurons use the time domain to encode sensory information. In this focused review, we summarize this recent work from our laboratory. We focus in particular on the mathematical methods that we developed for the quantification of how information is encoded by populations of neurons and on how we used these methods to investigate the encoding of complex naturalistic sounds in auditory cortex. We review how these methods revealed a complementary role of low frequency oscillations and millisecond precise spike patterns in encoding complex sounds and in making these representations robust to imprecise knowledge about the timing of the external stimulus. Further, we discuss challenges in extending this work to understand how large populations of neurons encode sensory information. Overall, this previous work provides analytical tools and conceptual understanding necessary to study the principles of how neural populations reflect sensory inputs and achieve a stable representation despite many uncertainties in the environment.

1. Introduction

Our sensory percept and our interaction with the environment arise from neural representations of the external world. An important question is therefore how the characteristics of external events, such as sensory stimuli, are represented by patterns of neural activity in the brain. Answering these questions amounts to determining the neural code [1–3], more formally defined as the smallest set of response patterns capable of encoding relevant stimulus parameters [4].

Two dimensions of neural representations are important for characterizing a neural code. The first is defined by space: sensory processing is based on spatially distributed populations of neurons, ranging from localized groups to populations of neurons spread across brain areas [5, 6].

The second dimension is defined by time: neuronal responses evolve over time, and the temporal structure of neural activity is often required to explain speeded reactions. Under most circumstances, neglecting the temporal dimension of neural activity results in a much impoverished representation of the sensory input [4, 7].

In this review, we focus on the recent work of our laboratory towards understanding the temporal dimension of neural codes in the auditory system. We first discuss our general mathematical approach, based on the principles of information theory, to evaluate the information content of different components of neural activity. We then discuss how this can be applied to neural data and to understand how auditory cortical neurons encode information about complex naturalistic sounds. In particular, we review our work showing that neural activity is patterned on multiple timescales carrying complementary information, ranging from millisecond precision spike patterns to slower oscillatory patterns.

The analysis of neural activity is a technically challenging problem. A typical analysis of the structure and information content of time-varying spike trains starts by aligning the spikes with sensory events (e.g., with the stimulus onset, or a reference point during the stimulus time course). Then, spike trains are partitioned into representative time intervals. These steps are necessary for even just plotting the data, or for any subsequent analysis, such as those attempting to decode the information carried by the temporal structure of the spike train. The experimenter conducts these procedures using measurements from a laboratory-based computer clock that registers stimuli and neural activity with supreme accuracy. Likewise, if a decoding mechanism in the brain uses information encoded in temporally precise codes, it may be able do so only after obtaining precise knowledge about the timing of sensory events and having access to a representation of time intervals with a reasonable degree of precision.

This raises a crucial question: how can the brain decode the information carried by the temporal variations of neural responses, given that the brain does not have access to the laboratory computer clock with its exact measures of time intervals and time of stimulus presentation [8–10]? We hence phrase the problem of interpreting and deciphering neural activity in the context of a decoding perspective; hence how a higher-level brain area (or an experimenter) can make best sense of the spiking activity observed in sensory cortices.

In this review, we focus on the problem of how decoders may extract information from spike times using different reference frames. We first describe relevant analytical approaches to address this problem and we then review recent studies investigating intrinsic reference frames derived from local network activity.

2. Information Theoretic Tools Available to Estimate and Compare Different Codes and Reference Frames

To study the role of spike timing in sensory decoding, it is necessary to have quantitative tools to assess the amount of information carried by different putative coding schemes. Shannon information, abbreviated hereafter as information, offers a rigorous measure to compute single-trial stimulus discriminability:

$$I(S; \mathbf{R}) = \sum_{\mathbf{r},s} P(\mathbf{r}, s) \log_2 \frac{P(\mathbf{r}, s)}{P(\mathbf{r}) P(s)}, \qquad (1)$$

where $P(\mathbf{r}, s)$ is the joint probability of presenting a stimulus s and observing a response $\mathbf{r}$ and $P(\mathbf{r})$ is the probability of observing the response $\mathbf{r}$ across all stimuli and $P(s)$ is the probability of each stimulus. Information quantifies the reduction of uncertainty (i.e., the gain in knowledge) about the stimuli obtained when the neural response of a single trial is observed (averaged over stimuli and responses). It is measured in bits, where one bit of information indicates

that on average the uncertainty is reduced by a factor of two. Information provides an upper bound on the amount of knowledge about stimuli that can be extracted by any algorithm extracting knowledge from neural responses. The fact that mutual information quantifies single trial stimulus knowledge is particularly appealing because neural systems usually must discriminate or identify stimuli on a single encounter.

One can evaluate the capacity of different candidate neural codes $\mathbf{r}$ by computing the information carried by the neural codes based on different response aspects (e.g., the timing or total number of spikes) and defined relative to different reference frames. For example, in previous work, we determined whether precise spike times carry significant information by comparing the information obtained from responses $\mathbf{r}$ quantified using different timing precisions. We then evaluated the extent to which the information present in spike timing can be decoded based on reference frames intrinsically available to the brain by comparing the information that can be extracted from responses $\mathbf{r}$ defined using the experimenter's clock with responses defined using an internal reference.

Information can be calculated by means of the stimulus-response probabilities: $P(\mathbf{r})$, $P(\mathbf{r}, s)$, and $P(s)$. Determining information by means of these probabilities is the so-called direct method for calculating information [3]. In an idealized case, these could be measured precisely. However, for experimental data, these probabilities need to be estimated from limited available data, such as a finite (and often small) number of trials. As a consequence, a systematic error (bias) is present in the estimated probabilities and hence the derived information values. The correction of this bias has been the subject of extensive research (see [11, 12] for reviews). An important consideration is that in general more complex codes defined by many parameters (such as, for example, finely timed sequences of spike times) tend to have a larger upward bias than simpler codes defined by a smaller number of parameters (such as, for example, those based on spike counts or on coarse measures of spike times). This means that, in a naïve analysis, the more complex codes may artificially appear to have higher information than in reality. Considerable work of our group has concentrated on trying to estimate and remove this upward bias as precisely as possible and in developing classes of information estimators that have a tendency for being biased downward (rather than upward) when using more complex codes (see [11, 12] for reviews). These downward biased estimators are important for the questions about the nature of the neural code, as they allow conservative conclusions about the role of spike timing in comparison to methods that may overestimate the significance of a specific code.

When using very high dimensional neural responses, it becomes impossible to correct the bias of the direct information measures defined by (1). Given a typically available number of stimulus repeats (~30–60 trials), this is the case for codes characterized by a cardinality of 50–100 or more elements, corresponding, for example, to either spike time computed in 6-7 or more subsequent small time bins, the population rate of 5 neurons or more, or a mixture thereof.

In such cases, information metrics are often computed using an intermediate decoding step. In this approach, the most likely stimulus s^p that elicited a given response $\mathbf{r}$ is determined using a cross-validated decoding algorithm [13, 14]. Then, the information extracted through the stimulus reconstruction scheme can be quantified as follows [14–16]:

$$I\left(S; S^P\right) = \sum_{s, s^P} Q\left(s^P, s\right) \log_2 \frac{Q\left(s^P, s\right)}{Q\left(s^P\right) Q\left(s\right)}, \quad (2)$$

where in the above $Q(s^P, s)$ is the joint probability that in a trial the decoding procedure reports that the stimulus s^P was presented when the true presented stimulus is s. The decoded information $I(S; S^P)$ quantifies (in bits) the average knowledge gained, per trial, when predicting the stimulus using a specific algorithm and takes into account both the fraction of correct decoding and the spread of the decoding errors.

Information depends on both the choice of the stimulus set and of the quantification of the neural response. Stimulus set here refers to both the stimulus material used for the experimental paradigm (e.g., simple tones versus natural sounds) and how the presented material is grouped or divided into the stimulus dimension s used for the information theoretic analysis. In our work, we mostly concentrated on studying how neurons encode time-varying natural sounds or video clips. Such stimulus material is difficult to analyze in terms of sensory coding because they contain many different feature dimensions that vary continuously at different time scales. To create the stimulus set S for analysis, we used a feature agnostic approach: we divided the presentation time of the dynamic stimulus material presented in the experiment into different segments of length T (a parameter that was varied in the range from few ms to several seconds) and each segment was considered as a different stimulus s for the analysis (see schematic in Figure 1). We then computed the information about which stimulus segment elicited the considered response. This procedure has several advantages. The first is that it is simple to apply and it lends itself to comparisons between different experimental datasets and between experimental and theoretical studies. The second is that it does not make any assumption as to which specific features of the dynamic stimulus triggered the neural response and so can potentially capture information about all possible dynamical stimulus features presented experimentally [17].

2.1. Precise Spike Times Encode Stimulus Information. Here, we summarize our investigation on the role of spike timing in encoding complex time-varying stimuli. The work in this subsection is a summary of the work previously reported in [18, 19] to which we refer for full details.

We recorded responses of single neurons in the caudal auditory cortex of passively listening macaque monkeys. In a first experiment, we recorded the responses to a sequence of pseudorandom tones (so-called "random chords"), a stimulus with short correlation time scale, hence rapid dynamic content. Because of this short intrinsic time scale, and

given the debate about whether there could be a precise temporal encoding in the absence of response locking to fast sequences of stimulus presentations [20], such stimuli are particularly suited to determine whether precise spike timing can contribute to the encoding of complex sounds within a rich acoustic background.

We thus used Shannon information ($I(S; \mathbf{R})$; see (1)) to directly quantify the information carried by temporal spike patterns sampled at different temporal precisions. Shannon information was computed from many (average 55) repeats of the same stimulus sequence using the direct method [3]. We computed the stimulus information carried by spike patterns characterized as "binary" (spike/no spike) sequences sampled in fine (1 ms) time bins and used a temporal shuffling procedure to compare the stimulus information encoded at different "effective" response precisions (Figure 2(a)). This shuffling procedure entailed shuffling spikes in nearby time bins and can be used to progressively degrade the effective precision of a spike train without affecting the statistical dimensionality of the data. We considered the randomly selected epochs from the long stimulus sequence as "stimuli," and the resulting information estimates (averaged across many selections of stimulus epochs), hence indicating how well these different sounds can be discriminated given the observed responses.

Estimating stimulus information from responses at effective precisions coarser than 1 ms resulted in a considerable information loss. Across the population of neurons, the dependency of stimulus information on response precision was quantified by normalizing information values at coarser precisions by the information derived from the original (1 ms precision) response (Figure 2(b)). Across neurons, the information loss amounted to 5%, 11%, and 20% (median) for effective precisions of 4, 6, and 12 ms, respectively, demonstrating that a considerable fraction of the encoded stimulus information is discarded when sampling the same response at coarser temporal resolution.

In a second experiment, we further tested the importance of reading responses at millisecond precision using an additional set of neurons recorded during the presentation of natural sounds. This stimulus comprised a continuous sequence of environmental sounds, animal vocalizations, and conspecific macaque vocalizations, and the information values hence indicate the relevance of finely timed activity to discriminate natural sounds occurring within a context of similar sounds. Across the entire sample of neurons, the proportional information lost by reducing the effective temporal precision was smaller than the results obtained during stimulation with random chords (Figure 2(c)). Importantly, however, a subset of neurons carried considerable stimulus information at high temporal precision and revealed a significant information loss when ignoring the temporal response precision. The fraction of neurons with significant information loss (bootstrap test; $P < 0.05$) was 11% and 17% at 6 and 12 ms, respectively. For those with significant loss at 12 ms the information transmitted per spike dropped from 3.8 bit/spike at 1 ms to 3.2 and 2.7 bit/spike (median) at 6 and 12 ms precision, respectively. This demonstrates that

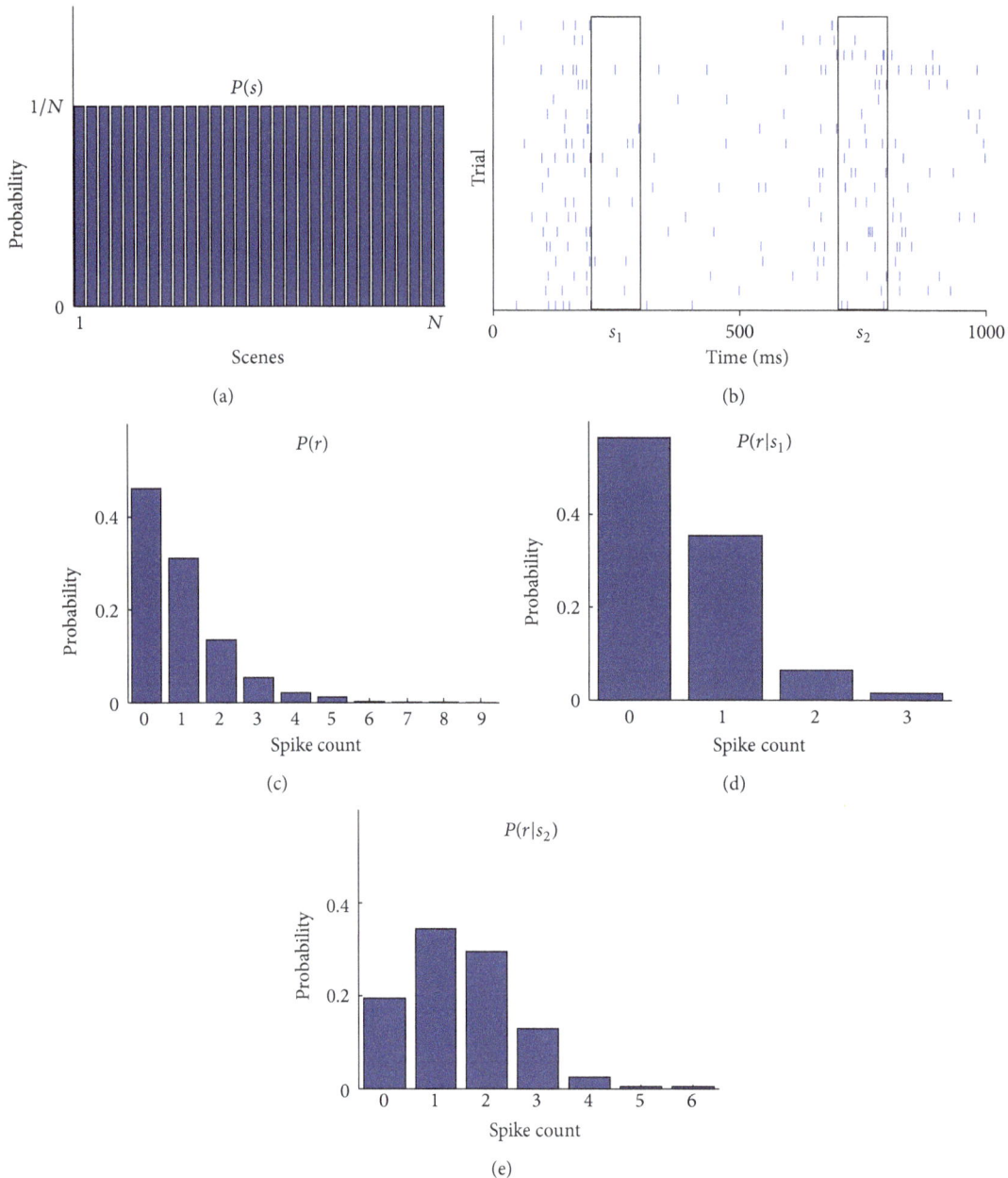

FIGURE 1: Schematic representation of the computation of the mutual information carried by spikes about which part of a dynamic stimulus was shown. The figure illustrates how we obtain different probabilities needed to compute (through (1)) the information about a movie carried by the spike responses (spike counts in this illustration). (a) First the stimulus presentation time is portioned into nonoverlapping windows, each considered a different stimulus s (a "scene"). The set of stimuli is the set of different scenes, each of which is presented once every trial, so the probability of each scene is the inverse of the number N of the scenes presented. (b) The raster plot shows a cartoon with simulated spike times across all trials and movie scenes. From these data we compute (c) probability distribution of the spike counts across all trials and scenes, (d) and (e) probability distribution of the spike counts across trials given the presented scenes s_1 and s_2, respectively. Computing probability distributions of the spike counts across trials for all scenes, using them to calculate the joint probability of spike counts and scenes, and then applying (1), we obtain the actual value of the mutual information.

millisecond precise spike timing can also carry additional information about natural sounds that cannot be recovered from the spike count on the scale of about 10 ms or coarser. Recent work by other groups corroborates these results using similar studies and analysis methods in the auditory inferior colliculus [21] and the rat auditory cortex [22].

3. A Candidate Intrinsic Indicator of Stimulus Onset: Stereotyped Neurons

In the analysis presented above, information is analyzed by aligning spikes and sensory events using a reference frame such as a laboratory-based computer clock. This procedure

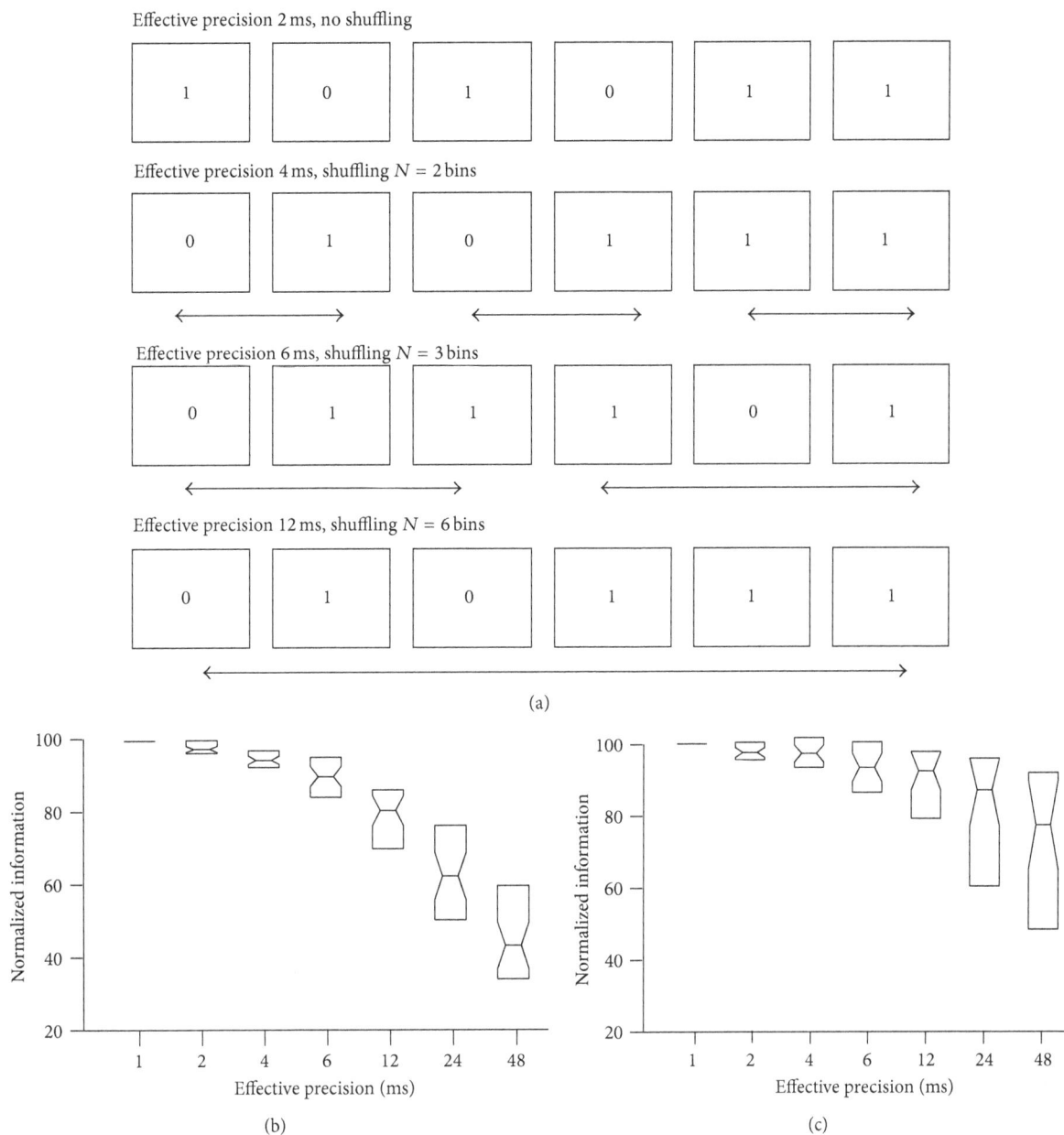

FIGURE 2: Stimulus information obtained from responses of auditory cortex neurons at different effective precisions. (a) Procedure to modify the effective response precision. We shuffled spikes (independently across trials and stimuli) across N neighboring time bins. Illustration shows time bins with $\Delta t = 2$ ms. Effective precision was degraded to 4 ms by shuffling spikes in neighboring bins ($N = 2$), degraded to 6 ms by using three neighboring bins for shuffling ($N = 3$) or degraded to 12 ms by shuffling spikes in all six bins of the pattern ($N = 6$). (b) Normalized stimulus information from responses to random chords. For each neuron, the absolute information values were normalized to the value at 1 ms precision. The median and 25th and 75th percentile across neurons are shown by boxplots. Information values from 1 to 6 ms were calculated by using $\Delta t = 1$ ms bins, whereby the effective precisions of 2, 3, and 6 ms were obtained by shuffling spikes in two, three, and six neighboring bins; values for 12, 24, and 48 ms precision were calculated by using bins of $\Delta t = 2$, 4, and 8 ms, respectively, and by shuffling spikes in six neighboring bins. (c) like (b), except for responses to natural sounds. Figure redrawn from data presented in [19].

is typical for the vast majority of analyses about the information content of spike times, but problematic. It raises the question of how the brain may succeed in interpreting the information carried by the temporal variations of neural responses without the benefit of a computer clock measuring perfect time intervals and providing the exact time of stimulus presentation [8–10]. In "active sampling," situations

where the motor system actively initiates or modulates the sampling of external information [10, 23, 24], sensory systems may receive a motor efference copy that reduces temporal uncertainty about stimulus timing [25–27]. However, in more general situations (e.g., when sampling is not actively initiated or when the stimulus appears at unpredictable times), such efference mechanisms are not available. Under such conditions, the system must have an intrinsic temporal reference or an otherwise intrinsic mechanism deriving a signature of stimulus occurrence in a stimulus-derived, hence bottom-up manner.

One possibility is that a neural population event could provide an estimate of the time of the stimulus, which could then be used to measure the relative timing of subsequent spikes. For a population event to act as a plausible "clock" that indicates the stimulus onset, the event must enable the extraction of information about complex natural stimulus features in an alert animal with sufficient robustness across trials, without needing to rely on any external predictive clues about stimulus timing. We investigated the feasibility of a relative coding scheme and its robustness with regard to these requirements in the auditory cortex of awake primates [28]. Using a paradigm that minimizes predictive cues about stimulus onset, we recorded the responses of single neurons from primary auditory cortex to naturalistic sounds made of conspecific vocalizations and vocalizations or noises of other animals (Figure 3(a)). In this section, we review this work, following what we summarized in [29].

We started the analysis by measuring the single-trial response latencies of the recorded neurons using a statistical algorithm. Then, for each neuron, we computed the standard deviation of the response latency across all trials of each stimulus as well as the average response latency over all stimuli. This was useful to characterize the trial-to-trial variability in the response latency of the neuron. We found a clear dichotomy in the population with respect to the response latency variability. Some neurons exhibited very low variability in their response latency, while many others displayed higher variability. Based on this finding, we applied a threshold on the latency variability (Figure 3(b)) and divided the population into two distinct groups, which we named as "stereotyped" neurons and "modulated" neurons. Neurons that were classified into the stereotyped group (approximately one-fourth of the population) had very low latency variability. Modulated neurons on the other hand had larger variability in their latencies. Example responses of one stereotyped and one modulated neuron are shown in Figure 3(b). When we observed the response characteristics of neurons in the two groups, we found two other distinctions. Stereotyped neurons responded to all tested sounds, while modulated neurons responded only to some sounds. In addition, stereotyped neurons exhibited much shorter mean response latencies (21.7 ± 0.8 ms) compared to modulated neurons (72.0 ± 4.6 ms; two-sample t-test $P < 10^{-7}$).

Stereotyped neurons are thus distinctive from modulated neurons due to their fast, reliable, and nonspecific responses. This suggests that stereotyped neurons may provide an intrinsic reference signal of the stimulus time. This reference signal could enable a putative downstream neuron to extract the information carried by the time-varying responses of stimulus-modulated neurons. We tested this hypothesis in the following way. We defined the stimulus onset using two alternative reference frames, one being the precise stimulus time as measured by the laboratory clock (external reference) and the other being the response onset of a simultaneously recorded stereotyped neuron (internal reference). We formulated two candidate codes **r** by aligning the spike trains of the modulated neurons to either one of the two references. We found that when the responses of the modulated neurons were aligned with respect to the stimulus onset using the extremely precise external reference, the responses showed temporally precise stimulus modulated spike patterns (Figure 3(c)) indicating that information is conveyed in the auditory cortex through precise spike timing [19, 30]. When the responses of the modulated neurons were aligned using the internal reference provided by the single-trial onsets of a simultaneously recorded stereotyped neuron, these temporal response patterns were largely preserved (Figure 3(c)). We then computed the information carried by each of these codes. We found that only little of the information about the sound identity carried by the externally referenced time-varying neural responses was lost when computing information with the internally referenced time-varying neural responses (Figure 3(d)). This is due to the temporal reliability of stereotyped neurons. Importantly, when we used the response onset time of a modulated neuron as the reference point of stimulus onset, the temporal response patterns were highly degraded (Figure 3(c)) and resulted in a higher information loss (Figure 3(d)).

We finally investigated whether the selective pooling of stereotyped neurons could act as a reliable indicator of stimulus onset. By using a computational modelling approach, we estimated that more than 95% of the full information that is contained in the spike times measured with respect to the precise stimulus onset could be recovered when the reference point for stimulus onset is calculated by pooling the responses of about 25 stereotyped neurons [28].

Previous studies have shown that the relative timing of neural responses can carry considerable sensory information and sometimes even more than the absolute timing relative to the stimulus [9, 31, 32]. Our results show that the relative timing of neural responses to an intrinsically defined population event can constitute a highly informative code also in the alert animal and for complex and suddenly appearing stimuli.

4. A Candidate Intrinsic Mechanism to Partition Spike Sequences: Network Oscillations

Access to information in temporally precise codes by the brain requires not only the existence of intrinsic indicators of stimulus onset, but also the existence of internal mechanisms to partition neural responses into precisely defined time intervals. The problem of maintaining a precise representation of time intervals is likely more difficult when considering the partitioning of long-lasting neural responses, such as those generated during presentation of a long-lasting stimuli. The auditory system is often exposed to continuous stimuli such as a speech and has to represent individual sound objects within the evolving stimulus stream [33, 34], for example, representing individual words in the speech. Based on these considerations, we conducted a study to investigate which temporal aspects of the activity of the primary cortical

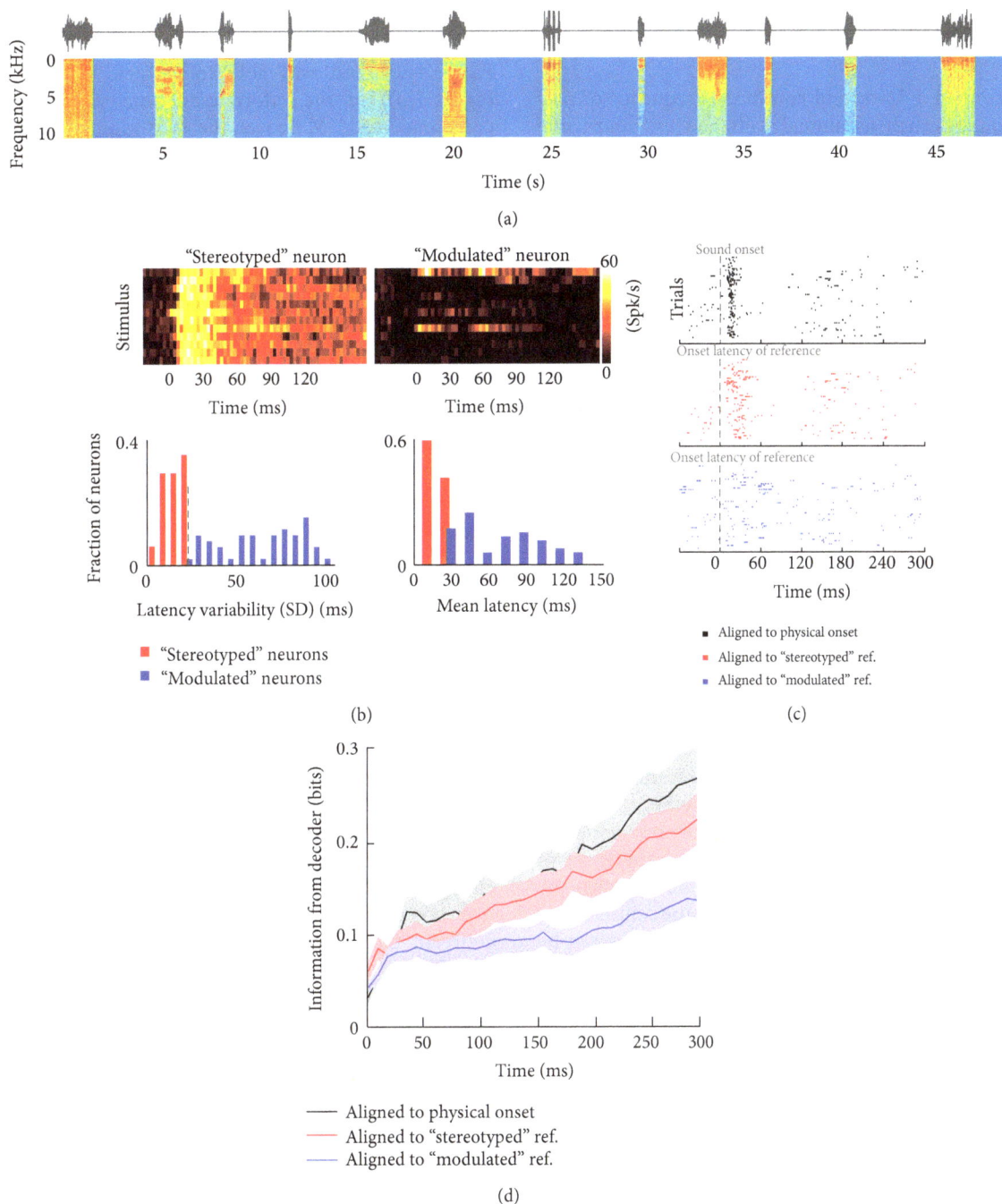

FIGURE 3: Stereotyped neurons may act as reference for stimulus onset in auditory cortex. (a) Sound wave and spectrogram for the auditory stimulus sequence on one example trial. Twelve different natural sounds (stimuli) were presented in pseudorandom sequence and with random intersound intervals (blue periods) on each trial. The sound wave is shown above the spectral representation (red colors indicate high power). (b) Top: time course of trial-averaged responses to all 12 stimuli (each row represents a different stimulus) for one stereotyped (left) and one modulated (right) neuron. Time $t = 0$ corresponds to sound onset. Bottom: distribution of the latency variability (standard deviation across trials) and mean latency across neurons. Stereotyped and modulated neurons are color-coded in red and blue, respectively, and the dashed line in the left histogram indicates the threshold used to separate (i.e., define) the two groups. (c) Example response from one modulated neuron after being aligned to different reference frames. Top: spike raster when aligned to stimulus onset time ($t = 0$). Middle: the same response but with each trial aligned to the response onset of a simultaneously recorded stereotyped reference neuron (here $t = 0$ corresponds to the onset latency of the reference neuron). Bottom: the same response aligned to the onset of a modulated neuron. While the stereotyped reference preserves the temporal shape of the stimulus locked response, the use of a modulated neuron as reference results in a much more dispersed spike raster. (d) Information about stimulus identity obtained using the three considered reference frames in progressively longer time windows (starting at $t = 0$ and ending at each indicated time point). Lines denote the mean and shaded areas denote the standard error (SEM) across the population ($n = 48$) of modulated neurons. Information was computed with a linear decoder and (2). Figure and caption re-elaborated from [28, 29] and reproduced with permission from [29].

auditory network could act as a temporal frame that provides an informative partitioning of long spike trains into finer time intervals.

We presented a 52-second continuous sequence of naturalistic sounds, such as animal calls and environmental sounds (Figure 4(a)) and recorded the responses of neurons from monkey primary auditory cortex [18, 32]. In this section, we review this work, following what we summarized in [29].

We first defined the stimulus set by randomly selecting sets of 10 epochs from the long sound sequence (Figure 4(a)). The response of one example neuron across trials is shown in Figure 4(b). Previous work on the data (see e.g., [19]) had revealed that the spike patterns encoded information with high temporal precision (in the range of few milliseconds) when the spike trains were stimulus aligned and partitioned into equally spaced time bins based on the laboratory clock (*time-partitioned* spike trains, Figure 4(c)).

In the present study, we investigated whether we could use a reference frame purely based on intrinsic network activity to partition responses into informative spike patterns. We considered slow oscillatory network activity, which has previously been suggested as a potential reference signal for neural processing [35]. Rhythms with cycle lengths of 100 ms or longer, such as delta or theta bands are often observed in sensory cortices during naturalistic stimulation [18, 36, 37].

We asked whether the phase of the network oscillation permits partitioning long spike sequences. In natural sounds, low frequency components in the theta (2–6 Hz) frequency range contain important acoustic information that is crucial for speech comprehension [38]. Slow rhythmic network activity in the auditory cortex entrains to the presentation of natural sounds [18, 34, 36, 39, 40]. This causes the phase of the oscillation to be reliably time-locked to the stimulus. The phase may then indicate salient points along the continuously varying stimulus [41]. As a result, phase differences can be used as a surrogate measure of time intervals during stimulation, at least so on the order of few tens of milliseconds. Thus, we used the phase of the theta band of local field potential (LFP) as an oscillatory reference to partition spikes trains (Figure 4(c)). Specifically, we divided the full phase cycle of the oscillation into phase ranges (or phase bins) and allocated each spike in a spike train to the corresponding phase bin based on the instantaneous phase of the oscillation at the time of the spike (*phase-partitioned* spike trains, Figure 4(c)). This is an alternative way of assigning spikes into representative intervals, using the oscillatory phase as a virtual time axis. Note that the phase epochs may not be equally spaced in time as a result of natural variability in network rhythms.

We found that the phase-partitioned spike trains still had clear stimulus dependence (Figure 4(b)). For comparison, we formulated a time-partitioned spike code, where time intervals were defined using the laboratory clock, and a spike count based code, which takes the sum of all spikes without considering the time structure. Then, we estimated the information in each of the three coding schemes about the defined stimulus set (where different sections of the long sound sequence were defined as stimuli). We evaluated the viability of the phase-partitioned code by comparing its information with those in the other two coding schemes.

The phase-partitioned code had a large information gain compared to the spike count (40%, population mean, Figure 4(d)) and was able to recover almost all (86%, Figure 4(d)) of the information conveyed by the time-partitioned code. Moreover, the excess information in either partitioning scheme over the spike count was highly correlated across neurons (Spearman's rank correlation r = 0.87). Therefore, good stimulus discrimination displayed by one partitioning scheme implies good discrimination performance from the other. Notably, the information recovered by the phase-partitioned code in some of the neurons was higher than that for the time-partitioned code. This suggests that the oscillatory phase during which these neurons fire was more reliable and stimulus specific than the precise timing to the stimulus itself [32].

An important question is where these oscillations come from, or how they are generated. To address this we performed additional modelling studies [42–44]. Results from these studies and experimental data [36, 39, 40] show that low frequency oscillations are generated by entrainment of cortical activity to the low frequency components of dynamics of the stimulus. These low frequency variations are a very prominent component of natural stimuli. In naturalistic movies, the power spectrum of most visual features decreases proportionally to the square of the frequency [45], meaning that the components of natural movies with higher amplitudes are those at low temporal frequencies. Similar results apply to the auditory domain [46].

Notably, an oscillatory reference frame based on the oscillatory phase arises from the intrinsic network activity and is likely to be directly accessible within local cortical network [47, 48]. This is because low frequency LFPs reflect changes in neuronal excitability that are spatially coherent over several millimeters [49, 50] and often accompanied by coherent fluctuations of neural membrane potentials [51] whose low frequency phase provides an effective reference signal for decoding spike information [52]. Given that the majority of synapses are made within local networks [53], pre- and postsynaptic neurons likely have access to the same slow rhythm for the majority of cortical connections.

In sum, our investigations suggest that network oscillations may be able to act as a highly effective, biologically plausible, and purely internal reference frame to generate informative spike patterns.

5. Characterizing the Role of Response Timing in Population Activity: Results, Challenges, and Ideas for Future Work

The studies discussed the above focused mostly on how the timing of single neurons encoded information. An important question is how these results generalize to populations of neurons, or, in other words, how to include the spatial dimension of neural codes along with the temporal dimension. This is particularly difficult because of the combinatorial problem of considering many space-time parameters. The number of possible spike patterns grows exponentially with the number of neurons and the number of time bins. This is known as

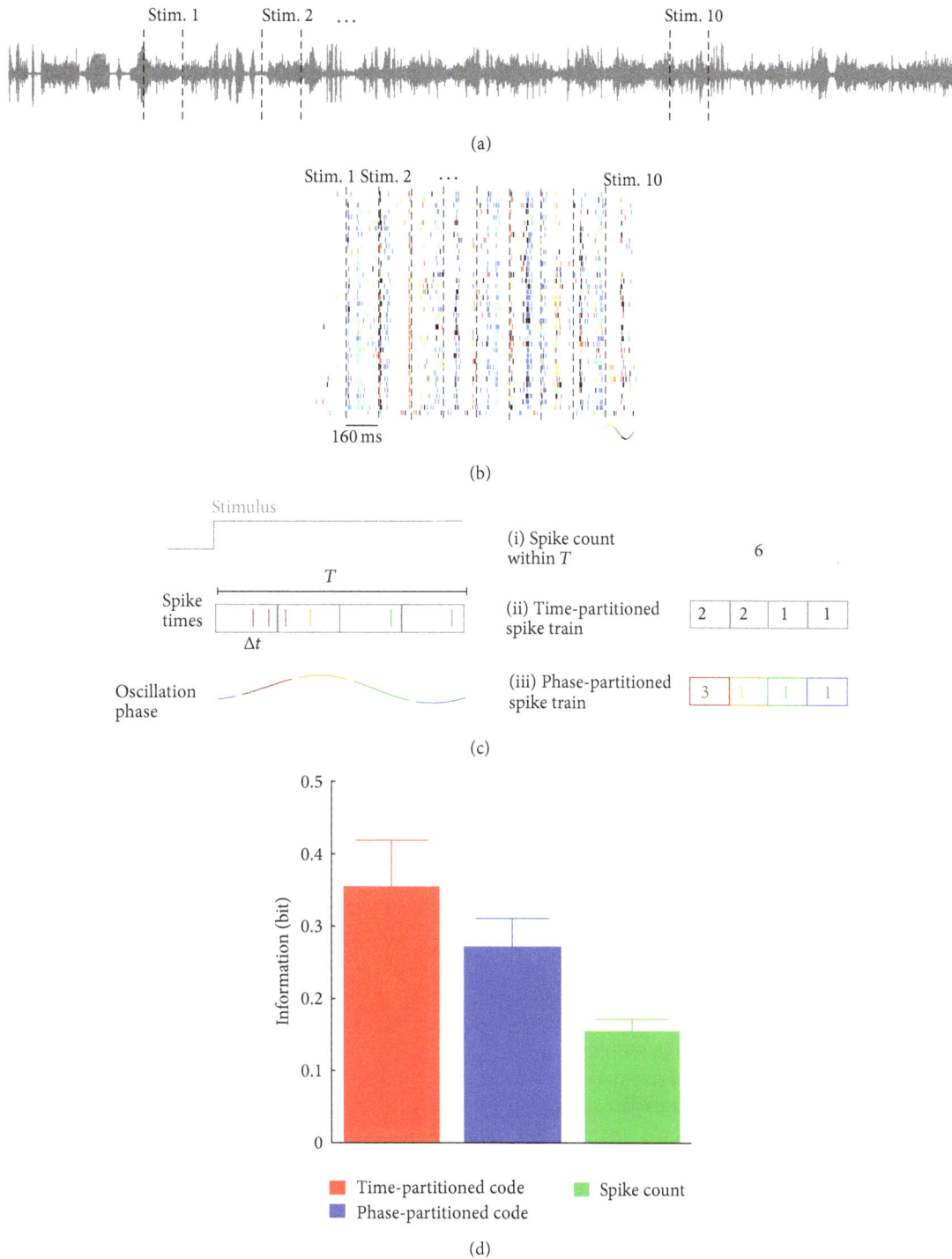

FIGURE 4: Using network oscillations to partition spike sequences in auditory cortex. (a) Sound wave of the 52 s sequence comprising natural and environmental sounds presented during the experiment. Dashed lines illustrate the random selection of 10 stimulus epochs used for the decoding analysis (stimulus epoch duration not to scale). (b) Spike raster from one example neuron with spikes color-coded according to the phase of the concurrently recorded 2–6 Hz LFP during multiple repetitions of each stimulus epoch. (c) Schematic illustration of the different partitioning schemes within a stimulus epoch of width T. The timing of spikes can be measured by temporal binning relative to stimulus onset. This "time-partitioned code" is defined as the vector consisting of the number of spikes per time bin. Alternatively, the timing can be measured relative to an intrinsic slow oscillatory signal. Here, the phase of such an oscillation was divided into four-phase quadrants and spikes are color-coded by their respective phase angle. This "phase-partitioned" code is defined as the vector consisting of the number of spikes per phase range. For comparison, a "spike count" code was defined as the total number of spikes within the window T. (d) Stimulus information provided by each code across neurons sampled in auditory cortex (mean ± SEM; $n = 40$). Figure and caption adapted redrawn from [29, 32] and reproduced with permission from [29].

the curse of dimensionality and is fundamental and, in its general form, unsolved problem of computation and sampling [54]. As noted above, for the specific case of information estimates from neural data, the curse of dimensionality problem arises primarily because of the limited amount of data that can be collected from a neural system (especially from behaving subjects), rather than from computation time issues (see [11, 12] for recent reviews). The limited amount of experimental neural data that can be collected limits severely the size of the neural populations that can be analyzed and ultimately requires additional techniques to study high dimensional activity patterns.

One possible scenario is that sensory areas in the brain process information using not only small but also high informative ensembles; hence they effectively rely on a subset of the many available neurons. If this was true, analysis could be limited to those "relevant" ensembles and the combinatorial space-time problem of large populations could be possibly avoided altogether. Noteworthy, in a recent study on the encoding of natural sounds in primate auditory cortex, we found strong evidence for this to be possible [55]. We found that a small fraction of cells carried the vast majority of information available in a much larger sample of recorded neurons. Hence, rather than using all neurons to decode stimulus identity, similar or sometimes even more information could be recovered when studying only a selected subset of neurons. Moreover, we could determine optimal subpopulations by the encoding timescales of the neurons in the pool of recorded cells, thereby providing a plausible way to identify and readout optimal populations in biologically realistic circuits.

Another possibility is that the information available in precisely timed spike patterns of some neurons is replaceable by the information provided by the spike counts of other neurons in the population. This would reduce the complexity of the combinatorial problem tremendously by reducing the temporal granularity of the response readout. However, in our study, we found that the informative subpopulations carried their information by means of temporally precise spiking [55]. This means that in order to readout these populations optimally (i.e., to achieve best possible performance), time could not be replaced by space. In other words, the additional information provided by temporal response patterns was not encoded by the spike counts of other neurons. This suggests that the code by which auditory cortical neurons carry information is therefore genuinely made of space and time.

When considering very large populations of neurons, a typical procedure is to reduce the dimensionality of the considered problem to overcome the curse of dimensionality. Several techniques are available to search for structure in the neural interactions that allows simplifying the representation of the data. One possibility is to make assumptions about the coding characteristics within pools of neurons like, for instance, disregarding the identity of which neuron fires a spike and to compute a so-called pooled code [56]. Another possibility is to preprocess the data with a general dimensionality reduction technique. Many techniques for dimensionality reduction with different constraints and objectives are available. One example is nonnegative matrix factorization (NMF), which is particularly suitable for nonnegative data such as neural responses. This technique factorizes data into approximate nonnegative components with a resulting data representation that is parts-based and sparse [57].

Recently, Delis and colleagues developed a variant of NMF called sample-based nonnegative matrix trifactorization [58]. Originally, the method was proposed for the analysis of muscle synergies. What makes this method potentially interesting for the space-time problem of neural population responses is its ability to decompose its input into space-by-time components in a data-driven way. The method is illustrated in Figure 5. A nonnegative input matrix which may consist of time-varying responses of a population of neurons is decomposed into three components: temporal modules, spatial modules, and activation coefficients. Temporal modules are temporal activity patterns in the data while spatial modules are groups of neurons that are active in fixed proportions. Temporal and spatial modules are constant across trials whereas activation coefficients are trial dependent. By using spatial and temporal modules that are fixed across trials, the method reduces the dimensionality of the data considerably under the assumption that the composition of coactive neurons is stimulus-driven and reliable within the dataset. The method thereby identifies functional units in space and time that can be further analyzed with regard to stimulus information or other properties of interest. Although these methods were not yet applied to neural data, they have the potential to tackle long-standing problems in the analysis of large-scale populations and to facilitate future studies of very large populations of neurons.

Last, when considering population codes the correlation structure between responses of different neurons becomes an important determining factor on how independent or synergistic different neurons reflect the sensory environment. In our study [55], we found that correlations between neurons of subpopulations did not have a strong impact on information and could be safely ignored. But this may not always be the case. Several methods were developed to analyze the impact of correlations on information and to construct models that take correlations into account [59, 60]. For small ensembles of neurons and a rate coding assumption, the information theoretic importance of taking detailed correlations into account can be tested within a maximum entropy framework [61] and, if necessary, models of detailed population dependencies can be constructed [62, 63]. Moreover, detailed interactions in the spike timing of populations can be investigated in terms of the rate of synchronous discharge [56]. The techniques developed in these studies are useful to study neural populations in the presence of strong correlations and to test the implications of such correlations in a principled and analytical framework.

6. Discussion

The quest for the neural code has been going on for several decades and is still an open question that raises heated discussions among neuroscientists [4, 64–66]. Our contribution to

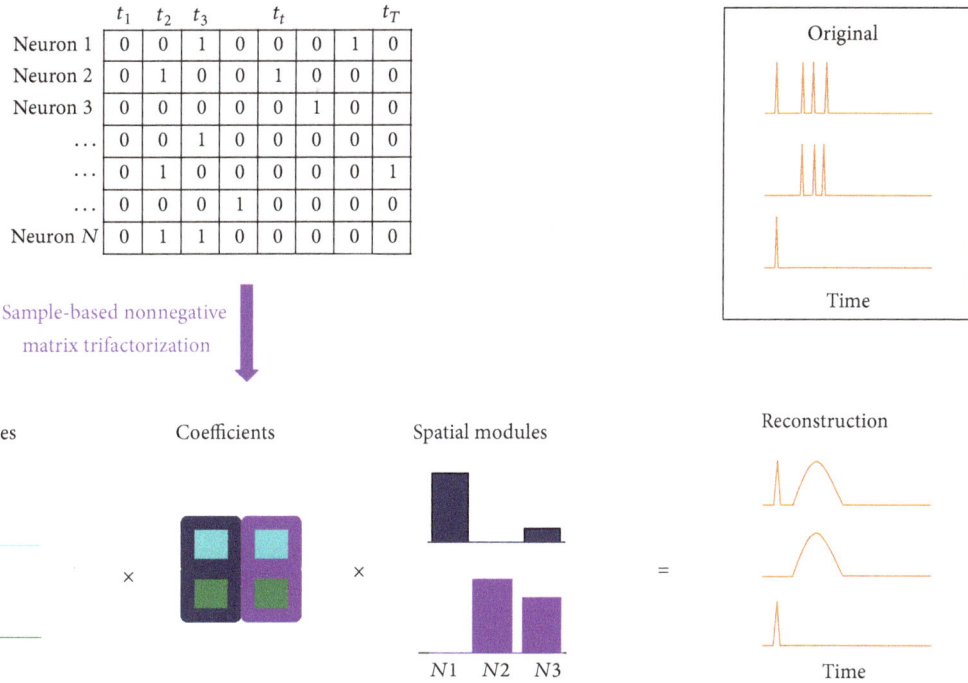

FIGURE 5: Schematic illustration of the sample-based nonnegative matrix trifactorization algorithm. The algorithm [58] factorizes the full spatiotemporal matrix into three matrices: a temporal module matrix, a spatial module matrix, and a coefficient matrix. The temporal module matrix contains temporal activity patterns that are present in the data. The spatial module matrix contains groups of neurons that fired together in fixed proportions. The coefficient matrix specifies the strength of activation of each temporal activity pattern by each spatial group of neurons during individual trials. Each column of the coefficient matrix corresponds to a spatial module and the values in each column specify the strength of each temporal activity pattern shown by the neurons of that spatial module during a particular trial. Therefore, once sample-based nonnegative matrix trifactorization is applied, the full spatiotemporal matrix can be collapsed into a lower dimensional representation that is contained in the coefficient matrix. To obtain an approximation to the activity of one trial, the coefficients of the respective trial are multiplied with the temporal and spatial module matrices as shown.

the understanding of this question has been to develop methods, based on the principles of information, for the unbiased quantification of the information carried by different kinds of neural codes. These methods have the advantage that they can be applied likewise to any kind of stimulus material including complex and naturalistic stimuli, thereby making it possible to investigate neural representations in conditions closer to real life. Importantly, our methods allow the investigation of how different coding schemes complement each other and cooperate. This helped to unite previous somewhat contradicting results by showing that auditory cortical neurons may multiplex sensory information across multiple response time scales [18].

We feel that the opportunities offered by the information theoretic formalism introduced here for understanding how different coding mechanisms and different scales cooperate are very significant. We therefore see the further development of these methods (in particular, to be able to consider the information provided by many spatial and temporal scales simultaneously), as an important area for progress in computational neuroscience for the next years. The ideas for information rich dimensionality reduction of neural

population responses discussed in the previous section may be instrumental to this progress.

Evidence for information that is represented by temporal spike patterns does not imply that the nervous system can make use of such temporally precise codes. It is commonly criticized that spike timing information encoded in variables such as poststimulus latency, which are defined with respect to external events such as stimulus onset, cannot be utilized by a downstream neuron because a biological system is not able to measure such variables. Therefore, identification of intrinsic temporal reference frames that enable direct decoding of spike trains without reference to external frameworks is crucial to link temporally precise spike codes to behavior. Studies over the last few years began to investigate this problem, and the results reviewed here provide a series of useful insights.

One insight from recent work is that the population activity of the network itself can generate a sufficient reference frame for reconstructing informative spike patterns. As we reviewed in this paper, considerable sensory information can be recovered even under challenging conditions, including natural stimuli whose presentation timing cannot be predicted from stimulus regularities [28], or long stretches of natural stimuli [32]. In visual cortex, Shriki and colleagues [67] studied the encoding of visual orientation and also reported a subpopulation of stereotyped neurons with reliable nonstimulus-selective response latency. Similar to our results in the auditory system, these visual neurons with invariant robust latencies could be used to compute informative spike times from other neurons with longer and stimulus-selective latencies [67]. In some cases, internally referenced codes may outperform externally referenced ones [9, 31, 32]. This may, for example, happen when variations in spike timing are coordinated across neurons due to a common covarying factor. In this case, spike timing relative to the stimulus is more adversely affected than the relative timing between neurons [68].

Another insight is that distinct populations within a single area separately encode the stimulus timing and the stimulus identity [28, 67]. While some neurons show time-dependent stimulus-selective responses, other neurons exhibit short-latency and unselective responses that reflect stimulus occurrence [28]. It is possible that the neurons showing unselective responses may have been systematically ignored in previous work. These neurons could act as "saliency detector" neurons and may have the function to ensure that the early poststimulus part of neural responses (which is the most informative one in many cases [4, 20, 69, 70]) is not missed out. Future work needs to elucidate whether and how these neurons interact with slow network rhythms to collectively form reliable and precise intrinsic temporal reference frames for neural coding.

The work reviewed here does not tell about how the computations needed for decoding spike timing information may be implemented in real neural networks at the biophysical level. However, some insights about these mechanisms may be gained using computational models [71]. Sensitivity to temporal spike patterns at different scales, for example, can arise from synaptic mechanisms like short-term depression or facilitation [72, 73]. Recent work has suggested that downstream learning and decoding of temporal patterns of spikes may rely upon spike timing-dependent plasticity (STDP). If downstream neural networks are with STPD, then they can easily localize a repeating spatiotemporal spike pattern embedded in equally dense background spike trains [74]. Such plasticity of decoding mechanisms may be facilitated by the fact that internally referenced patterns of neural activity show a degree of robustness in their coarse structure across stimulation conditions and during spontaneous activity [75]. Model neurons equipped with STDP robustly detect a pattern of spikes encoded by the phase of a subset of afferents, even so when these patterns are presented at unpredictable intervals [76] and even when only a fraction of afferents are organized according to the phase [76].

Together, the observations reviewed in this paper support the view that transmitting, learning, and decoding spike timing information based on internal temporal frames are computational capabilities of the microcircuitry of cortical sensory structures [71, 77]. Thus, precise spike timing of individual neurons and neural populations may play an important role in the neural cortical encoding of sensory signals.

Conflict of Interests

The authors declare that there is no conflict of interests regarding the publication of this paper.

Acknowledgments

The authors acknowledge the financial support of the VISUALISE and SICODE projects of the Future and Emerging Technologies (FET) Programme within the Seventh Framework Programme for Research of the European Commission (FP7-ICT-2011.9.11) under Grant Agreement nos. FP7-600954 and FP7-284553 and the European Community's Seventh Framework Programme FP7/2007-2013 under Grant Agreement no. PITN-GA-2011-290011. This work was further supported by the Max Planck Society and was part of the research program of the Bernstein Center for Computational Neuroscience, Tübingen, funded by the German Federal Ministry of Education and Research (BMBF; FKZ: 01GQ1002). The funders had no role in study design, data collection and analysis, decision to publish, or preparation of the paper.

References

[1] D. Ferster and N. Spruston, "Cracking the neuronal code," *Science*, vol. 270, no. 5237, pp. 756–757, 1995.

[2] C. F. Stevens and A. Zador, "The enigma of the brain," *Current Biology*, vol. 5, no. 12, pp. 1370–1371, 1995.

[3] F. Rieke, *Spikes: Exploring the Neural Code*, The MIT Press, Cambridge, Mass, USA, 1999.

[4] S. Panzeri, N. Brunel, N. K. Logothetis, and C. Kayser, "Sensory neural codes using multiplexed temporal scales," *Trends in Neurosciences*, vol. 33, no. 3, pp. 111–120, 2010.

[5] W. B. Kristan Jr. and B. K. Shaw, "Population coding and behavioral choice," *Current Opinion in Neurobiology*, vol. 7, no. 6, pp. 826–831, 1997.

[6] A. Pouget, P. Dayan, and R. Zemel, "Information processing with population codes," *Nature Reviews Neuroscience*, vol. 1, no. 2, pp. 125–132, 2000.

[7] J. D. Victor, "How the brain uses time to represent and process visual information," *Brain Research*, vol. 886, no. 1-2, pp. 33–46, 2000.

[8] G. Foffani, J. K. Chapin, and K. A. Moxon, "Computational role of large receptive fields in the primary somatosensory cortex," *Journal of Neurophysiology*, vol. 100, no. 1, pp. 268–280, 2008.

[9] T. Gollisch and M. Meister, "Rapid neural coding in the retina with relative spike latencies," *Science*, vol. 319, no. 5866, pp. 1108–1111, 2008.

[10] R. Shusterman, M. C. Smear, A. A. Koulakov, and D. Rinberg, "Precise olfactory responses tile the sniff cycle," *Nature Neuroscience*, vol. 14, no. 8, pp. 1039–1044, 2011.

[11] S. Panzeri, R. Senatore, M. A. Montemurro, and R. S. Petersen, "Correcting for the sampling bias problem in spike train information measures," *Journal of Neurophysiology*, vol. 98, no. 3, pp. 1064–1072, 2007.

[12] R. A. A. Ince, R. Senatore, E. Arabzadeh, F. Montani, M. E. Diamond, and S. Panzeri, "Information-theoretic methods for studying population codes," *Neural Networks*, vol. 23, no. 6, pp. 713–727, 2010.

[13] I. Nelken and G. Chechik, "Information theory in auditory research," *Hearing Research*, vol. 229, no. 1-2, pp. 94–105, 2007.

[14] R. Q. Quiroga and S. Panzeri, "Extracting information from neuronal populations: information theory and decoding approaches," *Nature Reviews Neuroscience*, vol. 10, no. 3, pp. 173–185, 2009.

[15] C. E. Shannon, "The mathematical theory of communication," *The Bell System Technical Journal*, vol. 27, pp. 379–423, 623–656, 1948.

[16] J. D. Victor and K. P. Purpura, "Nature and precision of temporal coding in visual cortex: a metric-space analysis," *Journal of Neurophysiology*, vol. 76, no. 2, pp. 1310–1326, 1996.

[17] R. R. D. R. van Steveninck, G. D. Lewen, S. P. Strong, R. Koberle, and W. Bialek, "Reproducibility and variability in neural spike trains," *Science*, vol. 275, no. 5307, pp. 1805–1808, 1997.

[18] C. Kayser, M. A. Montemurro, N. K. Logothetis, and S. Panzeri, "Spike-phase coding boosts and stabilizes the information carried by spatial and temporal spike patterns," *Neuron*, vol. 61, no. 4, pp. 597–608, 2009.

[19] C. Kayser, N. K. Logothetis, and S. Panzeri, "Millisecond encoding precision of auditory cortex neurons," *Proceedings of the National Academy of Sciences of the United States of America*, vol. 107, no. 39, pp. 16976–16981, 2010.

[20] S. Panzeri, R. S. Petersen, S. R. Schultz, M. Lebedev, and M. E. Diamond, "The role of spike timing in the coding of stimulus location in rat somatosensory cortex," *Neuron*, vol. 29, no. 3, pp. 769–777, 2001.

[21] J. A. Garcia-Lazaro, L. A. Belliveau, and N. A. Lesica, "Independent population coding of speech with sub-millisecond precision," *The Journal of Neuroscience*, vol. 33, no. 49, pp. 19362–19372, 2013.

[22] C. A. Perez, C. T. Engineer, V. Jakkamsetti, R. S. Carraway, M. S. Perry, and M. P. Kilgard, "Different timescales for the neural coding of consonant and vowel sounds," *Cerebral Cortex*, vol. 23, no. 3, pp. 670–683, 2013.

[23] M. E. Diamond, M. von Heimendahl, and E. Arabzadeh, "Whisker-mediated texture discrimination," *PLoS Biology*, vol. 6, article e220, 2008.

[24] M. E. Diamond and E. Arabzadeh, "Whisker sensory system—from receptor to decision," *Progress in Neurobiology*, vol. 103, pp. 28–40, 2013.

[25] K. P. Purpura, S. F. Kalik, and N. D. Schiff, "Analysis of perisaccadic field potentials in the occipitotemporal pathway during active vision," *Journal of Neurophysiology*, vol. 90, no. 5, pp. 3455–3478, 2003.

[26] C. E. Schroeder, D. A. Wilson, T. Radman, H. Scharfman, and P. Lakatos, "Dynamics of active sensing and perceptual selection," *Current Opinion in Neurobiology*, vol. 20, no. 2, pp. 172–176, 2010.

[27] J. D. Moore, M. Deschênes, T. Furuta et al., "Hierarchy of orofacial rhythms revealed through whisking and breathing," *Nature*, vol. 497, no. 7448, pp. 205–210, 2013.

[28] R. Brasselet, S. Panzeri, N. K. Logothetis, and C. Kayser, "Neurons with stereotyped and rapid responses provide a reference frame for relative temporal coding in primate auditory cortex," *Journal of Neuroscience*, vol. 32, no. 9, pp. 2998–3008, 2012.

[29] S. Panzeri, R. A. Ince, M. E. Diamond, and C. Kayser, "Reading spike timing without a clock: intrinsic decoding of spike trains," *Philosophical Transactions of the Royal Society of London Series B, Biological Sciences*, vol. 369, no. 1637, 2014.

[30] C. T. Engineer, C. A. Perez, Y. H. Chen et al., "Cortical activity patterns predict speech discrimination ability," *Nature Neuroscience*, vol. 11, no. 5, pp. 603–608, 2008.

[31] S. M. Chase and E. D. Young, "First-spike latency information in single neurons increases when referenced to population onset," *Proceedings of the National Academy of Sciences of the United States of America*, vol. 104, no. 12, pp. 5175–5180, 2007.

[32] C. Kayser, R. A. A. Ince, and S. Panzeri, "Analysis of slow (theta) oscillations as a potential temporal reference frame for information coding in sensory cortices," *PLoS Computational Biology*, vol. 8, no. 10, Article ID e1002717, 2012.

[33] S. A. Shamma, M. Elhilali, and C. Micheyl, "Temporal coherence and attention in auditory scene analysis," *Trends in Neurosciences*, vol. 34, no. 3, pp. 114–123, 2011.

[34] A. Giraud and D. Poeppel, "Cortical oscillations and speech processing: emerging computational principles and operations," *Nature Neuroscience*, vol. 15, no. 4, pp. 511–517, 2012.

[35] J. Lisman, "The theta/gamma discrete phase code occuring during the hippocampal phase precession may be a more general brain coding scheme," *Hippocampus*, vol. 15, no. 7, pp. 913–922, 2005.

[36] H. Luo and D. Poeppel, "Phase patterns of neuronal responses reliably discriminate speech in human auditory cortex," *Neuron*, vol. 54, no. 6, pp. 1001–1010, 2007.

[37] M. A. Montemurro, M. J. Rasch, Y. Murayama, N. K. Logothetis, and S. Panzeri, "Phase-of-firing coding of natural visual stimuli in primary visual cortex," *Current Biology*, vol. 18, no. 5, pp. 375–380, 2008.

[38] T. M. Elliott and F. E. Theunissen, "The modulation transfer function for speech intelligibility," *PLoS Computational Biology*, vol. 5, no. 3, Article ID e1000302, 2009.

[39] C. Chandrasekaran, H. K. Turesson, C. H. Brown, and A. A. Ghazanfar, "The influence of natural scene dynamics on auditory cortical activity," *The Journal of Neuroscience*, vol. 30, no. 42, pp. 13919–13931, 2010.

[40] J. Gross, N. Hoogenboom, G. Thut et al., "Speech rhythms and multiplexed oscillatory sensory coding in the human brain," *PLoS Biology*, vol. 11, Article ID e1001752, 2013.

[41] F. D. Szymanski, N. C. Rabinowitz, C. Magri, S. Panzeri, and J. W. H. Schnupp, "The laminar and temporal structure of stimulus information in the phase of field potentials of auditory cortex," *Journal of Neuroscience*, vol. 31, no. 44, pp. 15787–15801, 2011.

[42] A. Mazzoni, S. Panzeri, N. K. Logothetis, and N. Brunel, "Encoding of naturalistic stimuli by local field potential spectra in networks of excitatory and inhibitory neurons," *PLoS Computational Biology*, vol. 4, no. 12, Article ID e1000239, 2008.

[43] A. Mazzoni, K. Whittingstall, N. Brunel, N. K. Logothetis, and S. Panzeri, "Understanding the relationships between spike rate and delta/gamma frequency bands of LFPs and EEGs using a local cortical network model," *NeuroImage*, vol. 52, no. 3, pp. 956–972, 2010.

[44] S. Cavallari, S. Panzeri, and A. Mazzoni, "Comparison of the dynamics of neural interactions between current-based and conductance-based integrate-and-fire recurrent networks," *Frontiers in Neural Circuits*, vol. 8, article 12, 2014.

[45] D. W. Dong and J. J. Atick, "Statistics of natural time-varying images," *Network: Computation in Neural Systems*, vol. 6, pp. 345–358, 1995.

[46] H. Attias and C. Schreiner, "Temporal low-order statistics of natural sounds," in *Advances in Neural Information Processing Systems*, pp. 27–33, MIT Press, Cambridge, Mass, USA, 1997.

[47] A. T. Schaefer, K. Angelo, H. Spors, and T. W. Margrie, "Neuronal oscillations enhance stimulus discrimination by ensuring action potential precision," *PLoS Biology*, vol. 4, no. 6, article e163, 2006.

[48] J. Kwag, D. McLelland, and O. Paulsen, "Phase of firing as a local window for efficient neuronal computation: tonic and phasic mechanisms in the control of theta spike phase," *Frontiers in Human Neuroscience*, vol. 5, article 3, 2011.

[49] A. Arieli, D. Shoham, R. Hildesheim, and A. Grinvald, "Coherent spatiotemporal patterns of ongoing activity revealed by real-time optical imaging coupled with single-unit recording in the cat visual cortex," *Journal of Neurophysiology*, vol. 73, no. 5, pp. 2072–2093, 1995.

[50] J. B. M. Goense and N. K. Logothetis, "Neurophysiology of the BOLD fMRI signal in awake monkeys," *Current Biology*, vol. 18, no. 9, pp. 631–640, 2008.

[51] M. Okun, A. Naim, and I. Lampl, "The subthreshold relation between cortical local field potential and neuronal firing unveiled by intracellular recordings in awake rats," *Journal of Neuroscience*, vol. 30, no. 12, pp. 4440–4448, 2010.

[52] A. Alenda, M. Molano-Mazón, S. Panzeri, and M. Maravall, "Sensory input drives multiple intracellular information streams in somatosensory cortex," *Journal of Neuroscience*, vol. 30, no. 32, pp. 10872–10884, 2010.

[53] V. Braintenberg and A. Schuetz, *Cortex: Statistics and Geometry of Neuronal Connectivity*, Springer, Berlin, Germany, 1998.

[54] J. D. Fitzgerald, R. J. Rowekamp, L. C. Sincich, and T. O. Sharpee, "Second order dimensionality reduction using minimum and maximum mutual information models," *PLoS Computational Biology*, vol. 7, no. 10, Article ID e1002249, 2011.

[55] R. A. Ince, S. Panzeri, and C. Kayser, "Neural codes formed by small and temporally precise populations in auditory cortex," *The Journal of Neuroscience*, vol. 33, no. 46, pp. 18277–18287, 2013.

[56] F. Montani, R. A. Ince, R. Senatore, E. Arabzadeh, M. E. Diamond, and S. Panzeri, "The impact of high-order interactions on the rate of synchronous discharge and information transmission in somatosensory cortex," *Philosophical Transactions A: Mathematical, Physical and Engineering Sciences*, vol. 367, no. 1901, pp. 3297–3310, 2009.

[57] D. D. Lee and H. S. Seung, "Learning the parts of objects by non-negative matrix factorization," *Nature*, vol. 401, no. 6755, pp. 788–791, 1999.

[58] I. Delis, S. Panzeri, T. Pozzo, and B. Berret, "A unifying model of concurrent spatial and temporal modularity in muscle activity," *Journal of Neurophysiology*, vol. 111, pp. 675–693, 2014.

[59] J. H. Macke, P. Berens, A. S. Ecker, A. S. Tolias, and M. Bethge, "Generating spike trains with specified correlation coefficients," *Neural Computation*, vol. 21, no. 2, pp. 397–423, 2009.

[60] A. S. Ecker, P. Berens, A. S. Tolias, and M. Bethge, "The effect of noise correlations in populations of diversely tuned neurons," *The Journal of Neuroscience*, vol. 31, no. 40, pp. 14272–14283, 2011.

[61] A. Onken, V. Dragoi, and K. Obermayer, "A maximum entropy test for evaluating higher-order correlations in spike counts," *PLoS Computational Biology*, vol. 8, no. 6, Article ID e1002539, 12 pages, 2012.

[62] A. Onken, S. Grunewalder, M. H. J. Munk, and K. Obermayer, "Analyzing short-term noise dependencies of spike-counts in Macaque prefrontal cortex using copulas and the flashlight transformation," *PLoS Computational Biology*, vol. 5, no. 11, Article ID e1000577, e1000577, 13 pages, 2009.

[63] B. Staude, S. Rotter, and S. Grün, "CuBIC: cumulant based inference of higher-order correlations in massively parallel spike trains," *Journal of Computational Neuroscience*, vol. 29, no. 1-2, pp. 327–350, 2010.

[64] M. N. Shadlen and J. A. Movshon, "Synchrony unbound: a critical evaluation of the temporal binding hypothesis," *Neuron*, vol. 24, no. 1, pp. 67–77, 111–125, 1999.

[65] C. von der Malsburg, "The what and why of binding: the modeler's perspective," *Neuron*, vol. 24, no. 1, pp. 95–104, 1999.

[66] S. H. Nirenberg and J. D. Victor, "Analyzing the activity of large populations of neurons: how tractable is the problem?" *Current Opinion in Neurobiology*, vol. 17, no. 4, pp. 397–400, 2007.

[67] O. Shriki, A. Kohn, and M. Shamir, "Fast coding of orientation in primary visual cortex," *PLoS Computational Biology*, vol. 8, no. 6, Article ID e1002536, 2012.

[68] T. Masquelier, "Neural variability, or lack thereof," *Frontiers in Computational Neuroscience*, vol. 7, 2013.

[69] S. Furukawa, L. Xu, and J. C. Middlebrooks, "Coding of sound-source location by ensembles of cortical neurons," *Journal of Neuroscience*, vol. 20, no. 3, pp. 1216–1228, 2000.

[70] S. Junek, E. Kludt, F. Wolf, and D. Schild, "Olfactory coding with patterns of response latencies," *Neuron*, vol. 67, no. 5, pp. 872–884, 2010.

[71] A. Kumar, S. Rotter, and A. Aertsen, "Spiking activity propagation in neuronal networks: reconciling different perspectives on neural coding," *Nature Reviews Neuroscience*, vol. 11, no. 9, pp. 615–627, 2010.

[72] M. V. Tsodyks and H. Markram, "The neural code between neocortical pyramidal neurons depends on neurotransmitter release probability," *Proceedings of the National Academy of Sciences of the United States of America*, vol. 94, no. 2, pp. 719–723, 1997.

[73] R. Gütig and H. Sompolinsky, "The tempotron: a neuron that learns spike timing-based decisions," *Nature Neuroscience*, vol. 9, no. 3, pp. 420–428, 2006.

[74] T. Masquelier, R. Guyonneau, and S. J. Thorpe, "Spike timing dependent plasticity finds the start of repeating patterns in continuous spike trains," *PLoS ONE*, vol. 3, no. 1, Article ID e1377, 2008.

[75] A. Luczak, P. Bartho, and K. D. Harris, "Gating of sensory input by spontaneous cortical activity," *Journal of Neuroscience*, vol. 33, no. 4, pp. 1684–1695, 2013.

[76] T. Masquelier, E. Hugues, G. Deco, and S. J. Thorpe, "Oscillations, phase-of-firing coding, and spike timing-dependent plasticity: an efficient learning scheme," *Journal of Neuroscience*, vol. 29, no. 43, pp. 13484–13493, 2009.

[77] D. V. Buonomano and W. Maass, "State-dependent computations: spatiotemporal processing in cortical networks," *Nature Reviews Neuroscience*, vol. 10, no. 2, pp. 113–125, 2009.

14

Neck Flexion Induces Larger Deformation of the Brain Than Extension at a Rotational Acceleration, Closed Head Trauma

Hans-Arne Hansson,[1] Ulrika Krave,[2] Svante Höjer,[3] and Johan Davidsson[2]

[1] *Institute of Biomedicine, Sahlgren Academy, University of Gothenburg, P.O. Box 440, 40530 Gothenburg, Sweden*
[2] *Department of Applied Mechanics, Chalmers University of Technology, 41296 Gothenburg, Sweden*
[3] *GU Holding, University of Gothenburg, 40530 Gothenburg, Sweden*

Correspondence should be addressed to Hans-Arne Hansson; hans-arne.hansson@gu.se

Academic Editor: John B. Redell

A closed head trauma induces incompletely characterized temporary movement and deformation of the brain, contributing to the primary traumatic brain injury. We used the pressure patterns recorded with light-operated miniature sensors in anaesthetized adult rabbits exposed to a sagittal plane rotational acceleration of the head, lasting 1 ms, as a measure of brain deformation. Two exposure levels were used and scaled to correspond to force levels reported to cause mild and moderate diffuse injury in an adult man, respectively. Flexion induced transient, strong, extended, and predominantly negative pressures while extension generated a short positive pressure peak followed by a minor negative peak. Low level flexion caused as strong, extended negative pressures as did high level extension. Time differences were demonstrated between the deformation of the cerebrum, brainstem, and cerebellum. Available X-ray and MRI techniques do not have as high time resolution as pressure recordings in demonstrating complex, sequential compression and stretching of the brain during a trauma. The exposure to flexion caused more protracted and extensive deformation of the brain than extension, in agreement with a published histopathological report. The severity and extent of the brain deformation generated at a head trauma thus related to the direction at equal force.

1. Introduction

A closed head trauma may result in traumatic brain injury (TBI), and its consequences constitute a large burden for the victims, their families, and the society [1–5]. The relation between the external loading of the head and the response in the brain, resulting in damage, during an impact lasting just milliseconds needs further clarification. Inertial shearing deformation of the brain is considered to be a primary cause of injury [6–14] and generates temporary pressures in the brain parenchyma, as demonstrated in, for example, post-mortem human subjects and in nonhuman primates [15–17]. Anderson et al. [18] reported correlations between applied force, dynamic pressures, and histopathological changes at a lateral head impact. The forces applied at a closed head impulse have been proposed to possibly induce cavitation at interfaces [19–23].

The aim of the present study was to elucidate the importance of the direction of a sagittal plane rotational acceleration trauma to the head and neck for the deformation of the brain, which thereby induces brain concussion, also named mild traumatic brain injury (TBI) [10, 12–14, 17]. We consider that the direction of the force at a head trauma is likely to influence the resulting primary brain damage, which is generated during as short time as just a few milliseconds [6, 7, 24–27]. Pudenz and Shelden [28] were the first to demonstrate that at a trauma the brain moves within the skull and is deformed, as subsequently repeatedly confirmed [6, 7, 10, 11, 29, 30]. A number of approaches have been reported to further characterize the movement and deformation of the brain at the exposure to a trauma by, for example, high speed photography of the brain through a window in the calvarium, the use of flash X-ray of implanted lead particles, or advanced biplanar X-ray system combined with embedded

TABLE 1: Number of animals, exposures and results.

Impact condition, number of animals[1]	Acceleration (krad/s²)			Location of transducer	Animals, n	Tests, n	Peak Pressure (bar)	
	Mean	Std. dev.[4]	n[2]				Mean[4]	Std. dev.[4]
High Flexion[3] n = 4	208,0	n.a.	1	Brainstem	1	1	−0,47	n.a.
				Basal ganglia	1	1	n.a	n.a.
Low Flexion n = 8	96,3	15,0	52	Brainstem	7	48	−0,38	0,20
				Basal ganglia	6	30	−0,49	0,16
				Paraflocculus	1	3	−0,20	0,05
				Cerebellum	1	1	−0,15	n.a
				Angled in Basal ganglia	1	12	—	—
High Extension n = 10	−184,5	14,5	20	Brainstem	3	6	0,29	0,10
				Basal ganglia	4	8	0,34	0,18
				Hippocampus	6	13	0,62	0,24
				Parieto-temporal cortex	5	12	0,48	0,34
Low Extension n = 12	−95,0	6,6	37	Brainstem	4	8	0,51	0,15
				Basal ganglia	4	18	0,30	0,16
				Hippocampus	8	24	0,25	0,14
				Parieto-temporal cortex	8	23	0,33	0,19

[1] The total number of animals exposed to sagittal rotational acceleration impulses was 24. Three animals were exposed to a single high level flexion tests, one animal was exposed to multiple low and high level flexion tests and four animals were exposed to multiple low level flexion tests. Three animals were exposed to multiple low level extension tests, six animals were exposed to multiple low and high level extension tests, three animals were exposed to a single high level extension test and one animal was exposed to multiple high level extension tests. Finally, three animals were exposed to multiple low level flexion and extension tests.

[2] The total number of experiments that provided useful data was 110.

[3] The three animals that were exposed to a single high level flexion tests did not provide peak pressure data. All transducers installed bottomed out; the underpressure was as least in the range of −0.45 bar. As such these test confirm the data provided by the single test that provided brainstem pressure data.

[4] n.a.: not available.

neutral-density particles as well as with the aid of MRI [6, 7, 11, 13, 28–32]. Finite element analyses indicate that head impacts induce complex displacement and deformation resulting in compression and strain in the brain [12, 23, 33]. We have used a different approach to elucidate what happens in the brain parenchyma during the very short time, usually in the order of milliseconds, when a sagittal plane closed head rotational acceleration impulse forces the brain to transiently move and be deformed, thereby contributing to the primary brain injury [34, 35]. High speed recordings of the pressures generated by the mechanical events taking place in the brain parenchyma at a head and neck trauma were used by utilizing sensitive and flexible miniature pressure sensors, operated by light, and enabling high sampling rate and resolution. At neck flexion, the brain and spinal cord will initially be stretched and then after a short lag, perhaps including oscillations, regain the position in the skull and spine. In contrast, at extension of the neck, the frontal and temporal brain lobes especially will be compressed, and the brainstem, the cerebellum, and the spinal cord are as well affected. Another goal was to investigate whether the inertial displacement and deformation of the brain and spinal cord in an intact cranium and vertebral column, lasting just milliseconds, generated complex pressure patterns differing for flexion versus extension. Further, we aimed to elucidate if differences could be demonstrated between the cerebrum, brainstem, and cerebellum as judged from the recorded pressure patterns.

2. Materials and Methods

2.1. Ethical Considerations. The experiments were approved by the Regional Animal Experiments Ethics Committee and performed in accordance with Swedish and European Union guidelines (Directive 2010/63/EU). Care was taken to minimize the number of animals and their suffering.

2.2. Test Procedure. Two sagittal rotational acceleration rates were used at flexion, 96.3 ± 15.0 krad·s^{-2} and 208 krad·s^{-2}, and at extension, -95.0 ± 6.6 krad·s^{-2} and -184.5 ± 14.5 krad·s^{-2}, termed low level and high level, respectively (Table 1). These exposure conditions were scaled to match peak accelerations in an adult man, as previously described in detail [34–36]. The high acceleration level for a rabbit corresponded for an adult man to 11 krad·s^{-2}, considered sufficient to induce a moderate TBI [25, 37]. The low exposure level was equivalent to 6 krad·s^{-2} for an adult man, likely to cause a mild TBI, and of the same magnitude as the calculated average rotational acceleration of the head of professional American football players at concussions. Each animal was repeatedly exposed to either flexion or extension, or both, at low and high acceleration levels (Table 1). Data from previously reported extension experiments were included for comparison [34].

2.3. Animals and Exposure System. Adult New Zealand albino rabbits (2.3–3 kg) were kept anaesthetized throughout

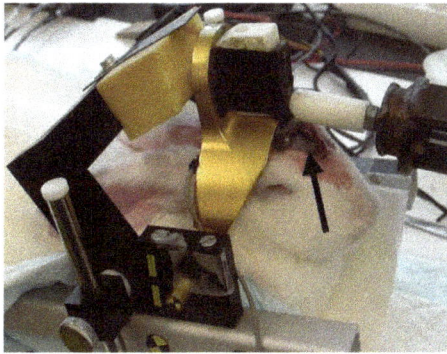

FIGURE 1: The model system. The setup is shown with an anaesthetized rabbit in position for exposure to a closed head sagittal rotational acceleration. The arrow points to the glass fiber reinforced plastic helmet, glued to the cranium. A piston, attached to a pneumatic cylinder and driven by compressed air, was used to deliver the force to the moving (golden) arc to which the rabbit head was attached, as was an accelerometer.

the experiment by injections of Dormicum (Roche) and Hypnorm (Janssen). A helmet of glass fiber reinforced epoxy plastic was glued to the exposed calvarium, providing a broad-based, firm attachment between the rabbit head and a bar, which rotated around a horizontal axis at exposure (Figure 1) [34]. The animals were not restrained except for the attachment of the head. The position of the anaesthetized animals at flexion and extension in the exposure equipment only differed with regard to the orientation of the longitudinal axis [35]. The angular displacement of the head was for both flexion and extension set to 21°, based on pilot experiments, to limit mechanical deformation of the cervical spinal cord and the brainstem. The center of rotation was approximated to the center-of-gravity of the head, located inferior to the brain, and close to the pituitary [36] to minimize the risk for spinal cord damage. The bar, when struck by a piston driven by compressed air, forced the head to rotate in sagittal plane while the acceleration was recorded [35, 36].

Further, 3 animals were sham-exposed and 4 naïve controls used for comparison. In all, 42 animals were used in the present study.

2.4. Pressure Recording System.
Pressures generated by the brain deformation were recorded with a fiber optical miniaturized pressure transducer (FOPT), connected to a control unit (Samba 3200; Samba Sensors AB, Sweden; Figure 2) and a computer. The FOPT was inserted in a 0.9 mm (outer diameter) polytetrafluoroethylene (PTFE) tube to protect the sensor from direct mechanical influence by the brain tissue. The pressure range was −0.8 to 5.5 bars, relative to the continuously recorded ambient atmospheric air pressure, and the average resolution 0.008 bar. Two pressure sensors were used concomitantly and supplied an analogue signal updated at 15 kHz (filtered signal) and were acquired with the acceleration signal with a DataBRICK system (GMH Eng. Inc., Orem, UT, USA) at 12.8 kHz. No filters were applied to these signals to facilitate proper resolution in

time. Aliasing was avoided for the pressure recordings as the oscillation frequency provided by the Samba unit was lower than the sampling frequency. The recorded accelerations were identical with an antialiasing filter set at 2500 Hz as compared to those without. System performance was checked prior to each test. The factory calibrated pressure sensors were additionally calibrated prior to and after use by immersion in a water-filled glass cylinder. Care was taken to keep the sensors clean.

2.5. Implantation of Pressure Transducers and Assessment of Structural Brain Injury.
Two FOPTs, enclosed by PTFE tubes, were during each experiment inserted perpendicular to the rotation direction in the brain parenchyma through tightly fitting holes drilled in the skull [34]. The anterior FOPT, designated the parietotemporal one, was inserted through the parietal bone (8 mm lateral to the midline; 6 mm posterior to the bregma) and directed coronally toward the basal ganglia [38]. The posterior FOPT, named the occipital one, was positioned ipsilaterally through the occipital bone 6 mm behind the first one and directed towards the brainstem. The sensing tips were positioned 6–16 mm below the dura mater. Great care was taken to ensure that the sensors were positioned at the same locations during flexion as extension. The FOPTs were not sealed to the skull, except in one low level flexion experiment in which they were secured to the bone by dental glue. The FOPT cables were kept perpendicular to the rotation plane of the head. The FOPTs were in one set of experiments inserted at a 45-degree angle relative to the plane of rotation and thereby positioned close to each other, one angled rearward and the other angled forward. In other experiments, the two transducers were inserted in opposite brain hemisphere with the sensors facing each other. Holes were further drilled for recordings in the cerebellum.

Additional animals (Table 1; $n = 6$) were exposed to a low level sagittal rotational acceleration flexion impulse to investigate the function of the blood-brain barrier (BBB) 15 min after an intravenous injection of the marker Evans blue (1% in buffered saline; 1 mL/kg b.w.) as the BBB is considered to remain essentially intact at a mild TBI. One h later, the animal was fixed by transcardial perfusion with buffered formalin after an initial rinsing with buffered saline. The brains were inspected macroscopically for extravasation of the dye-protein complex and thin sections prepared for fluorescence microscopy and examined for BBB dysfunction. Further animals ($n = 5$) had a single low level flexion exposure prior to fixation by transcardial perfusion to elucidate effects on blood vessels in the subarachnoid and Virchow-Robin spaces. Sham-exposed ($n = 3$) and naïve control animals ($n = 4$) were investigated as well (Table 1).

All animals were at the end of the experiments euthanized by overdose of Dormicum and Hypnorm. The FOPT tracks were inspected visually and with an operating microscope. The position of the sensor was thereby checked and named according to a rabbit brain atlas [38].

2.6. Analysis of Pressure Recordings.
Differences in peak pressures (positive peak pressures recorded in extension trauma

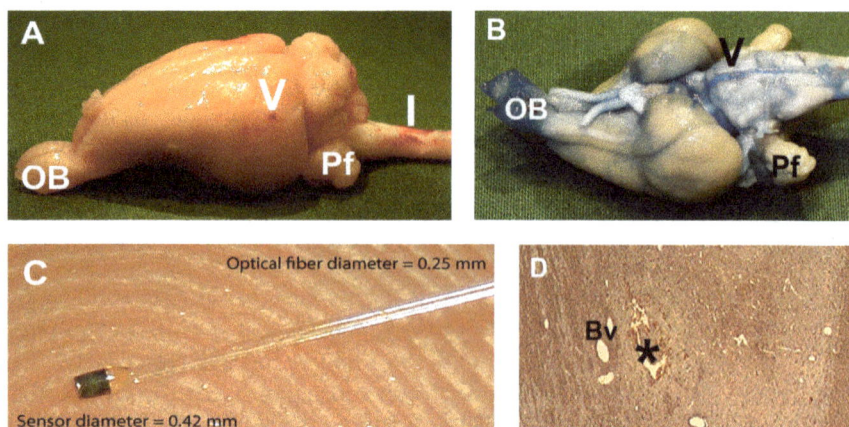

FIGURE 2: Effects on brain by exposures. A rabbit brain after a single exposure to a low level sagittal flexion closed head rotational acceleration (A). There are small hemorrhages in the leptomeninges and on the dorsal surface of the medulla and uppermost cervical cord (marked I). The track after a FOPT used in this special exposure indicated by an arrowhead. Paraflocculus (Pf) and the olfactory bulbs (OB) marked. The brain has no signs of contusion or distortion. (B) shows that there was no blood-brain barrier dysfunction but in the olfactory bulbs (OB), as revealed by Evans blue staining after a low level flexion exposure. The arrowhead points to a stained segment of the basilar artery. Note the staining along the vessels in the subarachnoid spaces. (C) shows the design of a FOPT, resting on a fingertip. The sensor is to the left at the tip of the glass fiber conducting LED light. Note the small dimensions and the absence of mechanical parts and electric leads. (D) Light micrograph of a stained section of brain parenchyma with a tiny hole (∗) constituting the track formed by a FOPT after two exposures to a high level extension. Blood vessel marked Bv.

and negative peak pressure recorded in flexion trauma) between flexion and extension trauma for measurements in one region of the brain and between different measurement sites for different trauma levels were analysed using a one-way analysis of variance (ANOVA) blocked by sample and a post hoc test at a 5% significance level. All differences analysed with aforementioned statistical methods were assessed for the first peak; the second peak that appeared in some extension tests was neglected.

3. Results

3.1. Macroscopically Visible Injuries. Rabbits exposed to either a low level flexion or low or high level extension sagittal rotational acceleration, closed head impulse had no skeletal fractures or dislocations; all breathed spontaneously and none had any apnea (all survived). In contrast, all rabbits exposed to a high level flexion suffered lasting apnea and died at the exposure but had neither any skeletal fractures or dislocations nor any deformation of the head and neck. The carotids and their main branches and the vertebral arteries were inspected and found to be intact in all exposed animals. Sham-exposed animals were unaffected as were the naïve controls.

Autopsy of three rabbits that succumbed at the exposure to a single high level flexion disclosed scattered parenchymal and extensive meningeal hemorrhages, extending to the cervical spinal cord, but no skeletal fractures, contusions, lacerations, or torn structures. In contrast, animals exposed to a low level flexion rarely showed rupture of cerebral cortical veins, thin hemorrhages in the leptomeninges and along Virchow-Robins spaces, and leptomeningeal hemorrhages at the transition between the cervical spinal cord and the

brainstem (Figure 2 A). No focal injuries or hemorrhages were demonstrable in the brain parenchyma, not even underlying the helmet or at the countercoup position. The C1 and occasionally the C2 dorsal roots were teased but never ruptured. The spinal cord appeared macroscopically intact. The olfactory bulbs were partly detached from the cribriform plates and petechiae recognized. The BBB was as expected at a mild TBI intact except for regarding the olfactory bulbs (Figure 2 B). However, the leptomeninges looked slightly blue as did parts of the basilar artery and some leptomeningeal vessels, most evidently in the subarachnoid and Virchow-Robins spaces, indicating slight dysfunction of the vascular barriers but without prevalence of hemorrhages or meningeal ruptures.

Brains from rabbits exposed to a closed head extension trauma at either low or high level looked at autopsy like those from sham-exposed animals and naïve controls, that is, macroscopically uninjured.

Small hemorrhages were observed in immediate connection to and along the tracks formed by the FOPTs, especially after multiple runs (C and D in Figure 2).

3.2. Pressure Measurements at Head Flexion. At a low level flexion rotational acceleration, negative pressures (also named underpressures in this report and related to ambient air pressure) dominated (Figures 3(a) and 3(b); Table 1). The acceleration recordings are shown in Figures 3(a) and 3(c). The posterior FOPT, positioned in the upper brainstem, showed an initial deep pressure drop lasting approximately 2 ms, sometimes followed by a transient positive pressure (also named overpressure and related to ambient air pressure). The anterior FOPT, positioned in the basal ganglia, similarly disclosed an initial pressure drop lasting about 2 ms

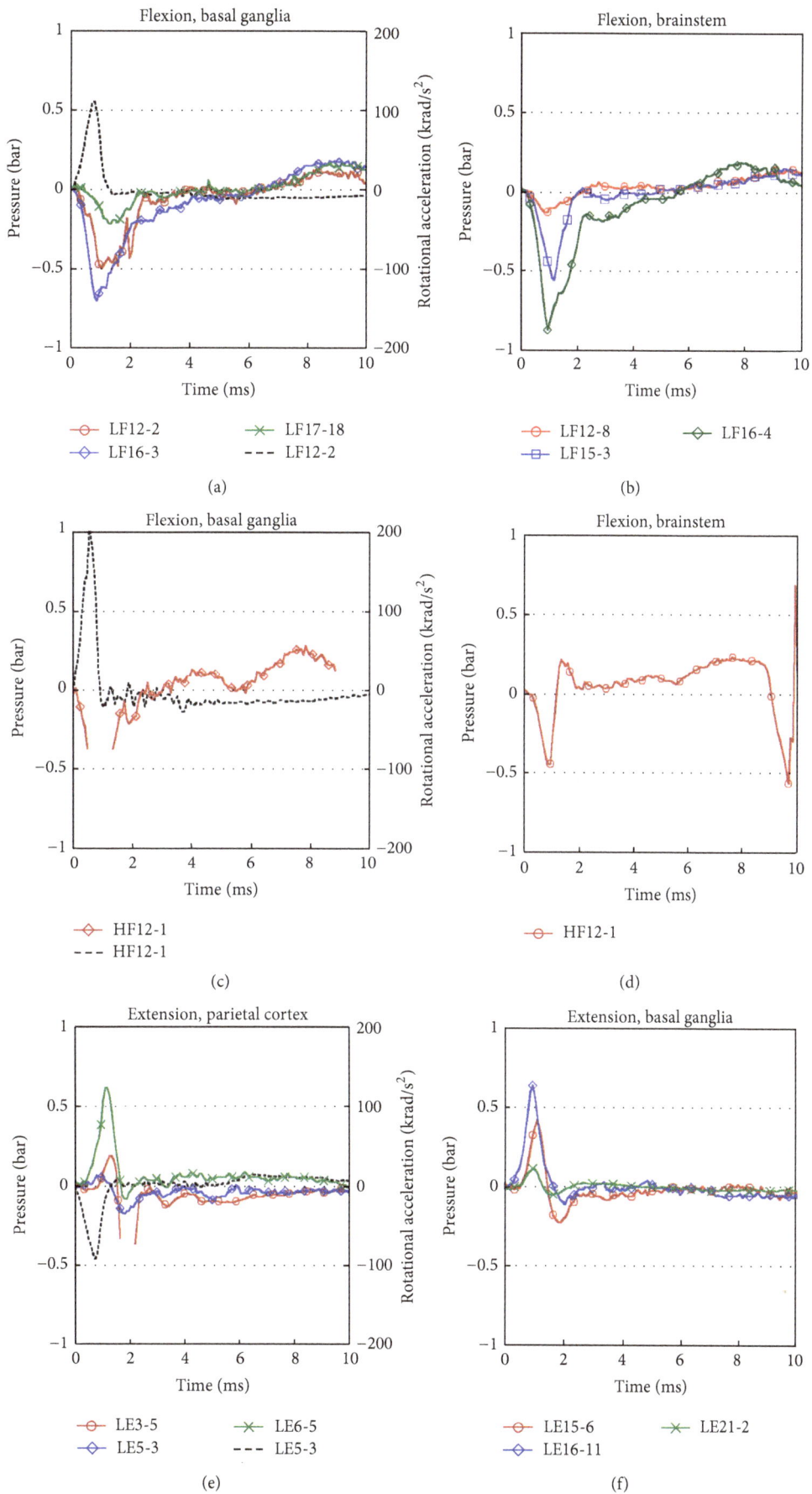

FIGURE 3: Continued.

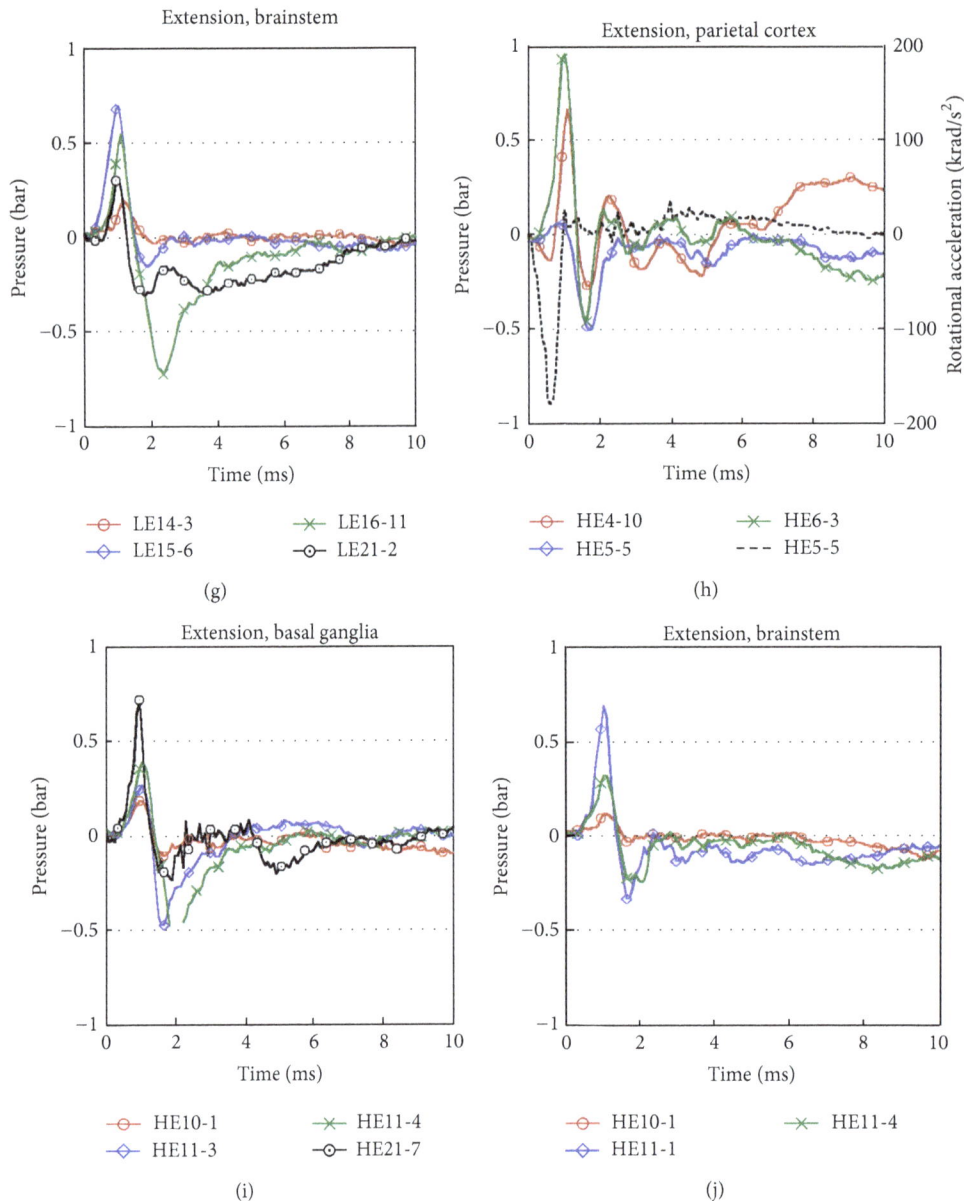

FIGURE 3: Sagittal closed head rotational acceleration and pressure recordings in indicated regions of the brain during low and high level flexion ((a)–(d)) and extension ((e)–(j)), respectively. The recorded sagittal rotational acceleration rate is indicated by the black dashed line and the scale to the right in (a), (c), (e), and (h). (a) and (b) demonstrate that a low level flexion initially induced a strong underpressure, followed by slight overpressure. (c) and (d) show the strong pressures recorded at a high level flexion. Extension at a low level ((e)–(g)) generated initially overpressure followed by underpressure, thus strikingly differing from the pressure patterns induced by flexion at the same level ((a) and (b)). Pressure patterns at high level extensions are presented in (h)–(j). Three experiments were performed in 3 different animals, except for high level flexion. The largest change in peak pressures, the least change in pressure, and representative pressure time histories are presented. See Figure 8 for statistical analyses.

and then ambient pressure, sometimes after a transient, slight overpressure.

All animals exposed to a high level flexion sagittal rotational acceleration impulse died at the exposure. The pressures mostly exceeded the sensors measuring range (Figures 3(c) and 3(d); Table 1).

Consecutive low level flexion exposures in the same animal showed acceptable pressure repeatability (Figures 4(a)–4(d)). The recorded negative peak pressure varied when all tests were studied (Figures 3 and 4), but the pressure patterns were similar, indicating reproducibility.

Implantation of two pressure sensors just a few mm apart at the same depth in the brain parenchyma resulted in small differences in the pressure patterns.

A sensor in the paraflocculus of the cerebellum disclosed that a low level flexion induced positive and negative pressure peaks divergent from those concomitantly recorded by a second sensor in the brainstem (Figures 5(a) and 5(b)).

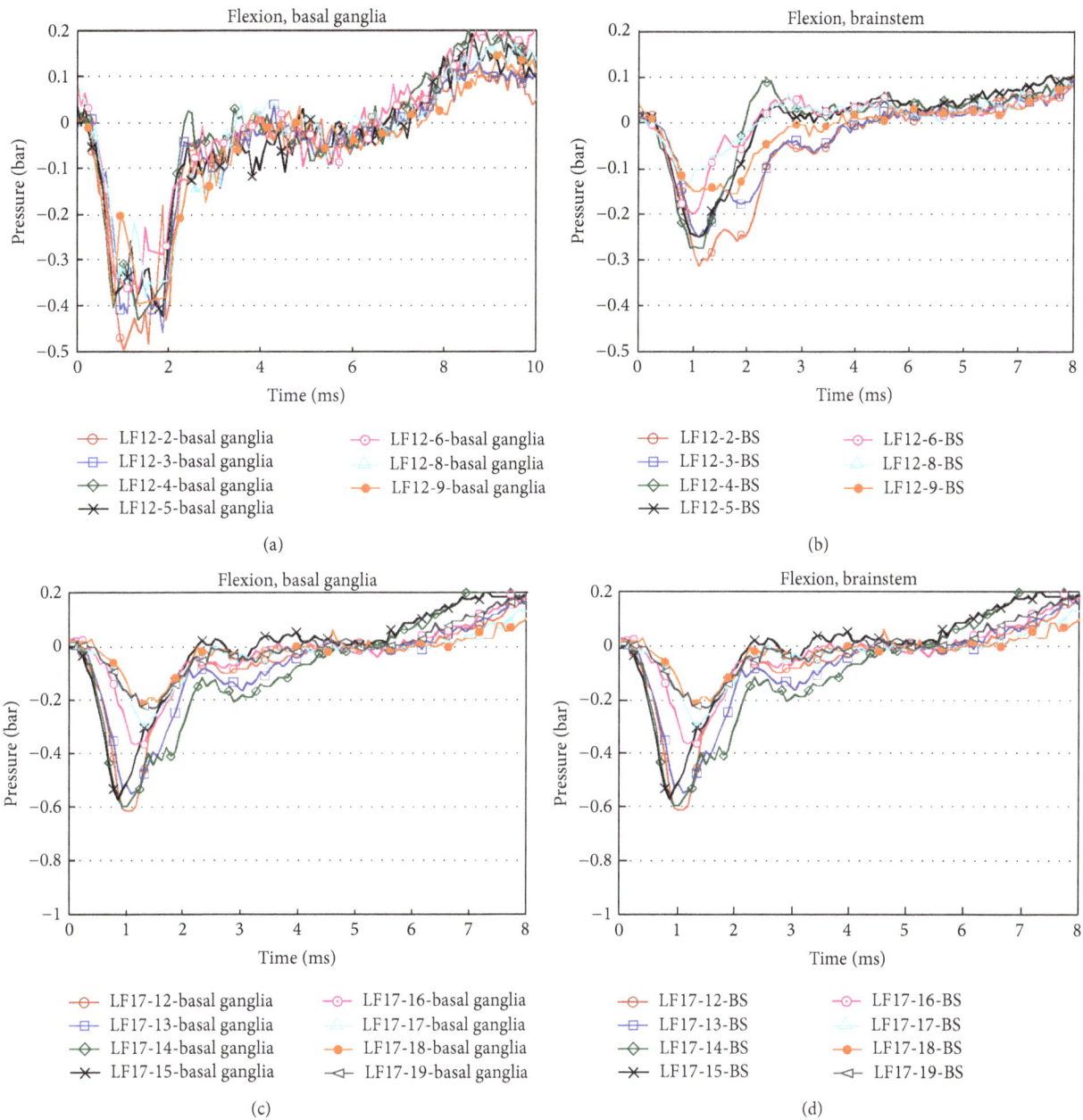

FIGURE 4: Repeated pressure recordings in animal number 12 ((a), (b)) and animal number 17 ((c), (d)) with sensors kept at the same locations in the brain parenchyma throughout a series of repeated consecutive low level sagittal plane flexion rotational acceleration exposures. Recordings from the basal ganglia (left) and the brainstem (BS; right). Close to the same pressure, patterns are recorded, but larger amplitudes are obtained at the first exposures. See Figure 8 for statistical analyses.

An initial positive peak was recorded by the paraflocculus sensor and followed by a negative peak. There was ~0.5 ms time difference between the two sensors as the pressure changes occurred later in the paraflocculus than in the brainstem (Figure 5(a)). A sensor deep in the cerebellum recorded at a low level flexion a pressure pattern similar to that in paraflocculus (Figure 5(b)). A time delay was consistently demonstrable between the pressures in the different parts of the cerebellum as compared to those in the cerebrum and brainstem.

3.3. Pressure Measurements at Head Extension.
At low level extension, an initial positive pressure peak was followed by a brief negative one (Figures 3(e)–3(j)). The accelerometer readings are shown in Figures 3(e) and 3(h). These recordings were similar to those previously reported [34]. For a high level extension, the pressure drop was more prominent in the basal ganglia as compared to that in the rostral brainstem (Figures 3(f), 3(g), and 5(c)).

A sensor inserted in the border between the pons and medulla oblongata, that is, in caudal parts of the brainstem, at

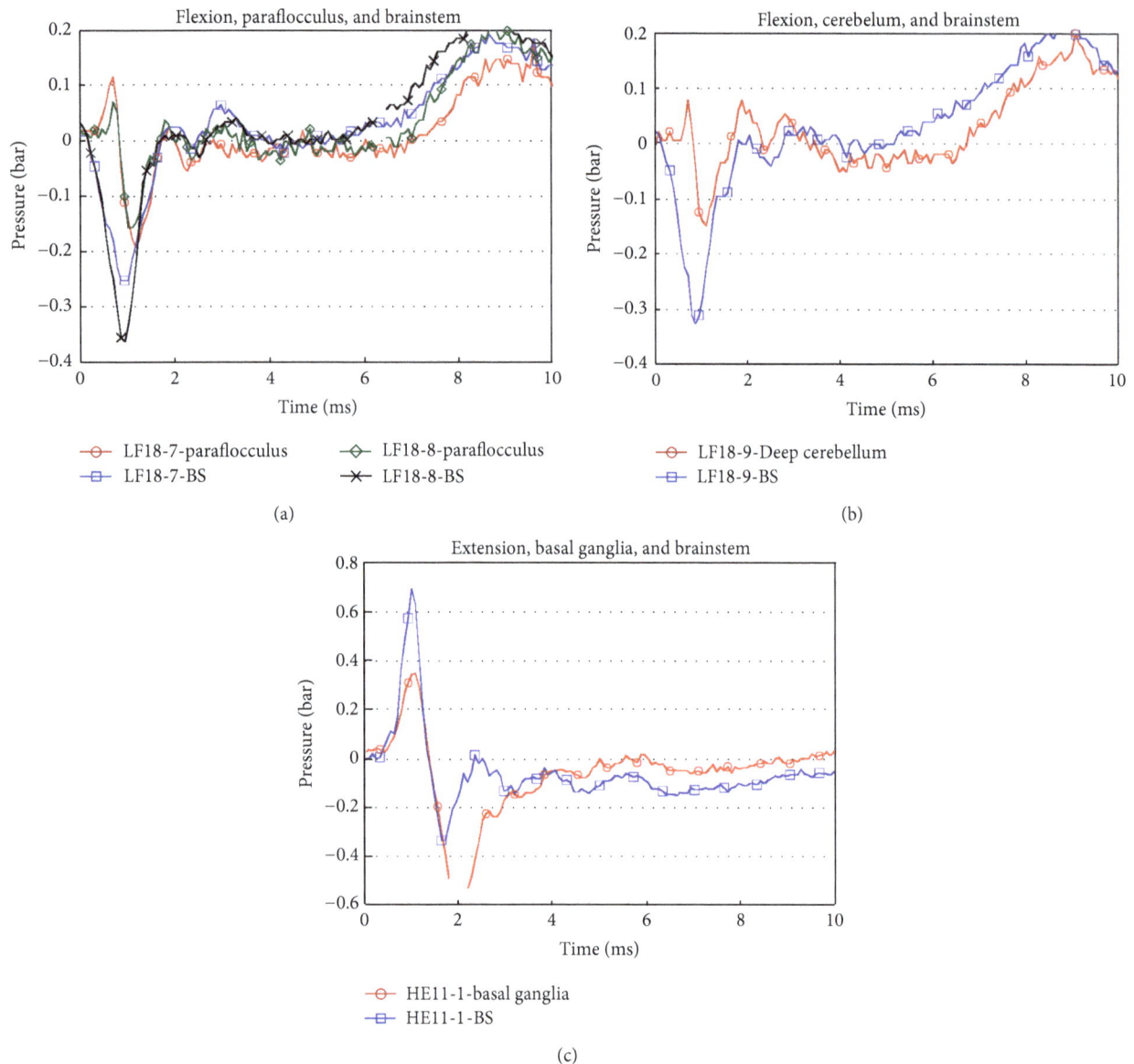

FIGURE 5: Two consecutive pressure recordings in the same animal at two locations, brainstem (BS) and paraflocculus cerebelli (a), and a subsequent one with one sensor in the brainstem and the second one deep in the cerebellum (b) at a low level sagittal plane flexion rotational acceleration. Note the difference in time between the appearance of pressure changes in the brainstem and in the cerebellum. A high level sagittal extension trauma (c) induced strong pressure amplitudes, initially overpressure followed by underpressure, with one sensor positioned in deep in the caudate head (basal ganglia) and the other one in the pons portion of the brainstem. The sensor in the brainstem indicates extended, persistent underpressure due to extensive deformation.

a high level extension closed head exposure recorded a strong overpressure followed by underpressure, while the anterior FOPT, placed in the basal ganglia, revealed an even stronger pressure drop (Figure 5(c)). The pons sensor recorded a sustained negative pressure for a prolonged time as compared with the sensor in the caudate head of the basal ganglia (Figure 5(c)).

3.4. Pressure Measurements to Elucidate the Importance of Direction and Anchoring of the Sensors. Two sensors, implanted in mirror positions in either brain hemisphere,

revealed similar pressure patterns at both flexion and extension rotational accelerations (Figures 6(a) and 6(b)) with small differences, likely due to variations in sensor positions.

Attaching the PTFE tube to the skull bone with glue had no measureable effects on the pressure recordings at exposure to low level flexion, in concordance with our previous report on extension [34].

The insertion of the sensors in deep brain structures at an angle of approximately 45 degrees relative to the plane of rotation, with the anterior FOPT angled in a posterior direction and the posterior one angled anteriorly, had little or no effect on the recorded pressures (Figures 7(a) and 7(b)).

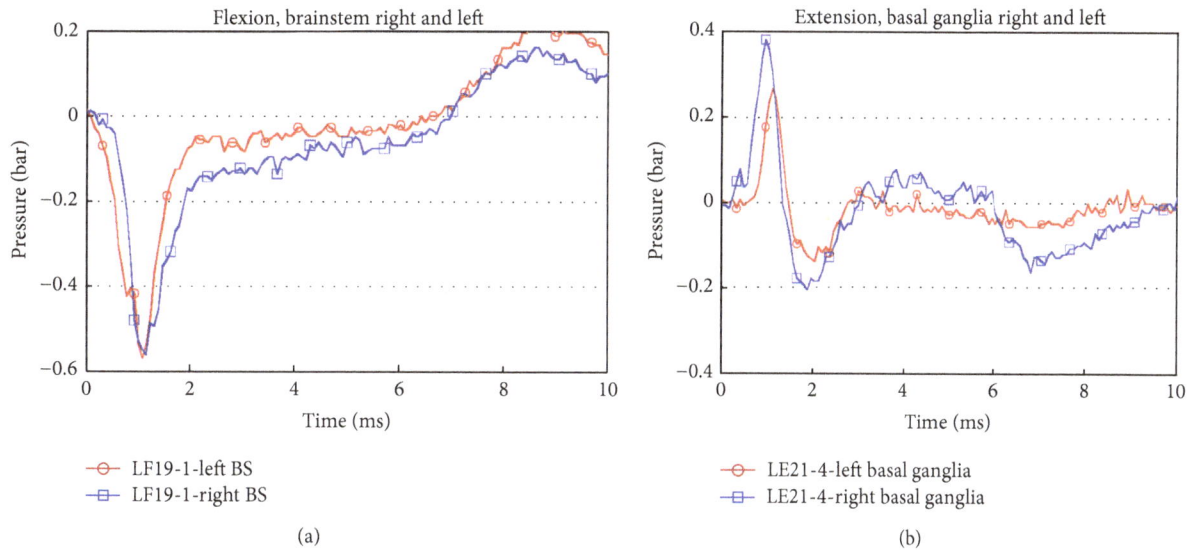

FIGURE 6: Two FOPTs in opposite brain hemispheres from the right and the left side, facing each other, recorded the pressure in the left or right side of the brainstem (BS) at a low level flexion (a) and basal ganglia at a low level extension (b). Similar pressure recordings were obtained for both the brainstem and the basal ganglia, respectively, at either exposure direction. The variations reflect minor differences in sensor positions.

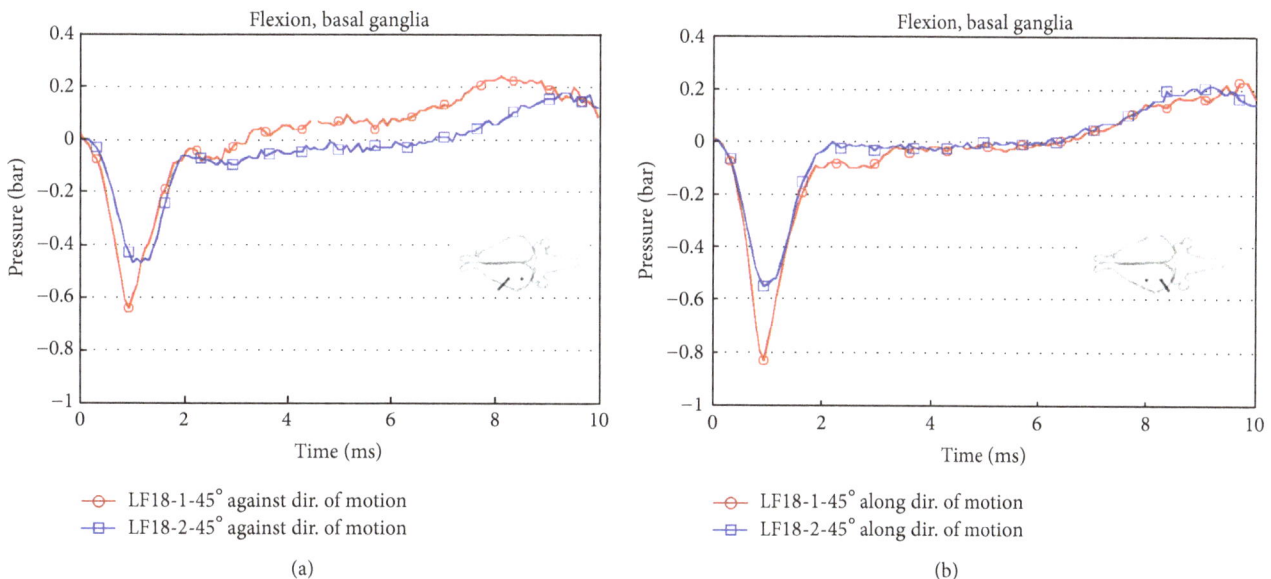

FIGURE 7: Repeated recordings at a low level sagittal flexion closed head rotational acceleration with the sensors in basal ganglia. One FOPT was inserted through the hole in the parietotemporal bone and directed at an angle of 45° rearward (a), while the one through the occipital bone was directed at an angle of 45° forward (b). Thereby the sensor tips were positioned only a few mm apart during the exposure. Similar pressure patterns were obtained whether the sensor was aligned against or along the direction of the sagittal rotational acceleration. The sensors are thus likely to record dynamic pressures generated in the brain parenchyma at the exposure. No obvious indication suggesting that the pressures were related to movements of the FOPTs in the brain tissue.

3.5. *Assessment of Structural Brain Injury Caused by the Two FOPTs and by the Exposure.* The tracks formed by the FOPTs were traced visually and by light microscopy to map the positions of the transducers. Light microscopy of stained brain sections disclosed that a FOPT track generated a collapsed channel (Figure 2 D). Hemorrhages and tissue contusions were rarely observed after a single exposure but

after multiple exposures and when the FOPT position was changed.

In a published report, we have characterized the histopathological changes demonstrable in exposed animals surviving one week after an exposure to sagittal plane rotational acceleration impulse as described above. Diffuse brain injuries were demonstrable in the brains of rabbits exposed to a sagittal plane low level flexion rotational acceleration impulse as could be shown for animals exposed to high or low level extension [35]. The animals exposed to a high level flexion suffered brain contusions and none survived, and therefore no corresponding histopathological data are available. These histopathological investigations on animals exposed to a low level flexion and a high or low level extension thus demonstrate that the used exposure levels are to be considered causing mild TBI according to commonly used criteria [10, 18, 20, 22, 39].

3.6. Statistical Analysis of the Results. The statistical analysis of the achieved results is presented in Figure 8.

4. Discussion

A major result was that strikingly differing pressure patterns were generated in the brain depending on the direction of movement of a head at a sagittal closed head rotational acceleration impulse and equal force lasting close to 1 ms [Figure 8]. Flexion resulted in pressures with longer duration and larger amplitudes than did extension. A low level flexion induced prominent negative, prolonged pressures in contrast to extension, which resulted in a short positive pressure peak followed by a small negative one (Figure 3). Pudenz and Shelden [28] reported that the brain moves and may be deformed at a closed head trauma, as subsequently repeatedly confirmed [6, 7, 10, 17, 29, 30]. The recorded pressures were generated by deformation of the brain and spinal cord on exposure to a sagittal plane rotational acceleration. The pressure pattern and its duration constitute a measure of the inertial twisting and strain at the deformation of the brain. We conclude that flexion caused more extensive mechanical trauma to the brain than did extension at the same force, in agreement with what has previously been demonstrated histopathologically [35]. At a low level flexion, there were macroscopically no visible hemorrhages, contusions, or tearing of the brain parenchyma and spinal cord, but histopathologically demonstrable diffuse brain injuries [35]. Consistent findings were mechanical damage to the olfactory bulbs, hemorrhages in the leptomeninges and along the Virchow-Robins space, and deformation of the C1/C2 nerve roots (Figures 1 and 2). The exposure to flexion thus likely overstretched the brain and spinal cord. Unexpectedly, we did not observe any apnoea, considered a sensitive marker of brainstem damage, except at a high level flexion. The paraflocculus, which in rabbits is largely enclosed by bone, showed the same pressure pattern as deep central parts of the cerebellum (Figure 5). The cerebellum was histopathologically damaged but less than the olfactory bulbs [35], which in parts detached from their normal anchoring to the cribriform plates. Extension, similarly limited to 21°, likely compressed the brain but caused no macroscopic signs of damage [34, 35]. The prevalence, distribution, and severity of brain and spinal injuries are known from other types of exposures to be direction dependent [6, 7, 9, 10, 15, 24, 27]. Our published histopathological investigations have disclosed that flexion caused much more extensive damage than did extension

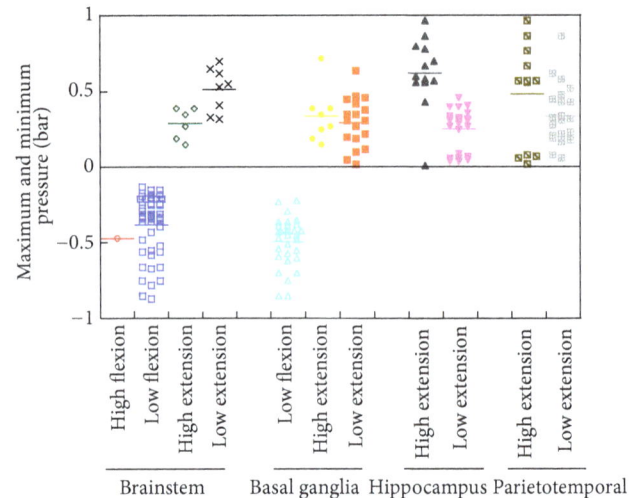

FIGURE 8: The ANOVA of the pressure data provided the following results: for pressure measurements in the brainstem: low flexion was significantly different from low extension. Pressure in the brainstem was not significantly different between low and high extension. For pressure measurements in the basal ganglia: low flexion was significantly different from low extension. Pressure in the basal ganglia was not significantly different between low and high extension. For pressure measurements in the hippocampus: low extension was significantly different from high extension. For pressure measurements in the parietotemporal cortex: low extension was not significantly different from high extension. For pressure measurements in low extension trauma: only the peak pressure in the hippocampus was significantly different from the peak pressure in the brainstem. All other combinations of pressure recordings in the brainstem, basal ganglia, hippocampus, and parietotemporal cortex were found not to be significantly different from each other when exposed to a low extension trauma. For pressure measurements in high extension trauma: only the peak pressure in the hippocampus was significantly different from the peak pressure in the brainstem and basal ganglia. All other combinations of pressure recordings in the brainstem, basal ganglia, hippocampus, and parietotemporal cortex were found not significantly different from each other when exposed to a high extension trauma. For pressure measurements in low flexion trauma: peak pressures in the brainstem and basal ganglia regions were found not to be significantly different from each other.

at the same force [35]. It must however be stressed that in either case the diffuse brain injury demonstrated must be classified as fulfilling the criteria for being mild TBI as there was no evidence indicating any contusion, tearing, or parenchymal hemorrhages. We conclude that the increased magnitude and duration of the recorded transient pressures at flexion as compared to extension movements in the brain parenchyma correlated with the macroscopically and histopathologically more extensive brain damage [35]. Case reports in the forensic medicine indicate that flexion may be more deleterious than extension also to human subjects, but to our knowledge no systematic investigation is available [20, 22].

Our presented results elucidated the importance of rapid, transient vibrations and movements of a head at impact for the severity of the resulting brain damage. In our initial experiments [36], the force delivering helmet was attached to the cranium with individually glued titanium pins, which enabled movements of the cranium and thus of the head as less than 40% of the calvaria was anchored to the helmet. In contrast, in the present experiments, the entire calvaria was firmly attached with glue to a fitting helmet [34], restricting head movements. Further, the glue formed a continuous layer firmly bridging the calvarial bone and the shaped helmet of glass fiber reinforced epoxy, thereby minimizing any mechanical deformation of the skull. The head movements allowed by our previous system strikingly increased the severity of the damage as reflected by, for example, brain hemorrhages, widespread diffuse brain injury, elevated levels of excitotoxic amino acids, and extensive gliosis [36, 40, 41]. At simulated traffic accidents, brain damage may be avoided if head and neck movements are limited [14]. We conclude that restricting the head movements and deformation of the skull, as done in the present study, reduced the extent and severity of the induced TBI [35], in agreement with considerations in clinical and experimental reports [14, 20, 22, 28, 42].

We asked whether the recorded transitory pressure changes at a rotational acceleration, closed head impulse could add to the injury in the anisotropic brain. Support is gained from studies based on finite element modeling and blast-induced TBI at pressures of similar magnitude and duration [19, 43–47]. Distant high energy missile hind leg impact to animals induces positive and negative pressure waves in the brain as well as histopathologically demonstrable brain damage [48]. Pressure waves of similar magnitude and duration are injurious to cultured neurons [49]. Detailed mapping of the deformation and pressure patterns at a sagittal rotational acceleration is required to derive firm statements about whether the induced pressure waves per se added to the diffuse brain injury.

The brain lacks conventional lymphatics [50–54]. Instead, the cerebrospinal fluid (CSF) and the interstitial (extracellular) fluid (ISF) are drained along paravascular pathways and nerves. It is essential for the brain to have a proper turnover of fluid, nutrients, and waste products. A main pathway for the ISF flow constitutes the Virchow-Robin space (VRS) and further along brain blood vessels, draining fluid eventually to, for example, cervical lymph nodes. A closed head sagittal rotational acceleration trauma as in the present study resulted in mechanical displacement and deformation of the brain, including blood vessels and meninges, which may impair the blood flow and the traffic of CSF and ISF. Rabbits exposed to a flexion impulse had hemorrhages preferentially localized perivascularly in the subarachnoid space (A and B in Figure 2) and along the VRS. Histopathological investigation of exposed, surviving animals disclosed posttraumatic reactive gliosis along cortical arteries in the VRS [35]. In our opinion, a closed head trauma not only deforms the brain but in addition may impair the trafficking of fluid, metabolites, and waste products by paravascular routes, adding to the primary brain injury.

One limitation is that the achieved results are not readily applicable to humans, whose neuraxis has a sharp angle between the main part of the brain and the spinal cord while the neuraxis in rabbits is slightly S-shaped, as judged by the position at the exposures in the present study. Further, the human cerebrum is gyrencephalic, having distinct sulci and gyri, while the rabbit brain is lissencephalic, that is, smooth surfaced, likely to influence the outcome [51, 55]. However, the cerebellum both in humans and in animals has an elaborated system of fissures and folia which are injured more often than generally anticipated both in humans and in animals [22, 30, 35, 39].

5. Conclusions

Our approach to use the dynamic pressure patterns at a sagittal plane rotational acceleration trauma enables evaluation of the induced deformation of the brain. The information achieved with our approach supplements other available methods in assessing the movements and structural alterations going on in the brain at the exposure to a closed head trauma at a very high time resolution. Further, we could demonstrate the prevalence of time differences in displacement and deformation of different parts of the brain, as were revealed by the timing of the pressure patterns. We further conclude that a closed head sagittal flexion rotational acceleration impulse caused more extensive deformation of the brain and spinal cord than extension, generating stronger pressures of longer duration and aggravation of the induced TBI. Different parts of the brain are displaced and deformed in a noncoherent manner, which likely explain differences in extent of the resulting TBI. The events in the leptomeninges and Virchow-Robin spaces deserve elucidation with regard to likely importance for the generation of primary and secondary brain damages.

Conflict of Interests

The authors declare that they have no conflict of interests regarding the publication of this paper. Svante Höjer was initially an employee of Samba Sensor AB, but subsequently working at the University of Gothenburg.

Acknowledgments

This work was supported by grants from VINNOVA, SAFER, the W. and M. Lundgren Foundation, Lantmännen AS-Faktor AB, Gothenburg Medical Society, the Swedish Federal Government, and the Sahlgren's University Hospital. The authors thank Per Lövsund and Margareta Rosenkvist for support, advice, and help.

References

[1] J. A. Langlois Orman, J. F. Kraus, E. Zaloshnja, and T. Miller, "Epidemiology," in *Textbook of Traumatic Brain Injury*, J. M. Silver, T. W. Mcalister, and S. C. Yudofsky, Eds., pp. 3–22, American Psychiatric Publishing Inc, Washington, DC, USA, 2nd edition, 2011.

[2] V. G. Coronado, L. Xu, S. V. Basaravaju et al., "Surveillance for traumatic brain injury-related deaths—United States, 1997–2007," *Morbidity and Mortality Weekly Report—Surveillance Summaries*, vol. 60, no. 5, pp. 1–32, 2011.

[3] V. L. Feigin, A. Theadom, S. Barker-Collo et al., "Incidence of traumatic brain injury in New Zealand: a population-based study," *The Lancet Neurology*, vol. 12, no. 1, pp. 53–64, 2013.

[4] F. Tagliaferri, C. Compagnone, M. Korsic, F. Servadei, and J. Kraus, "A systematic review of brain injury epidemiology in Europe," *Acta Neurochirurgica*, vol. 148, no. 3, pp. 255–267, 2006.

[5] A. Kay and G. Teasdale, "Head injury in the United Kingdom," *World Journal of Surgery*, vol. 25, no. 9, pp. 1210–1220, 2001.

[6] W. N. Hardy, C. D. Foster, M. J. Mason, K. H. Yang, A. I. King, and S. Tashman, "Investigation of head injury mechanisms using neutral density technology and high-speed biplanar X-ray," *Stapp Car Crash Journal*, vol. 45, pp. 337–368, 2001.

[7] W. N. Hardy, M. J. Mason, C. D. Foster et al., "A study of the response of the human cadaver head to impact," *Stapp Car Crash Journal*, vol. 51, pp. 17–80, 2007.

[8] E. D. Bigler and W. L. Maxwell, "Neuropathology of mild traumatic brain injury: relationship to neuroimaging findings," *Brain Imaging and Behavior*, vol. 6, no. 2, pp. 108–136, 2012.

[9] A. K. Ommaya, W. Goldsmith, and L. Thibault, "Biomechanics and neuropathology of adult and paediatric head injury," *British Journal of Neurosurgery*, vol. 16, no. 3, pp. 220–242, 2002.

[10] P. Reilly and R. Bullock, *Head Injury—Pathophysiology and Management*, Hodder Arnold, London, UK, 2nd edition, 2005.

[11] A. A. Sabet, E. Christoforou, B. Zatlin, G. M. Genin, and P. V. Bayly, "Deformation of the human brain induced by mild angular head acceleration," *Journal of Biomechanics*, vol. 41, no. 2, pp. 307–315, 2008.

[12] D. F. Meaney and D. H. Smith, "Biomechanics of concussion," *Clinics in Sports Medicine*, vol. 30, no. 1, pp. 19–31, 2011.

[13] M. E. Shenton, H. M. Hamoda, J. S. Schneiderman et al., "A review of magnetic resonance imaging and diffusion tensor imaging findings in mild traumatic brain injury," *Brain Imaging and Behavior*, vol. 6, no. 2, pp. 137–192, 2012.

[14] D. R. Namjoshi, C. Good, W. H. Cheng et al., "Towards clinical management of traumatic brain injury: a review of models and mechanisms from a biomechanical perspective," *Disease Models & Mechanisms*, vol. 6, no. 6, pp. 1325–1338, 2013.

[15] S. S. Margulies, L. E. Thibault, and T. A. Gennarelli, "Physical model simulations of brain injury in the primate," *Journal of Biomechanics*, vol. 23, no. 8, pp. 823–836, 1990.

[16] G. S. Nusholtz, P. S. Kaiker, and W. S. Gould, "Two factors critical in the pressure response of the impacted head," *Aviation, Space, and Environmental Medicine*, vol. 58, no. 12, pp. 1157–1164, 1987.

[17] L. Zhang, K. H. Yang, and A. I. King, "Biomechanics of neurotrauma," *Neurological Research*, vol. 23, no. 2-3, pp. 144–156, 2001.

[18] R. W. G. Anderson, C. J. Brown, P. C. Blumbergs, A. J. McLean, and N. R. Jones, "Impact mechanics and axonal injury in a sheep model," *Journal of Neurotrauma*, vol. 20, no. 10, pp. 961–974, 2003.

[19] J. Goeller, A. Wardlaw, D. Treichler, J. O'Bruba, and G. Weiss, "Investigation of cavitation as a possible damage mechanism in blast-induced traumatic brain injury," *Journal of Neurotrauma*, vol. 29, no. 10, pp. 1970–1981, 2012.

[20] J. E. Leestma, *Forensic Neuropathology*, CRC Press, Boca Raton, Fla, USA, 2nd edition, 2008.

[21] G. S. Nusholtz, E. B. Wylie, and L. G. Glascoe, "Internal cavitation in simple head impact model," *Journal of Neurotrauma*, vol. 12, no. 4, pp. 707–714, 1995.

[22] M. Oehmichen, R. N. Auer, and H. G. König, *Forensic Neuropathology and Associated Neurology*, Springer, Heidelberg, Germany, 2009.

[23] M. B. Panzer, B. S. Myers, B. P. Capehart, and C. R. Bass, "Development of a finite element model for blast brain injury and the effects of CSF cavitation," *Annals of Biomedical Engineering*, vol. 40, no. 7, pp. 1530–1544, 2012.

[24] S. A. Eucker, C. Smith, J. Ralston, S. H. Friess, and S. S. Margulies, "Physiological and histopathological responses following closed rotational head injury depend on direction of head motion," *Experimental Neurology*, vol. 227, no. 1, pp. 79–88, 2011.

[25] E. J. Pellman, D. C. Viano, A. M. Tucker et al., "Concussion in professional football: reconstruction of game impacts and injuries," *Neurosurgery*, vol. 53, no. 4, pp. 799–814, 2003.

[26] S. Rowson and S. M. Duma, "Brain injury prediction: assessing the combined probability of concussion using linear and rotational head acceleration," *Annals of Biomedical Engineering*, vol. 41, no. 5, pp. 873–882, 2013.

[27] A. A. Weaver, K. A. Danelson, and J. D. Stitzel, "Modeling brain injury response for rotational velocities of varying directions and magnitudes," *Annals of Biomedical Engineering*, vol. 40, no. 9, pp. 2005–2018, 2012.

[28] R. H. Pudenz and C. H. Shelden, "The lucite calvarium-a method for direct observation of the brain; cranial trauma and brain movement," *Journal of Neurosurgery*, vol. 3, no. 6, pp. 487–505, 1946.

[29] Y. Feng, T. M. Abney, R. J. Okamoto, R. B. Pless, G. M. Genin, and P. V. Bayly, "Relative brain displacement and deformation during constrained mild frontal head impact," *Journal of the Royal Society Interface*, vol. 7, no. 53, pp. 1677–1688, 2010.

[30] E. B. Yan, V. P. A. Johnstone, D. S. Alwis, M.-C. Morganti-Kossmann, and R. Rajan, "Characterising effects of impact velocity on brain and behaviour in a model of diffuse traumatic axonal injury," *Neuroscience*, vol. 248, pp. 17–29, 2013.

[31] V. R. Hodgson, E. S. Gurdjian, and L. M. Thomas, "Experimental skull deformation and brain displacement demonstrated by flash x-ray technique," *Journal of Neurosurgery*, vol. 25, no. 5, pp. 549–552, 1966.

[32] H. Zou, J. P. Schmiedeler, and W. N. Hardy, "Separating brain motion into rigid body displacement and deformation under low-severity impacts," *Journal of Biomechanics*, vol. 40, no. 6, pp. 1183–1191, 2007.

[33] R. K. Gupta and A. Przekwas, "Mathematical models of blast-induced TBI: current status, challenges, and prospects," *Frontiers in Neurology*, vol. 4, pp. 1–21, 2013.

[34] U. Krave, S. Höjer, and H.-A. Hansson, "Transient, powerful pressures are generated in the brain by a rotational acceleration impulse to the head," *European Journal of Neuroscience*, vol. 21, no. 10, pp. 2876–2882, 2005.

[35] U. Krave, M. Al-Olama, and H.-A. Hansson, "Rotational acceleration closed head flexion trauma generates more extensive diffuse brain injury than extension trauma," *Journal of Neurotrauma*, vol. 28, no. 1, pp. 57–70, 2011.

[36] E. Gutierrez, Y. Huang, K. Haglid et al., "A new model for diffuse brain injury by rotational acceleration: I. model, gross appearance, and astrocytosis," *Journal of Neurotrauma*, vol. 18, no. 3, pp. 247–257, 2001.

[37] S. Rowson, S. M. Duma, J. G. Beckwith et al., "Rotational head kinematics in football impacts: An injury risk function for concussion," *Annals of Biomedical Engineering*, vol. 40, no. 1, pp. 1–13, 2012.

[38] J. W. Shek, G. Y. Wen, and H. M. Wisniewski, *Atlas of the Rabbit Brain and Spinal Cord*, Karger, Basel, Switzerland, 1986.

[39] P. Blumbergs, P. Reilly, and R. Vink, "Trauma," in *Greenfields Neuropathology*, S. Love, D. N. Louis, and D. W. Ellison, Eds., pp. 733–832, Arnold, London, UK, 8th edition, 2008.

[40] A. Hamberger, Y.-L. Huang, H. Zhu et al., "Redistribution of neurofilaments and accumulation of β-amyloid protein after brain injury by rotational acceleration of the head," *Journal of Neurotrauma*, vol. 20, no. 2, pp. 169–178, 2003.

[41] M. Runnerstam, F. Bao, Y.-L. Huang et al., "A new model for diffuse brain injury by rotational acceleration: II. Effects on extracellular glutamate, intracranial pressure, and neuronal apoptosis," *Journal of Neurotrauma*, vol. 18, no. 3, pp. 259–273, 2001.

[42] L. E. Goldstein, A. M. Fisher, C. A. Tagge et al., "Chronic traumatic encephalopathy in blast-exposed military veterans and a blast neurotrauma mouse model," *Science Translational Medicine*, vol. 4, no. 134, Article ID 134ra60, 2012.

[43] M. S. Chafi, G. Karami, and M. Ziejewski, "Biomechanical assessment of brain dynamic responses due to blast pressure waves," *Annals of Biomedical Engineering*, vol. 38, no. 2, pp. 490–504, 2010.

[44] A. Säljö, F. Bao, K. G. Haglid, and H.-A. Hansson, "Blast exposure causes redistribution of phosphorylated neurofilament subunits in neurons of the adult rat brain," *Journal of Neurotrauma*, vol. 17, no. 8, pp. 719–726, 2000.

[45] A. Säljö, Y.-L. Huang, and H.-A. Hansson, "Impulse noise transiently increased the permeability of nerve and glial cell membranes, an effect accentuated by a recent brain injury," *Journal of Neurotrauma*, vol. 20, no. 8, pp. 787–794, 2003.

[46] R. C. Turner, Z. J. Naser, A. F. Logsdon et al., "Modeling clinically relevant blast parameters based on scaling principles produces functional & histological deficits in rats," *Experimental Neurology*, vol. 248, pp. 520–529, 2013.

[47] C. Giordano, R. J. H. Cloots, J. A. W. van Dommelen, and S. Kleiven, "The influence of anisotropy on brain injury prediction," *Journal of Biomechanics*, vol. 47, no. 5, pp. 1052–1059, 2014.

[48] A. Suneson, H.-A. Hansson, and T. Seeman, "Pressure wave injuries to the nervous system caused by high-energy missile extremity impact: Part II. Distant effects on the central nervous system—a light and electron microscopic study of pigs," *Journal of Trauma*, vol. 30, no. 3, pp. 295–306, 1990.

[49] A. Suneson, H. A. Hansson, E. Lycke, and T. Seeman, "Pressure wave injuries to rat dorsal root ganglion cells in culture caused by high-energy missiles," *Journal of Trauma*, vol. 29, no. 1, pp. 10–18, 1989.

[50] J. J. Iliff, M. Wang, Y. Liao et al., "A paravascular pathway facilitates CSF flow through the brain parenchyma and the clearance of interstitial solutes, including amyloid β," *Science Translational Medicine*, vol. 4, no. 147, Article ID 147ra111, 2012.

[51] J. Nolte, *The Human Brain*, Mosby, St. Louis, Mo, USA, 6th edition, 2008.

[52] M. L. Rennels, T. F. Gregory, O. R. Blaumanis, K. Fujimoto, and P. A. Grady, "Evidence for a paravascular fluid circulation in the mammalian central nervous system, provided by the rapid distribution of tracer protein throughout the brain from the subarachnoid space," *Brain Research*, vol. 326, no. 1, pp. 47–63, 1985.

[53] V. R. Thrane, A. S. Thrane, B. A. Plog et al., "Paravascular microcirculation facilitates rapid lipid transport and astrocyte signaling in the brain," *Scientific Reports*, vol. 3, article 2582, 2013.

[54] R. O. Weller, E. Djuanda, H.-Y. Yow, and R. O. Carare, "Lymphatic drainage of the brain and the pathophysiology of neurological disease," *Acta Neuropathologica*, vol. 117, no. 1, pp. 1–14, 2009.

[55] J. Ho and S. Kleiven, "Can sulci protect the brain from traumatic injury?" *Journal of Biomechanics*, vol. 42, no. 13, pp. 2074–2080, 2009.

15

The Potentiation of Associative Memory by Emotions: An Event-Related FMRI Study

David Luck,[1,2,3] **Marie-Eve Leclerc,**[2,3] **and Martin Lepage**[1,4]

[1] *Douglas Mental Health University Institute, Verdun, QC, Canada H4H 1R3*
[2] *Institut Universitaire en Santé Mentale de Montréal, Montreal, QC, Canada H1N 3M5*
[3] *Department of Psychiatry, University of Montreal, Montreal, QC, Canada H3T 1J4*
[4] *Department of Psychiatry, McGill University, Montreal, QC, Canada H3A 2T5*

Correspondence should be addressed to Martin Lepage; martin.lepage@mcgill.ca

Academic Editor: Jan Gläscher

Establishing associations between pieces of information is related to the medial temporal lobe (MTL). However, it remains unclear how emotions affect memory for associations and, consequently, MTL activity. Thus, this event-related fMRI study attempted to identify neural correlates of the influence of positive and negative emotions on associative memory. Twenty-five participants were instructed to memorize 90 pairs of standardized pictures during a scanned encoding phase. Each pair was composed of a scene and an unrelated object. Trials were neutral, positive, or negative as a function of the emotional valence of the scene. At the behavioral level, participants exhibited better memory retrieval for both emotional conditions relative to neutral trials. Within the right MTL, a functional dissociation was observed, with entorhinal activation elicited by emotional associations, posterior parahippocampal activation elicited by neutral associations, and hippocampal activation elicited by both emotional and neutral associations. In addition, emotional associations induced greater activation than neutral trials in the right amygdala. This fMRI study shows that emotions are associated with the performance improvement of associative memory, by enhancing activity in the right amygdala and the right entorhinal cortex. It also provides evidence for a rostrocaudal specialization within the MTL regarding the emotional valence of associations.

1. Introduction

Episodic memory refers to the capacity to recollect individual events [1], which include perceptive dimensions of physical objects as well as the time and the place in which they occurred. All this disparate information has to be bound to create a unique coherent representation in memory [2]. This ability to bind and integrate disparate elements is an essential feature of episodic memory and has been referred to as associative memory [3].

It is now generally accepted that the medial temporal lobe (MTL) is involved in processing episodic events, but the exact nature of the contribution of its different parts is still a matter of debate. The MTL is composed of the amygdala, the hippocampus, and surrounding cortices (i.e., the perirhinal, the entorhinal, and the parahippocampal

cortices). In nonhuman primates, the perirhinal and parahippocampal cortices, and to a lesser extent the entorhinal cortex, receive projections from unimodal and polymodal sensory cortices. In turn, MTL cortices, and mainly the entorhinal cortex, provide inputs to the hippocampus [4–7]. Guided by these neuroanatomical considerations, it has been proposed that the MTL mediates different associative networks [5]. One hypothesis is that the hippocampus is required in the processing of associations between multiple stimuli, such as words [8–12], objects [13, 14], faces, and names [15–17]. Given their connections with sensory cortices, perirhinal and parahippocampal cortices are implicated in the processing of objects and scenes, respectively [16, 18–26].

Most of studies on associative memory were conducted using neutral materials, limiting their ecological validity, as people encounter multiple emotional stimuli and experience various affective states in their live. To overcome this limitation, emotion must be taken into account [12]. Emotion generally increases the likelihood that single information is remembered, and this effect reflects in part the influence of the amygdala on encoding and consolidation processes occurring in the hippocampus and MTL cortices [27–29].

Most neuroimaging studies that have investigated the effects of emotion on memory were limited to item memory [30]. Remembering discrete items is an important aspect of memory; however, remembering items associated with others or items placed in a context is another important aspect that also needs to be considered, since it better reflects what is experienced by individuals [30, 31]. Indeed, it is rare that people encounter information presented in isolation in everyday life. The effects of emotion on memory for discrete stimuli have been demonstrated in numerous studies [30]. Nonetheless, the effects of emotion on an individual's capacity to associate information remain unclear, since results of studies are contradictory [32]. Some studies report enhanced remembering, whereas others report impaired performance, and some report no effect of emotion [30].

In the current study, we used fMRI to investigate the neural correlates of the effects of emotion on associative memory. In light of previous work, we systematically examined MTL activations, as well as the interactions between amygdala activity and both hippocampal and MTL cortical activity.

2. Material and Methods

2.1. Subjects. Twenty-five participants (16 males; 18–29 years) were recruited by means of advertisements placed in local newspapers. All were right-handed as established by the Edinburgh Inventory (91.44 ± 7.78%). The participants were examined with the Non-Patient Edition of the Structured Clinical Interview for DSM-IV Axis I Disorders (SCID-I/NP) to rule out current or past Axis I psychiatric disorder.

The ethics board of the Montreal Neurological Institute (MNI) approved the study. Each participant signed an informed consent form prior to the experiment and received financial compensation for their participation.

2.2. Procedure. Prior to scanning, participants were provided with a detailed description of the task and instructions. Participants were instructed to memorize pairs of images. They were explicitly asked to memorize both images and also their pairing. Then, a short practice session was administered in order to familiarize participants with the experimental task.

The experimental task was adapted from that initially developed by Touryan et al. [33]. A graphical representation of the procedure is presented in Figure 1. During the scanned encoding session, participants had to memorize 90 pairs of standardized images. Each trial began with the presentation of a fixation cross (3000 ms), followed by a pair of pictures (3000 ms). These parameters were in line with our previous fMRI studies using emotional stimuli [34–36]. Each pair was composed of a picture depicting a complex scene (e.g.,

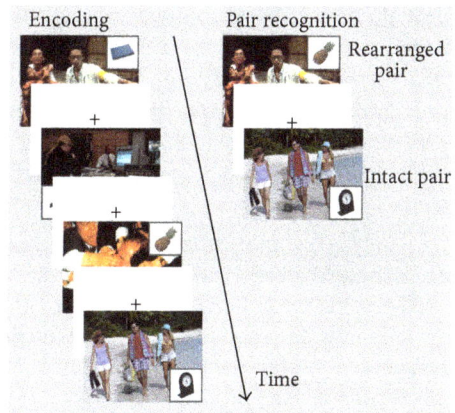

FIGURE 1: Illustration of the behavioral task. The left part represents a segment of the encoding session, with pairs composed of a scene and an unrelated common object presented in one of the four corners. The right part represents the pair recognition test during which intact and rearranged pairs were presented.

smiling people walking on the beach, a robbery in the subway) and a common object (e.g., a screwdriver). The scenes were selected from various sources (for more details, see [34]). Of these scenes, 30 were negatively valenced , 30 were positively valenced, and 30 were neutral. To minimize the potential confounding effect of arousal level differences between positive and negative pictures, we excluded pictures known to trigger high arousal (based on previous pictures rating from the IAPS), such as pictures presenting erotic scenes or mutilated bodies. The objects were selected from the BOSS standardized database [37] and were conceptually unrelated to the pictures with which they were presented. Each object was placed in a white box delimited by gray borders to dissociate the object from the scene. The corner designated for object location was equally distributed among the four corners, across valence. The order of stimulus presentation during the encoding phase was pseudorandom, with no more than three consecutive positive, negative, or neutral pictures. On each encoding trial, subjects had to indicate with a fiberoptic response pad whether the object was located on the left or on the right side, regardless of whether it was located at the top or the bottom of the screen. This task, in combination with associative-encoding instructions, ensured that subjects focused on both stimuli during their presentation. In other words, associative encoding is intentional.

Approximately 10 minutes after completing the encoding session, participants were required to make a pair recognition judgment. No functional scanning was conducted during the associative recognition test. Participants were presented with 90 consecutive trials (45 intact pairs and 45 rearranged pairs) and were instructed to indicate whether pairs were intact (objects and scenes presented in the same pairing as in the encoding session) or rearranged (pictures previously studied but presented in a new pairing). For rearranged pairs, the object was located in the same corner as during encoding to control for potential source memory effects. Additionally, a given object, if presented at encoding with a negative scene, was rearranged with another negative scene at recognition and not with a positive or neutral scene. The use of rearranged pairs as lures is designed to avoid judgment based on the familiarity of items. Thus, accurately rejecting rearranged pairs requires explicit knowledge of stimuli as well as their association.

Approximately 30 minutes after completing the recognition session, a cued recall test and a valence rating task were administered outside the scanner. We included a cued recall test to determine how an emotional stimulus (i.e., the scene) influences the between-stimuli binding of a neutral stimulus (i.e., the object). We also included a valence rating task since we were interested in confirming that the participants considered the emotional pictures as emotional and the neutral pictures as neutral. In both the cued recall test and the valence rating task, the central scenes were presented again but without any objects. In the cued recall test, participants were asked to (i) recall from memory the object that was presented with the scene during encoding; and (ii) indicate in which corner it was presented, even if they could not recall the objects themselves. During the valence rating task, participants were asked to rate the emotional valence of each visual scene using a 9-point Likert scale ranging from 1 (extremely negative) to 9 (extremely positive), with 5 indicating a neutral valence. The order of these two tasks was fixed, with the cued-recall test first and the valence task second.

2.3. FMRI Scanning Protocol. Scanning was carried out on a whole-body 1.5T Siemens Sonata System, using gradient-echo EPI sequences. The head was stabilized with a moldable vacuum cushion to minimize head movements. First a localizer scan was acquired followed by the functional run consisting of 214 T_{2^*}-weighted images acquired with a blood oxygenation level-dependent contrast (TR = 2540 ms; TE = 50 ms; Flip angle = 90°; 30 interleaved slices; voxel size 4 × 4 × 4 mm). Functional scans were acquired parallel to the anterior-posterior commissural plane. After completing the functional run, a 3D-T_1 MDEFT sequence was used for the acquisition of anatomical images (voxel size 1 × 1 × 1 mm).

2.4. Data Analysis

2.4.1. Behavioral Analyses. Behavioral performance was analyzed using Statistica 6.0 (Statsoft). In order to estimate pair recognition accuracy separately from response bias, a primary recognition index was examined using the Two-High Threshold Theory [38]. The Pr index (hits-false alarms) provides an unbiased estimate of recognition accuracy and reflects the participant's ability to discriminate between intact and rearranged pairs. Recall performance was scored by the proportion of correct responses. A response was considered correct when the object and its location were correctly recalled.

In all behavioral analyses, the alpha level was set at 0.05.

2.4.2. Neuroimaging Analyses. Functional images acquired during memory encoding were pretreated with SPM5 (http://www.fil.ion.ucl.ac.uk/spm/software/spm5/). The T_{2^*} images were first realigned to the 29th image in their respective run and normalized to the Echo Planar Imaging (EPI) template. Images were then spatially smoothed with an 8-mm full width half maximum (FWHM) isotropic Gaussian kernel. Prior to individual analyses, the movement correction logs were examined to ensure that none of the participants presented movements greater the 5 mm or 5°.

To assess the effects of emotion on associative memory, four event types were modeled: positive, negative, and neutral associations and the fixation cross (baseline). Positive and negative trials were pooled into a single condition named "emotional" condition, as analyses revealed no significant differences between positive and negative valence conditions for either behavioral performance ($t_{24} = 0.63$; $P = 0.78$) for the recognition test and ($t_{24} = 0.12$; $P = 0.13$) for the recall test or brain activations ([Positive-Negative]) analysis threshold at $P < 0.001$ uncorrected. Functional images were analyzed in two steps. In a first-level analysis, a general linear model was created for [Emotional-baseline], [Neutral-baseline], [Emotional-Neutral], and [Neutral-Emotional] contrasts, for each subject. In a second-level analysis, [Emotional-Neutral] and [Neutral-Emotional] contrasts were pooled for main effects into one-sample t-tests of within-group effects (random effect analysis). Main effects were assessed at the whole-brain level. Activations were considered significant with a voxel extent threshold of 10 or more voxels, with $P < 0.001$ (uncorrected for multiple comparisons). [Emotional-baseline] and [Neutral-baseline] contrasts were used to conduct a conjunction analysis ($P < 0.001$ uncorrected) [Emotional ∩ Neutral] in order to determine cerebral areas activated by both emotional and neutral associations. Lastly, restricted analyses focusing on the MTL were conducted using a small-volume correction implemented in SPM5. To that end, masks were obtained using the Automated Anatomical Labeling (AAL) atlas [39], included as a subset of regions of interest into the PickAtlas toolbox [40]. Masks comprised bilateral hippocampi, parahippocampal gyri, and amygdala. The threshold for these restricted analyses was lowered based on a priorihypotheses of the involvement of the hippocampus and its surrounding cortices in associative memory and the amygdala in emotion. Accordingly, analyses were thresholded at $P < 0.005$ (uncorrected), with a voxel extent threshold of >10 voxels.

3. Results

3.1. Behavioral Analyses

3.1.1. Recognition and Recall Tests. Data are summarized in Table 1. The analysis of the Pr index showed that participants were significantly more accurate in recognizing emotional associations than neutral associations ($t_{24} = -2.20$; $P = 0.04$). Similarly, the analysis of recall performance showed that participants better recalled the object and its location when it was associated with emotional scenes than with neutral scenes ($t_{24} = -2.45$; $P = 0.02$).

Table 1: Mean (and SEM) proportions of hits (H), false alarms (FA), Pr index, and recall score as a function of emotional associations and neutral associations conditions.

	Recognition			Recall
	H	FA	Pr	
Emotional associations	0.80 (0.03)	0.15 (0.04)	0.63 (0.04)	0.33 (0.04)
Neutral associations	0.79 (0.04)	0.20 (0.03)	0.57^* (0.06)	0.28^{**} (0.04)

*P value significant at 0.04 (for the emotional versus neutral associations comparison).
**P value significant at 0.02 (for the emotional versus neutral associations comparison).

3.1.2. Emotional Valence. T-tests showed that the ratings of positive (mean: 7.02; SEM: 0.15) and negative (mean: 2.90; SEM: 0.13) pictures significantly differed from 5 ($t_{24} = 13.05$; $P < 0.001$ and $t_{24} = -16.05$; $P < 0.001$ for positive and negative pictures, resp.) but that the ratings of neutral pictures (mean: 5.09; SEM: 0.09) did not differ from 5 ($t_{24} = 1.77$; $P = 0.10$). The ratings of positive pictures significantly differed from the rating of negative pictures ($t_{24} = 15.54$; $P < 0.001$). Together, these results confirmed that participants considered the positive and negative pictures as positive and negative, respectively, and the neutral pictures as neutral. As a result, they validate the appropriateness of stimuli for an emotional task.

3.2. Functional Neuroimaging Analyses. Two participants were excluded from fMRI analyses as they failed to reach criterion for performance during the encoding phase (<75% correct responses for the object-location judgment). The 23 remaining participants achieved above 96% correct responses (mean: 99%; SEM: 0.22), a performance level clearly indicative of full attention during stimulus presentation.

Whole brain analyses revealed that emotional associations activated predominately posterior regions, relative to neutral associations. Activations were observed in occipital (inferior and middle gyri), cuneus, parietal (postcentral, supramarginal gyri, and precuneus), temporal (middle, superior and fusiform gyri, entorhinal cortex), frontal (precentral superior frontal gyri, cingulate), and subcortical (substantia nigra and reticular formation) areas. Conversely, neutral associations elicited greater activations than emotional associations, predominately in anterior regions, including the cingulate (posterior and anterior gyri), temporal (superior and parahippocampal gyri), and frontal (middle and inferior gyri) areas. The conjunction analysis revealed that both emotional and neutral associations induced activations in the left premotor cortex and in the left anterior cingulate cortex, as well as in the right caudate nucleus, fusiform gyrus, culmen, and the hippocampus. Details about all these activations are reported in Table 2.

Restricted analyses focusing on the MTL showed that emotional associations induced greater activations in the right entorhinal cortex (26/−12/−32; $Z = 3.65$; 40 voxels) and the right amygdala (30/4/−26; $Z = 2.86$; 11 voxels). Conversely, greater activations were observed in the posterior part of the right parahippocampal gyrus (24/−42/−6; $Z = 3.63$; 50 voxels) for neutral associations relative to emotional associations (levels of activation were estimated in these

three clusters to ensure that entorhinal and amygdala activations were due to greater activity for emotional associations and that parahippocampal activation was due to greater activity for neutral associations. To that end, the peak of the entorhinal and amygdala clusters for the [emotional-baseline] contrast and the parahippocampal cluster for the [neutral-baseline] contrast were determined as the center of a 5 mm diameter sphere. Activation levels were then estimated. Paired t-tests showed significantly greater levels of activation for emotional than neutral associations in entorhinal ($t_{22} = 3.43$; $P = 0.002$) and the amygdala ($t_{22} = 2.76$; $P = 0.01$) clusters. Conversely, significantly greater levels of activations were observed for neutral than emotional associations in the parahippocampal cluster ($t_{22} = 3.22$; $P = 0.004$)) . Finally, activations were observed in the hippocampus (32/−28/−12; $Z = 2.62$; 10 voxels) for both emotional and neutral associations. Activations are illustrated in Figure 2. Here we considered that the cluster is located in the right entorhinal cortex. However, it should be mentioned that it remains difficult to straightforwardly determine whether the anterior parahippocampal activations arise from entorhinal or perirhinal cortex.

The mean activation level in each of these four clusters was then evaluated. Using the amygdala modulatory hypothesis as a model to explore MTL interregional covariation in activity [41, 42], correlations between amygdala activation and the other three MTL clusters were evaluated. The mean activity of each cluster for each participant was assessed for the [Emotional-Neutral] contrast and then correlations based on individual differences were calculated. The data of two participants were removed, as their individual activation levels in the entorhinal and in the parahippocampal clusters were more than 2 S.D. lower than the mean activation levels in these clusters. After removing these two outliers, correlation analyses showed that amygdala activity significantly covaried with entorhinal activity ($r = 0.51$; $P = 0.02$) and posterior parahippocampal activity ($r = -0.60$; $P = 0.008$) but not with hippocampal activity ($r = -0.25$; $P = 0.25$).

4. Discussion

This event-related fMRI study yielded three main results. First, participants had better memory performance for emotional than for neutral associations. This enhancement was observed for both recognition and recall test modalities. Second, rostrocaudal dissociation within the medial temporal lobe was observed as a function of the emotional valence of associations: greater activations were found in the

TABLE 2: Activations elicited by encoding when contrasting the emotional and neutral conditions.

Cerebral domain	BA	Z score	Stereotaxic coordinates			Cluster size (voxels)
			x	y	z	
Emotional > neutral						
Middle occipital gyrus (R)	19	4.54	48	−76	0	231
Postcentral gyrus (L)	3	4.51	−52	−26	58	73
Cuneus (R)	18/19	4.30	12	−88	14	150
Inferior occipital gyrus (L)	18	3.96	−38	−86	−18	25
Fusiform gyrus (R)	37	3.94	36	−52	−22	66
Posterior cingulate gyrus (L)	31	3.86	−14	−42	42	42
Inferior occipital gyrus (R)	17	3.85	28	−96	−6	43
Middle temporal gyrus (L)	19	3.81	−52	−72	14	75
Culmen		3.76	16	−66	−12	26
Superior frontal gyrus (R)	8	3.71	24	40	52	35
Entorhinal cortex (R)	28	3.65	26	−12	−32	15
Precuneus (L)	19	3.63	−2	−78	38	53
Inferior occipital gyrus (L)	18	3.62	−28	−98	−10	24
Posterior cingulate gyrus (R)	30	3.56	4	−48	18	84
Supramarginal gyrus (L)	40	3.55	−50	−46	32	19
Substantia nigra		3.55	12	−12	−8	12
Superior temporal gyrus (R)	22	3.50	54	−60	14	16
Pons (reticular formation)		3.49	−2	−28	−36	13
Precentral gyrus (L)	6	3.47	−52	6	38	27
Precuneus (R)	7	3.46	12	−58	30	41
Fusiform gyrus (R)	19	3.37	32	−78	−12	12
Pulvinar		3.32	−10	−30	12	13
Neutral > emotional						
Parahippocampal gyrus (R)	36	4.28	16	−36	−16	24
Middle frontal gyrus (R)	46	4.19	32	44	16	17
Superior temporal gyrus (R)	22	3.96	50	−6	−4	22
Inferior frontal gyrus (L)	46	3.73	−34	34	12	21
Parahippocampal gyrus (R)	36	3.63	24	−42	−6	12
Posterior cingulate gyrus (R)	23	3.48	22	−32	28	13
Anterior cingulate gyrus (R)	33	3.41	10	12	22	15
Emotional ∩ neutral						
Caudate nucleus (R)		4.26	22	20	18	65
Fusiform gyrus (R)	37	3.86	34	−56	−10	168
Anterior cingulate gyrus (L)	24	3.44	−20	−2	34	33
Precentral gyrus (L)	6	3.44	−48	−8	22	41
Precentral gyrus (L)	4	3.05	−22	−18	50	10
Culmen		2.85	30	−40	−28	12
Hippocampus (R)	36	2.62	32	−28	−12	10

L: left, R: right, and BA: Brodmann area.

entorhinal cortex for emotional associations while greater activations were found in the posterior parahippocampal gyrus for neutral associations. In addition, amygdala activity had an opposite effect on entorhinal and parahippocampal activity. Third, emotional and neutral associations shared common cerebral areas, comprising the hippocampus and other regions belonging to an attentional network.

As previously mentioned, the behavioral effects of emotion on associative memory are mixed [32]. The attention-narrowing hypothesis and priority-binding theory illustrate the discrepancy observed in the literature. According to the attention-narrowing hypothesis [43], emotions have an impact on memory by selectively modulating attention. Itsuggests that an arousing stimulus would narrow the focus of attention, which directs the attention to this same specific stimulus and therefore more details of this item are retrieved [44]. Indeed, the amount of attention available for surrounding information is decreased, leading to a lack of attentional resources for remembering the association between the concomitant information. Accordingly, associations comprising emotional stimuli are more poorly remembered relative to associations composed of neutral stimuli. Alternately, the priority-binding theory stated by MacKay and colleagues [45, 46] suggests that arousing stimuli evoke emotional

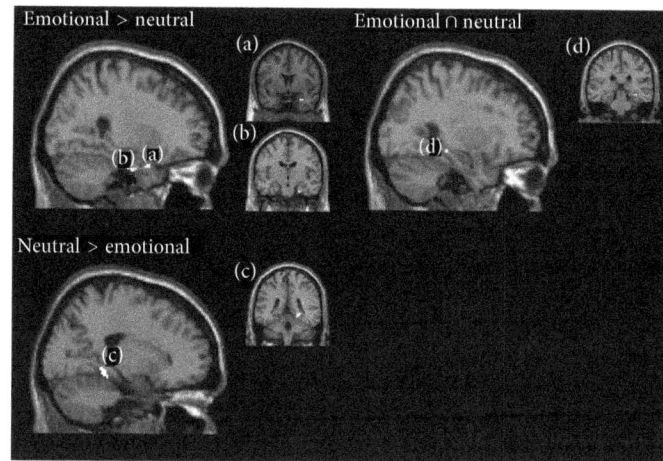

FIGURE 2: Illustration of activations revealed by ROI analyses. Emotional associations induced greater activations than neutral associations in (a) the right amygdala ($x = 30$; $y = 4$; $z = -26$) and (b) the right entorhinal cortex ($x = 26$; $y = -12$; $z = -32$). Conversely, neutral associations induced greater activations in the posterior part of (c) the right parahippocampal gyrus ($x = 24$; $y = -42$; $z = -6$). Emotional and neutral associations both induced activations in (d) the right hippocampus ($x = 32$; $y = -28$; $z = -12$).

reactions that give priority to the binding mechanisms, strengthening the association between emotional stimuli and associated nonemotional stimuli. As a result, associations between emotional information and neutral information are better remembered than associations between solely neutral information.

In our study, participants were more accurate in recognizing emotional associations than neutral associations. Similarly, participants better recalled objects and their location when these were associated with emotional scenes than neutral scenes. These results converge with many previous findings [45–48] and are also consistent with the priority-binding theory [46]. However, our results are in sharp contrast with other studies [12, 33] reporting lower performance for emotional (i.e., negative associations) relative to neutral associations. At the current stage, various factors may explain these discrepancies, such as the fact that results of memory performance may be a function of parametric differences. For instance, the nature of the stimuli (words, pictures, and object), the presentation modality (visual versus auditory) or their duration of presentation (3 s versus 6 s), the length of the delay between study and test (whether the task is administered as a working memory or long-term memory task), the way associative recognition is assessed (intact/rearranged pair recognition test versus cued associative test), and encoding instructions (intentional versus incidental associative encoding) vary among all studies and are important to consider because they alter the manner in which the information is held and how it is retained [49]. Furthermore, the way in which the emotion is induced and manipulated, the valence, and arousal levels of stimuli may also strongly influence the way the information is retained [49]. Further studies are required to examine the contribution of each of these factors. The use of emotional images, for example, compared to words, may potentially induce a greater effect of emotions on associative memory, as they are more elaborated and

might have the ability to evoke stronger emotions. Also, participants were explicitly instructed to encode both items and their association, whereas in other studies, such as that of Touryan et al. [33], they had to remember as much about each stimulus as possible. It has been established that instructions determine encoding and/or retrieval strategies [50, 51].

Within the right MTL, we observed a functional specialization along the longitudinal axis: encoding emotional associations led to enhanced activations in the entorhinal cortex, whereas encoding neutral associations led to enhanced activations in the posterior parahippocampal cortex. Such rostrocaudal dissociation has already been demonstrated with IAPS pictures [27] and words [52]. Our study confirms the role of MTL cortices in the processing of scenes but also examines their respective role. It may thus be hypothesized that the entorhinal cortex is implicated in the processing of emotional scenes, while the posterior parahippocampal cortex is implicated in the processing of neutral scenes. This dissociation may result from amygdala influence, as revealed by the correlation analyses. More precisely, amygdala activity positively covaried with entorhinal activity but negatively covaried with posterior parahippocampal activity. This modulation effect fits well with anatomical connections, given that amygdala shares strong connections with these MTL cortices [53–57].

Previous hypotheses with respect to rostrocaudal dissociation of medial temporal function have been proposed. For instance, a meta-analysis of experimentally induced changes in blood flow ("activation") in positron emission tomography (PET) studies of memory revealed such functionally dissociation between rostral and caudal regions of the hippocampal formation [54]. The authors observed that rostral regions were strongly activated during encoding tasks, while caudal regions were highly activated during retrieval tasks. Lepage and colleagues refer to this general pattern as the HIPER (hippocampal encoding/retrieval) model [54]. Our results are not compatible with this model, given that we observed activations in the right medial temporal lobe only (Lepage and colleagues pooled activations in both hemispheres) and that clusters were more rostral and caudal when compared to Lepage's report. Our results may also be consistent with another model proposing that the anterior part of the MTL is associated with semantic information and the posterior part with perceptual information [58]. With respect to this model, it has been suggested that greater activity in the entorhinal cortex reflects enhanced semantic and relational processing for emotional stimuli, whereas greater activity in the posterior parahippocampal cortex reflects enhanced perceptual processing of neutral stimuli [27]. However, there is currently no demonstration validating this hypothesis and future research is needed to clarify the specific mechanism involved in processing emotional/semantic and neutral/perceptual information.

In parallel with the functional specialization of MTL cortices, the conjunction analysis revealed that the right hippocampus was activated by both emotional and neutral associations, regardless of amygdala activity. This result is consistent with the proposal that the hippocampus binds distinct elements of an event into an integrated representation [59–62]. Guided by neuroanatomical knowledge reviewed in the Introduction, our results support the view of different associative networks within the MTL. A first associative network comprises MTL cortices. Given that they share strong connections with unimodal and polymodal sensory cortices, MTL cortices may bind multiple sensory information, composing IAPS scenes into an integrated representation [16, 20, 23–26]. This may explain why we observed the same pattern of activations in MTL cortices as Dolcos et al. [27], as both studies used IAPS scenes. Another associative network is composed of the hippocampus, which receives convergent inputs from MTL cortices, and may thus mediate encoding processes associating scenes and concomitant objects.

In addition to the hippocampal activation, greater activations were also induced by both emotional and neutral associations in various areas subserving attentional processing. For instance, common activations were found in the premotor cortex, the posterior part of the fusiform gyrus, and the dorsal part of the anterior cingulate gyrus. This pattern of activations has been consistently found in tasks demanding spatial attention [63–65]. Finally, activations in the caudate nucleus may be related to ocular movements essential to focusing spatial attention [66, 67]. Spatial attention is needed to establish associations between multiple stimuli and to maintain these associations in memory [68–70].

One limitation of this study is that interactions between amygdala activity and hippocampal and MTL cortices activity rely on correlation analyses, which do not indicate the direction of these interactions. Further analyses examining effective connectivity should be performed to overcome this limitation. Another limitation of this study is the lack of a condition assessing the processing of individual stimuli. At the current level, it remains difficult to straightforwardly conclude that the results were driven by associative processes per se, rather than by emotions. Lastly, the subsequent memory effect, which represents the difference during encoding between brain activity for items that are subsequently remembered and brain activity for items that are subsequently forgotten [27], could not be evaluated. This limits the understanding of neural mechanisms that predict encoding success depending on the emotional valence of associations. A comparison between successfully and unsuccessfully encoded associations was not possible because of an insufficient number of "miss" trials by most participants. Future studies would benefit from a modified design that might induce a greater number of misses by participants. For instance, the delay between encoding and recognition sessions might be increased, as well as the number of studied associations. All of these parameters would be expected to increase the number of forgotten associations, thus allowing the estimation of the subsequent memory effect. Future studies may also benefit from scanning both the encoding and recognition sessions, in order to investigate effects of emotion on retrieval processes.

With respect to previously published data, our results confirm that the hippocampus, in concert with attentional network regions, participates in the encoding of associations in memory. Our results also extend past findings by demonstrating that emotions are associated with the performance improvement of associative memory. This potentiation may result from enhanced activity in the right entorhinal cortex by the right amygdala. Future research may consider functional connections among these cerebral structures to elucidate the neural mechanisms assuming their respective functions.

Conflict of Interests

The authors declare that there is no conflict of interests regarding the publication of this paper.

Acknowledgments

This study was supported by an operating grant from NSERC. Drs. Lepage Martin and Luck David are supported by a salary award from the *Fonds de recherche en santé du Québec*. The authors thank Thomas Howells for his helpful corrections on English language regarding the paper.

References

[1] E. Tulving, *Elements of Episodic Memory*, Oxford University Press, New York, NY, USA, 1983.

[2] H. Zimmer, A. Mecklinger, and U. Lindenberger, *Handbook of Binding and Memory*, Oxford University Press, New York, NY, USA, 2006.

[3] B. H. Pierce and E. A. Kensinger, "Effects of emotion on associative recognition: valence and retention interval matter," *Emotion*, vol. 11, no. 1, pp. 139–144, 2011.

[4] D. G. Amaral and M. P. Witter, "The three-dimensional organization of the hippocampal formation: a review of anatomical data," *Neuroscience*, vol. 31, no. 3, pp. 571–591, 1989.

[5] P. Lavenex and D. G. Amaral, "Hippocampal-neocortical interaction: a hierarchy of associativity," *Hippocampus*, vol. 10, pp. 420–430, 2000.

[6] P. Lavenex, W. A. Suzuki, and D. G. Amaral, "Perirhinal and parahippocampal cortices of the macaque monkey: projections

to the neocortex," *Journal of Comparative Neurology*, vol. 447, no. 4, pp. 394–420, 2002.

[7] P. Lavenex, W. A. Suzuki, and D. G. Amaral, "Perirhinal and parahippocampal cortices of the macaque monkey: intrinsic projections and interconnections," *Journal of Comparative Neurology*, vol. 472, no. 3, pp. 371–394, 2004.

[8] M. Lepage, R. Habib, H. Cormier, S. Houle, and A. R. McIntosh, "Neural correlates of semantic associative encoding in episodic memory," *Cognitive Brain Research*, vol. 9, no. 3, pp. 271–280, 2000.

[9] O. Jackson III and D. L. Schacter, "Encoding activity in anterior medial temporal lobe supports subsequent associative recognition," *NeuroImage*, vol. 21, no. 1, pp. 456–462, 2004.

[10] S. Köhler, S. Danckert, J. S. Gati, and R. S. Menon, "Novelty responses to relational and non-relational information in the hippocampus and the parahippocampal region: a comparison based on event-related fMRI," *Hippocampus*, vol. 15, no. 6, pp. 763–774, 2005.

[11] J. A. Meltzer and R. T. Constable, "Activation of human hippocampal formation reflects success in both encoding and cued recall of paired associates," *NeuroImage*, vol. 24, no. 2, pp. 384–397, 2005.

[12] K. Onoda, Y. Okamoto, and S. Yamawaki, "Neural correlates of associative memory: the effects of negative emotion," *Neuroscience Research*, vol. 64, no. 1, pp. 50–55, 2009.

[13] A. M. Achim, M.-C. Bertrand, A. Montoya, A. K. Malla, and M. Lepage, "Medial temporal lobe activations during associative memory encoding for arbitrary and semantically related object pairs," *Brain Research*, vol. 1161, pp. 46–55, 2007.

[14] A. M. Achim and M. Lepage, "Neural correlates of memory for items and for associations: an event-related functional magnetic resonance imaging study," *Journal of Cognitive Neuroscience*, vol. 17, no. 4, pp. 652–667, 2005.

[15] R. A. Sperling, J. F. Bates, A. J. Cocchiarella, D. L. Schacter, B. R. Rosen, and M. S. Albert, "Encoding novel face-name associations: a functional MRI study," *Human Brain Mapping*, vol. 14, no. 3, pp. 129–139, 2001.

[16] C. B. Kirwan and C. E. L. Stark, "Medial temporal lobe activation during encoding and retrieval of novel face-name pairs," *Hippocampus*, vol. 14, no. 7, pp. 919–930, 2004.

[17] E. F. Chua, D. L. Schacter, E. Rand-Giovannetti, and R. A. Sperling, "Evidence for a specific role of the anterior hippocampal region in successful associative encoding," *Hippocampus*, vol. 17, no. 11, pp. 1071–1080, 2007.

[18] M. D. Barense, T. J. Bussey, A. C. H. Lee et al., "Functional specialization in the human medial temporal lobe," *Journal of Neuroscience*, vol. 25, no. 44, pp. 10239–10246, 2005.

[19] M. D. Barense, D. Gaffan, and K. S. Graham, "The human medial temporal lobe processes online representations of complex objects," *Neuropsychologia*, vol. 45, no. 13, pp. 2963–2974, 2007.

[20] M. D. Barense, R. N. A. Henson, A. C. H. Lee, and K. S. Graham, "Medial temporal lobe activity during complex discrimination of faces, objects, and scenes: effects of viewpoint," *Hippocampus*, vol. 20, no. 3, pp. 389–401, 2010.

[21] P. S. F. Bellgowan, E. A. Buffalo, J. Bodurka, and A. Martin, "Lateralized spatial and object memory encoding in entorhinal and perirhinal cortices," *Learning and Memory*, vol. 16, no. 7, pp. 433–438, 2009.

[22] E. A. Buffalo, P. S. F. Bellgowan, and A. Martin, "Distinct roles for medial temporal lobe structures in memory for objects and

their locations," *Learning & Memory*, vol. 13, no. 5, pp. 638–643, 2006.

[23] H. Eichenbaum, "The hippocampus and declarative memory: cognitive mechanisms and neural codes," *Behavioural Brain Research*, vol. 127, no. 1-2, pp. 199–207, 2001.

[24] R. Epstein, A. Harris, D. Stanley, and N. Kanwisher, "The parahippocampal place area: recognition, navigation, or encoding?" *Neuron*, vol. 23, no. 1, pp. 115–125, 1999.

[25] R. Epstein and N. Kanwisher, "A cortical representation the local visual environment," *Nature*, vol. 392, no. 6676, pp. 598–601, 1998.

[26] R. A. Epstein and J. S. Higgins, "Differential parahippocampal and retrosplenial involvement in three types of visual scene recognition," *Cerebral Cortex*, vol. 17, no. 7, pp. 1680–1693, 2007.

[27] F. Dolcos, K. S. LaBar, and R. Cabeza, "Interaction between the amygdala and the medial temporal lobe memory system predicts better memory for emotional events," *Neuron*, vol. 42, no. 5, pp. 855–863, 2004.

[28] F. Dolcos, K. S. Labar, and R. Cabeza, "Remembering one year later: role of the amygdala and the medial temporal lobe memory system in retrieving emotional memories," *Proceedings of the National Academy of Sciences of the United States of America*, vol. 102, no. 7, pp. 2626–2631, 2005.

[29] J. L. McGaugh, "The amygdala modulates the consolidation of memories of emotionally arousing experiences," *Annual Review of Neuroscience*, vol. 27, pp. 1–28, 2004.

[30] Y.-C. Chiu, F. Dolcos, B. D. Gonsalves, and N. J. Cohen, "On opposing effects of emotion on contextual or relational memory," *Frontiers in Psychology*, vol. 4, article 103, 2013.

[31] M. Mather and K. Nesmith, "Arousal-enhanced location memory for pictures," *Journal of Memory and Language*, vol. 58, no. 2, pp. 449–464, 2008.

[32] M. Mather, "Emotional arousal and memory binding: an object-based framework," *Perspectives on Psychological Science*, vol. 2, pp. 33–52, 2007.

[33] S. R. Touryan, D. E. Marian, and A. P. Shimamura, "Effect of negative emotional pictures on associative memory for peripheral information," *Memory*, vol. 15, no. 2, pp. 154–166, 2007.

[34] P. O. Harvey, P. Fossati, and M. Lepage, "Modulation of memory formation by stimulus content: specific role of the medial prefrontal cortex in the successful encoding of social pictures," *Journal of Cognitive Neuroscience*, vol. 19, no. 2, pp. 351–362, 2007.

[35] P.-O. Harvey, J. Pruessner, Y. Czechowska, and M. Lepage, "Individual differences in trait anhedonia: a structural and functional magnetic resonance imaging study in non-clinical subjects," *Molecular Psychiatry*, vol. 12, no. 8, pp. 767–775, 2007.

[36] M. Roy, P.-O. Harvey, M. T. Berlim et al., "Medial prefrontal cortex activity during memory encoding of pictures and its relation to symptomatic improvement after citalopram treatment in patients with major depression," *Journal of Psychiatry and Neuroscience*, vol. 35, no. 3, pp. 152–162, 2010.

[37] M. B. Brodeur, E. Dionne-Dostie, T. Montreuil, and M. Lepage, "The bank of standardized stimuli (BOSS), a new set of 480 normative photos of objects to be used as visual stimuli in cognitive research," *PLoS ONE*, vol. 5, no. 5, Article ID e10773, 2010.

[38] J. G. Snodgrass and J. Corwin, "Perceptual identification thresholds for 150 fragmented pictures from the Snodgrass and Vanderwart picture set," *Perceptual and Motor Skills*, vol. 67, no. 1, pp. 3–36, 1988.

[39] N. Tzourio-Mazoyer, B. Landeau, D. Papathanassiou et al., "Automated anatomical labeling of activations in SPM using a macroscopic anatomical parcellation of the MNI MRI single-subject brain," *NeuroImage*, vol. 15, no. 1, pp. 273–289, 2002.

[40] J. A. Maldjian, P. J. Laurienti, R. A. Kraft, and J. H. Burdette, "An automated method for neuroanatomic and cytoarchitectonic atlas-based interrogation of fMRI data sets," *NeuroImage*, vol. 19, no. 3, pp. 1233–1239, 2003.

[41] J. L. McGaugh, "Memory—a century of consolidation," *Science*, vol. 287, no. 5451, pp. 248–251, 2000.

[42] J. L. McGaugh, C. K. McIntyre, and A. E. Power, "Amygdala modulation of memory consolidation: interaction with other brain systems," *Neurobiology of Learning and Memory*, vol. 78, no. 3, pp. 539–552, 2002.

[43] J. A. Easterbrook, "The effect of emotion on cue utilization and the organization of behavior," *Psychological Review*, vol. 66, no. 3, pp. 183–201, 1959.

[44] T. Sharot and E. A. Phelps, "How arousal modulates memory: disentangling the effects of attention and retention," *Cognitive, Affective and Behavioral Neuroscience*, vol. 4, no. 3, pp. 294–306, 2004.

[45] D. G. MacKay and M. V. Ahmetzanov, "Emotion, memory, and attention in the taboo stroop paradigm an experimental analogue of flashbulb memories," *Psychological Science*, vol. 16, no. 1, pp. 25–32, 2005.

[46] D. G. MacKay, M. Shafto, J. K. Taylor, D. E. Marian, L. Abrams, and J. R. Dyer, "Relations between emotion, memory, and attention: evidence from taboo Stroop, lexical decision, and immediate memory tasks," *Memory and Cognition*, vol. 32, no. 3, pp. 474–488, 2004.

[47] S. Doerksen and A. P. Shimamura, "Source memory enhancement for emotional words," *Emotion*, vol. 1, no. 1, pp. 5–11, 2001.

[48] R. Guillet and J. Arndt, "Taboo words: the effect of emotion on memory for peripheral information," *Memory and Cognition*, vol. 37, no. 6, pp. 866–879, 2009.

[49] H. C. Bergmann, M. Rijpkema, G. Fernández, and R. P. C. Kessels, "The Effects of Valence and Arousal on Associative Working Memory and Long-Term Memory," *PLoS ONE*, vol. 7, no. 12, Article ID e52616, 2012.

[50] N. E. Noldy, R. M. Stelmack, and K. B. Campbell, "Event-related potentials and recognition memory for pictures and words: the effects of intentional and incidental learning," *Psychophysiology*, vol. 27, no. 4, pp. 417–428, 1990.

[51] A. A. Rodrigues and S. L. Marques, "Influence of the instructions on the performance and establishment of memorization strategies in space judgments," *Spanish Journal of Psychology*, vol. 9, no. 2, pp. 312–320, 2006.

[52] S. Dougal, E. A. Phelps, and L. Davachi, "The role of medial temporal lobe in item recognition and source recollection of emotional stimuli," *Cognitive, Affective and Behavioral Neuroscience*, vol. 7, no. 3, pp. 233–242, 2007.

[53] K. M. Kerr, K. L. Agster, S. C. Furtak, and R. D. Burwell, "Functional neuroanatomy of the parahippocampal region: the lateral and medial entorhinal areas," *Hippocampus*, vol. 17, no. 9, pp. 697–708, 2007.

[54] K. Majak and A. Pitkänen, "Projections from the periamygdaloid cortex to the amygdaloid complex, the hippocampal formation, and the parahippocampal region: a PHA-L study in the rat," *Hippocampus*, vol. 13, no. 8, pp. 922–942, 2003.

[55] A. Pitkänen, J. L. Kelly, and D. G. Amaral, "Projections from the lateral, basal, and accessory basal nuclei of the amygdala to the entorhinal cortex in the macaque monkey," *Hippocampus*, vol. 12, no. 2, pp. 186–205, 2002.

[56] A. Pitkänen, M. Pikkarainen, N. Nurminen, and A. Ylinen, "Reciprocal connections between the amygdala and the hippocampal formation, perirhinal cortex, and postrhinal cortex in rat," *Annals of the New York Academy of Sciences*, vol. 911, pp. 369–391, 2000.

[57] M. P. Witter, P. Room, H. J. Groenewegen, and A. H. M. Lohman, "Connections of the parahippocampal cortex in the cat. V. Intrinsic connections; comments on input/output connections with the hippocampus," *Journal of Comparative Neurology*, vol. 252, no. 1, pp. 78–94, 1986.

[58] R. Cabeza, S. M. Rao, A. D. Wagner, A. R. Mayer, and D. L. Schacter, "Can medial temporal lobe regions distinguish true from false? An event-related functional MRI study of veridical and illusory recognition memory," *Proceedings of the National Academy of Sciences of the United States of America*, vol. 98, no. 8, pp. 4805–4810, 2001.

[59] L. Davachi, J. P. Mitchell, and A. D. Wagner, "Multiple routes to memory: distinct medial temporal lobe processes build item and source memories," *Proceedings of the National Academy of Sciences of the United States of America*, vol. 100, no. 4, pp. 2157–2162, 2003.

[60] R. A. Diana, A. P. Yonelinas, and C. Ranganath, "Imaging recollection and familiarity in the medial temporal lobe: a three-component model," *Trends in Cognitive Sciences*, vol. 11, no. 9, pp. 379–386, 2007.

[61] H. Eichenbaum, G. Schoenbaum, B. Young, and M. Bunsey, "Functional organization of the hippocampal memory system," *Proceedings of the National Academy of Sciences of the United States of America*, vol. 93, no. 24, pp. 13500–13507, 1996.

[62] H. Eichenbaum, A. P. Yonelinas, and C. Ranganath, "The medial temporal lobe and recognition memory," *Annual Review of Neuroscience*, vol. 30, pp. 123–152, 2007.

[63] S. M. Courtney, L. G. Ungerleider, K. Keil, and J. V. Haxby, "Object and spatial visual working memory activate separate neural systems in human cortex," *Cerebral Cortex*, vol. 6, pp. 39–49, 1996.

[64] D. R. Gitelman, A. C. Nobre, T. B. Parrish et al., "A large-scale distributed network for covert spatial attention: further anatomical delineation based on stringent behavioural and cognitive controls," *Brain*, vol. 122, part 6, pp. 1093–1106, 1999.

[65] R. I. Schubotz and D. Y. von Cramon, "Functional organization of the lateral premotor cortex: fMRI reveals different regions activated by anticipation of object properties, location and speed," *Cognitive Brain Research*, vol. 11, no. 1, pp. 97–112, 2001.

[66] A. D. Baddeley, *Working Memory*, University Press, Oxford, UK, 1986.

[67] B. R. Postle, C. Idzikowski, S. Della Sala, R. H. Logie, and A. D. Baddeley, "The selective disruption of spatial working memory by eye movements," *Quarterly Journal of Experimental Psychology*, vol. 59, no. 1, pp. 100–120, 2006.

[68] A. Baddeley, "The episodic buffer: a new component of working memory?" *Trends in Cognitive Sciences*, vol. 4, no. 11, pp. 417–423, 2000.

[69] N. Cowan, "The magical number 4 in short-term memory: a reconsideration of mental storage capacity," *Behavioral and Brain Sciences*, vol. 24, no. 1, pp. 87–114, 2001.

[70] N. Cowan, *Working Memory Capacity*, Psychology Press, London, UK, 2005.

Permissions

List of Contributors

André Aleman
Department of Neuroscience, University Medical Center Groningen, University of Groningen, 9700 RB Groningen, The Netherlands
Department of Psychology, University of Groningen, 9712 CP Groningen, The Netherlands

Rui Nouchi
Human and Social Response Research Division, International Research Institute of Disaster Science, Tohoku University, 4-1 Seiryo-cho, Aoba-ku, Sendai 980-8575, Japan
Department of Advanced Brain Science, Smart Ageing International Research Center, Institute of Development, Aging and Cancer, Tohoku University, 4-1 Seiryo-cho, Aoba-ku, Sendai 980-8575, Japan

Ryuta Kawashima
Department of Advanced Brain Science, Smart Ageing International Research Center, Institute of Development, Aging and Cancer, Tohoku University, 4-1 Seiryo-cho, Aoba-ku, Sendai 980-8575, Japan
Department of Functional Brain Imaging, Institute of Development, Aging and Cancer, Tohoku University, 4-1 Seiryo-cho, Aoba-ku, Sendai 980-8575, Japan

Alan Percy
Civitan International Research Center, University of Alabama at Birmingham, 1720 2nd Avenue South, CIRC 320E, Birmingham, AL 35294-0021, USA

Deepak Khuntia
Varian Medical Systems, 3100 HansenWay, E-175, Palo Alto, CA 94340, USA

Michael I. Posner, Mary K. Rothbart and Pascale Voelker
University of Oregon, Eugene, OR 97403, USA

Brad E. Sheese
IllinoisWesleyan University, Bloomington, IL 61701, USA

David Rudrauf
Laboratory of Functional Imaging (LIF), INSERM U678S, 91 Boulevard de l'Hôpital, 75013 Paris, France

Stefania Ferri
Department of Neuroscience, Università di Parma, Via Volturno 39/E, 43100 Parma, Italy

Cristina Meini
Department of Humanistic Studies, Università del Piemonte Orientale, Via Manzoni 8, 13100 Vercelli, Italy

Giorgio Guiot
Associazione Cantabile, Via Campana 2, 10125 Turin, Italy

Daniela Tagliafico
Department of Philosophy, Università Degli Studi di Torino, Via Sant'Ottavio 20, 10125 Turin, Italy

Gabriella Gilli
Department of Psychology, Università Cattolica del Sacro Cuore, 20123 Milan, Italy

Cinzia Di Dio
Department of Neuroscience, Università di Parma, Via Volturno 39/E, 43100 Parma, Italy
Department of Psychology, Università Cattolica del Sacro Cuore, 20123 Milan, Italy

Mustapha Shehu Muhammad
Department of Human Physiology, College of Medical Sciences, Gombe State University, Gombe 760214, Nigeria

Rabiu Abdussalam Magaji, Aliyu Mohammed and Ahmed-Sherif Isa
Department of Human Physiology, Faculty of Medicine, Ahmadu Bello University, Zaria 810001, Nigeria

Mohammed Garba Magaji
Department of Pharmacology and Therapeutics, Faculty of Pharmaceutical Sciences, Ahmadu Bello University, Zaria 810001, Nigeria

Diego Kaski and Adolfo M. Bronstein
Division of Brain Sciences, Imperial College London, Charing Cross Hospital, LondonW6 8RF, UK

Gabriella D'Arcangelo
Department of Cell Biology and Neuroscience, Rutgers, The State University of New Jersey, Piscataway, NJ 08854, USA

Henry H. Yin
Department of Psychology and Neuroscience and Department of Neurobiology, Center for Cognitive Neuroscience, Duke University, P.O. Box 91050, Durham, NC 27708, USA

Marc Fakhoury and Sergio Domínguez López
Department of Neuroscience, Faculty of Medicine, University of Montreal, Montreal, QC, Canada H2V 2S9

Arno Onken and Stefano Panzeri
Center for Neuroscience and Cognitive Systems @UniTn, Istituto Italiano di Tecnologia, Via Bettini 31, 38068 Rovereto, Italy

P. P. Chamanthi R. Karunasekara
Center for Neuroscience and Cognitive Systems @UniTn, Istituto Italiano di Tecnologia, Via Bettini 31, 38068 Rovereto, Italy
Doctoral School in Cognitive and Brain Sciences, University of Trento, Via Bettini 31, 38068 Rovereto, Italy

Christoph Kayser
Institute of Neuroscience and Psychology, University of Glasgow, Glasgow G12 8QB, UK
Max Planck Institute for Biological Cybernetics, Spemannstraße 38, 72076 Tübingen, Germany
Bernstein Centre for Computational Neuroscience, 72076 Tübingen, Germany

Hans-Arne Hansson
Institute of Biomedicine, Sahlgren Academy, University of Gothenburg, P.O. Box 440, 40530 Gothenburg, Sweden

Ulrika Krave and Johan Davidsson
Department of Applied Mechanics, Chalmers University of Technology, 41296 Gothenburg, Sweden

Svante Höjer
GU Holding, University of Gothenburg, 40530 Gothenburg, Sweden

David Luck
Douglas Mental Health University Institute, Verdun, QC, Canada H4H 1R3
Institut Universitaire en Santé Mentale de Montréal, Montreal, QC, Canada H1N 3M5
Department of Psychiatry, University of Montreal, Montreal, QC, Canada H3T 1J4

Marie-Eve Leclerc
Institut Universitaire en Santé Mentale de Montréal, Montreal, QC, Canada H1N 3M5
Department of Psychiatry, University of Montreal, Montreal, QC, Canada H3T 1J4

Martin Lepage
Douglas Mental Health University Institute, Verdun, QC, Canada H4H 1R3
Department of Psychiatry, McGill University, Montreal, QC, Canada H3A 2T5

www.ingramcontent.com/pod-product-compliance
Lightning Source LLC
Chambersburg PA
CBHW070153240326
41458CB00126B/4527